facts and comparisons

patient drug information

a companion to Nurses Drug Facts™

1997

facts and comparisons

In Collaboration With

ANA

AMERICAN NURSES ASSOCIATION

Patient Drug Information, a companion to Nurses Drug Facts™ 1997 Edition

ISBN 1-57439-001-5

ISBN 1-57439-002-3 (*Nurses Drug Facts* Reference Set)
ISBN 1-57439-000-7 *(Nurses Drug Facts)*

Printed in the United States of America

Published by
Facts and Comparisons
111 West Port Plaza, Suite 300
St. Louis, Missouri 63146-3098
314/878-2515
Toll free customer service 800/223-0554

President	**C. Sue Sewester**
Publisher-Healthcare	**Paul S. Heirendt**
Director, Drug Information	**Bernie R. Olin, PharmD**
Business Development	**Heidi L. Meredith**
Editorial Development	**Cathy H. Reilly**
Print Products	**Noël A. Shamleffer**
Quality Control Editor	**Kirsten K. Novak**
Assistant Editors	**Stephanie Hug** **Tim O'Brien**
Reviewers	**David S. Tatro, PharmD** Drug Information Consultant San Francisco, CA
	Larry R. Borgsdorf, PharmD, FCSHP Pharmacist Specialist Ambulatory Care Kaiser Permanente Bakersfield, CA
	Julio R. Lopez, PharmD Director of Drug Information VA Medical Center Martinez, CA

Table of Contents

Introduction vi

Monographs A to Z 1

Use of Aerosol Metered Sprays 645

Use of Ophthalmic Products 646

Use of Oral Contraceptives 647

Use of Otic Products 649

Use of Rectal Products 650

Use of Rectal Suppositories 651

Use of Respiratory Nebulizers 652

Use of Topical Products 653

Use of Transdermal Patches 654

Use of Vaginal Creams 655

Use of Vaginal Suppositories 656

Index 657

Introduction

Patient Drug Information is the patient counseling companion to *Nurses Drug Facts*. The single page drug information monographs are designed to be photocopied and sent home with the patient and/or family member. Enlarging to 140% will fit an 8½" x 11" page. These monographs are cross-referenced in *Nurses Drug Facts*, creating a comprehensive drug information reference set for use by nurses in their daily practice.

The book is organized alphabetically by generic drug name. If a drug is used for different indications or if there are different doseforms, more than one monograph may be included. Monographs have *not* been included for drugs used only in situations where patient counseling is not appropriate (eg, emergency or surgical settings).

The drug monographs are written in lay terms that the patient will understand, at approximately an 8th grade reading level. The monographs focus on usage guidelines that will help ensure that the patient understands how and why to take their medication.

Patient Drug Information uses the format and icons found in *Nurses Drug Facts*, simplifying access to the information. The information is standardized and organized according to the patient's level of understanding. The following sections are included:

Drug Name: Generic drug name and common synonyms are listed in each monograph header. A slash between drug names indicates a combination product.

Phonetic Pronunciation: A guide is provided for generic drug names. Pronunciations for commonly used terms, such as acid, have not been given. The pronunciations are based on the USAN Council officially designated pronunciations. The syllable in capital letters receives the emphasis.

Trade Name: U.S. trade names are listed for each drug. These are italicized and organized alphabetically. Some drugs are available only as a generic, for those no trade names appear.

General information: Indications, contraindications, precautions and side effects are included whenever appropriate. This information has been simplified for the non-professional. Specific guidelines for use that the patient will understand are also provided.

A section of general use guidelines for a variety of doseforms and oral contraceptives follows the drug monographs. These are designed to help the patient in using metered sprays, topicals, suppositories, transdermal patches, nebulizer sprays, ophthalmic products, otic products and oral contraceptives.

Acarbose

(A-car-bose)

Precose

To treat Type II (non-insulin-dependent) diabetes in adults whose blood sugar levels cannot be managed by diet alone. This medicine may be taken in combination with a sulfonylurea (other oral diabetes medication).

Precautions

DO NOT USE if you are allergic to this medicine; have severe liver disease; inflammatory bowel disease; rectal bleeding; bowel or intestinal obstruction (blockage); certain digestive disorders or diabetic ketoacidosis.

BEFORE USING THIS MEDICINE, tell your healthcare provider if you are pregnant or breastfeeding; if you are taking, will be taking or stop taking any prescription or nonprescription medicine; or if you have any other medical conditions.

Side Effects

Every medicine can cause side effects, but many people have no, or minor, side effects. Tell your healthcare provider if any of the following occurs: stomach pain; diarrhea; gas. These symptoms usually lessen over time.

Guidelines for Use

USE EXACTLY AS PRESCRIBED.

Take this medicine 3 times daily at the start (with the first bite) of each main meal.

Do not change the dose without checking with your healthcare provider.

If a dose is missed at the beginning (first bite) of a meal, take it during the meal. Do not take it after the meal has been fully eaten. Do not take a dose if you are going to skip a meal. If more than one dose is missed, contact your healthcare provider.

Be sure to follow the diet, exercise and testing of urine or blood glucose programs prescribed by your helathcare provider.

Lab tests/exams are required to monitor treatment; keep appointments.

This medicine alone does not cause hypoglycemia (low blood sugar levels), but it may increase the hypoglycemic activity (lowering of blood sugar) of sulfonylureas or insulin. Because this medicine prevents the breakdown of table (cane) sugar, be sure to use glucose (dextrose), not sugar or fruits, to treat symptoms of low blood sugar (fatigue, excessive hunger, profuse sweating, numbness in arms or legs). Contact your healthcare provider if these symptoms occur.

Store below 77°F in a tightly sealed bottle. Protect from moisture.

Acebutolol Hydrochloride

(ass-cee-BYOO-toe-lahl HIGH-droe-KLOR-ide)

Sectral

A beta blocker medicine used to lower high blood pressure and to treat angina and heart attack.

Precautions

DO NOT USE if you are allergic to this medicine or its relatives, or if you are breastfeeding.

BEFORE USING THIS MEDICINE, tell your healthcare provider if you are pregnant; or if you are taking, will be taking or stop taking any prescription or nonprescription medicine; or if you have any other medical conditions.

Side Effects

Every medicine can cause side effects, but many people have no, or minor, side effects. Tell your healthcare provider if any of the following occurs: nausea; vomiting; stomach ache; diarrhea; constipation; appetite changes; indigestion; depression; anxiety; hallucinations; short-term memory loss; behavior changes; disorientation; fainting; dizziness; lightheadedness; tiredness; sleep disturbances; decreased concentration; headache; nightmares; emotional instability; changes in heart rate; chest pain; chills; cold or numb extremities; pounding in the chest; difficulty breathing; cough; nasal congestion; rash; hives; fluid retention; flushing or paleness; increased pigmentation; itching; hair loss; sweating; dry skin; psoriasis; painful and aching joints and muscles; painful, frequent or difficult urination; blurred vision; dry, burning or irritated eyes; ringing in the ears; taste changes; sore throat; dry mouth; slurred speech; fever; weight gain; changes in blood sugar levels.

Guidelines for Use

USE EXACTLY AS PRESCRIBED.

Ask your healthcare provider before using other medicines including nasal decongestants, diet aids or nonprescription cold preparations.

Do not stop this medicine suddenly, it could cause a worsening of disease including worse angina (chest pain), irregular heartbeats and increased risk of heart attack and death.

Withdraw this medicine slowly over 1 to 2 weeks by gradually decreasing the dose.

Diabetes — These products can mask signs of low blood sugar and change blood sugar levels. It may be necessary for your healthcare provider to change your dose of diabetic medications.

Use caution while driving or performing other tasks requiring mental alertness, coordination and dexterity.

Dizziness or lightheadedness when rising quickly from a seated or lying position may occur. Avoid sudden changes in posture.

Hypertension (high blood pressure) is a long-term or life-long disease. This medication is not a cure for hypertension, but helps to control it. Do not discontinue or change your dose, even if you don't feel any different, without your healthcare provider's consent. It is important not to miss any doses, and to follow your healthcare provider's instructions to monitor your condition at home. You may be asked to monitor your diet, weight and/or sodium intake.

Acetaminophen

(ass-cet-ah-MEE-noe-fen)

Acephen, Apacet, Arthritis Pain Formula Aspirin Free, Banesin, Children's Feverall, Dapa, Datril Extra-Strength, Dolanex, Genapap Extra Strength, Genebs, Halenol, Liquiprin, Meda Cap, Myapap, Oraphen-PD, Panadol, Panex, Phenaphen, Snaplets-FR, Tapanol Extra Strength, Tempra, Tylenol

A medicine used to relieve pain and reduce fever.

Precautions

DO NOT USE if you are allergic to this medicine.

BEFORE USING THIS MEDICINE, tell your healthcare provider if you are pregnant or breastfeeding; or if you are taking, will be taking or stop taking any prescription or nonprescription medicine; or if you have any other medical conditions.

Side Effects

Every medicine can cause side effects, but many people have no, or minor, side effects. Tell your healthcare provider if any of the following occurs: hives; yellowing of the skin or eyes; fainting; allergic reaction--difficulty breathing, rash, fever.

Guidelines for Use

USE EXACTLY AS PRESCRIBED.

Severe or recurrent pain or high or continued fever may indicate serious illness. If pain persists for more than 10 days, if redness is present, or in arthritic and rheumatic conditions affecting children under 12 years old, consult your healthcare provider immediately.

Do not exceed the recommended dosage. Consult your healthcare provider for use in children under 3 years of age or in oral use longer than 10 days.

Poisoning or overdose may cause few early symptoms, but requires immediate medical treatment.

Store suppositories below 80 degrees F.

Acetaminophen with Codeine Phosphate

(ass-cet-ah-MEE-noe-fen with KOE-deen FOSS-fate)

Aceta w/Codeine, APAP w/Codeine, Capital w/Codeine, Codaphen, Phenaphen w/Codeine No. 2, Phenaphen w/Codeine No. 3, Phenaphen w/Codeine No. 4, Phenaphen-650 w/Codeine, Ty-Tab #3, Tylenol w/Codeine, Tylenol w/Codeine #2, Tylenol w/Codeine #3, Tylenol w/Codeine #4

A nonaspirin pain reliever plus a narcotic pain reliever for relief of mild to moderate pain.

Precautions

DO NOT USE if you are allergic to either of these medications. Long-term use may be habit forming or lead to physical tolerance.

BEFORE USING THIS MEDICINE, tell your healthcare provider if you are pregnant or breastfeeding; or if you are taking, will be taking or stop taking any prescription or nonprescription medicine; or if you have any other medical conditions.

Side Effects

Every medicine can cause side effects, but many people have no, or minor, side effects. Tell your healthcare provider if any of the following occurs: drowsiness; dizziness; blurred vision; urinary retention; nausea; vomiting; constipation; shortness of breath; difficulty breathing; yellowing of the skin or gums.

Guidelines for Use

USE EXACTLY AS PRESCRIBED.

Take with food.

Avoid drinking alcohol and use caution with other drowsiness-causing medicines (eg, sleeping pills, antihistamines).

This medicine may cause drowsiness; use caution while driving or performing any tasks requiring mental alertness, coordination and dexterity.

If pain is severe, persistent or recurrent, contact your healthcare provider. Wait 30 to 60 minutes for the medicine to take effect before deciding if more is needed.

If a dose is missed, you do not need to make it up.

If constipation becomes a problem, a stool softener or bulk laxative may help.

Overdosage with this medicine can be very dangerous. If this occurs, contact your healthcare provider or poison control center immediately.

Acetazolamide

(uh-seet-uh-ZOLE-uh-mide)

AK-Zol, Dazamide, Diamox, Diamox Sequels, Storzolamide

A diuretic (water pill) that increases urine flow and reduces fluid pressure in the inner eye. It is used to treat glaucoma and to prevent Mountain Sickness in climbers. It also is used to reduce fluid accumulation and swelling. It may occasionally be prescribed for other reasons.

Precautions

DO NOT USE if you are allergic to this medicine or sulfa drugs (eg, *Gantrisin*).

BEFORE USING THIS MEDICINE, tell your healthcare provider if you are pregnant or breastfeeding; or if you are taking, will be taking or stop taking any prescription or nonprescription medicine; or if you have any other medical conditions.

Side Effects

Every medicine can cause side effects, but many people have no, or minor, side effects. Tell your healthcare provider if any of the following occurs: loss of appetite; nausea; vomiting; constipation; dark or bloody stools; weakness; nervousness; drowsiness; depression; dizziness; confusion; difficulty walking or performing other tasks; headache; tingling or tremors in the hands or feet; rash; hives; frequent or painful urination; flank or loin pain; blood or sugar in urine; fever; weight loss; nearsightedness; ringing in the ears.

Guidelines for Use

USE EXACTLY AS PRESCRIBED.

If stomach upset occurs, take with food.

May cause drowsiness. Use caution while driving or performing other tasks requiring alertness.

Taking larger than recommended doses does not increase the diuretic (water pill) activity of the drug. However, it will increase the risk of side effects.

Diabetes — This product may change blood or urine sugar levels. It may be necessary for your healthcare provider to change your dose of diabetic medications.

Acetohexamide

(uh-seet-uh-HEX-uh-mide)

Dymelor

An oral antidiabetic medicine that lowers blood sugar. It is used only in patients with non-insulin-dependent diabetes mellitus (Type II) who cannot manage blood sugar levels by diet and exercise alone.

Precautions

DO NOT USE if you have an allergy to this medicine or sulfa drugs.

BEFORE USING THIS MEDICINE, tell your healthcare provider if you are pregnant or breastfeeding; or if you are taking, will be taking or stop taking any prescription or nonprescription medicine; or if you have any other medical conditions.

Side Effects

Every medicine can cause side effects, but many people have no, or minor, side effects. Tell your healthcare provider if any of the following occurs: nausea; vomiting; heartburn; diarrhea; fever; sore throat; rash; itching; weakness; unusual bruising or bleeding.

Guidelines for Use

USE EXACTLY AS PRESCRIBED.

Take 30 minutes before a meal. Take with food if nausea or stomach upset occurs.

Consult your healthcare provider before consuming alcohol-containing beverages or medicines.

Monitor blood sugar levels daily. Notify your healthcare provider if low blood sugar develops (eg, fatigue, nausea, confusion, agitation, excessive hunger, profuse sweating, numbness or tingling of lips, tongue or extremities) or if excessive thirst or urination, or other symptoms of high blood sugar levels occur (glucose or ketones in the urine or blood).

Proper diet and exercise are important.

To prevent low blood sugar: 1. Know the symptoms of low blood sugar. 2. Keep track of your blood sugar levels. 3. Keep a source of quick-acting sugar with you at all times. 4. Maintain an adequate diet. 5. Know how diet and exercise affect your blood sugar level. Acute illness (eg, physical trauma, infection, fever, surgery) may require the temporary administration of insulin.

Acetylcysteine

(ASS-cee-till-SIS-teen)

Mucomyst, Mucosil-10, Mucosil-20

A medicine used to treat abnormally thick mucous secretions in chronic emphysema; emphysema with bronchitis; chronic asthmatic bronchitis; tuberculosis; bronchiectasis (chronic dilation of the airways); pneumonia; bronchitis; respiratory complications of cystic fibrosis; and other conditions involving excess mucus accumulation in the lung that is significant enough to effect breathing. It also has been given orally as an antidote to acetaminophen poisoning. It may occasionally be prescribed for other reasons.

Precautions

DO NOT USE if you are allergic to this medicine.

BEFORE USING THIS MEDICINE, tell your healthcare provider if you are pregnant or breastfeeding; or if you are taking, will be taking or stop taking any prescription or nonprescription medicine; or if you have any other medical conditions.

Side Effects

Every medicine can cause side effects, but many people have no, or minor, side effects. Tell your healthcare provider if any of the following occurs: rash; inflammation of the mouth; nausea; vomiting; runny nose; spasm of breathing passageways (tightness in the chest); drowsiness; clamminess; fever; coughing; blood in sputum; disagreeable odor.

Guidelines for Use

USE EXACTLY AS PRESCRIBED.

Use should be administered, supervised or directed by a respiratory therapist or healthcare provider. Special equipment is required.

It must be given as soon as possible, but within 24 hours as an antidote to acetaminophen poisoning.

May initially produce a slight disagreeable odor that soon disappears. The face mask may cause stickiness on the face after nebulization; remove with water.

Acyclovir

(A-SIKE-low-vihr)

Zovirax

An antiviral medicine used to treat genital herpes infections, herpes zoster (shingles) and chickenpox. It may occasionally be prescribed for other reasons.

Precautions

DO NOT USE if you are allergic to this medicine.

BEFORE USING THIS MEDICINE, tell your healthcare provider if you are pregnant or breastfeeding; if you are taking, will be taking or stop taking any prescription or nonprescription medicine; or if you have any other medical conditions.

Side Effects

Every medicine can cause side effects, but many people have no, or minor, side effects. Tell your healthcare provider if any of the following occurs: nausea; vomiting; diarrhea; headache; abnormal skin sensations; rash; weakness; numbness or tingling; general body discomfort; burning; itching; stinging (ointment only).

Guidelines for Use

USE EXACTLY AS PRESCRIBED.

Do not exceed recommended dosage, frequency or length of treatment.

Suspension: Shake well before using.

Ointment: Do not use in or near eyes. For external use only. Begin therapy as early as possible following the onset of symptoms. Apply to all lesions (sores) every 3 hours, 6 times per day for 7 days. A ½ inch ribbon of ointment generally will cover about 4 square inches. Ointment must thoroughly cover all lesions. To reduce the risk of spreading the infection, use a finger cot or rubber glove to apply the ointment.

If a dose is missed, take or apply it as soon as possible. If several hours have passed or if it is nearing time for the next dose, do not double the dose to catch up, unless advised by your healthcare provider. If more than one dose is missed, contact your healthcare provider.

This medicine is not a cure for herpes simplex infections.

Avoid sexual intercourse when lesions (sores) are present to prevent infecting your partner.

Notify your healthcare provider if lesions appear more frequently or become worse.

Patient information from the manufacturer is included with product.

Albuterol

(al-BYOO-ter-ahl)

Proventil, Proventil Repetabs, Ventolin, Ventolin Rotacaps

A medicine that makes breathing easier by widening breathing passages of the lung and by removing (expectorating) mucus and other debris causing congestion in the lungs. It may be used to treat or prevent asthma.

Precautions

DO NOT USE if you have an allergy to this medicine or heart rhythm disturbances associated with a rapid heart rate.

BEFORE USING THIS MEDICINE, tell your healthcare provider if you are pregnant or breastfeeding; or if you are taking, will be taking or stop taking any prescription or nonprescription medicine; or if you have any other medical conditions.

Side Effects

Every medicine can cause side effects, but many people have no, or minor, side effects. Tell your healthcare provider if any of the following occurs: nausea; vomiting; loss of appetite; heartburn; nervousness; restlessness; dizziness; lightheadedness; headache; anxiety; tension; tremor; drowsiness; weakness; sleeplessness; chest pain; pounding in chest (palpitations); breathing problems; coughing; flushing; sweating; hives; muscle cramps; unusual or bad taste in mouth; drying or irritation of mouth; stomach ache; diarrhea; teeth discoloration; nosebleeds; hyperactivity; feeling of a whirling motion.

Guidelines for Use

USE EXACTLY AS PRESCRIBED.

Tell your healthcare provider if palpitations, chest pain, muscle tremors, dizziness, headache, flushing or difficult urination occurs, or if breathing difficulty or nervousness persists.

Do not exceed recommended dosage. Excessive use may lead to side effects or loss of effectiveness. Do not stop or adjust the dose except on the recommendation of your healthcare provider.

If a dose is missed, take it as soon as possible. If several hours have passed, or if it is nearing time for the next dose, do not double the dose to "catch up," unless advised by your healthcare provider. If more than one dose is missed, contact your healthcare provider.

If you do not get the usual relief from your normal dose, do not increase your dose, but call your healthcare provider immediately.

Extended Release Tablets and Repetabs: Do not crush or chew this medicine.

Aerosol, Capsules for Inhalation, and Solution for Inhalation: Patient instructions are available with products. Shake well before using. Administer pressurized inhalation during the second half of breath intake. The usual dose is 1–2 inhalations (puffs) every 4 hours. If more than one inhalation per dose is necessary, wait at least one full minute between doses. (Administer second inhalation at 3 to 5 minutes.)

Do not spray in eyes.

Do not use epinephrine or other inhaled bronchodilators while using this medicine.

Store at room temperature. Medicine does not work as well when cold. Store away from heat and cold, out of reach of children.

Alendronate Sodium

(al-LEN-droe-nate SO-dee-um)

Fosamax

A hormone used to treat adults with Paget's disease of the bone and osteoporosis in post-menopausal women.

Precautions

DO NOT USE if you are allergic to this medicine or its relatives (bisphosphonates); have low calcium blood levels; active stomach problems (eg, esophagitis, gastritis, ulcers); difficulty swallowing or inability to stand/sit upright for at least 30 minutes.

BEFORE USING THIS MEDICINE, tell your healthcare provider if you are pregnant; or if you are taking, will be taking or stop taking any prescription or nonprescription medicine; or if you have any other medical conditons.

Side Effects

Every medicine can cause side effects, but many people have no, or minor, side effects. Tell your healthcare provider if any of the following occurs: gas; heartburn; stomach pain; nausea; vomiting; constipation; diarrhea; ulcer; difficulty swallowing; bloating; headache; muscle pain or cramps; appetite loss.

Guidelines for Use

USE EXACTLY AS PRESCRIBED.

Follow the patient instructions provided with the medicine exactly.

Take each tablet first thing in the morning with a full glass of water (6-8 oz), at least 30 minutes before the first food, beverage or medication of the day.

Taking this medicine with orange juice or coffee can decrease its effectiveness.

Do not chew or suck on the tablet.

After taking this medicine, remain upright (sitting/standing) for 30 minutes. Do not lie down until after eating.

Do not take at bedtime.

Do not take at the same time as other medicines (including aspirin), antacids or calcium supplements.

If a dose is missed, do not take it later in the day. The next day, continue your usual schedule of 1 tablet once a day. Continue use of this medicine.

Contact your healthcare provider if any throat or swallowing problems occur.

Do not change the dose or discontinue therapy unless advised to do so by your healthcare provider.

May cause stomach upset, nausea or diarrhea. Patients should maintain adequate nutrition, particularly an adequate intake of calcium and vitamin D. Supplemental calcium and vitamin D may be required. Avoid cigarette smoking and alcohol, which deplete calcium from bones. Consider weight-bearing exercises to increase the calcium density of bones.

Lab tests may be required to monitor treatment. Keep appointments.

Store at room temperature (59-86°F), in a tightly sealed container.

Allopurinol

(AL-oh-PURE-ee-nahl)

Lopurin, Zyloprim

A medicine used to treat various types of gout; to manage the increased uric acid blood levels associated with leukemia, lymphoma and other malignancies; to manage some types of kidney stones.

Precautions

DO NOT USE if you are allergic to this medicine.

BEFORE USING THIS MEDICINE, tell your healthcare provider if you are pregnant or breastfeeding; or if you are taking, will be taking or stop taking any prescription or nonprescription medicine; or if you have any other medical conditions.

Side Effects

Every medicine can cause side effects, but many people have no, or minor, side effects. Tell your healthcare provider if any of the following occurs: stomach upset; diarrhea; nausea; vomiting; abdominal pain; drowsiness; headache; chills; rash; unusual bleeding or bruising; yellowing of the skin and eyes; fever; muscle aches; painful urination; blood in the urine; tingling and numbness of legs and arms; acute gouty attacks.

Guidelines for Use

USE EXACTLY AS PRESCRIBED.

May cause stomach upset; take with food or milk.

Gouty attacks may not decrease for 2 to 6 weeks.

Drink plenty of fluids while taking this medication, at least 10 to 12 full (8 oz glasses) a day.

May cause drowsiness. Use caution while driving or performing other tasks requiring mental alertness. Call your healthcare provider at the first sign of a rash.

Large doses of vitamin C may increase the possibility of kidney stone formation and should be avoided. It is important to keep appointments with your healthcare provider.

Lab tests, including blood, kidney and liver tests, will be required during treatment with this medicine.

Alprazolam

(al-PRAY-zoe-lam)

Xanax

A benzodiazepine medicine used to treat anxiety disorders and panic attacks.

Precautions

DO NOT USE if you are allergic to this medicine or its relatives or are breastfeeding.

BEFORE USING THIS MEDICINE, tell your healthcare provider if you are pregnant; or if you are taking, will be taking or stop taking any prescription or nonprescription medicine; or if you have any other medical conditions.

Side Effects

Every medicine can cause side effects, but many people have no, or minor, side effects. Tell your healthcare provider if any of the following occurs: stomach upset; constipation; diarrhea; change in appetite; vomiting; confusion; depression; nervousness; memory loss; drowsiness; fatigue; dizziness; crying; disorientation; vivid dreams; headache; seizures; changes in heart rate; pounding in the chest; itching; rash; hair growth; yellowing of skin or eyes; visual or hearing disturbances; slurred speech; loss of bladder function; change in sex drive; urine retention; menstrual problems; dry mouth; fever; tremors/uncontrollable muscle movement; difficult breathing; swelling; excessive perspiration; joint pain; weight gain or loss; dehydration; fainting.

Guidelines for Use

USE EXACTLY AS PRESCRIBED.

May be taken with food or water if stomach upset occurs.

If a dose is missed, take it as soon as possible. If several hours have passed or if it is nearing time for the next dose, do not double the dose to "catch up," unless advised by your healthcare provider. If more than one dose is missed, contact your healthcare provider.

This medication can be addictive if used in large doses or for a long time. Discuss overuse with your healthcare provider.

May cause drowsiness. Use caution while driving or performing other tasks requiring mental alertness, coordination and dexterity.

Consult your healthcare provider before comsuming alcohol or alcohol-containing beverages or medicines.

Excitement, stimulation and acute rage have been reported. If these symptoms occur, tell your healthcare provider.

Patients on long-term or high dosage therapy may have withdrawal symptoms if therapy is suddenly stopped.

Alprostadil Injection

(al-PRAHST-ud-dill)

Caverject

Used to treat erectile dysfunction (impotence) in adult males. It may also be used with tests to diagnose erectile difficulties.

Precautions

DO NOT USE if you are allergic to this medicine; have sickle cell anemia, bone marrow tumors or leukemia; have a deformed penis or a penile implant; or if advised not to engage in sexual activity. Do not use in women, children or newborns.

BEFORE USING THIS MEDICINE, tell your healthcare provider if you are taking, will be taking or stop taking any prescription or non-prescription medicine; or if you have any other medical conditions.

Side Effects

Every medicine can cause side effects, but many people have no, or minor, side effects. Tell your healthcare provider if any of the following occurs: injection site bruising/bleeding; erections over 1 hour; difficult urination; prostate disorder or pain; penile pain; itching, redness, rash, swelling, hardening, or discoloration of the skin; yeast infection; headache; dizziness; respiratory infection; flu syndrome; sinus infection; nasal congestion; cough; back pain.

Guidelines for Use

USE EXACTLY AS PRESCRIBED.

Carefully follow the preparation and injection instructions included in each package. Proper use can eliminate certain side effects.

Examine each vial for discoloration or particles. Discard such vials.

Do not shake the contents of the reconstituted (mixed) vial. Use the solution immediately. Discard any unused solution immediately; do not store or freeze mixed solution.

Do not change the dose without asking your healthcare provider.

Properly discard needle after each use. Do not re-use or share needles or syringes. Do not allow anyone else to access or use your medicine.

Erections usually occur within 5 to 20 minutes after injection and last about 1 hour. If an erection lasts longer than 6 hours, contact your healthcare provider immediately.

Do not use this medicine more than 3 times per week; wait at least 24 hours between each use.

If penile redness, swelling, tenderness, pain, hardening of the skin or curving of erect penis occurs, contact your healthcare provider immediately.

This medicine offers no protection from the transmission of sexually transmitted diseases such as HIV (the virus that causes AIDS).

A small amount of bleeding at the injection site may occur. This can increase the risk of transmitting serious diseases between partners.

Regular medical checkups are necessary to monitor treatment.

Store below 77°F for up to 3 months. Do not freeze, store in checked luggage during air travel or leave in a closed automobile.

Altretamine

(ahl-TRETT-uh-meen)

Hexalen

A medicine used to treat ovarian cancer.

Precautions

DO NOT USE if you are allergic to this medicine.

BEFORE USING THIS MEDICINE, tell your healthcare provider if you are pregnant or breastfeeding; or if you are taking, will be taking or stop taking any prescription or nonprescription medicine; or if you have any other medical conditions.

Side Effects

Every medicine can cause side effects, but many people have no, or minor, side effects. Tell your healthcare provider if any of the following occurs: appetite loss; diarrhea; constipation; stomach pain; nausea; vomiting; dizziness; mood disorders; disorders of consciousness; anxiety; fatigue; weakness; feeling of whirling motion; seizures; severe bleeding; hair loss; itching; redness; skin disorders; allergic reaction; inflammation of mucous membranes; abnormal vision; blood in urine; speech problems.

Guidelines for Use

USE EXACTLY AS PRESCRIBED.

The use of birth control is recommended during therapy with this medication. Notify your healthcare provider immediately if you suspect you are pregnant.

May cause drowsiness or dizziness. Use caution while driving or performing other tasks requiring alertness.

Do not have immunizations without your healthcare provider's approval.

Practice good oral hygiene and have regular dental checkups.

Be careful when using a regular toothbrush, dental floss and toothpicks. Your healthcare provider may recommend other ways to clean teeth and gums.

Check with your healthcare provider before having any dental work done.

Be careful not to cut yourself and use caution when using sharp objects (razor, nail clippers). Avoid situations such as sports, where injury or bruising could occur.

Lab tests will be required during treatment. Be sure to keep appointments.

Neurologic exams should be performed regularly during therapy.

Aluminum Salts

(uh-LOO-min-uhm salts)

AlternaGel, Alu-Cap, Alu-Tab, Amphojel, Basaljel, Dialume, Rolaids

Used to treat upset stomach due to too much acid secretion (eg, heartburn, acid indigestion and sour stomach); to treat irritation associated with peptic ulcers. It may occasionally be prescribed for other reasons.

Precautions

DO NOT USE if you are allergic to this medicine.

BEFORE USING THIS MEDICINE, tell your healthcare provider if you are pregnant or breastfeeding; or if you are taking, will be taking or stop taking any prescription or nonprescription medicine; or if you have any other medical conditions.

Side Effects

Every medicine can cause side effects, but many people have no, or minor, side effects. Tell your healthcare provider if any of the following occurs: nausea; vomiting; stomach pain; constipation; muscular weakness; lack of energy; headache; confusion; irritability.

Guidelines for Use

USE EXACTLY AS PRESCRIBED.

Antacids reduce acidity for about 30 minutes when taken on an empty stomach. Acidity is reduced for about 3 hours when antacids are taken 1 hour after meals.

Do not take other medications within 1 to 2 hours of taking this medicine.

Tell your healthcare provider if coffee-ground vomiting or black, tar-like stools occur.

Taking too much of these products can cause the stomach to secrete excess stomach acid. Talk to your healthcare provider about the appropriate dose.

Chewable tablets--Chew thoroughly before swallowing. Follow with a glass of water.

Suspension--Shake well before using.

Amantadine Hydrochloride

(uh-MAN-tuh-deen HIGH-droe-KLOR-ide)

Symadine, Symmetrel

A medicine used to treat influenza A (the flu); it also is used for the treatment of Parkinson's disease. It may occasionally be prescribed for other reasons.

Precautions

DO NOT USE if you are allergic to this medicine or its relatives.

BEFORE USING THIS MEDICINE, tell your healthcare provider if you are pregnant or breastfeeding; or if you are taking, will be taking or stop taking any prescription or nonprescription medicine; or if you have any other medical conditions.

Side Effects

Every medicine can cause side effects, but many people have no, or minor, side effects. Tell your healthcare provider if any of the following occurs: seizures (in epileptics); constipation; dizziness; lightheadedness; insomnia; depression; anxiety; hallucinations; confusion; headache; fatigue; visual disturbances; difficulty breathing; edema (fluid retention); dry mouth; urinary retention; vomiting; slurred speech.

Guidelines for Use

USE EXACTLY AS PRESCRIBED.

May cause blurred vision. Use caution when driving or performing other tasks requiring mental alertness.

Do not get up quickly after sitting or lying down as this may cause fainting or dizziness. Notify your healthcare provider if this occurs.

Tell your healthcare provider if mood or mental changes, swelling of the extremities, difficult urination or shortness of breath occurs.

If a dose is missed, take it as soon as possible. If several hours have passed or if it is nearing time for the next dose, do not double the dose to catch up, unless advised by your healthcare provider. If more than one dose is missed, contact your healthcare provider.

Amifostine

(am-ih-FOSS-teen)

Ethyol

A medicine used to reduce damage to the kidneys in patients given repeated courses of cisplatin for advanced ovarian cancer.

Precautions

DO NOT USE if you are allergic to aminothiol compounds or mannitol.

BEFORE USING THIS MEDICINE, tell your healthcare provider if you are pregnant or breastfeeding; or if you are taking, will be taking or stop taking any prescription or nonprescription medicine (especially high blood pressure medicine); or if you have any other medical conditions (especially high or low blood pressure).

Side Effects

Every medicine can cause side effects, but many people have no, or minor, side effects. Tell your healthcare provider if any of the following occurs: nausea; vomiting; flushing/feeling of warmth; chills/feeling of coldness; dizziness; somnolence; hiccoughs; sneezing; rapid heartbeat.

Guidelines for Use

USE EXACTLY AS PRESCRIBED.

This medicine is given once daily as a 15 minute IV infusion, starting within 30 minutes before the chemotherapy treatment.

If you experience low blood pressure, this medicine may be stopped until your blood pressure has reutrned to normal. The medicine can then be restarted.

This medicine can cause nausea and possibly severe vomiting. Medicines to help control this are often given along with amifostine.

Blood pressure will be monitored frequently while receiving this medicine.

Lab tests may be required; be sure to keep appointments.

Amiloride Hydrochloride

(uh-MILL-oh-ride HIGH-droe-KLOR-ide)

Midamor

A potassium-sparing diuretic or water pill. It is generally used to treat fluid accumulation and swelling, high blood pressure and to prevent or treat low potassium levels.

Precautions

DO NOT USE if you are allergic to this medicine or its relatives, or are breastfeeding.

BEFORE USING THIS DRUG, tell your healthcare provider if you are pregnant or breastfeeding; or if you are taking, will be taking or stop taking any prescription or nonprescription medicine; or if you have any other medical conditions.

Side Effects

Every medicine can cause side effects, but many people have no, or minor, side effects. Tell your healthcare provider if any of the following occurs: stomach or intestinal pain; nausea; vomiting; diarrhea; constipation; gas; heartburn; loss of appetite; weakness, fatigue; drowsiness; confusion; tingling or numbness of hands or feet; depression; headache; dizziness or lightheadedness when arising from a seated or lying position; sleeplessness; nervousness; chest pain; shortness of breath; cough; nasal congestion; rash; itching; yellowing of the skin or eyes; hair loss; muscle weakness or cramping; ringing in the ears; visual disturbances; changes in sex drive; dry mouth.

Guidelines for Use

USE EXACTLY AS PRESCRIBED.

If a single dose is prescribed, generally take it in the morning.

May cause stomach upset. Take with food.

Use caution while driving or performing other tasks requiring alertness.

Avoid large quantities of potassium-rich food or salt substitutes.

Patients being treated for high blood pressure often feel tired for a few weeks. It takes time for the body to adjust to lowered blood pressure. Continue taking your medication and check with your healthcare provider regarding any new symptoms to assure that they are a normal consequence of changes in blood pressure.

Hypertension (high blood pressure) is a long-term or life-long disease. This medication is not a cure for high blood pressure, but helps to control it. Do not discontinue or change your dose, even if you feel well or do not feel any different without your healthcare provider's consent. It is important not to miss any doses, and to follow you healthcare provider's instructions to monitor your condition at home. You may be asked to monitor your diet, weight and/or sodium intake.

Dizziness or lightheadedness when rising quickly from a seated or lying positon may occur. Avoid sudden changes in posture.

Aminocaproic Acid

(uh-mee-no-kuh-PRO-ik acid)

Amicar

A medicine used to treat excessive bleeding resulting from certain conditions (systemic hyperfibrinolysis and urinary fibrinolysis). It may occasionally be prescribed for other reasons.

Precautions

DO NOT USE if you are allergic to this medicine or benzyl alcohol.

BEFORE USING THIS MEDICINE, tell your healthcare provider if you are pregnant or breastfeeding; or if you are taking, will be taking or stop taking any prescription or nonprescription medicine; or if you have any other medical conditions.

Side Effects

Every medicine can cause side effects, but many people have no, or minor, side effects. Tell your healthcare provider if any of the following occurs: nausea; cramps; diarrhea; general body discomfort; weakness; fatigue; dizziness; ringing in the ears; headache; hallucinations; seizures; excessive tearing; nasal congestion; skin rash; difficulty urinating.

Guidelines for Use

USE EXACTLY AS PRESCRIBED.

Lab tests may be required during treatment with this medicine.

Contact your healthcare provider if unusual bleeding or bruising, reddish-brown colored urine, chest or leg pain or difficulty breathing occurs.

Hemophilia — There have been some reports of dry ejaculation during the period of treatment. This occurred after undergoing dental surgical procedures. Symptoms cleared up within 24 to 48 hours.

Brush teeth with a soft toothbrush.

This medicine may cause drowsiness or dizziness. Use caution while driving or performing other tasks requiring mental alertness, coordination and dexterity.

Aminophylline

(am-in-AHF-ih-lin)

Phyllocontin, Somophyllin, Somophyllin-DF, Truphylline

A medicine used to prevent and relieve symptoms of bronchial asthma, and to treat chronic bronchitis and emphysema. It may occasionally be prescribed for other reasons.

Precautions

DO NOT USE if you are allergic to this medicine or any xanthine (eg, caffeine, chocolate).

BEFORE USING THIS MEDICINE, tell your healthcare provider if you are pregnant or breastfeeding; or if you are taking, will be taking or stop taking any prescription or nonprescription medicine; or if you have any other medical conditions.

Side Effects

Every medicine can cause side effects, but many people have no, or minor, side effects. Tell your healthcare provider if any of the following occurs: nausea; vomiting; severe stomach pain; diarrhea; loss of appetite; sleeplessness; jitteriness; headache; rash; restlessness; convulsions; irregular heartbeat.

Guidelines for Use

USE EXACTLY AS PRESCRIBED.

Take at regular intervals around the clock.

Avoid large amounts of caffeine-containing food or beverages, such as tea, coffee, cocoa and cola drinks or large amounts of chocolate because these products may increase side effects.

It is important to keep regular appointments with your healthcare provider.

Do not change the dose of your medication without consulting your healthcare provider.

Do not use this medicine for an acute asthma attack.

If a dose is missed, take it as soon as possible. If several hours have passed or if it is nearing time for the next dose, do not double the dose to "catch up," unless advised by your healthcare provider. If more than one dose is missed, contact your healthcare provider.

Tablets and liquids: If stomach upset occurs, take with food.

Timed release tablets: Swallow whole; do not crush or chew.

Suppositories: If you do not know the proper way to insert a suppository, ask your healthcare provider.

Aminosalicylate Sodium

(uh-MEE-no-suh-LIS-ih-late SO-dee-uhm)

Sodium P.A.S.

A medicine used with other medicines to treat tuberculosis infections.

Precautions

DO NOT USE if you have an allergy to this medicine or to salicylates (eg, aspirin).

BEFORE USING THIS MEDICINE, tell your healthcare provider if you are pregnant or breastfeeding; if you are taking, will be taking or stop taking any prescription or nonprescription medicine; or if you have any other medical conditions.

Side Effects

Every medicine can cause side effects, but many people have no, or minor, side effects. Tell your healthcare provider if any of the following occurs: nausea; vomiting; appetite loss; diarrhea; stomach pain; dizziness; unusual tiredness; weakness; drowsiness; rash; itching; hives; headache; vision problems; fever; general body discomfort; goiter; unusual bleeding or bruising; skin reactions; yellowing of skin or eyes.

Guidelines for Use

USE EXACTLY AS PRESCRIBED.

Take as directed. Avoid missing doses.

May cause stomach upset. Take with food or meals.

Do not use if the tablets are brown or purple in color.

This medicine will not work if it becomes wet or is left in extreme heat or direct sunlight. Therefore, do not store in the kitchen or bathroom cabinet.

Do not stop taking this medicine before consulting your healthcare provider.

If a dose is missed, take it as soon as possible. If several hours have passed or if it is nearing time for the next dose, do not double the dose in order to "catch up," unless advised to do so by your healthcare provider. If more than one dose is missed, contact your healthcare provider.

Contact your healthcare provider if fever, sore throat, yellowing of skin or eyes, unusual bleeding or bruising or skin rash occurs.

Amiodarone

(A-MEE-oh-duh-rone)

Cordarone

A heart medicine (antiarrhythmic) used to treat certain serious heart rhythm disturbances.

Precautions

DO NOT USE if you are allergic to this medicine or if you are breastfeeding.

BEFORE USING THIS MEDICINE, tell your healthcare provider if you are pregnant; or if you are taking, will be taking or stop taking any prescription or nonprescription medicine; or if you have any other medical conditions.

Side Effects

Every medicine can cause side effects, but many people have no, or minor, side effects. Tell your healthcare provider if any of the following occurs: appearance of halos around lights; sensitivity to light; blurred vision; dry eye; other vision problems; nausea; vomiting; constipation; loss of appetite; abdominal pain; tremors; twitches; fatigue; unsteady walking; dizziness; numbness and tingling in hands and feet; difficulty with sleep; headache; slowing of heartbeat (rhythm); worsening of irregular heart rhythm; difficult breathing; coughing; sensitivity to sunlight; blue-gray skin color; rash; dermatitis; bruising; hair loss; flushing; disturbances in thyroid, respiratory and liver function (cirrhosis, hepatitis); abnormal taste and smell; fluid retention; abnormal salivation; loss of sex drive.

Guidelines for Use

USE EXACTLY AS PRESCRIBED.

Take with meals, especially if stomach upset occurs.

Daily doses may vary depending on individual needs. Do not adjust the dose without consulting your healthcare provider.

A worsening of heart rhythm irregularities is unusual while under treatment but can occur. This medicine can also cause slow heart rates or occasional pauses in the heart rhythm.

Sensitivity of the skin to sunlight and to ultraviolet light may occur. During long-term treatment, exposed skin may appear blue-gray. Risk is increased in patients with a fair complexion and in those with excessive exposure to the sun. Use sunscreens and wear protective clothing.

Amitriptyline Hydrochloride

(am-ee-TRIP-tih-leen HIGH-droe-KLOR-ide)

Elavil, Endep, Enovil

A mood elevating medicine usually used for the relief of depression. It may occasionally be prescribed for other reasons.

Precautions

DO NOT USE if you are allergic to this medicine or its relatives, or if you are using monoamine oxidase inhibitors (MAOIs, eg, *Nardil, Parnate*).

BEFORE USING THIS MEDICINE, tell your healthcare provider if you are pregnant or breastfeeding; or if you are taking, will be taking or stop taking any prescription or nonprescription medicine; or if you have any other medical conditions.

Side Effects

Every medicine can cause side effects, but many people have no, or minor, side effects. Tell your healthcare provider if any of the following occurs: dry mouth; blurred vision; increased heart rate; impaired coordination; difficult urination; excessive sedation; seizures.

Guidelines for Use

USE EXACTLY AS PRESCRIBED.

Take as directed with a full glass of water, with or without food.

If a dose is missed, take it as soon as possible. If several hours have passed or if it is nearing time for the next dose, do not double the dose to catch up, unless advised by your healthcare provider. If more than one dose is missed, contact your healthcare provider.

This medicine may not be effective for 2 to 3 weeks.

May cause drowsiness or blurred vision. Use caution while driving or performing other tasks requiring mental alertness.

Using this medicine with alcohol or other central nervous system depressants (eg, pain relievers, sedatives, antihistamines) may cause added drowsiness.

May cause sensitivity to sunlight. Avoid prolonged exposure to the sun. Use sunscreens and wear protective clothing until tolerance is determined.

Taking this medicine at bedtime may help reduce side effects (eg, daytime drowsiness). Discuss this possibility with your healthcare provider.

Amlodipine

(am-LOW-dih-PEEN)

Norvasc

A calcium channel blocker medicine that is used to treat various types of angina and high blood pressure. It may occasionally be prescribed for other reasons.

Precautions

DO NOT USE if you are allergic to this medicine.

BEFORE USING THIS MEDICATION, tell your healthcare provider if you are pregnant or breastfeeding; or if you are taking, will be taking or stop taking any prescription or non-prescription medicine; or if you have any other medical conditions.

Side Effects

Every medicine can cause side effects, but many people have no, or minor, side effects. Tell your healthcare provider if any of the following occurs: irregular heartbeat; increased frequency/severity of angina (may occur at the start of therapy or when dose is increased); shortness of breath; swelling of hands and feet; dizziness; constipation; nausea; low blood pressure or symptoms of drug allergy (eg, itching, rash, hives, difficult breathing); flushing; headache; fatigue; gum enlargement; unusual bruising or bleeding.

Guidelines for Use

USE EXACTLY AS PRESCRIBED.

May be taken without regard to meals.

If a dose is missed, take it as soon as possible. If several hours have passed or if it is nearing time for the next dose, do not double the dose to catch up unless advised by your healthcare provider. If more than one dose is missed, contact your healthcare provider.

Do not suddenly stop taking this medicine as this may cause serious chest pains. This risk can be minimized if the medicine is slowly reduced by your healthcare provider.

Low blood pressure may occur (usually as dizziness or lightheadedness). Tell your healthcare provider if this occurs.

It is important to brush and floss your teeth and see your dentist regularly.

Amobarbital Sodium

(am-oh-BAR-bih-tahl SO-dee-uhm)

Amytal Sodium

A barbiturate central nervous system depressant that can produce mild sedation, sleep and up to deep coma. Usually used to treat insomnia, to calm agitated people and to treat certain seizure disorders.

Precautions

DO NOT USE if you are allergic to this medicine or its relatives. This medicine may be habit-forming. Tolerance and dependence may occur, especially following prolonged use of high doses. Withdrawal symptoms can be severe.

BEFORE USING THIS MEDICINE, tell your healthcare provider if you are pregnant or breastfeeding; or if you are taking, will be taking or stop taking any prescription or nonprescription medicine; or if you have any other medical conditions.

Side Effects

Every medicine can cause side effects, but many people have no, or minor, side effects. Tell your healthcare provider if any of the following occurs: sleepiness; tired feeling; nausea; vomiting; morning hangover.

Guidelines for Use

USE EXACTLY AS PRESCRIBED.

Take only the amount of medicine prescribed by your healthcare provider.

May decrease alertness or physical ability. Use caution when driving or performing tasks requiring mental alertness.

Avoid alcohol and other mental depressants (eg, narcotics, tranquilizers, antihistamines) while you are taking this medicine.

Use as an aid to sleep is limited; generally not for use longer than 2 weeks.

Seizure control — Do not stop therapy suddenly.

Amobarbital/Secobarbital

(am-oh-BAR-bih-tahl/see-koe-BAR-bih-tahl)

Tuinal Pulvules

A barbiturate combination that can produce mild sedation, sleep and even deep coma. Usually used to treat insomnia, to calm agitated people and to treat certain seizure disorders.

Precautions

DO NOT USE if you are allergic to this medicine or barbiturates or if you have drug abuse tendencies. This medicine may be habit-forming. Tolerance and dependence may occur, especially following prolonged use of high doses. Withdrawal symptoms can be severe.

BEFORE USING THIS MEDICINE, tell your healthcare provider if you are pregnant or breastfeeding; or if you are taking, will be taking or stop taking any prescription or nonprescription medicine; or if you have any other medical conditions.

Side Effects

Every medicine can cause side effects, but many people have no, or minor, side effects. Tell your healthcare provider if any of the following occurs: nausea; vomiting; constipation; diarrhea; drowsiness; agitation; confusion; nightmares; hangover feeling; nervousness; hallucinations; sleeplessness; headache; difficulty breathing; nosebleeds; unusual behavior; dizziness; incoordination; skin rash; hives.

Guidelines for Use

USE EXACTLY AS PRESCRIBED.

Take only the amount of medicine prescribed by your healthcare provider.

This medicine may cause drowsiness or dizziness. Use caution while driving or performing other tasks requiring mental alertness, coordination and dexterity.

Avoid alcohol and other mental depressants (eg, narcotics, tranquilizers, antihistamines) while you are taking this medicine.

Use as an aid to sleep is limited; generally not for use longer than two weeks. Discuss with your healthcare provider if the medicine seems to be less effective with repeated use.

Amoxapine

(am-OX-uh-peen)

Asendin

A mood elevating medicine usually used for the relief of depression. It may occasionally be prescribed for other reasons.

Precautions

DO NOT USE if you are allergic to this medicine or its relatives, or if you are using monoamine oxidase inhibitors (eg, *Nardil*, *Parnate*).

BEFORE USING THIS MEDICINE, tell your healthcare provider if you are pregnant or breastfeeding; or if you are taking, will be taking or stop taking any prescription or nonprescription medicine; or if you have any other medical conditions.

Side Effects

Every medicine can cause side effects, but many people have no, or minor, side effects. Tell your healthcare provider if any of the following occurs: dry mouth; blurred vision; increased heart rate; impaired coordination; difficult urination; excessive sedation; seizures.

Guidelines for Use

USE EXACTLY AS PRESCRIBED.

Take as directed with a full glass of water, with or without food.

If a dose is missed, take it as soon as possible. If several hours have passed or if it is nearing time for the next dose, do not double the dose to "catch up," unless advised by your healthcare provider. If more than one dose is missed, contact your healthcare provider.

This medicine may not be effective for 2 to 3 weeks.

Using this medicine with alcohol or other central nervous system depressants (eg, pain relievers, sedatives, antihistamines) may cause added drowsiness.

May cause drowsiness or blurred vision. Use caution while driving or performing other tasks requiring mental alertness.

May cause sensitivity to sunlight. Avoid prolonged exposure to the sun. Use sunscreens and wear protective clothing until tolerance is determined.

Taking this medicine at bedtime may help reduce side effects (eg, daytime drowsiness). Discuss this possibility with your healthcare provider.

Amoxicillin

(a-MOX-ih-sil-in)

Amoxil, Amoxil Pediatric, Biomox, Polymox, Trimox, Wymox

A penicillin antibiotic used to treat infections caused by certain bacteria.

Precautions

DO NOT USE if you are allergic to any cephalosporin or penicillin.

BEFORE USING THIS MEDICINE, tell your healthcare provider if you are pregnant or breastfeeding; or if you are taking, will be taking or stop taking any prescription or nonprescription medicine; or if you have any other medical conditions.

Side Effects

Every medicine can cause side effects, but many people have no, or minor, side effects. Tell your healthcare provider if any of the following occurs: rash; itching; hives; severe diarrhea; shortness of breath; wheezing; dizziness; black tongue; sore throat; nausea; vomiting; fever; swollen joints; or any unusual bleeding or bruising.

Guidelines for Use

USE EXACTLY AS PRESCRIBED.

May be taken without regard to meals.

Take at evenly spaced intervals throughout the day.

If a dose is missed, take it as soon as possible. If several hours have passed or if it is nearing time for the next dose, do not double the dose to catch up, unless advised by your healthcare provider. If more than one dose is missed, contact your healthcare provider.

Continue until all the prescribed medicine has been taken. Failure to take a full course of therapy may cause a relapse of the infection.

Suspension: Shake well before using. Keep refrigerated; discard after 10 days.

Amoxicillin/Potassium Clavulanate

(a-MOX-ih-sil-in/poe-TASS-ee-uhm CLAV-you-lon-ate)

Augmentin

A penicillin antibiotic used to treat infections caused by certain bacteria.

Precautions

DO NOT USE if you are allergic to any penicillin or cephalosporin.

BEFORE USING THIS MEDICINE, tell your healthcare provider if you are pregnant or breastfeeding; or if you are taking, will be taking or stop taking any prescription or nonprescription medicine; or if you have any other medical conditions.

Side Effects

Every medicine can cause side effects, but many people have no, or minor, side effects. Tell your healthcare provider if any of the following occurs: rash; itching; hives; severe diarrhea; shortness of breath; wheezing; dizziness; black tongue; sore throat; nausea; vomiting; fever; swollen joints; unusual bleeding or bruising.

Guidelines for Use

USE EXACTLY AS PRESCRIBED.

May be taken without regard to meals.

Take at evenly spaced intervals throughout the day.

If a dose is missed, take it as soon as possible. If several hours have passed or if it is nearing time for the next dose, do not double the dose to "catch up," unless advised by your healthcare provider. If more than one dose is missed, contact your healthcare provider.

Continue to take until all the prescribed medicine is gone. Failure to take a full course of therapy may cause a relapse of the infection.

Suspension: Keep refrigerated; discard after 10 days. Shake well before using.

Amphetamine

(am-FET-uh-meen)

Lannett

A medicine that is used to treat narcolepsy, attention deficit disorder in children (hyperactivity) and as a short-term addition in a weight reduction program.

Precautions

DO NOT USE if you are allergic to this medicine or if you are taking a monoamine oxidase inhibitor (MAOI, eg, *Parnate*).

BEFORE USING THIS MEDICINE, tell your healthcare provider if you are pregnant or breastfeeding; or if you are taking, will be taking or stop taking any prescription or nonprescription medicine; if you have any other medical conditions; or if you are allergic to tartrazine.

Side Effects

Every medicine can cause side effects, but many people have no, or minor, side effects. Tell your healthcare provider if any of the following occurs: diarrhea; constipation; dry mouth; headache; anxiety; tension; nervousness; dizziness; depression or fatigue (between doses or after stopping); inability to sleep; excessive restlessness; irritability; pounding in the chest (palpitations); rash; flushing; sweating; hives; fever; muscle tremor or twitching; sexual problems; weight loss; rapid breathing/panting; unpleasant taste.

Guidelines for Use

USE EXACTLY AS PRESCRIBED.

Take early in the day to avoid nighttime sleep loss.

Do not increase dosage, except on the advice of your healthcare provider.

This medicine may impair your ability to drive or perform other tasks requiring mental alertness.

It may mask extreme fatigue and cause dizziness.

It may cause nervousness, restlessness, sleeplessness, dizziness, appetite loss, dry mouth and digestive tract disturbances. Contact your healthcare provider if these effects become pronounced.

Attention deficit disorder in children - Your healthcare provider may occasionally interrupt therapy to determine if there is a need for continued use.

Weight control — Appropriate lifestyle changes (eg, diet and exercise) should be made while on therapy. Use beyond 8 to 12 weeks is not encouraged.

Use of this medicine to improve athletic skills, mental alertness or to stay awake is dangerous and illegal. Never share medicine with others.

Amphotericin B Injection

(am-foe-TER-ih-sin B)

Fungizone Intravenous

Used to treat a variety of fungal infections.

Side Effects

Every medicine can cause side effects, but many people have no, or minor, side effects. Tell your healthcare provider if any of the following occurs: fever (sometimes with severe chills); headache; loss of appetite; general body discomfort; generalized pain, including muscle and joints; nausea; vomiting; upset stomach; diarrhea; cramping; weight loss; pain or infection at the injection site.

Amphotericin B Topical

(am-foe-TER-ih-sin B)

Fungizone

Used for the treatment of skin infections caused by Candida sp.

Precautions

DO NOT USE if you are allergic to this medicine.

BEFORE USING THIS MEDICINE, tell your healthcare provider if you are pregnant or breastfeeding; or if you are taking, will be taking or stop taking any prescription or nonprescription medicine; or if you have any other medical conditions.

Side Effects

Every medicine can cause side effects, but many people have no, or minor, side effects. Tell your healthcare provider if any of the following occurs: irritation; drying of the skin.

Guidelines for Use

USE EXACTLY AS PRESCRIBED.

For external use only; avoid contact with the eyes.

Cleanse affected area(s) of skin prior to application.

Apply a generous amount to lesions and rub in gently.

Redness, itching or burning also may occur, particularly in skin folds. Tell your healthcare provider if these effects become bothersome, if skin rash develops or if the condition being treated worsens.

Any discoloration of fabrics from the cream or lotion may be removed by hand washing the fabric with soap and warm water.

Any fabric discoloration from the ointment may be removed by applying a standard cleaning fluid.

Use for the full treatment time, even if symptoms improve.

Tell your healthcare provider if there is no improvement after 5–7 days.

Cream--May cause drying and slight discoloration of the skin.

Lotion and ointment--May cause staining of nail lesions, but not skin, if thoroughly rubbed in.

Ampicillin

(am-pih-SILL-in)

D-Amp, Omnipen, Omnipen-N, Polycillin, Polycillin-N, Polycillin Pediatric, Polycillin-PRB (with probenecid), Principen, Probampacin (with probenecid), Totacillin, Totacillin-N

A penicillin antibiotic used to treat infections caused by certain bacteria.

Precautions

DO NOT USE if you are allergic to any penicillin or cephalosporin.

BEFORE USING THIS MEDICINE, tell your healthcare provider if you are pregnant or breastfeeding; or if you are taking, will be taking or stop taking any prescription or nonprescription medicine; or if you have any other medical conditions.

Side Effects

Every medicine can cause side effects, but many people have no, or minor, side effects. Tell your healthcare provider if any of the following occurs: rash; itching; hives; severe diarrhea; shortness of breath; wheezing; dizziness; black tongue; sore throat; nausea; vomiting; fever; swollen joints; or any unusual bleeding or bruising.

Guidelines for Use

USE EXACTLY AS PRESCRIBED.

Take on an empty stomach approximately 30 minutes to one hour before meals or two hours after a meal.

Take at evenly spaced intervals throughout the day.

If a dose is missed, take it as soon as possible. If several hours have passed or if it is nearing time for the next dose, do not double the dose to "catch up", unless advised by your healthcare provider. If more than one dose is missed, contact your healthcare provider.

Continue until all the prescribed medicine has been taken. Failure to take a full course of therapy may cause a relapse of the infection.

Suspension: Shake well before using. Store in the refrigerator; discard after 10 days.

Ampicillin Sodium/Sulbactam Sodium

(am-pih-SILL-in SO-dee-uhm/sull-BAK-tam SO-dee-uhm)

Unasyn

Used in the treatment of infections due to susceptible microorganisms.

Side Effects

Every medicine can cause side effects, but many people have no, or minor, side effects. Tell your healthcare provider if any of the following occurs: pain at the injection or IV site; diarrhea; rash.

Amyl Nitrite

(A-mill NYE-trite)

Amyl Nitrite Aspirols, Amyl Nitrite Vaporole

This medicine is used to treat angina attacks. It should be taken before events or activities that are likely to provoke an attack. It also is used to treat congestive heart failure associated with heart attacks.

Precautions

DO NOT USE if you are allergic to this medicine or its relatives or if you are pregnant or breastfeeding.

BEFORE USING THIS MEDICINE, tell your healthcare provider if you are taking, will be taking or stop taking any prescription or nonprescription medicine; or if you have any other medical conditions.

Side Effects

Every medicine can cause side effects, but many people have no, or minor, side effects. Tell your healthcare provider if any of the following occurs: persistent headache; faintness; apprehension; restlessness; dizziness; muscle twitching; weakness; chest pain; pounding in the chest (palpitations); flushing; fever; involuntary passing of urine or feces; itching; rash.

Guidelines for Use

USE EXACTLY AS PRESCRIBED.

It is important to maintain the prescribed dosing schedule while on this medicine.

The effect of inhalation is almost instantaneous, causing lightheadedness, dizziness and euphoria.

Headache is a common side effect. Aspirin or acetaminophen often relieves the headaches.

Dizziness or lightheadedness may occur if you stand up too fast from a lying or sitting position. If this occurs, get up slowly and avoid sudden changes in posture.

Alcohol may worsen this effect. Chronic misuse can cause bronchial irritation and a blood disorder.

Highly flammable; do not use near where it might be ignited.

Use in a well ventilated area.

Use when lying down.

Crush capsule and wave under nose while inhaling; 1-6 inhalations from the capsule are usually sufficient.

Anastrozole

(an-ASS-troe-zole)

Arimidex

A chemotherapy (anticancer) drug used to treat advanced breast cancer in postmenopausal women following therapy with tamoxifen.

Precautions

DO NOT USE if you are allergic to this medicine.

BEFORE USING THIS MEDICINE, tell your healthcare provider if you are pregnant or breastfeeding; if you are taking, will be taking or stop taking any prescription or nonprescription medicine; or if you have any other medical conditions.

Side Effects

Every medicine can cause side effects, but many people have no, or minor, side effects. Tell your healthcare provider if any of the following occurs: nausea; vomiting; diarrhea; appetite change; constipation; dry mouth; weight gain; abnormal vaginal bleeding or dryness; hot flushes; back, bone, muscle, joint, pelvic, stomach or chest pain; difficulty breathing; cough; sore throat; headache; weakness; dizziness; depression; rash; sweating; tingling or swelling in hands, feet or lower legs.

Guidelines for Use

USE EXACTLY AS PRESCRIBED.

Take one tablet on an empty stomach at the same time once daily.

If a dose is missed, take it as soon as possible. If several hours have passed or if it is nearing time for the next dose, do not double the dose to "catch up," unless advised by your healthcare provider. If more than one dose is missed, contact your healthcare provider.

Inform your healthcare provider if you are pregnant, become pregnant or are planning to become pregnant.

Store at room temperature.

Ascorbic Acid (Vitamin C)

(ASS-kor-bik acid)

Ascorbicap, Cebid Timecelles, Cecon, Cetane, Cevalin, Cevi-Bid, Ce-Vi-Sol, Dull-C, Flavorcee, N'ice Vitamin C Drops, Vita-C

Used to prevent and treat scurvy.

Side Effects

Every medicine can cause side effects, but many people have no, or minor, side effects. Tell your healthcare provider if any of the following occurs: increased urination; diarrhea; mouth sores; nausea; vomiting; stomach upset.

Guidelines for Use

USE EXACTLY AS PRESCRIBED.

Most people on a balanced diet do not need vitamin supplements.

Use with caution in diabetes, history of kidney stones, salt-restricted diet and during oral anticoagulant therapy.

Common sources of vitamin C--Strawberries, citrus fruit, tomatoes, potatoes, leafy vegetables, meat, fish, poultry, eggs and dairy products.

Total vitamin C intake includes the amounts taken in the diet, plus supplements. This total should not exceed the Recommended Dietary Allowance (RDA) unless your healthcare provider has been consulted.

RDA--Adults: 60 mg; Pregnancy and lactation: 70 to 95 mg.

Aspirin

(ASS-pihr-in)

Ascriptin A/D, Aspergum, Bayer Children's, Bufferin, Cama Arthritis Pain Reliever, Easprin, Ecotrin, Empirin, Genprin, Genuine Bayer, ½ Halfprin, Magnaprin, ZORprin

A medicine used to relieve mild to moderate pain, reduce fever and reduce inflammation, redness and swelling. Also given to decrease the chance of having a heart attack. It may occasionally be prescribed for other reasons.

Precautions

DO NOT USE if you are allergic to this medicine, any other salicylates, any nonsteroidal anti-inflammatory medicine or to tartrazine. Do not use during pregnancy. Aspirin should never be given to children under the age of 18 for any reason.

BEFORE USING THIS MEDICINE, tell your healthcare provider if you are pregnant or breastfeeding; or if you are taking, will be taking or stop taking any prescription or nonprescription medicine; or if you have any other medical conditions.

Side Effects

Every medicine can cause side effects, but many people have no, or minor, side effects. Tell your healthcare provider if any of the following occurs: stomach upset; nausea; vomiting; appetite loss; indigestion; heartburn; diarrhea; dizziness; weakness; confusion; headache; ringing in the ears; difficulty hearing; thirst; sweating; black or bloody stools; rapid breathing; dim vision; rash; fever; hives; allergic reaction--difficulty breathing and inflammation in the nose may occur in people with a history of nasal polyps or asthma.

Guidelines for Use

USE EXACTLY AS PRESCRIBED.

May cause stomach upset. Take with food or after meals.

Take with a full glass of water to reduce the risk of lodging medicine in the throat.

Tell your healthcare provider if ringing in the ears or persistent stomach pain occurs.

Do not use if a strong vinegar-like odor is present.

Do not place or dissolve on an oral lesion (eg, canker sore, cold sore) or directly on an aching tooth. A serious inflammatory reaction could occur.

Sustained release—Do not crush or chew preparations.

Astemizole

(ASS-TEM-ih-zole)

Hismanal

A medicine (antihistamine) used for relief of seasonal allergy symptoms and symptoms associated with some types of hives and skin rash with mild to moderate itching.

Precautions

DO NOT USE if you are allergic to this medicine or its relatives; are breastfeeding; or are taking erythromycin or monoamine oxidase inhibitors (MAOIs, eg, *Nardil, Parnate*).

BEFORE USING THIS MEDICINE, tell your healthcare provider if you are pregnant, or if you are taking, will be taking or stop taking any prescription or nonprescription medicine; or if you have any other medical conditions.

Side Effects

Every medicine can cause side effects, but many people have no, or minor, side effects. Tell your healthcare provider if any of the following occurs: drowsiness; dizziness; dry mouth; stomach upset; constipation; blurred vision; difficult urination; confusion; fainting; irregular heart beats.

Guidelines for Use

USE EXACTLY AS PRESCRIBED.

Take on an empty stomach, one hour before or two hours after the evening meal.

Do not eat for at least 1 hour after taking the medicine.

Avoid alcohol and drowsiness-causing medicines.

Use caution while driving or performing tasks requiring mental alertness or coordination.

Use alone when sneezing and runny nose exist but nasal congestion is slight. When nasal congestion occurs with sneezing and runny nose, an oral or topical decongestant also may be used.

Do not take for several days before allergy skin testing.

Atenolol

(ah-TEN-oh-lahl)

Tenormin

A beta blocker medicine used to lower high blood pressure and to treat angina and heart attack.

Precautions

DO NOT USE if you are allergic to this medicine or its relatives, or if you are breastfeeding.

BEFORE USING THIS MEDICINE, tell your healthcare provider if you are pregnant; or if you are taking, will be taking or stop taking any prescription or nonprescription medicine; or if you have any other medical conditions.

Side Effects

Every medicine can cause side effects, but many people have no, or minor, side effects. Tell your healthcare provider if any of the following occurs: nausea; vomiting; stomach ache; diarrhea; constipation; appetite changes; indigestion; depression; anxiety; hallucinations; short-term memory loss; behavior changes; disorientation; fainting; dizziness; lightheadedness; tiredness; sleep disturbances; decreased concentration; headache; nightmares; emotional instability; changes in heart rate; chest pain; chills; cold or numb extremities; pounding of the chest; difficulty breathing; cough; nasal congestion; rash; hives; fluid retention; flushing or paleness; increased pigmentation; itching; hair loss; sweating; dry skin; psoriasis; painful and aching joints and muscles; painful, frequent or difficult urination; blurred vision; dry, burning or irritated eyes; ringing in the ears; taste changes; sore throat; dry mouth; slurred speech; fever; weight gain; changes in blood sugar levels.

Guidelines for Use

USE EXACTLY AS PRESCRIBED.

Ask your healthcare provider before using other medicines including nasal decongestants, diet aids or nonprescription cold preparations.

Do not stop this medicine suddenly; it could cause a worsening of disease including worse angina (chest pain), irregular heartbeats and increased risk of heart attack and death. Withdraw these medications slowly over one to two weeks by gradually decreasing the dose.

Diabetes — These products can mask signs of low blood sugar and change blood sugar levels. It may be necessary for your healthcare provider to change your dose of diabetic medications.

Use caution while driving or performing other tasks requiring mental alertness, coordination and dexterity.

Atenolol/Chlorthalidone

(ah-TEN-oh-lahl/klor-THAL-ih-dohn)

Tenoretic

A combination of a beta-blocking agent and diuretic (water pill) used to lower high blood pressure.

Precautions

DO NOT USE if you are allergic to thiazides, beta blockers, oral diabetic medicine or sulfa antibiotics; or if you are breastfeeding.

BEFORE USING THIS MEDICINE, tell your healthcare provider if you are pregnant; or if you are taking, will be taking or stop taking any prescription or nonprescription medicines; or if you have any medical conditions.

Side Effects

Every medicine can cause side effects, but many people have no, or minor, side effects. Tell your healthcare provider if any of the following occurs: difficult breathing, especially on exertion or when lying down; night cough; swelling of the extremities; slow pulse rate; dizziness; confusion or depression; rash; fever; sore throat; unusual bleeding or bruising. May cause gout attacks. Contact your healthcare provider if sudden significant joint pain occurs.

Guidelines for Use

USE EXACTLY AS PRESCRIBED.

Increases urination, therefore take early in the day.

May cause stomach upset. May be taken with food or milk.

If signs of low potassium occur (weakness, cramps, nausea, dizziness, etc), contact your healthcare provider.

Diabetes — May increase blood sugar levels.

Discontinuing therapy: If discontinued suddenly, beta-blockers may cause rebound withdrawal symptoms some of which may be serious. Withdraw these medications slowly over one to two weeks only with healthcare provider supervision.

Diuretics are usually given as a single daily dose in the morning.

Atovaquone

(uh-TOE-vuh-KWONE)

Mepron

A medicine used to treat mild to moderate *Pneumocystis carinii* pneumonia.

Precautions

DO NOT USE if you are allergic to this medicine. Use with caution in the elderly.

BEFORE USING THIS MEDICINE, tell your healthcare provider if you are pregnant; or if you are taking, will be taking or stop taking any prescription or nonprescription medicines; or have any other medical conditions.

Side Effects

Every medicine can cause side effects, but many people have no, or minor, side effects. Tell your healthcare provider if any of the following occurs: nausea; diarrhea; vomiting; constipation; stomach pain; appetite loss; indigestion; headache; sleeplessness; weakness; dizziness; anxiety; cough; sinus inflammation; congestion; rash; itching; sweating; fever; pain; taste changes; low blood sugar; low blood pressure; oral fungal infection.

Guidelines for Use

USE EXACTLY AS PRESCRIBED.

Take daily doses with meals.

Atropine Sulfate Ophthalmic

(AT-troe-peen)

Atropine-1, Atropine Care, Atropine Sulfate S.O.P., Atropisol, Isopto Atropine

A pupil dilator used when there is eye inflammation or when an eye exam is performed. It works by relaxing the muscles of the eye to cause the pupil to dilate (widen) and prevent the eye from focusing.

Precautions

DO NOT USE if you are allergic to this medicine or its relatives.

BEFORE USING THIS MEDICINE, tell your healthcare provider if you are pregnant or breastfeeding; or if you are taking, will be taking or stop taking any prescription or nonprescription medicine; if you have any other medical conditions; or if you are allergic to sulfite preservatives.

Side Effects

Every medicine can cause side effects, but many people have no, or minor, side effects. Tell your healthcare provider if any of the following occurs: stinging; redness; swelling; sensitivity to light; blurred vision; headache; drowsiness; slurred speech; loss of coordination; incoherent speech; restlessness; hallucinations; hyperactivity; seizures; disorientation; flushing; dryness; rash; lack of sweating; dryness of mouth and nose; fever.

Guidelines for Use

USE EXACTLY AS PRESCRIBED.

For topical ophthalmic use only.

May produce drowsiness, loss of coordination, blurred vision or sensitivity to light (due to dilated pupils).

Use caution while driving or performing other tasks requiring mental alertness.

If eye pain occurs, stop using the medicine and contact your healthcare provider.

Atropine Sulfate Oral

(AT-troe-peen)

Sal-Tropine

A medicine used to treat various stomach and intestinal disorders.

Precautions

DO NOT USE if you are allergic to this medicine or if you have asthma. This medicine can cause excitement, agitation, drowsiness and other mental reactions in older patients.

BEFORE USING THIS MEDICINE, tell your healthcare provider if you are pregnant or breastfeeding; or if you are taking, will be taking or stop taking any prescription or nonprescription medicine; if you have any other medical conditions; or if you are allergic to tartrazine.

Side Effects

Every medicine can cause side effects, but many people have no, or minor, side effects. Tell your healthcare provider if any of the following occurs: nausea; vomiting; bloating; heartburn; constipation; confusion; excitement; restlessness; tremors; hallucinations; delirium; uncoordinated walking; seizures; headache; nervousness; drowsiness; dizziness; inability to sleep; pounding in the chest; difficulty breathing; nasal congestion; rash; itching; flushing; decreased sweating; difficult urination; eye pain; fever; muscle weakness or loss of muscle function; dry mouth; altered taste perception; difficult swallowing; urine retention; impotence; blurred vision; sensitivity to light; reduced breast milk production and flow; thirst; widening pupils.

Guidelines for Use

USE EXACTLY AS PRESCRIBED.

Take 30 minutes before meals.

May cause drowsiness. Use caution when driving or performing other tasks requiring alertness.

Notify your healthcare provider if skin rash, flushing or eye pain occurs.

May cause dry mouth, difficulty in urinating, constipation or increased sensitivity to light. Notify your healthcare provider if these effects persist or become severe.

This medicine can reduce sweating, which can cause heat prostration, fever and heatstroke during hot weather.

This medicine can cause drying of the eyes. Contact lens wearers should use a lubricating solution while taking this medicine.

Atropine Sulfate/Scopolamine Hydrobromide/ Hyoscyamine Sulfate/Phenobarbital

(AT-troe-peen SULL-fate/skoe-POLE-uh-meen HIGH-droe-BROE-mide/high-oh-SIGH-uh-meen/fee-no-BAR-bih-tahl)

Donnatal, Malatal, Spasmolin

A combination medicine used to treat various stomach and intestinal disorders.

Precautions

DO NOT USE if you are allergic to any component of this medicine.

BEFORE USING THIS MEDICINE, tell your healthcare provider if you are pregnant or breastfeeding; or if you are taking, will be taking, or stop taking any prescription or nonprescription medicine; or if you have any other medical conditions.

Side Effects

Every medicine can cause side effects, but many people have no, or minor, side effects. Tell your healthcare provider if any of the following occurs: nausea; vomiting; bloating; heartburn; constipation; sleepiness; tired feeling; feeling of morning hangover; confusion; excitement; restlessness; tremors; hallucinations; delirium; uncoordinated walking; drowsiness; dizziness; pounding in the chest (palpitations); difficulty breathing; nasal congestion; rash; itching; flushing; decreased sweating; muscle weakness; dry mouth; altered taste perception; difficult swallowing; difficult urination; urine retention; impotence; eye pain; blurred vision; sensitivity of eyes to light; reduced breast milk production and flow.

Guidelines for Use

USE EXACTLY AS PRESCRIBED.

Take 30 minutes before meals.

This medicine may cause drowsiness, dizziness or blurred vision. Use caution while driving or performing other tasks requiring mental alertness, coordination and dexterity.

Notify your healthcare provider if skin rash, flushing or eye pain occurs.

May cause dry mouth, difficult urination, constipation or increased sensitivity of eyes to light. Contact your healthcare provider if these effects persist or become severe.

This medicine can reduce sweating, which can cause heat prostration, fever and heatstroke during hot weather. Use caution in hot weather.

This medicine can cause drying of the eyes. Contact lens wearers should use a lubricating solution while taking this medicine.

Avoid alcohol and other mental depressants (eg, narcotics, tranquilizers, antihistamines) while you are taking this medicine.

Auranofin

(or-RAIN-oh-fin)

Ridaura

This medicine is used to treat active adult and juvenile rheumatoid arthritis that are not adequately controlled by other therapies. It may occasionally be prescribed for other reasons.

Precautions

DO NOT USE if you are allergic to this medicine.

BEFORE USING THIS MEDICINE, tell your healthcare provider if you are pregnant or breastfeeding; or if you are taking, will be taking or stop taking any prescription or nonprescription medicine; or if you have any other medical conditions.

Side Effects

Every medicine can cause side effects, but many people have no, or minor, side effects. Tell your healthcare provider if any of the following occurs: indigestion; nausea; vomiting; diarrhea; constipation; stomach cramps; gas; rash; hives; itching; sores in the mouth; yellowing of skin or eyes; confusion; hallucinations; dizziness; fainting; weakness; fever; cough; shortness of breath; itching; hives; swelling; flushing; redness; sweating; easy bruising; blood in urine; sore mouth or throat; swollen gums or tongue; nosebleeds; metallic taste; hair loss; loss of fingernails; flushing; gray-to-blue skin; sensitivity to light.

Guidelines for Use

USE EXACTLY AS PRESCRIBED.

Read the patient package insert provided with the product.

Notify your healthcare provider if any of the following occurs: rash; sore mouth; indigestion; metallic taste; easy bruising or nosebleeds; itching.

A gray-to-blue discoloration of the skin may occur, especially on exposed areas. Minimize exposure to sunlight or artificial ultraviolet light.

It is important to brush and floss your teeth and see your dentist on a regular basis.

Regular follow-up with your healthcare provider is needed to monitor for side effects.

Azathioprine

(AZE-uh-THIGH-oh-preen)

Imuran

This medicine is used to prevent rejection of kidney transplants and to treat severe rheumatoid arthritis that does not respond to other therapies. It may occasionally be prescribed for other reasons.

Precautions

DO NOT USE if you are allergic to this medicine or if you are pregnant.

BEFORE USING THIS MEDICINE, tell your healthcare provider if you are breastfeeding; or if you are taking, will be taking or stop taking any prescription or nonprescription medicine; or if you have any other medical conditions.

Side Effects

Every medicine can cause side effects, but many people have no, or minor, side effects. Tell your healthcare provider if any of the following occurs: stomach pain; nausea; vomiting; diarrhea; pale stools; rash; itching; unusual bleeding or bruising; hair loss; fever; sore throat; mouth sores; infection; darkened urine; joint pain; yellowing of skin or eyes.

Guidelines for Use

USE EXACTLY AS PRESCRIBED.

May cause stomach upset. Take in divided doses or take with food or milk.

If a dose is missed, take it as soon as possible. If several hours have passed or if it is nearing time for the next dose, do not double the dose to catch up, unless advised by your healthcare provider. If more than one dose is missed, contact your healthcare provider.

Contact your healthcare provider if any of the following occurs: unusual bleeding or bruising; fever; sore throat; mouth sores; signs of infection; pale stools or darkened urine; yellowing of skin or eyes.

Lab tests will be required during treatment with this medicine.

Serious infections are a constant hazard for patients on chronic immunosuppression, especially transplant recipients. Avoid contact with persons who have active infections.

Long-term use of this medication may increase the risk of developing tumors. Talk with your healthcare provider about this possibility.

May cause nausea, vomiting, rash, fever, joint pain and diarrhea. Contact your healthcare provider if these persist or become bothersome.

Avoid pregnancy while taking this medication. If you suspect you may be pregnant, notify your healthcare provider immediately.

Azithromycin

(UHZ-ith-row-MY-sin)

Zithromax

An antibiotic used to treat infections caused by certain bacteria.

Precautions

DO NOT USE if you are allergic to this medicine, erythromycin or its relatives.

BEFORE USING THIS MEDICINE, tell your healthcare provider if you are pregnant or breastfeeding; or if you are taking, will be taking or stop taking any prescription or nonprescription medicine; or if you have any other medical conditions

Side Effects

Every medicine can cause side effects, but many people have no, or minor, side effects. Tell your healthcare provider if any of the following occurs: vomiting; diarrhea; stomach cramps; unusual tiredness; severe abdominal pain; yellowing of skin or eyes; rash; itching; hives; dark urine; pale stools; headache; indigestion; vaginal infection; sensitivity to sunlight; difficulty breathing.

Guidelines for Use

USE EXACTLY AS PRESCRIBED.

Suspension: Shake well before using.

Take on an empty stomach, 1 hour before or 2 hours after meals.

If stomach upset occurs, take with food.

Do not take aluminum or magnesium-containing antacids with this product.

Take each dose with an adequate amount of fluid (preferably 6 to 8 ounces).

Take at evenly spaced intervals throughout the day, preferably around the clock.

If diarrhea occurs, contact your healthcare provider immediately. This could be a symptom of a severe side effect (pseudomembranous colitis) requiring immediate medical attention.

If a dose is missed, take it as soon as possible. If several hours have passed or if it is nearing time for the next dose, do not double the dose to "catch up," unless advised by your healthcare provider. If more than one dose is missed, contact your healthcare provider.

Continue use until all the prescribed medicine has been taken. Failure to take all of the medicine may prevent complete elimination of bacteria, causing the infection to return.

Discontinue this medicine and contact your healthcare provider if any of the following occur: Rash, hives, itching, difficulty breathing.

May cause sensitivity to sunlight. Avoid prolonged exposure to the sun. Use sunscreens and wear protective clothing until tolerance is determined.

Store below 86°F.

Baclofen

(BACK-low-fen)

Lioresal

A skeletal muscle relaxant used to relieve the pain from muscle spasms due to multiple sclerosis in adults and children over 12 years of age. It may occasionally be prescribed for other reasons.

Precautions

DO NOT USE if you are allergic to this medicine. Children: Safety and effectiveness in children under 12 have not been established.

BEFORE USING THIS MEDICINE, tell your healthcare provider if you are pregnant or breastfeeding; or if you are taking, will be taking or stop taking any prescription or nonprescription medicine; or if you have any other medical conditions.

Side Effects

Every medicine can cause side effects, but many people have no, or minor, side effects. Tell your healthcare provider if any of the following occurs: frequent urination; difficult or painful urination; blood in urine; difficult erection; difficult ejaculation; nausea; constipation; loss of appetite; change in taste; abdominal pain; vomiting; diarrhea; blood in stool; drowsiness; dizziness; weakness; tiredness; confusion; headache; difficulty sleeping; palpitations (pounding in chest); chest pain; rash; itching; excessive sweating; visual disturbances; dry mouth; edema (ankle swelling); weight gain; nasal congestion; fainting; shortness of breath.

Guidelines for Use

USE EXACTLY AS PRESCRIBED.

May cause drowsiness, dizziness and tiredness. Use caution when driving or performing other tasks requiring mental alertness, coordination and dexterity.

Avoid alcohol and medicines that cause drowsiness during therapy.

Sudden discontinuation of this medicine can result in hallucinations. Discontinue only under your healthcare provider's supervision.

Diabetes — This medicine can cause changes in blood sugar levels.

Beclomethasone Dipropionate Aerosol

(BEK-low-METH-uh-zone die-PRO-pee-oh-NATE)

Beclovent, Vanceril

A medicine used to prevent or reduce the frequency and severity of bronchial asthma attacks. It is not to treat a severe asthma attack.

Precautions

DO NOT USE if you have an allergy to this medicine or if you are breastfeeding.

BEFORE USING THIS MEDICINE, tell your healthcare provider if you are pregnant; are taking, will be taking or stop taking any prescription or nonprescription medicines; or if you have any medical conditions.

Side Effects

Every medicine can cause side effects, but many people have no, or minor, side effects. Tell your healthcare provider if any of the following occurs: sore throat or mouth; cough; dry mouth; rash; facial swelling; difficult breathing.

Guidelines for Use

USE EXACTLY AS PRESCRIBED.

Read patient package insert carefully.

For preventive therapy only. Do NOT use for an acute asthma attack requiring rapid relief.

Use at regularly scheduled intervals as prescribed.

Do not exceed recommended dose.

Supplementary oral steroids may be necessary during periods of high stress or an asthma attack. Carry identification indicating this potential need.

If symptoms of steroid withdrawal occur when changing from oral to inhalant therapy (eg, joint or muscle pain, lack of energy, depression), contact your healthcare provider immediately for instructions.

This information is advisory only; it does not contain all information about this medicine. If you have any questions about your medicine, ask your healthcare provider.

Beclomethasone Nasal Spray

(BEK-low-METH-uh-zone)

Beconase, Beconase AQ, Vancenase, Vancenase AQ

A medicine used to treat allergy symptoms including itching, runny nose, nasal congestion, and sneezing in patients over 6 years of age and for nonallergic rhinitis (continual) in adults. It is also used in the prevention of nasal polyps.

Precautions

DO NOT USE if you are allergic to this medicine or its ingredients, have nasal infections or herpes infection near the eye.

BEFORE USING THIS MEDICINE, tell your healthcare provider if you are pregnant or breastfeeding; or if you are taking, will be taking or stop taking any prescription or nonprescription medicines; or if you have any other medical conditions.

Side Effects

Every medicine can cause side effects, but many people have no, or minor, side effects. Tell your healthcare provider if any of the following occurs: sneezing; nasal irritation or burning; nosebleed; runny nose; drying of the nasal tissues.

Guidelines for Use

USE EXACTLY AS PRESCRIBED.

Shake well before use.

Follow patient instructions exactly. Do not exceed recommended dosage.

Usual adult dose is 1 spray per nostril 2-4 times a day; children, 1 spray per nostril 3 times a day.

Effects are not immediate; benefit usually occurs in a few days.

Clear nasal passages prior to use by blowing nose. If nasal passages are blocked, use a decongestant to ensure penetration of the spray.

May be used alone, or with an antihistamine or decongestant.

Allergy symptoms (watering, itching eyes) are not cured by this spray. Use with caution if sores or injuries occur in the nasal passages (eg, frequent nosebleed).

This medicine may prevent or slow proper healing.

Infection of the nose and throat has been linked with long-term use. Such infection may require stopping this medicine.

If symptoms do not improve within 3 weeks, contact your healthcare provider. After the desired effect is obtained, reduce the maintenance dose to the smallest amount necessary to control the symptoms.

Benazepril Hydrochloride

(BEN-AZE-uh-prill HIGH-droe-KLOR-ide)

Lotensin

An angiotensin converting enzyme (ACE) inhibitor medicine generally used to lower high blood pressure.

Precautions

DO NOT USE if you are allergic to this medicine or if you are pregnant.

BEFORE USING THIS MEDICINE, tell your healthcare provider if you are pregnant or breastfeeding; or if you are taking, will be taking or stop taking any prescription or nonprescription medicine; or if you have any other medical conditions.

Side Effects

Every medicine can cause side effects, but many people have no, or minor, side effects. Tell your healthcare provider if any of the following occurs: stomach pain; vomiting; diarrhea; constipation; appetite loss; depression; headache; dizziness; nervousness; sleeping difficulties; fatigue; rapid or irregular heartbeat; dizziness/lightheadedness when rising quickly from a sitting or lying position; shortness of breath; cough; nasal congestion; bronchitis; sinus inflammation; rash; sweating; flushing; yellowing of skin or eyes; muscle cramps; weight loss; taste loss; dry mouth; decreased sex drive; back, joint and shoulder pain; urination changes; fever; vision disturbances; numbness/tingling of hands or feet.

Guidelines for Use

USE EXACTLY AS PRESCRIBED.

May be taken without regard to meals.

Patients starting treatment for high blood pressure may at first feel tired. It takes time for the body to adjust. Continue taking medication and check with your healthcare provider.

If a dose is missed, take it as soon as possible. If several hours have passed or if it is nearing time for the next dose, do not double the dose to catch up, unless advised by your healthcare provider. If more than one dose is missed, contact your healthcare provider.

Do not interrupt or stop medication without consulting your healthcare provider.

Do not use salt substitutes without telling your healthcare provider.

A persistent, dry, nonproductive cough may occur. Tell healthcare provider if this occurs. Recovery is rapid when the medicine is stopped.

Dizziness, fainting or lightheadedness is most likely after the first dose or in the first days of therapy; avoid sudden changes in posture. If fainting occurs, discontinue medicine until talking to your healthcare provider.

Benzphetamine

(benz-FET-uh-meen)

Didrex

A medicine that reduces appetite by suppressing the hunger center in the brain.

Precautions

DO NOT USE if you are pregnant; allergic to this medicine or if you have a history of drug abuse.

BEFORE USING THIS MEDICINE, tell your healthcare provider if you are breastfeeding; or if you are taking, will be taking or stop taking any prescription or nonprescription medicine; if you have any other medical conditions; or if you are allergic to tartrazine.

Side Effects

Every medicine can cause side effects, but many people have no, or minor, side effects. Tell your healthcare provider if any of the following occurs: nausea; vomiting; constipation; stomach pain; diarrhea; dry mouth; unpleasant taste; restlessness; tremor; nervousness; anxiety; tension; confusion; difficulty sleeping; excitement; depression; headache; aggressiveness; pounding in the chest; chest pain; hives; rash; menstrual changes; sexual problems; dizziness; blurred vision; eye irritation; problems urinating.

Guidelines for Use

USE EXACTLY AS PRESCRIBED.

Appetite suppressants are not a substitute for proper dieting. Make lifestyle changes (eg, diet and exercise) while on therapy. Use beyond 8 to 12 weeks is not encouraged.

Take on an empty stomach.

May cause insomnia. Avoid taking this medicine late in the day.

May produce dizziness or blurred vision. Use caution while driving or performing other tasks requiring mental alertness.

Use of this medicine to improve athletic skills or mental alertness or to stay awake is dangerous and illegal.

Never share medicines with others.

Interrupted courses of therapy supervised by a healthcare provider may be useful in the treatment of obesity.

Contact your healthcare provider immediately if chest pain, pounding in the chest, nervousness or dizziness occurs.

Avoid pregnancy while taking this medication. If you suspect you may be pregnant, notify your healthcare provider immediately.

May cause dry mouth and constipation; tell your healthcare provider if these become severe.

Benztropine Mesylate

(BENZ-troe-peen MEH-sih-LATE)

Cogentin

Used to treat the symptoms of Parkinsonism, and medicine-induced Parkinsonism-like disorders. This agent is not a cure for symptoms of Parkinsonism.

Precautions

DO NOT USE if you are allergic to this medicine or its relatives.

BEFORE USING THIS MEDICINE, tell your healthcare provider if you are pregnant or breastfeeding; or if you are taking, will be taking or stop taking any prescription or nonprescription medicine; or if you have any other medical conditions.

Side Effects

Every medicine can cause side effects, but many people have no, or minor, side effects. Tell your healthcare provider if any of the following occurs: nausea; vomiting; stomach pain; constipation; confusion; memory loss; hallucinations; lightheadedness; dizziness; weakness; agitation; nervousness; paranoia; delirium; excitement; depression; rapid heart rate; pounding in the chest (palpitations); lightheadedness and dizziness upon rising quickly from a lying position; rash; flushing; decreased sweating; hives; visual disturbances; eye pain; glaucoma; difficulty urinating; muscle weakness; cramping; dry mouth; fever; numbness of fingers; difficulty achieving or maintaining an erection; swollen glands.

Guidelines for Use

USE EXACTLY AS PRESCRIBED.

May cause drowsiness, dizziness or blurred vision. Use caution when driving or performing other tasks requiring mental alertness, coordination and dexterity.

Avoid alcohol and medicines (eg, tranquilizers, antihistamines, some pain medicines) that cause drowsiness.

Stomach upset may occur. Take with food.

Sucking on hard candy, drinking fluids or maintaining good dental hygiene can relieve dry mouth.

If constipation occurs, use stool softeners if necessary.

This medicine can reduce the ability to sweat, an important function by which overheating is prevented. Avoid excess sun or exercise, which may cause excessive sweating.

Betamethasone

(BAY-tuh-METH-uh-zone)

Celestone, Diprolene, Diprosone, Uticort

A topical anti-inflammatory agent used to treat rash and skin irritation.

Precautions

DO NOT USE near eyes or eyelids or if you have an allergy to this medicine.

BEFORE USING THIS MEDICINE, tell your healthcare provider if you are pregnant or breastfeeding; or if you are taking, will be taking, or stop taking any prescription or nonprescription medicine; or if you have any other medical conditions.

Side Effects

Every medicine can cause side effects, but many people have no, or minor, side effects. Tell your healthcare provider if any of the following occurs: burning; itching; irritation; redness; dryness; acne; streaks in skin; stinging and cracking; numbness of fingers.

Guidelines for Use

USE EXACTLY AS PRESCRIBED.

Apply sparingly as a thin film. Rub in lightly.

Wash or soak the affected area before application as this may increase medicine absorption.

Avoid contact with the eyes.

Avoid prolonged use, especially near the eyes, on the face, on genital and rectal areas, and in skin folds.

Do not use tight-fitting diapers or plastic pants on children being treated in the diaper area.

Do not wrap the treated area with bandages or tight-fitting clothing unless specifically directed by your healthcare provider. Skin infections may worsen. It may be necessary to stop the corticosteroid and treat the infection.

Skin wasting may occur in 3 to 4 weeks.

Do not mix this medicine with other products. Allergic reactions may occur.

If the condition being treated gets worse or irritation, burning, redness, swelling or stinging persists, contact your healthcare provider before reapplying medicine.

Alcohol-containing preparations may cause drying, burning or irritation of open lesions.

Betamethasone/Clotrimazole

(BAY-tuh-METH-uh-zone/kloe-TRIM-uh-zole)

Lotrisone

A corticosteroid and antifungal topical combination. Used to relieve inflamed and itching fungal skin conditions.

Precautions

DO NOT USE if you are allergic to this medicine.

BEFORE USING THIS MEDICINE, tell your healthcare provider if you are pregnant or breastfeeding; or if you are taking, will be taking or stop taking any prescription or nonprescription medicine; or if you have any other medical conditions.

Side Effects

Every medicine can cause side effects, but many people have no, or minor, side effects. Tell your healthcare provider if any of the following occurs: increased irritation (eg, redness, itching, burning, blisters).

Guidelines for Use

USE EXACTLY AS PRESCRIBED.

For external use only. Avoid contact with the eyes.

Apply after cleaning the affected area (unless directed otherwise).

Apply sparingly in a light film; rub in lightly.

Use for the full treatment time even though the symptoms may have improved.

Notify your healthcare provider if there is no improvement after 4 weeks of treatment.

Avoid prolonged use, especially near the eyes, in genital and rectal areas, on the face and in skin creases.

Notify your healthcare provider if the condition being treated persists or worsens.

Do not use occlusive (air-tight) dressings.

Do not use tight-fitting diapers or plastic pants on a child treated in the diaper area.

Betaxolol Ophthalmic

(BAY-TAX-oh-lahl)

Betoptic, Betoptic S

A beta-blocking agent used to treat glaucoma.

Precautions

DO NOT USE if you have an allergy to this medicine or its relatives.

BEFORE USING THIS MEDICINE, tell your healthcare provider if you are pregnant or breastfeeding; or if you are taking, will be taking or stop taking any prescription or nonprescription medicine; if you have any other medical conditions; or if you are allergic to sulfite preservatives.

Side Effects

Every medicine can cause side effects, but many people have no, or minor, side effects. Tell your healthcare provider if any of the following occurs: temporary stinging or pain when using drops; visual problems or irritation; browache; light sensitivity; depression; palpitations (pounding in the chest); stomach upset; nausea; breathing difficulty; rash.

Guidelines for Use

USE EXACTLY AS PRESCRIBED.

If a dose is missed, take it as soon as possible. If several hours have passed or if it is nearing time for the next dose, do not double the dose to catch up, unless advised by your healthcare provider. If more than one dose is missed, contact your healthcare provider.

May cause stinging or pain when first instilled in the eye.

Intraocular pressure must be monitored periodically by your healthcare provider to make sure the medicine is working properly.

Notify your healthcare provider if you are using these eye drops and plan to have surgery. You may have to temporarily stop using them.

Betaxolol Oral

(BAY-TAX-oh-lahl)

Kerlone

A beta-blocker medicine used to lower high blood pressure and to treat angina and heart attack.

Precautions

DO NOT USE if you are allergic to this medicine or its relatives, or if you are breastfeeding.

BEFORE USING THIS MEDICINE, tell your healthcare provider if you are pregnant or breastfeeding; or if you are taking, will be taking or stop taking any prescription or nonprescription medicine; or if you have any other medical conditions.

Side Effects

Every medicine can cause side effects, but many people have no, or minor, side effects. Tell your healthcare provider if any of the following occurs: nausea; vomiting; stomach ache; diarrhea; constipation; appetite changes; indigestion; depression; anxiety; hallucinations; short-term memory loss; behavior changes; disorientation; fainting; dizziness; lightheadedness; tiredness; sleep disturbances; decreased concentration; headache; nightmares; emotional instability; chest pain; chills; cold or numb extremities; pounding in the chest; difficulty breathing; cough; nasal congestion; rash; hives; fluid retention; flushing or paleness; increased pigmentation; itching; hair loss; sweating; dry skin; painful and aching joints and muscles; painful, frequent or difficult urination; blurred vision; dry, burning or irritated eyes; ringing in the ears; taste changes; sore throat; dry mouth; slurred speech; fever; weight gain.

Guidelines for Use

USE EXACTLY AS PRESCRIBED.

Ask your healthcare provider before using other medicines including nonprescription cold preparations.

Do not stop this medicine suddenly, it could cause a worsening of disease including worse angina (chest pain), irregular heartbeats and increase risk of heart attack and death.

Withdraw these medications slowly over one to two weeks by gradually decreasing the dose.

Diabetes — These products can mask signs of low blood sugar and change blood sugar levels. It may be necessary for your healthcare provider to change your dose of diabetic medications.

Use caution while driving or performing other tasks requiring mental alertness, coordination and dexterity.

Bethanechol Chloride

(beth-AN-ih-kole KLOR-ide)

Duvoid, Myotonachol, Urabeth

A medicine used to assist in urination after surgery or childbirth or in neurogenic atony. It may occasionally be prescribed for other reasons.

Precautions

DO NOT USE if you are allergic to this medicine or if you have asthma, epilepsy or high or low blood pressure.

BEFORE USING THIS MEDICINE, tell your healthcare provider if you are pregnant or breastfeeding; or if you are taking, will be taking or stop taking any prescription or nonprescription medicine; if you have any other medical conditions; or if you are allergic to tartrazine.

Side Effects

Every medicine can cause side effects, but many people have no, or minor, side effects. Tell your healthcare provider if any of the following occurs: belching; abdominal pain; diarrhea; cramps/discomfort; rumbling stomach; asthma attack; difficulty breathing; general body discomfort; urinary urgency; headache; sweating; flushing; facial warmth; visual disturbances; tearing of eyes; salivation.

Guidelines for Use

USE EXACTLY AS PRESCRIBED.

Take on an empty stomach. May cause nausea or vomiting if taken with food.

May cause increased salivation, sweating, flushing or stomach ache. Notify your healthcare provider if these symptoms persist or become severe.

May cause dizziness, lightheadedness or fainting, especially when rising from a seated or lying position. Avoid sudden changes in posture.

Biperiden

(by-PURR-ih-den)

Akineton

Used to treat the symptoms of parkinsonism, and medicine-induced parkinsonism-like disorders. This agent is not a cure for symptoms of parkinsonism.

Precautions

DO NOT USE if you are allergic to this medicine or its relatives.

BEFORE USING THIS MEDICINE, tell your healthcare provider if you are pregnant or breastfeeding; or if you are taking, will be taking or stop taking any prescription or nonprescription medicine; or if you have any other medical conditions.

Side Effects

Every medicine can cause side effects, but many people have no, or minor, side effects. Tell your healthcare provider if any of the following occurs: nausea; vomiting; stomach pain; constipation; confusion; memory loss; hallucinations; lightheadedness; dizziness; weakness; agitation; nervousness; paranoia; delirium; excitement; depression; pounding in the chest (palpitations); lightheadedness and dizziness upon rising quickly from a lying position; rash; flushing; decreased sweating; hives; visual disturbances; eye pain; difficulty urinating; muscle weakness; cramping; dry mouth; fever; numbness of fingers; difficulty achieving or maintaining an erection; swollen glands.

Guidelines for Use

USE EXACTLY AS PRESCRIBED.

May cause drowsiness, dizziness or blurred vision. Use caution when driving or performing other tasks requiring mental alertness.

Avoid alcohol and medicines that cause drowsiness (eg, tranquilizers, antihistamines, some pain medicines).

Stomach upset may occur. Take with food.

Sucking on hard candy, drinking fluids, and maintaining good dental hygiene can relieve dry mouth.

If constipation occurs, use stool softeners if necessary.

This medicine can reduce the ability to sweat, an important function by which overheating is prevented. Avoid excess sun or exercise, which may cause excessive sweating.

Bisacodyl

(BISS-uh-koe-dill)

Biscolax, Dulcagen, Dulcolax, Fleet

Used for short-term treatment of constipation and to clean out the bowel before bowel examinations or bowel surgery.

Precautions

DO NOT USE if you are allergic to this medicine.

BEFORE USING THIS MEDICINE, tell your healthcare provider if you are pregnant or breastfeeding; or if you are taking, will be taking or stop taking any prescription or nonprescription medicine; or if you have any other medical conditions.

Side Effects

Every medicine can cause side effects, but many people have no, or minor, side effects. Tell your healthcare provider if any of the following occurs: nausea; vomiting; stomach ache; bowel cramping; diarrhea; weakness; dizziness; fainting; facial swelling; redness and discomfort; rectal bleeding; muscle cramps or pain; irritation of the rectal area; sweating; pounding in the chest.

Guidelines for Use

USE EXACTLY AS PRESCRIBED.

Take with a full glass of water or juice.

Laxative use is only a temporary measure. When normal bowel habits return, stop use of these products.

Prolonged use may result in dependence or electrolyte imbalance.

Do not take within 1 hour before or after antacids or milk.

Frequent use of laxatives and inadequate fluid intake can cause an imbalance in fluid and electrolyte levels. Symptoms can include muscle cramps, muscle weakness and dizziness.

Effects will occur in 6 to 10 hours with most of these products.

Tablets--Take whole; do not crush.

Bismuth Subsalicylate

(Biss-muth sub-suh-LIS-uh-late)

Bismatrol, Bismatrol Extra Strength, Pepto-Bismol Maximum Strength, Pepto-Bismol, Pink Bismuth

A medicine used to treat indigestion (without causing constipation); nausea; to control diarrhea; to relieve gas pains and stomach cramps. It may occasionally be prescribed for other reasons.

Precautions

DO NOT USE if you are allergic to this medicine, aspirin or any other salicylate; or if you are pregnant or breastfeeding. This medicine should never be given to children under the age of 18 for any reason.

BEFORE USING THIS MEDICINE, tell your healthcare provider if you are pregnant or breastfeeding; or if you are taking, will be taking or stop taking any prescription or nonprescription medicine; or if you have any other medical conditions.

Side Effects

Every medicine can cause side effects, but many people have no, or minor, side effects. Tell your healthcare provider if any of the following occurs: severe constipation; darkening of the tongue; darkening of the stools; stomach upset; nausea; vomiting; appetite loss; indigestion; heartburn; diarrhea; dizziness; weakness; confusion; headache; ringing in the ears; difficulty hearing; thirst; sweating; black or bloody stools; rapid breathing; dim vision; rash; fever; hives; allergic reaction--difficulty breathing and inflammation in the nose may occur in people with a history of nasal polyps or asthma.

Guidelines for Use

USE EXACTLY AS PRESCRIBED.

Stools may temporarily appear gray-black.

Contact your healthcare provider if diarrhea is accompanied by high fever, or if diarrhea continues for more than 2 days.

Liquids--Shake well before using.

Tablets--Chew or allow to dissolve in mouth. Do not swallow whole.

Bisoprolol Fumarate

(bih-SO-pro-lahl FYU-mah-rate)

Zebeta

A beta-blocker medicine used to lower high blood pressure and to treat angina and heart attack.

Precautions

DO NOT USE if you are allergic to this medicine or its relatives, or if you are breastfeeding.

BEFORE USING THIS MEDICINE, tell your healthcare provider if you are pregnant or breastfeeding; or if you are taking, will be taking or stop taking any prescription or nonprescription medicine; or if you have any other medical conditions.

Side Effects

Every medicine can cause side effects, but many people have no, or minor, side effects. Tell your healthcare provider if any of the following occurs: nausea; vomiting; stomach ache; diarrhea; constipation; appetite changes; indigestion; depression; anxiety; hallucinations; short-term memory loss; behavior changes; disorientation; fainting; dizziness; lightheadedness; tiredness; sleep disturbances; decreased concentration; headache; nightmares; emotional instability; chest pain; chills; cold or numb extremities; pounding in the chest; difficulty breathing; cough; nasal congestion; rash; hives; fluid retention; flushing or paleness; increased pigmentation; itching; hair loss; sweating; dry skin; psoriasis; painful and aching joints and muscles; painful, frequent or difficult urination; blurred vision; dry, burning or irritated eyes; ringing in the ears; taste changes; sore throat; dry mouth; slurred speech; fever; weight gain; changes in blood sugar levels.

Guidelines for Use

USE EXACTLY AS PRESCRIBED.

May be taken without regard to meals.

Ask your healthcare provider before using other medicines including nasal decongestants, diet aids or nonprescription cold preparations.

Do not stop taking this medicine suddenly, it could cause a worsening of disease including worse angina (chest pain), irregular heartbeats and increased risk of heart attack and death.

Withdraw these medications slowly over one to two weeks by gradually decreasing the dose.

Diabetes — These products can mask signs of low blood sugar and change blood sugar levels. It may be necessary for your healthcare provider to change your dose of diabetic medications.

Use caution while driving or performing other tasks requiring mental alertness, coordination and dexterity.

Bitolterol Mesylate

(by-TOLE-ter-ole MEH-sih-LATE)

Tornalate

A medicine that makes breathing easier by widening breathing passages of the lung and by removing (expectorating) mucus and other debris causing congestion in the lungs. May be used to prevent asthma attacks.

Precautions

DO NOT USE if you have an allergy to this medicine or have heart rhythm disturbances associated with a rapid heart rate.

BEFORE USING THIS MEDICINE, tell your healthcare provider if you are pregnant or breastfeeding; or if you are taking, will be taking or stop taking any prescription or nonprescription medicine; or if you have any other medical conditions.

Side Effects

Every medicine can cause side effects, but many people have no, or minor, side effects. Tell your healthcare provider if any of the following occurs: nausea; vomiting; loss of appetite; heartburn; nervousness; restlessness; dizziness; lightheadedness; headache; anxiety; tension; tremor; drowsiness; weakness; sleeplessness; chest pain; pounding in the chest (palpitations); breathing problems; coughing; flushing; sweating; hives; muscle cramps; unusual or bad taste in mouth; drying or irritation of mouth; tingling of hands or feet; fatigue; increase in blood sugar.

Guidelines for Use

USE EXACTLY AS PRESCRIBED.

Solution for Inhalation — Follow preparation instructions included with this medicine. Prepare solution just prior to use. Do not store in nebulizer. Use this medicine 3 times per day over a 10–15 minute period, with at least 4 hours between doses. It can be increased to 4 times per day, if needed.

Aerosol — Shake well before using. To relieve breathing difficulties: 2 inhalations (puffs) at least 1–3 minutes apart, followed by a third inhalation, if needed. Take the 2 inhalations every 8 hours. Do not exceed 3 inhalations every 6 hours or 2 inhalations every 4 hours. Administer pressurized inhalation during the second half of breath intake. If more than one inhalation per dose is necessary, wait at least one full minute between doses.

Do not exceed recommended dosage. Excessive use may lead to side effects or loss of effectiveness. Do not stop or adjust the dose except on the recommendation of your healthcare provider.

If you do not get the usual relief from your normal dose, do not increase your dose, but call your healthcare provider immediately.

If a dose is missed, inhale it as soon as possible. If several hours have passed or if it is nearing time for the next dose, do not double the dose to "catch up," unless advised by your healthcare provider. If more than one dose is missed, contact your healthcare provider.

Do not use epinephrine or other bronchodilators while using this medicine.

Discontinue use and contact your healthcare provider if you notice an unusual smell or taste with this medicine.

Tell your healthcare provider if palpitations, chest pain, muscle tremors, dizziness, headache, flushing or difficult urination occurs, or if breathing difficulty or nervousness persists.

Store at room temperature. Do not spray in eyes; puncture container; store near heat, cold or open flame; or throw container into fire or incinerator.

Bromocriptine Mesylate

(BROE-moe-KRIP-teen MEH-sih-LATE)

Parlodel

A medicine used to treat some types of female infertility and menstrual irregularities; to treat acromegaly; or to treat Parkinson's disease.

Precautions

DO NOT USE if you are allergic to this medicine, its relatives or to the dye tartrazine.

BEFORE USING THIS MEDICINE, tell your healthcare provider if you are pregnant or breastfeeding; or if you are taking, will be taking or stop taking any prescription or nonprescription medicine; or if you have any other medical conditions.

Side Effects

Every medicine can cause side effects, but many people have no, or minor, side effects. Tell your healthcare provider if any of the following occurs: nausea; vomiting; blood-containing or coffee-ground vomit; stomach cramps; constipation; diarrhea; appetite loss; indigestion; seizures; psychological disturbances; visual hallucinations; sluggishness; confusion; fainting; depression; headache; dizziness; fatigue; dizziness or lightheadedness when arising from a seated or lying position; drowsiness; anxiety; nervousness; nightmares; changes in sleep patterns; slow or irregular pulse; shortness of breath; nasal congestion; rash; itching; hair loss; tingling of ears; numbness or tingling in hands or feet; difficulty walking; swelling of feet or ankles; frequent, uncontrolled or difficult urination; cold feet; muscle cramps in feet or legs; aggravation of Raynaud's syndrome; dry mouth; reduced tolerance to cold; spasms of eyelids.

Guidelines for Use

USE EXACTLY AS PRESCRIBED.

Take with food.

Lab tests may be required. Be sure to keep appointments.

Consult your healthcare provider if you experience a persistent runny nose.

May cause drowsiness. Use caution when driving or performing other tasks requiring alertness or coordination.

Use mechanical contraceptive measures (eg, diaphragm, condom) during treatment. Do not use oral contraceptives.

Take the first dose while lying down; dizziness or fainting may occur.

Brompheniramine

(brome-fen-AIR-uh-meen)

Bromphen, Codimal-A, Cophene-B, Dehist, Diamine T.D., Dimetane, Dimetane Extentabs, Histaject, Nasahist B

A medicine used to relieve symptoms associated with seasonal and year-round allergic runny nose; allergic conjunctivitis (watering, itching eyes); hives (mild and uncomplicated); and rash, insect bites and stings where there is mild to moderate itching and no complications.

Precautions

DO NOT USE if you are allergic to this medicine or if you are taking a monoamine oxidase inhibitor (MAOI, eg, *Parnate*).

BEFORE USING THIS MEDICINE, tell your healthcare provider if you are pregnant or breastfeeding; or if you are taking, will be taking or stop taking any prescription or nonprescription medicine; or if you have any other medical conditions.

Side Effects

Every medicine can cause side effects, but many people have no, or minor, side effects. Tell your healthcare provider if any of the following occurs: stomach ache; constipation; appetite changes; nausea; vomiting; diarrhea; drowsiness; dizziness; confusion; poor coordination; fatigue; headache; sleeplessness; sleepiness; pounding in the chest; dry nose, throat and mouth; thickening of mucus in the respiratory tract; wheezing; nasal stuffiness; sensitivity to light; difficult urination; sore throat; ringing in the ears; blurred and double vision; rash; hives; excessive perspiration; chills.

Guidelines for Use

USE EXACTLY AS PRESCRIBED.

May cause stomach upset; take with food.

May cause drowsiness or dizziness. Use caution while driving or performing tasks requiring mental alertness, coordination and dexterity. Avoid alcohol and medicines that cause drowsiness.

May cause dry mouth.

Use alone when sneezing and runny nose exist, but nasal congestion is slight. When nasal congestion accompanies sneezing and runny nose, an oral decongestant may be added.

Elderly patients are more likely to experience dizziness, sedation, decreased coordination, mental confusion and fainting when they take antihistamines.

May produce unexpected excitation, restlessness, irritability and insomnia in rare instances. This is most likely to occur in children and elderly patients.

Do not take for several days before having an allergy skin test.

Budesonide

(byoo-DESS-oh-nide)

Rhinocort

To relieve the symptoms of seasonal or continual allergies (eg, hay fever) in adults and children over 6 years of age; it also may be used by adults for nonallergic, simple nasal congestion.

Precautions

DO NOT USE if you are allergic to this medicine or if you have sores or injuries in the nose/nasal tissues (eg, recent nasal surgery, nosebleed).

BEFORE USING THIS MEDICINE, tell your healthcare provider if you are pregnant or breastfeeding; if you are taking, will be taking or stop taking any prescription or nonprescription medicine; or if you have any other medical conditions.

Side Effects

Every medicine can cause side effects, but many people have no, or minor, side effects. Tell your healthcare provider if any of the following occurs: nasal irritation; sore throat; increased cough; nosebleed; dry mouth; indigestion; sneezing.

Guidelines for Use

USE EXACTLY AS PRESCRIBED.

Shake well before use.

Read and follow patient instructions provided with this medicine.

Do not exceed recommended dosage. The maximum daily dose for all patients is two sprays per nostril each morning and evening, or four sprays per nostril each morning.

As the condition improves, slowly reduce dosage. Begin full treatment again if symptoms return.

Use this medicine on a daily basis for maximum benefit. It may take several (usually 3 to 7) days. If symptoms do not improve within 3 weeks, or if they worsen, contact your healthcare provider.

Clear nasal passages prior to use by blowing the nose. If nasal passages are blocked, use a decongestant just before use to allow the spray to fully enter the nose.

Exams may be necessary. Be sure to keep appointments.

Avoid exposure to chickenpox, measles or other infections; if exposed, contact your healthcare provider immediately.

Report any unusual fever, muscle/joint pain, weakness, sneezing, nasal irritation, depression or fluid retention to your healthcare provider.

Store with valve angled down.

Keep at room temperature, in a dry place, out of the reach of children.

Contents under pressure. Do not puncture or throw into a fire.

After opening the aluminum pouch, use medicine within 6 months.

Cleaning - Remove the aerosol container and wash the plastic parts regularly in warm water with mild detergent, if necessary. Allow parts to dry completely, then reassemble.

Bumetanide

(BYOO-MET-uh-nide)

Bumex

This medicine is used to treat serious fluid accumulation (edema) due to a variety of causes.

Precautions

DO NOT USE if you are allergic to this medicine or its relatives, oral diabetic medicines, sulfa antibiotics; or if you have severe kidney disease or loss of kidney function.

BEFORE USING THIS MEDICINE, tell your healthcare provider if you are pregnant or breastfeeding; or if you are taking, will be taking or stop taking any prescription or nonprescription medicine; or if you have any other medical conditions.

Side Effects

Every medicine can cause side effects, but many people have no, or minor, side effects. Tell your healthcare provider if any of the following occurs: thirst; irregular heartbeat; mental confusion; mood changes; nausea; vomiting; unusual tiredness; weakness; weak pulse; muscle cramps; appetite loss; stomach upset; bloating; diarrhea; constipation; dizziness; lightheadedness; headache; tingling of toes and fingers; blurred vision; nervousness; insomnia; chest pain; ringing in the ears; hearing loss (reversible); sun sensitivity; rash; hives; itching; dry skin; yellow skin or eyes; unusual bruising; difficult breathing; blood sugar imbalance; muscle cramps; joint pain; fever; chills; weight loss; nose bleeds; gout attack.

Guidelines for Use

USE EXACTLY AS PRESCRIBED.

Increases urination, therefore to avoid disruption of sleep at night take early in the day usually as a single dose.

May cause stomach upset. May be taken with food or milk.

May cause loss of potassium. If signs of potassium loss occur (weakness, cramps, nausea, dizziness, etc), contact your healthcare provider. Ask about foods high in potassium.

Diabetes — May increase blood sugar levels.

Dizziness or lightheadedness may occur if you stand up too fast from lying or sitting. Get up slowly, and notify healthcare provider if fainting occurs.

Sensitivity to sunlight may occur. Use sunscreen and wear protective clothing until tolerance is determined.

Your healthcare provider may want to periodically check your blood to ensure that your medicine is working properly.

Bupropion Hydrochloride

(byoo-PRO-pee-ahn HIGH-droe-KLOR-ide)

Wellbutrin

A mood elevating medicine used to treat depression.

Precautions

DO NOT USE if you are allergic to this medicine; if you have anorexia, bulimia, manic depression or a seizure disorder; or if you are using alcohol or a monoamine oxidase inhibitor (MAOI, eg, *Parnate*).

BEFORE USING THIS MEDICINE, tell your healthcare provider if you are pregnant or breastfeeding; or if you are taking, will be taking or stop taking any prescription or nonprescription medicine; or if you have any other medical conditions such as seizures.

Side Effects

Every medicine can cause side effects, but many people have no, or minor, side effects. Tell your healthcare provider if any of the following occurs: tremors; dry mouth; difficulty breathing; incoordination; nausea; vomiting; diarrhea; constipation; indigestion; seizures; dizziness; mood or personality changes; euphoria (exaggerated sense of well-being); confusion; agitation; hostility; disturbed concentration; restlessness; anxiety; sedation; sleep disturbances; fatigue; headache; pounding in chest (palpitations); rash; excessive sweating; blurred vision; frequent urination; urinary retention; menstrual problems; weight loss or gain; altered sex drive; fainting.

Guidelines for Use

USE EXACTLY AS PRESCRIBED.

Treatment often requires several months of therapy.

If a dose is missed, take it as soon as possible. If several hours have passed or if it is nearing time for the next dose, do not double the dose to catch up, unless advised by your healthcare provider. If more than one dose is missed, contact your healthcare provider.

Take in equally divided doses 3 or 4 times daily to minimize the risk of seizure.

Avoid alcohol use to reduce the risk of seizure.

May cause drowsiness or decreased judgment or alertness. Use caution while driving or performing other tasks requiring alertness.

Buspirone Hydrochloride

(byoo-SPY-rone HIGH-droe-KLOR-ide)

BuSpar

A medicine used to relieve nervousness and anxiety. It may occasionally be prescribed for other reasons.

Precautions

DO NOT USE if you are allergic to this medicine.

BEFORE USING THIS MEDICINE, tell your healthcare provider if you are pregnant or breastfeeding; or if you are taking, will be taking or stop taking any prescription or nonprescription medicine; or if you have any other medical conditions.

Side Effects

Every medicine can cause side effects, but many people have no, or minor, side effects. Tell your healthcare provider if any of the following occurs: dizziness; drowsiness; nervousness; headache; chronic abnormal movements.

Guidelines for Use

USE EXACTLY AS PRESCRIBED.

Take with a full glass of water as directed.

If a dose is missed, take it as soon as possible. If several hours have passed or if it is nearing time for the next dose, do not double the dose to catch up, unless advised by your healthcare provider. If more than one dose is missed, contact your healthcare provider.

Optimum results are generally achieved after 3 to 4 weeks of treatment. Some improvement may be seen in 7 to 10 days.

Avoid alcohol and other depressants (eg, antihistamines, narcotics, tranquilizers).

May cause drowsiness and dizziness. Use caution while driving or performing other tasks requiring mental alertness.

Busulfan

(byoo-SULL-fan)

Myleran

An anticancer medicine that controls, but does not cure, certain types of leukemia by slowing down the growth of white blood cells by the bone marrow.

Precautions

DO NOT USE if you are allergic to this medicine.

BEFORE USING THIS MEDICINE, tell your healthcare provider if you are pregnant or breastfeeding; or if you are taking, will be taking or stop taking any prescription or nonprescription medicine; or if you have any other medical conditions.

Side Effects

Every medicine can cause side effects, but many people have no, or minor, side effects. Tell your healthcare provider if any of the following occurs: diarrhea; appetite loss; nausea; vomiting; weakness; dizziness; confusion; fatigue; hair loss; darkening of skin; unusual bleeding or bruising; shortness of breath; lower back pain; joint pain; stomach pain; chills or sore throat.

Guidelines for Use

USE EXACTLY AS PRESCRIBED.

Take this medication at the same time every day.

Drink plenty of fluids.

If nausea or vomiting occurs, it may help to take the medicine on an empty stomach.

If a dose is missed, take it as soon as possible. If several hours have passed or if it is nearing time for the next dose, do not double the dose to catch up, unless advised by your healthcare provider. If more than one dose is missed, contact your healthcare provider.

Birth control is recommended while taking this medicine.

Butalbital/Acetaminophen/Caffeine

(BYOO-TAL-bih-tuhl/ass-cet-ah-MEE-noe-fen/kaff-EEN)

Amaphen, Anoquan, Arcet, Bucet, Butace, Endolor, Esgic, Esgic-Plus, Femcet, Fioricet, Medigesic, Repan, Tencet, Triad, Two-Dyne

A nonaspirin pain reliever plus a sedative for the relief of mild to moderate pain.

Precautions

DO NOT USE if you are allergic to any of these medications or have a history of porphyria. Long-term use may be habit-forming or lead to physical tolerance.

BEFORE USING THIS MEDICINE, tell your healthcare provider if you are pregnant or breastfeeding; or if you are taking, will be taking or stop taking any prescription or nonprescription medicine; or if you have any other medical conditions.

Side Effects

Every medicine can cause side effects, but many people have no, or minor, side effects. Tell your healthcare provider if any of the following occurs: drowsiness; dizziness; blurred vision; urinary retention; nausea; vomiting; constipation; shortness of breath; difficulty breathing; yellowing of the skin or gums; fever; sore throat; mouth sores; easy bruising or bleeding; nosebleed; tiny broken blood vessels under the skin.

Guidelines for Use

USE EXACTLY AS PRESCRIBED.

Take with food.

Avoid drinking alcohol and use caution with drowsiness-causing medicines (eg, sleeping pills, antihistamines).

This medicine may cause drowsiness; use caution while driving or performing any tasks requiring mental alertness, coordination and dexterity.

If pain is severe, persistent or recurrent, contact your healthcare provider.

Wait 30 to 60 minutes for the medicine to take effect before deciding if more is needed.

If a dose is missed, take it as soon as possible. If several hours have passed or it is nearing time for the next dose, do not double the dose to "catch up", unless advised to do so by your healthcare provider. If more than one dose is missed, tell your healthcare provider.

If constipation becomes a problem, a stool softener or bulk laxative may help.

Overdosage with this medicine can be very dangerous. If this occurs, contact your healthcare provider or poison control center immediately.

Butalbital/Acetaminophen/Caffeine/Codeine

(BYOO-TAL-bih-tuhl/ass-cet-ah-MEE-noe-fen/kaff-EEN/KOE-deen)

A nonaspirin pain reliever plus a sedative for the relief of mild to moderate pain.

Precautions

DO NOT USE if you are allergic to any of these medications or have a history of porphyria. Long-term use may be habit-forming or lead to physical tolerance.

BEFORE USING THIS MEDICATION, tell your healthcare provider if you are pregnant or breastfeeding; or if you are taking, will be taking or stop taking any prescription or non-prescription medicine; or if you have any other medical conditions.

Side Effects

Every medicine can cause side effects, but many people have no, or minor, side effects. Tell your healthcare provider if any of the following occurs: drowsiness; dizziness; blurred vision; urinary retention; nausea; vomiting; constipation; shortness of breath; difficulty breathing; yellowing of the skin or gums; fever; sore throat; mouth sores; easy bruising or bleeding; nosebleed; tiny broken blood vessels under the skin.

Guidelines for Use

USE EXACTLY AS PRESCRIBED.

Take with food.

Avoid drinking alcohol and use caution with other drowsiness-causing medicines (eg, sleeping pills, antihistamines).

This medicine may cause drowsiness; use caution while driving or performing other tasks requiring mental alertness, coordination and dexterity.

If pain is severe, persistent or recurrent, contact your healthcare provider. Wait 30 to 60 minutes for the medicine to take effect before deciding if more is needed.

If a dose is missed, you do not need to "make it up".

If constipation becomes a problem, a stool softener or bulk laxative may help.

Overdosage with this medicine is very dangerous. If this occurs, contact your healthcare provider or poison control center immediately.

Butalbital/Aspirin/Caffeine

(BYOO-TAL-bih-tuhl/ASS-pihr-in/kaff-EEN)

B-A-C, Fiorgen PF, Fiorinal, Isollyl Improved, Lanorinal, Marnal

Pain reliever plus a sedative for the relief of mild to moderate pain.

Precautions

DO NOT USE if you are allergic to any of these medications or nonsteroidal anti-inflammatory drugs (NSAIDS) or the dye tartrazine or if you have porphyria. May be habit-forming. Tolerance and dependence may occur.

BEFORE USING THIS MEDICINE, tell your healthcare provider if you are pregnant or breastfeeding; or if you are taking, will be taking or stop taking any prescription or nonprescription medicine; or if you have any other medical conditions.

Side Effects

Every medicine can cause side effects, but many people have no, or minor, side effects. Tell your healthcare provider if any of the following occurs: fever; sore throat; mouth sores; easy bruising or bleeding; nosebleed; tiny broken blood vessels under the skin; ringing in the ears; persistent stomach pain; diarrhea; dizziness; headache.

Guidelines for Use

USE EXACTLY AS PRESCRIBED.

May cause stomach upset; take with food or after meals.

Take with a full glass of water.

May decrease alertness and physical ability. Use caution while driving or performing other tasks requiring mental alertness.

Avoid alcohol and drowsiness-causing medicines (eg, narcotics, tranquilizers, antihistamines).

Do not increase the dose without consulting your healthcare provider.

Do not exceed the recommended dosage.

Do not use if there is a strong vinegar-like odor.

If pain persists for more than 10 days, if redness is present or in arthritic and rheumatic conditions affecting children under 12, consult your healthcare provider immediately.

Butalbital/Aspirin/Caffeine/Codeine Phosphate

(BYOO-TAL-bih-tuhl/ASS-pirh-in/Kaff-ENN/KOE-deen FOSS-fate)

Fiorinal with Codeine

Pain reliever plus a sedative for the relief of mild to moderate pain.

Precautions

DO NOT USE if you are allergic to any of these medications or nonsteroidal anti-inflammatory drugs (NSAIDS) or the dye tartrazine or have porphyria. May be habit-forming. Tolerance and dependence may occur.

BEFORE USING THIS MEDICINE, tell your healthcare provider if you are pregnant or breastfeeding; or if you are taking, will be taking or stop taking any prescription or nonprescription medicine; or if you have any other medical conditions.

Side Effects

Every medicine can cause side effects, but many people have no, or minor, side effects. Tell your healthcare provider if any of the following occurs: fever; sore throat; mouth sores; easy bruising or bleeding; nosebleed; tiny broken blood vessels under the skin; ringing in the ears; persistent stomach pain; diarrhea; dizziness; headache.

Guidelines for Use

USE EXACTLY AS PRESCRIBED.

May cause stomach upset; take with food or after meals.

Take with a full glass of water.

May decrease alertness and physical ability. Use caution while driving or performing other tasks requiring mental alertness.

Avoid alcohol and drowsiness-causing medicines (eg, narcotics, tranquilizers, antihistamines).

Do not increase the dose without consulting your healthcare provider.

Do not exceed the recommended dosage.

Do not use if there is a strong vinegar-like odor.

If pain persists for more than 10 days, if redness is present or in arthritic and rheumatic conditions affecting children under 12, consult your healthcare provider immediately.

Butoconazole Nitrate

(BYOO-toe-KOE-nuh-zole NYE-trate)

Femstat

A medicine used to treat vaginal candida (yeast) infections.

Precautions

DO NOT USE if you are allergic to this medicine.

BEFORE USING THIS MEDICINE, tell your healthcare provider if you are pregnant or breastfeeding; or if you are taking, will be taking or stop taking any prescription or nonprescription medicine; or if you have any other medical conditions.

Side Effects

Every medicine can cause side effects, but many people have no, or minor, side effects. Tell your healthcare provider if any of the following occurs: headache; body aches; local irritation; burning; itching; rash; sensitivity to light; vaginal discharge; soreness.

Guidelines for Use

USE EXACTLY AS PRESCRIBED.

Patient instructions for proper use are enclosed in each package.

Insert high into the vagina, except during pregnancy.

Complete a full course of therapy. Keep using, even during the menstrual period.

If the medicine causes burning or irritation, or if symptoms worsen, contact your healthcare provider.

Refrain from sexual intercourse during treatment or the male sexual partner should use a condom to avoid the risk of reinfection.

A sanitary napkin or mini-pad may be used to prevent staining of clothing due to seepage or leakage.

If infection recurs, other factors may be involved. Factors that increase the risk of infection include AIDS, diabetes, chronic antibiotic therapy, pregnancy, chronic steroid use and oral contraceptive use.

Butorphanol Tartrate

(byoo-TORE-fan-ahl TAR-trate)

Stadol, Stadol NS

A narcotic medicine used to relieve pain, including migraine and postoperative pain.

Precautions

DO NOT USE if you are allergic to this medicine or to benzethonium chloride; are dependent upon narcotics; or have recently used narcotic (opioid drugs).

BEFORE USING THIS MEDICINE, tell your healthcare provider if you are pregnant or breastfeeding; or if you are taking, will be taking or stop taking any prescription or nonprescription medicine; or if you have any other medical conditions.

Side Effects

Every medicine can cause side effects, but many people have no, or minor, side effects. Tell your healthcare provider if any of the following occurs: nausea; vomiting; appetite loss; constipation; stomach pain; dizziness; drowsiness; sleeplessness; headache; anxiety; confusion; exaggerated sense of well-being; floating feeling; nervousness; tingling/numbness; pounding in the chest; cough; difficulty breathing; nasal congestion/irritation; runny nose; sore throat; nosebleed; sinus/upper respiratory infection; sweating; clamminess; itching; sensation of heat; blurred vision; ear pain; ringing in ears; unpleasant taste; weakness; flushing; dry mouth; tremors; difficulty breathing.

Guidelines for Use

USE EXACTLY AS PRESCRIBED.

Read the package insert that comes with the product.

The usual starting dose is 1 spray in 1 nostril only. Your healthcare provider may increase the dose for added pain relief.

When taking a larger dose, you should be lying down in case you become sleepy or dizzy.

The risk of side effects is greater with an increased dose.

Maximum effects may not be reached for 1–2 hours.

Elderly patients may feel more side effects and require lower doses.

The pump should be primed prior to the first dose, or if the medicine has not been used for 48 hours or longer. When priming the pump, aim it away from people and animals.

This medicine may cause drowsiness or dizziness. Use caution while driving or performing other tasks requiring mental alertness.

Avoid alcohol and drowsiness-causing medications (eg, antihistamines).

Contact your healthcare provider if you experience any trouble breathing.

Give the medicine ample time to work before determining if more is needed.

This medicine has abuse potential. Dependence may develop upon repeated use.

Before throwing away the medicine, unscrew cap and rinse bottle.

Store below 86°F. Do not use if solution is discolored.

Calcitonin-Human Injection

(kal-sih-TOE-nin-human)

Cibacalcin

A hormone that is used to treat Paget's disease (moderate to severe), a condition of abnormal and accelerated bone formation and resorption. It is also used to lower high calcium levels in cancer, multiple myeloma or primary hyperparathyroidism.

Precautions

DO NOT USE if you are allergic to this medicine, or are pregnant.

BEFORE USING THIS MEDICINE, tell your healthcare provider if you are breastfeeding; or if you are taking, will be taking or stop taking any prescription or nonprescription medicine; or if you have any other medical conditions.

Side Effects

Every medicine can cause side effects, but many people have no, or minor, side effects. Tell your healthcare provider if any of the following occurs: nausea; vomiting; loss of appetite; diarrhea; abdominal pain and discomfort; weakness; headache; dizziness; nasal congestion; shortness of breath; pain at the injection site; flushing of face or hands; salty or metallic taste in mouth; itching of ear lobes; swelling of feet; rashes; tender palms and soles; increased urination; feverish sensation; eye pain; chills; chest pressure; tingling sensations; weight loss.

Patient Information

Doses vary according to the condition being treated. Do not adjust dose without consulting your healthcare provider.

Nausea, vomiting and flushing may be minimized by administering the injection at bedtime.

Supplemental vitamin D and calcium should be considered in those receiving this medicine to treat postmenopausal osteoporosis.

Calcitonin-Salmon

(kal-sih-TOE-nin-salmon)

Calcimar, Miacalcin, Osteocalcin, Salmonine

A hormone that is used to treat moderate to severe Paget's disease (a condition of abnormal and accelerated bone formation and resorption), to lower high calcium levels in cancer, multiple myeloma or primary hyperparathyroidism. It is also used to treat postmenopausal osteoporosis. May prevent the progressive loss of bone mass if taken with adequate calcium and vitamin D.

Precautions

DO NOT USE if you are allergic to this medicine.

BEFORE USING THIS MEDICINE, tell your healthcare provider if you are pregnant or breastfeeding; or if you are taking, will be taking or stop taking any prescription or nonprescription medicine; or if you have any other medical conditions.

Side Effects

Every medicine can cause side effects, but many people have no, or minor, side effects. Tell your healthcare provider if any of the following occurs: nausea; vomiting; loss of appetite; diarrhea; abdominal pain and discomfort; weakness; headache; dizziness; nasal congestion; shortness of breath; inflammation at the injection site; flushing of face or hands; salty or metallic taste in mouth; itching of ear lobes; swelling of feet; rashes; tender palms and soles; increased urination; feverish sensation; eye pain; chills; chest pressure; tingling sensations; weight loss; allergic reaction (shortness of breath, difficult breathing, hives, rash).

Guidelines for Use

USE EXACTLY AS PRESCRIBED.

Injection—Doses vary according to the condition being treated. Do not adjust dose without consulting your healthcare provider.

Nausea, vomiting and flushing may be minimized by administering the injection at bedtime.

Supplemental vitamin D and calcium should be considered in those receiving calcitonin to treat postmenopausal osteoporosis.

Nasal spray—Take one dose daily, alternating nostrils. It is necessary to activate the pump before the first dose. Refer to the patient information sheet for instructions on how to activate the pump.

Contact your healthcare provider if you experience significant nasal irritation.

Calcium Injectable

(KAL-see-uhm)

Used to treat low calcium levels; insect or spider bites or stings; muscle cramping; rash due to an allergic reaction; overdose of magnesium; high levels of potassium. Also used during open heart surgery to improve weak contractions of the heart. It may occasionally be prescribed for other reasons.

Precautions

DO NOT USE if you have an allergy to this medicine.

BEFORE USING THIS MEDICINE, tell your healthcare provider if you are pregnant or breastfeeding; or if you are taking, will be taking or stop taking any prescription or nonprescription medicine; of if you have any other medical conditions.

Side Effects

Every medicine can cause side effects, but many people have no, or minor, side effects. Tell your healthcare provider if any of the following occurs: tingling; metallic or chalky taste; weakness; nausea; vomiting; irritation at the injection site.

Calcium Oral

(KAL-see-uhm)

Alka-Mints, Amitone, Cal Carb-HD, Cal-Plus, Calci-Chew, Calci-Mix, Calciday-667, Calcium 600, Caltrate 600, Caltrate Jr., Chooz, Citracal, Dicarbosil, Equilet, Florical, Gencalc 600, Mallamint, Neo-Calglucon, Nephro-Calci, Os-Cal 500, Oysco 500, Oystercal 500, Rolaids Calcium Rich, Tums, Tums E-X Extra Strength

For use as a dietary supplement when calcium intake may be inadequate; in the treatment of calcium deficiency states; and for the treatment of upset stomach due to too much acid secretion; to treat irritation of the stomach associated with peptic ulcer.

Precautions

DO NOT USE if you are allergic to this medicine.

BEFORE USING THIS MEDICINE, ask your healthcare provider if you are pregnant or breastfeeding; or if you are taking, will be taking or stop taking any prescription or nonprescription medicine; of if you have any other medical condition.

Side Effects

Every medicine can cause side effects, but many people have no, or minor, side effects. Tell your healthcare provider if any of the following occurs: loss of appetite; nausea; vomiting; constipation; abdominal pain; dry mouth; thirst; increased urination; Carbonate: nausea; vomiting; stomach pain; diarrhea; muscle weakness; lack of energy; headache; confusion; irritability; constipation.

Guidelines for Use

USE EXACTLY AS PRESCRIBED.

Take with or after meals. Take with a large glass of water.

Calcium can interfere with the absorption of some medicines. Do not take other medicines within 2 hours of taking this medicine.

Recommended Dietary Allowance (RDA)--Adults: 150 mg. Common sources of calcium--dairy products, and some leafy, green vegetables (eg, broccoli).

Carbonate--Antacids reduce acidity for about 30 minutes when taken on an empty stomach. Acidity is reduced for about 3 hours when antacids are taken 1 hour after meals.

Taking too much of this medicine can cause the stomach to secrete excess stomach acid. Talk to your healthcare provider about the appropriate dose.

Long-term use--Do not take for longer than 2 weeks for the relief of indigestion. If discomfort continues, talk to your healthcare provider.

Chewable tablets--Chew thoroughly before swallowing. Follow with a glass of water.

Suspension--Shake well before using.

Capsaicin

(kap-SAY-uh-sin)

Zostrix, Zostrix-HP

A topical cream used for the temporary relief of pain from rheumatoid arthritis, osteoarthritis, painful diabetic neuropathy or following shingles (herpes zoster).

Precautions

DO NOT USE if you are allergic to this medicine or chili pepper. Do not apply to open wounds, damaged or irritated skin.

BEFORE USING THIS MEDICINE, tell your healthcare provider if you are pregnant or breastfeeding; or if you are taking, will be taking or stop taking any prescription or nonprescription medicine; or if you have any other medical conditions.

Side Effects

Every medicine can cause side effects, but many people have no, or minor, side effects. Tell your healthcare provider if any of the following occurs: burning sensation, stinging or redness upon application (usually temporary).

Guidelines for Use

USE EXACTLY AS PRESCRIBED.

For external use only.

Onset of relief may take several weeks.

Apply to affected area 3 to 4 times daily to achieve maximum pain relief. Thoroughly rub into the area so no residue is left on the skin surface. Wash hands after application.

Avoid contact with eyes or other mucous membranes. If contact occurs, flush the affected area thoroughly with water. Use caution when handling contact lenses after application; washing hands, wearing gloves or using an applicator may be useful.

Do not use on children under 2 unless directed by your healthcare provider.

Do not apply to open wounds, damaged or irritated skin. Do not bandage tightly.

If condition worsens or does not improve after 28 days, consult your healthcare provider.

Warm water or excessive sweating may intensify burning sensation.

Captopril

(KAP-toe-prill)

Capoten

An angiotensin converting enzyme (ACE) inhibitor medicine generally used to lower high blood pressure or treat heart failure.

Precautions

DO NOT USE if you are allergic to this medicine or if you are pregnant.

BEFORE USING THIS MEDICINE, tell your healthcare provider if you are breastfeeding; or if you are taking, will be taking or stop taking any prescription or nonprescription medicine; or if you have any other medical conditions.

Side Effects

Every medicine can cause side effects, but many people have no, or minor, side effects. Tell your healthcare provider if any of the following occurs: stomach pain; vomiting; diarrhea; constipation; appetite loss; depression; headache; dizziness; nervousness; sleeping difficulties; fatigue; dizziness/lightheadedness when rising quickly from a sitting or lying position; shortness of breath; cough; nasal congestion; bronchitis; sinus inflammation; rash; sweating; flushing; yellowing of skin or eyes; muscle cramps; weight loss; taste loss; dry mouth; decreased sex drive; back, joint and shoulder pain; urination changes; fever; vision disturbances; numbness/tingling of hands or feet.

Guidelines for Use

USE EXACTLY AS PRESCRIBED.

Take one hour before meals.

Patients starting treatment for high blood pressure may at first feel tired. It takes time for the body to adjust. Continue taking medication and check with your healthcare provider.

If a dose is missed, take it as soon as possible. If several hours have passed or if it is nearing time for the next dose, do not double the dose to catch up, unless advised by your doctor. If more than one dose is missed, contact your healthcare provider. Do not interrupt or stop medication without consulting your healthcare provider.

Do not use salt substitutes without telling your healthcare provider.

A persistent, dry, nonproductive cough may occur. Tell your healthcare provider. Recovery is rapid when the medicine is stopped.

Dizziness, fainting or lightheadedness is most likely after the first dose or in the first days of therapy; avoid sudden changes in posture. If fainting occurs, discontinue medicine until talking to your healthcare provider.

Carbamazepine Suspension

(KAR-bam-AZE-uh-peen)

Tegretol

A medicine that helps control epilepsy and seizures. It is also an analgesic (pain reliever) for certain types of nerve pain. This medicine is not a simple pain reliever and should not be used for the relief of minor aches and pains. It may occasionally be prescribed for other reasons.

Precautions

DO NOT USE if you are allergic to this medicine or certain antidepressants (eg, amitriptyline); or use monoamine oxidase inhibitors (eg, phenelzine, tranylcypromine).

BEFORE USING THIS MEDICINE, tell your healthcare provider if you are pregnant or breastfeeding; or if you are taking, will be taking or stop taking any prescription or nonprescription medicine; or if you have any other medical conditions.

Side Effects

Every medicine can cause side effects, but many people have no, or minor, side effects. Tell your healthcare provider if any of the following occurs: unusual bleeding or bruising; yellowing of skin or eyes; stomach pain or vomiting; pale stools; darkened urine; decreased sexual ability; nervous system disturbances; swelling; fever; chills; sore throat; ulcers in the mouth; dizziness; drowsiness; unsteadiness.

Guidelines for Use

USE EXACTLY AS PRESCRIBED.

Shake well before using.

May cause stomach upset. Take with food.

Do not stop taking this medication without talking to your healthcare provider. If you stop taking this medication suddenly, your seizures may return.

If a dose is missed, take it as soon as possible. If several hours have passed or if it is nearing time for the next dose, do not double the dose to catch up, unless advised by your healthcare provider. If more than one dose is missed, contact your healthcare provider.

May cause drowsiness, dizziness or blurred vision. Use caution when driving or performing other tasks requiring mental alertness.

Carry identification indicating you are using this medicine.

Keep lid tightly closed. Store in a cool, dry place. Avoid humidity. Failure to store properly could reduce the effectiveness of the medicine.

Carbamazepine Tablets

(KAR-bam-AZE-uh-peen)

Atretol, Depitol, Epitol, Tegretol Chewable, Tegretol

A medicine that helps control epilepsy and seizures. It is also an analgesic (pain reliever) for certain types of nerve pain. This medicine is not a simple pain reliever and should not be used for the relief of minor aches and pains. It may occasionally be prescribed for other reasons.

Precautions

DO NOT USE if you are allergic to this medicine or certain antidepressants (eg, amitriptyline); or use monoamine oxidase inhibitors (eg, phenelzine, tranylcypromine).

BEFORE USING THIS MEDICINE, tell your healthcare provider if you are pregnant or breastfeeding; or if you are taking, will be taking or stop taking any prescription or nonprescription medicine; or if you have any other medical conditions.

Side Effects

Every medicine can cause side effects, but many people have no, or minor, side effects. Tell your healthcare provider if any of the following occurs: unusual bleeding or bruising; yellowing of skin or eyes; stomach pain or vomiting; pale stools; darkened urine; decreased sexual ability; nervous system disturbances; swelling; fever; chills; sore throat; ulcers in the mouth; dizziness; drowsiness; unsteadiness.

Guidelines for Use

USE EXACTLY AS PRESCRIBED.

May cause stomach upset. Take with food.

Do not stop taking this medication without talking to your healthcare provider. If you stop taking this medication suddenly, your seizures may return.

If a dose is missed, take it as soon as possible. If several hours have passed or if it is nearing time for the next dose, do not double the dose to catch up, unless advised by your healthcare provider. If more than one dose is missed, contact your healthcare provider.

May cause drowsiness, dizziness or blurred vision. Use caution when driving or performing other tasks requiring mental alertness.

Carry identification indicating you are using this medicine.

Keep lid tightly closed. Store in a cool, dry place. Avoid humidity. Failure to store properly could reduce the effectiveness of the medicine.

Carbenicillin Indanyl Sodium

(car-BEN-ih-SILL-in IN-duh-nil SO-dee-uhm)

Geocillin

A penicillin antibiotic used to treat infections caused by certain bacteria.

Precautions

DO NOT USE if you are allergic to penicillins, cephalosporins or imipenem. Not used for certain severe infections.

BEFORE USING THIS MEDICINE, tell your healthcare provider if you are allergic to any penicillin (eg, ampicillin, amoxicillin) or cephalosporin; are pregnant or breastfeeding; or if you are taking, will be taking or stop taking any prescription or nonprescription medicine; or if you have any other medical conditions.

Side Effects

Every medicine can cause side effects, but many people have no, or minor, side effects. Tell your healthcare provider if any of the following occurs: rash; itching; hives; severe diarrhea; shortness of breath; wheezing; dizziness; black tongue; sore throat; nausea; vomiting; fever; swollen joints; or any unusual bleeding or bruising.

Guidelines for Use

USE EXACTLY AS PRESCRIBED.

Take on an empty stomach approximately 30 minutes to one hour before meals or two hours after a meal. Take at even intervals, preferably around the clock.

If a dose is missed, take it as soon as possible. If several hours have passed or if it is nearing time for the next dose, do not double the dose to catch up, unless advised by your healthcare provider. If more than one dose is missed, contact your healthcare provider.

Continue until all the prescribed medicine has been taken. Failure to take a full course of therapy may cause a relapse of the infection.

Carisoprodol

(car-eye-so-PRO-dole)

Rela, Sodol, Soma, Soprodol

A medicine used to relieve muscle discomfort due to strain and sprain.

Precautions

DO NOT USE if you are allergic to this medicine or its relatives (meprobamate) or if you are breastfeeding.

BEFORE USING THIS MEDICINE, tell your healthcare provider if you are pregnant; or if you are taking, will be taking or stop taking any prescription or nonprescription medicine; or if you have any other medical conditions.

Side Effects

Every medicine can cause side effects, but many people have no, or minor, side effects. Tell your healthcare provider if any of the following occurs: dizziness; drowsiness; incoordination; agitation; headache; depression; fainting; sleep disturbance; flushing; nausea; vomiting; hiccups; severe rash; hives; itching; difficulty breathing.

Guidelines for Use

USE EXACTLY AS PRESCRIBED.

May be taken with food if stomach upset occurs.

If a dose is missed, take it as soon as possible. If several hours have passed or if it is nearing time for the next dose, do not double the dose to catch up unless advised by your healthcare provider. If more than one dose is missed, contact your healthcare provider.

May cause drowsiness. Use caution while driving or performing other tasks requiring mental alertness, coordination and dexterity. Avoid alcohol and medication that cause drowsiness while taking this medicine (eg, sleeping pills, tranquilizers, antihistamines).

Patients on long-term or high dosage therapy may have withdrawal symptoms if therapy is suddenly stopped. Do not stop therapy abruptly or change dosage without asking your healthcare provider.

Carmustine

(CAR-muss-teen)

BiCNU

Used alone and in combination with other chemotherapeutic agents to treat certain brain tumors, multiple myeloma, Hodgkin's disease and non-Hodgkin's lymphomas.

Side Effects

Every medicine can cause side effects, but many people have no, or minor, side effects. Tell your healthcare provider if any of the following occurs: nausea and vomiting; burning at the injection site; flushing.

Patient Information

Contraceptive (birth control) measures are recommended during treatment.

Carteolol Hydrochloride Ophthalmic

(CAR-tee-oh-lahl HIGH-droe-KLOR-ide)

Ocupress

A beta blocking agent used to treat glaucoma.

Precautions

DO NOT USE if you have an allergy to this medicine or its relatives.

BEFORE USING THIS MEDICINE, tell your healthcare provider if you are pregnant or breastfeeding; or if you are taking, will be taking or stop taking any prescription or nonprescription medicine; if you have any other medical conditions; or if you are allergic to sulfites.

Side Effects

Every medicine can cause side effects, but many people have no, or minor, side effects. Tell your healthcare provider if any of the following occurs: eye irritation; burning; tearing; redness; swelling; blurred vision; decreased night vision; decreased heart rate; pounding in the chest; difficult breathing; headache; dizziness; insomnia; taste perversion.

Guidelines for Use

USE EXACTLY AS PRESCRIBED.

If a dose is missed, take it as soon as possible. If several hours have passed or if it is nearing time for the next dose, do not double the dose to catch up, unless advised by your healthcare provider. If more than one dose is missed, contact your healthcare provider.

May cause stinging or pain when first instilled in the eye.

Intraocular pressure must be monitored periodically by your healthcare provider to make sure the medicine is working properly.

Notify your healthcare provider if you are using these eye drops and plan to have surgery. You may have to temporarily stop using them.

Carteolol Hydrochloride Oral

(CAR-tee-oh-lahl HIGH-droe-KLOR-ide)

Cartrol

A beta blocker medicine used to lower high blood pressure and to treat angina and heart attack.

Precautions

DO NOT USE if you are allergic to this medicine or its relatives, or if you are breastfeeding.

BEFORE USING THIS MEDICINE, tell your healthcare provider if you are pregnant; or if you are taking, will be taking or stop taking any prescription or nonprescription medicine; or if you have any other medical conditions.

Side Effects

Every medicine can cause side effects, but many people have no, or minor, side effects. Tell your healthcare provider if any of the following occurs: nausea; vomiting; stomach ache; diarrhea; constipation; appetite changes; indigestion; depression; anxiety; hallucinations; short-term memory loss; behavior changes; disorientation; fainting; dizziness; lightheadedness; tiredness; sleep disturbances; decreased concentration; headache; nightmares; emotional instability; chest pain; chills; cold or numb extremities; pounding of the chest; difficulty breathing; cough; nasal congestion; rash; hives; fluid retention; flushing or paleness; increased pigmentation; itching; hair loss; sweating; dry skin; psoriasis; painful and aching joints and muscles; painful, frequent or difficult urination; blurred vision; dry, burning or irritated eyes; ringing in the ears; taste changes; sore throat; dry mouth; slurred speech; fever; weight gain.

Guidelines for Use

USE EXACTLY AS PRESCRIBED.

Ask your healthcare provider before using other medicines including nasal decongestants, diet aids or nonprescription cold preparations.

Do not stop this medicine suddenly; it could cause a worsening of disease including worse angina (chest pain), irregular heartbeats and increased risk of heart attack and death.

Withdraw these medications slowly over one to two weeks by gradually decreasing the dose.

Diabetes — These products can mask signs of low blood sugar and change blood sugar levels. It may be necessary for your healthcare provider to change your dose of diabetic medications.

Use caution while driving or performing other tasks requiring mental alertness, coordination and dexterity.

Castor Oil

(KASS-ter oil)

Emulsoil, Purge, Fleet Flavored Castor Oil

A medicine used for short-term treatment of constipation and to clean out the bowel before bowel examinations or bowel surgery.

Precautions

DO NOT USE if you are allergic to this medicine or if you are pregnant.

BEFORE USING THIS MEDICINE, tell your healthcare provider if you are breastfeeding; or if you are taking, will be taking or stop taking any prescription or nonprescription medicine; or if you have any other medical conditions.

Side Effects

Every medicine can cause side effects, but many people have no, or minor, side effects. Tell your healthcare provider if any of the following occurs: nausea; vomiting; stomach ache; bowel cramping; diarrhea; weakness; dizziness; fainting; facial swelling; redness and discomfort; rectal bleeding; muscle cramps or pain; irritation of the rectal area; sweating; pounding in the chest.

Guidelines for Use

USE EXACTLY AS PRESCRIBED.

Take with a full glass of water or juice.

Laxative use is only a temporary measure. When normal bowel habits return, stop use of this medicine.

Frequent use of laxatives and inadequate fluid intake can cause an imbalance in fluid and electrolyte levels. Symptoms can include muscle cramps, muscle weakness and dizziness.

Effects will occur in 2 to 6 hours.

Emulsions--Shake well before using.

Cefaclor

(SEFF-uh-klor)

Ceclor

A cephalosporin antibiotic used to treat infections caused by certain bacteria.

Precautions

DO NOT USE if you are allergic to cephalosporins or penicillins.

BEFORE USING THIS MEDICINE, tell your healthcare provider if you are pregnant or breastfeeding; or if you are taking, will be taking or stop taking any prescription or nonprescription medicine; or if you have any other medical conditions.

Side Effects

Every medicine can cause side effects, but many people have no, or minor, side effects. Tell your healthcare provider if any of the following occurs: skin rash; hives; itching; joint/muscle pain or swelling; fever; difficulty breathing; fluid retention; numbness; chills; nausea; vomiting; severe diarrhea; or unusual bleeding or bruising.

Guidelines for Use

USE EXACTLY AS PRESCRIBED.

May cause stomach upset; take with food or milk.

Take at evenly spaced intervals throughout the day.

If a dose is missed, take it as soon as possible. If several hours have passed or if it is nearing time for the next dose, do not double the dose to catch up, unless advised by your healthcare provider. If more than one dose is missed, contact your healthcare provider.

Continue use until all the prescribed medicine has been taken. Failure to take all of the medicine may prevent complete elimination of bacteria, causing the infection to return.

Diabetes-May interfere with urine tests for glucose and may give false test results.

Cefadroxil

(SEFF-uh-DROX-ill)

Duricef

A cephalosporin antibiotic used to treat infections caused by certain bacteria.

Precautions

DO NOT USE if you are allergic to any cephalosporins or penicillins.

BEFORE USING THIS MEDICINE, tell your healthcare provider if you are allergic to cephalosporins or penicillins; are pregnant or breastfeeding; or if you are taking, will be taking or stop taking any prescription or nonprescription medicine; or if you have any other medical conditions.

Side Effects

Every medicine can cause side effects, but many people have no, or minor, side effects. Tell your healthcare provider if any of the following occurs: skin rash; hives; itching; joint/muscle pain or swelling; fever; difficulty breathing; fluid retention; numbness; chills; nausea; vomiting; severe diarrhea or unusual bleeding or bruising.

Guidelines for Use

USE EXACTLY AS PRESCRIBED.

May cause stomach upset; take with food or milk.

Take at even intervals around the clock as prescribed.

If a dose is missed, take it as soon as possible. If several hours have passed or if it is nearing time for the next dose, do not double the dose to catch up, unless advised by your healthcare provider. If more than one dose is missed, contact your healthcare provider.

Continue use until all the prescribed medicine has been taken. Failure to take all of the medicine may prevent complete elimination of bacteria, causing the infection to return.

Liquid preparations-Store in refrigerator; do not freeze. Shake well before using and check expiration date; may be kept for 14 days.

Diabetes-May interfere with urine tests for glucose and may give false test results.

Cefamandole Nafate

(SEFF-uh-MAN-dahl NA-fate)

Mandol

A cephalosporin antibiotic used to treat a variety of infections.

Side Effects

Every medicine can cause side effects, but many people have no, or minor, side effects. Tell your healthcare provider if any of the following occurs: nausea; vomiting; diarrhea; loss of appetite; taste distortion; inflammation of the tongue; abdominal pain; gas; heartburn; stomach cramps; upset stomach; headache; dizziness; lethargy; fatigue; abnormal skin sensations; excessive sweating; flushing; irritation at the injection site; fever; difficulty breathing; vaginal discharge; mouth sores; loss of sleep; sleepiness; nervousness; insomnia; hyperactivity; confusion.

Patient Information

Tell your healthcare provider if you have experienced allergic reactions to any cephalosporins, penicillins or their relatives.

Tell you doctor of nausea, vomiting or diarrhea, especially if the diarrhea is severe or contains blood, mucus or pus.

Tell your healthcare provider if you are breastfeeding.

Diabetes — A false-positive reaction for urine glucose may occur with the nonspecific urine test. Use an enzyme-based test.

Cefazolin

(seff-UH-zoe-lin)

Ancef, Kefzol, Zolicef

A cephalosporin antibiotic used to treat a variety of infections.

Side Effects

Every medicine can cause side effects, but many people have no, or minor, side effects. Tell your healthcare provider if any of the following occurs: nausea; vomiting; diarrhea; loss of appetite; taste distortion; inflammation of the tongue; abdominal pain; gas; heartburn; stomach cramps; upset stomach; headache; dizziness; lethargy; fatigue; abnormal skin sensations; excessive sweating; flushing; irritation at the injection site; fever; difficulty breathing; vaginal discharge; mouth sores; loss of sleep; sleepiness; nervousness; insomnia; hyperactivity; confusion.

Patient Information

Tell your healthcare provider if you have experienced allergic reactions to any cephalosporins, penicillins or their relatives.

Tell your healthcare provider of nausea, vomiting or diarrhea, especially if the diarrhea is severe or contains blood, mucus or pus.

Tell your healthcare provider if you are breastfeeding.

Diabetes — A false-positive reaction for urine glucose may occur with the nonspecific urine test. Use an enzyme-based test.

Cefixime

(SEFF-IKS-eem)

Suprax

A cephalosporin antibiotic used to treat infections caused by certain bacteria.

Precautions

DO NOT USE if you are allergic to cephalosporins or penicillins.

BEFORE USING THIS MEDICINE, tell your healthcare provider if you are pregnant or breastfeeding; or if you are taking, will be taking or stop taking any prescription or nonprescription medicine; or if you have any other medical conditions.

Side Effects

Every medicine can cause side effects, but many people have no, or minor, side effects. Tell your healthcare provider if any of the following occurs: skin rash; hives; itching; joint/muscle pain or swelling; fever; difficulty breathing; fluid retention; numbness; chills; nausea; vomiting; severe diarrhea; unusual bleeding or bruising.

Guidelines for Use

USE EXACTLY AS PRESCRIBED.

May cause stomach upset; take with food or milk.

Take at even intervals around the clock as prescribed.

If a dose is missed, take it as soon as possible. If several hours have passed or if it is nearing time for the next dose, do not double the dose to catch up, unless advised by your healthcare provider. If more than one dose is missed, contact your healthcare provider.

Continue use until all the prescribed medicine has been taken. Failure to take all of the medicine may prevent complete elimination of bacteria, causing the infection to return.

Shake well before using.

Check expiration date. May be kept for 14 days.

Diabetes-May interfere with urine tests for glucose and may give false test results.

Cefmetazole

(seff-MET-uh-zole)

Zefazone

A cephalosporin antibiotic used to treat a variety of infections.

Side Effects

Every medicine can cause side effects, but many people have no, or minor, side effects. Tell your healthcare provider if any of the following occurs: nausea; vomiting; diarrhea; loss of appetite; taste distortion; inflammation of the tongue; abdominal pain; gas; heartburn; stomach cramps; upset stomach; headache; dizziness; lethargy; fatigue; abnormal skin sensations; excessive sweating; flushing; irritation at the injection site; fever; difficulty breathing; vaginal discharge; mouth sores; loss of sleep; sleepiness; nervousness; insomnia; hyperactivity; confusion.

Patient Information

Tell your healthcare provider if you have experienced allergic reactions to any cephalosporins, penicillins or their relatives.

Tell your healthcare provider of nausea, vomiting or diarrhea, especially if the diarrhea is severe or contains blood, mucus or pus.

Tell your healthcare provider if you are breastfeeding.

Diabetes — A false-positive reaction for urine glucose may occur with the nonspecific urine test. Use an enzyme-based test.

Cefonicid

(seh-FAHN-ih-SID)

Monocid

A cephalosporin antibiotic used to treat a variety of infections.

Side Effects

Every medicine can cause side effects, but many people have no, or minor, side effects. Tell your healthcare provider if any of the following occurs: nausea; vomiting; diarrhea; loss of appetite; taste distortion; inflammation of the tongue; abdominal pain; gas; heartburn; stomach cramps; upset stomach; headache; dizziness; lethargy; fatigue; abnormal skin sensations; excessive sweating; flushing; irritation at the injection site; fever; difficulty breathing; vaginal discharge; mouth sores; loss of sleep; sleepiness; nervousness; insomnia; hyperactivity; confusion.

Patient Information

Tell your healthcare provider if you have experienced allergic reactions to any cephalosporins, penicillins or their relatives.

Tell your healthcare provider of nausea, vomiting or diarrhea, especially if the diarrhea is severe or contains blood, mucus or pus.

Tell your healthcare provider if you are breastfeeding.

Diabetes — A false-positive reaction for urine glucose may occur with the nonspecific urine test. Use an enzyme-based test.

Cefoperazone Sodium

(SEFF-oh-PURR-uh-zone SO-dee-uhm)

Cefobid

A cephalosporin antibiotic used to treat a variety of infections.

Side Effects

Every medicine can cause side effects, but many people have no, or minor, side effects. Tell your healthcare provider if any of the following occurs: nausea; vomiting; diarrhea; loss of appetite; taste distortion; inflammation of the tongue; abdominal pain; gas; heartburn; stomach cramps; upset stomach; headache; dizziness; lethargy; fatigue; abnormal skin sensations; excessive sweating; flushing; irritation at the injection site; fever; difficulty breathing; vaginal discharge; mouth sores; loss of sleep; sleepiness; nervousness; insomnia; hyperactivity; confusion.

Patient Information

Tell your healthcare provider if you have experienced allergic reactions to any cephalosporins, penicillins or their relatives.

Tell your healthcare provider of nausea, vomiting or diarrhea, especially if the diarrhea is severe or contains blood, mucus or pus.

Tell your healthcare provider if you are breastfeeding.

Diabetes — A false-positive reaction for urine glucose may occur with the nonspecific urine test. Use an enzyme-based test.

Cefotaxime Sodium

(seff-oh-TAX-eem SO-dee-uhm)

Claforan

A cephalosporin antibiotic used to treat a variety of infections.

Side Effects

Every medicine can cause side effects, but many people have no, or minor, side effects. Tell your healthcare provider if any of the following occurs: nausea; vomiting; diarrhea; loss of appetite; taste distortion; inflammation of the tongue; abdominal pain; gas; heartburn; stomach cramps; upset stomach; headache; dizziness; lethargy; fatigue; abnormal skin sensations; excessive sweating; flushing; irritation at the injection site; fever; difficulty breathing; vaginal discharge; mouth sores; loss of sleep; sleepiness; nervousness; insomnia; hyperactivity; confusion.

Patient Information

Tell your healthcare provider if you have experienced allergic reactions to any cephalosporins, penicillins or their relatives.

Tell your healthcare provider of nausea, vomiting or diarrhea, especially if the diarrhea is severe or contains blood, mucus or pus.

Tell your healthcare provider if you are breastfeeding.

Diabetes — A false-positive reaction for urine glucose may occur with the nonspecific urine test. Use an enzyme-based test.

Cefotetan Disodium

(SEFF-oh-tee-tan die-SO-dee-uhm)

Cefotan

A cephalosporin antibiotic used to treat a variety of infections.

Side Effects

Every medicine can cause side effects, but many people have no, or minor, side effects. Tell your healthcare provider if any of the following occurs: nausea; vomiting; diarrhea; loss of appetite; taste distortion; inflammation of the tongue; abdominal pain; gas; heartburn; stomach cramps; upset stomach; headache; dizziness; lethargy; fatigue; abnormal skin sensations; excessive sweating; flushing; irritation at the injection site; fever; difficulty breathing; vaginal discharge; mouth sores; loss of sleep; sleepiness; nervousness; insomnia; hyperactivity; confusion.

Patient Information

Tell your healthcare provider if you have experienced allergic reactions to any cephalosporins, penicillins or their relatives.

Tell your healthcare provider of nausea, vomiting or diarrhea, especially if the diarrhea is severe or contains blood, mucus or pus.

Tell your healthcare provider if you are breastfeeding.

Diabetes — A false-positive reaction for urine glucose may occur with the nonspecific urine test. Use an enzyme-based test.

Cefoxitin Disodium

(seff-OX-ih-tin die-SO-dee-uhm)

Mefoxin

A cephalosporin antibiotic used to treat a variety of infections.

Side Effects

Every medicine can cause side effects, but many people have no, or minor, side effects. Tell your healthcare provider if any of the following occurs: nausea; vomiting; diarrhea; loss of appetite; taste distortion; inflammation of the tongue; abdominal pain; gas; heartburn; stomach cramps; upset stomach; headache; dizziness; lethargy; fatigue; abnormal skin sensations; excessive sweating; flushing; irritation at the injection site; fever; difficulty breathing; vaginal discharge; mouth sores; loss of sleep; sleepiness; nervousness; insomnia; hyperactivity; confusion.

Patient Information

Tell your healthcare provider if you have experienced allergic reactions to any cephalosporins, penicillins or their relatives.

Tell your healthcare provider of nausea, vomiting or diarrhea, especially if the diarrhea is severe or contains blood, mucus or pus.

Tell your healthcare provider if you are breastfeeding.

Diabetes — A false-positive reaction for urine glucose may occur with the nonspecific urine test. Use an enzyme-based test.

Cefpodoxime Proxetil

(SEF-pode-OX-eem PROX-uh-til)

Vantin Suspension

A cephalosporin antibiotic used to treat infections caused by certain bacteria.

Precautions

DO NOT USE if you are allergic to any cephalosporin or penicillin.

BEFORE USING THIS MEDICINE, tell your healthcare provider if you are pregnant or breastfeeding; or if you are taking, will be taking or stop taking any prescription or nonprescription medicine; or if you have any other medical conditions.

Side Effects

Every medicine can cause side effects, but many people have no, or minor, side effects. Tell your healthcare provider if any of the following occurs: skin rash; hives; itching; joint/muscle pain or swelling; fever; difficulty breathing; fluid retention; numbness; chills; vomiting; nausea; severe diarrhea; vaginal infections; unusual bleeding or bruising.

Guidelines for Use

USE EXACTLY AS PRESCRIBED.

May cause stomach upset. Take with food to increase effectiveness.

Do not take this medicine with antacids. Take this medicine at least 2 hours before or after antacids.

Take at even intervals around the clock as prescribed.

If a dose is missed, take it as soon as possible. If several hours have passed or if it is nearing time for the next dose, do not double the dose to catch up, unless advised by your healthcare provider. If more than one dose is missed, contact your healthcare provider.

Continue use until all the prescribed medicine has been taken. Failure to take all of the medicine may prevent complete elimination of bacteria, causing the infection to return.

Store in refrigerator; do not freeze. Shake well before using and check expiration date; may be kept for 14 days.

Diabetes-May interfere with urine tests for glucose and may give false test results.

Cefprozil

(SEFF-pro-zil)

Cefzil

A cephalosporin antibiotic used to treat infections caused by certain bacteria.

Precautions

DO NOT USE if you are allergic to any cephalosporin or penicillin.

BEFORE USING THIS MEDICINE, tell your healthcare provider if you are pregnant or breastfeeding; or if you are taking, will be taking or stop taking any prescription or nonprescription medicine; or if you have any other medical conditions.

Side Effects

Every medicine can cause side effects, but many people have no, or minor, side effects. Tell your healthcare provider if any of the following occurs: skin rash; hives; itching; joint/muscle pain or swelling; fever; difficulty breathing; fluid retention; numbness; chills; nausea; vomiting; severe diarrhea; or unusual bleeding or bruising.

Guidelines for Use

USE EXACTLY AS PRESCRIBED.

May cause stomach upset; take with food or milk.

Take at even intervals around the clock as prescribed.

If a dose is missed, take it as soon as possible. If several hours have passed or if it is nearing time for the next dose, do not double the dose to catch up, unless advised by your healthcare provider. If more than one dose is missed, contact your healthcare provider.

Continue use until all the prescribed medicine has been taken. Failure to take all of the medicine may prevent complete elimination of bacteria, causing the infection to return.

Diabetes-May interfere with urine tests for glucose and may give false test results.

Suspension-Shake well before using.

Store in refrigerator; do not freeze.

Check expiration date; may be kept for 14 days.

Ceftazidime

(seff-TAZE-ih-deem)

Ceptaz, Fortaz, Tazicef, Tazidime

A cephalosporin antibiotic used to treat a variety of infections.

Side Effects

Every medicine can cause side effects, but many people have no, or minor, side effects. Tell your healthcare provider if any of the following occurs: nausea; vomiting; diarrhea; loss of appetite; taste distortion; inflammation of the tongue; abdominal pain; gas; heartburn; stomach cramps; upset stomach; headache; dizziness; lethargy; fatigue; abnormal skin sensations; excessive sweating; flushing; irritation at the injection site; fever; difficulty breathing; vaginal discharge; mouth sores; loss of sleep; sleepiness; nervousness; insomnia; hyperactivity; confusion.

Patient Information

Tell your healthcare provider if you have experienced allergic reactions to any cephalosporins, penicillins or their relatives.

Tell your healthcare provider of nausea, vomiting or diarrhea, especially if the diarrhea is severe or contains blood, mucus or pus.

Tell your healthcare provider if you are breastfeeding.

Diabetes — A false-positive reaction for urine glucose may occur with the nonspecific urine test. Use an enzyme-based test.

Ceftibuten

(seff-TIE-byoo-ten)

Cedax

A cephalosporin antibiotic used in adults and children over 6 months old to treat throat, tonsil, ear and bronchial infections.

Precautions

DO NOT USE if you are allergic to this medicine or any other cephalosporin antibiotics. Tell your healthcare provider if you are allergic to penicillin.

BEFORE USING THIS MEDICINE, tell your healthcare provider if you are pregnant or breastfeeding; or if you are taking, will be taking or stop taking any prescription or nonprescription medicine; or if you have any other medical conditions.

Side Effects

Every medicine can cause side effects, but many people have no, or minor, side effects. Tell your healthcare provider if any of the following occurs: nausea; vomiting; diarrhea; appetite loss; stomach pain or cramps; gas; inflammation of the colon; difficult/painful urination; kidney problems; blood in the urine; bleeding; yellowing of the skin or eyes; allergic reaction; severe skin problems; rash; multiple joint pains; fever; yeast infection.

Guidelines for Use

USE EXACTLY AS PRESCRIBED.

Shake suspension well before using.

The suspension should be taken on an empty stomach at least 2 hours before or 1 hour after a meal.

Tell your healthcare provider if you have experienced allergic reactions to any cephalosporins, penicillins or their relatives.

If a dose is missed, take it as soon as possible. If several hours have passed or if it is nearing time for the next dose, do not double the dose to "catch up," unless advised by your healthcare provider. If more than one dose is missed, contact your healthcare provider.

Continue to use until all of the prescribed medicine has been taken. Failure to take all of the medicine may prevent complete elimination of the becteria, causing the infection to return. Do not stop the therapy without asking your healthcare provider.

Contact your healthcare provider if signs of an allergic reaction occur or if nausea, vomiting or diarrhea occurs; especially if the diarrhea is severe or contains blood, mucus or pus.

Suspension — After mixing, store in a tightly-closed container in the refrigerator for up to 14 days.

Throw away any unused portion after 14 days.

Ceftizoxime Sodium

(SEFF-tih-ZOX-eem SO-dee-uhm)

Cefizox

A cephalosporin antibiotic used to treat a variety of infections.

Side Effects

Every medicine can cause side effects, but many people have no, or minor, side effects. Tell your healthcare provider if any of the following occurs: nausea; vomiting; diarrhea; loss of appetite; taste distortion; inflammation of the tongue; abdominal pain; gas; heartburn; stomach cramps; upset stomach; headache; dizziness; lethargy; fatigue; abnormal skin sensations; excessive sweating; flushing; irritation at the injection site; fever; difficulty breathing; vaginal discharge; mouth sores; loss of sleep; sleepiness; nervousness; insomnia; hyperactivity; confusion.

Patient Information

Tell your healthcare provider if you have experienced allergic reactions to any cephalosporins, penicillins or their relatives.

Tell your healthcare provider of nausea, vomiting or diarrhea, especially if the diarrhea is severe or contains blood, mucus or pus.

Tell your healthcare provider if you are breastfeeding.

Diabetes — A false-positive reaction for urine glucose may occur with the nonspecific urine test. Use an enzyme-based test.

Ceftriaxone Sodium

(SEFF-TRY-AXE-own SO-dee-uhm)

Rocephin

A cephalosporin antibiotic used to treat a variety of infections.

Side Effects

Every medicine can cause side effects, but many people have no, or minor, side effects. Tell your healthcare provider if any of the following occurs: nausea; vomiting; diarrhea; loss of appetite; taste distortion; inflammation of the tongue; abdominal pain; gas; heartburn; stomach cramps; upset stomach; headache; dizziness; lethargy; fatigue; abnormal skin sensations; confusion; excessive sweating; flushing; irritation at the injection site; fever; difficulty breathing; vaginal discharge; mouth sores; loss of sleep; sleepiness; nervousness; insomnia; hyperactivity; confusion.

Patient Information

Tell your healthcare provider if you have experienced allergic reactions to any cephalosporins, penicillins or their relatives.

Tell your healthcare provider of nausea, vomiting or diarrhea, especially if the diarrhea is severe or contains blood, mucus or pus.

Tell your healthcare provider if you are breastfeeding.

Diabetes — A false-positive reaction for urine glucose may occur with the nonspecific urine test. Use an enzyme-based test.

Cefuroxime Injection

(SEFF-yur-OX-eem)

Zinacef

A cephalosporin antibiotic used to treat a variety of infections.

Side Effects

Every medicine can cause side effects, but many people have no, or minor, side effects. Tell your healthcare provider if any of the following occurs: nausea; vomiting; diarrhea; loss of appetite; abdominal pain; gas; heartburn; stomach cramps; upset stomach; headache; dizziness; lethargy; fatigue; abnormal skin sensations; excessive sweating; flushing; irritation at the injection site; fever; difficulty breathing; vaginal discharge; mouth sores; loss of sleep; sleepiness; nervousness; insomnia; hyperactivity; confusion.

Patient Information

Tell your healthcare provider if you have experienced allergic reactions to any cephalosporins, penicillins or their relatives.

Tell your healthcare provider of nausea, vomiting or diarrhea, especially if the diarrhea is severe or contains blood, mucus or pus.

Tell your healthcare provider if you are breastfeeding.

Diabetes — A false-positive reaction for urine glucose may occur with the nonspecific urine test. Use an enzyme-based test.

Cefuroxime Oral

(SEFF-yur-OX-eem)

Ceftin, Kefurox, Zinacef

A cephalosporin antibiotic used to treat infections caused by certain bacteria.

Precautions

DO NOT USE if you are allergic to any cephalosporin or penicillin.

BEFORE USING THIS MEDICINE, tell your healthcare provider if you are pregnant or breastfeeding; or if you are taking, will be taking or stop taking any prescription or nonprescription medicine; or if you have any other medical conditions.

Side Effects

Every medicine can cause side effects, but many people have no, or minor, side effects. Tell your healthcare provider if any of the following occurs: skin rash; hives; itching; joint/muscle pain or swelling; fever; difficulty breathing; fluid retention; numbness; chills; nausea; vomiting; severe diarrhea; or unusual bleeding or bruising.

Guidelines for Use

USE EXACTLY AS PRESCRIBED.

May cause stomach upset; take with food or milk.

Take at evenly spaced intervals throughout the day.

If a dose is missed, take it as soon as possible. If several hours have passed or if it is nearing time for the next dose, do not double the dose to "catch up," unless advised by your healthcare provider. If more than one dose is missed, contact your healthcare provider.

Continue use until all the prescribed medicine has been taken. Failure to take all of all of the medicine may prevent complete elimination of bacteria, causing the infection to return.

Diabetes--May interfere with urine tests for glucose and may give false test results.

Suspension--Shake well before using. Store in the refrigerator; do not freeze. Discard after 14 days.

Cephalexin

(seh-fuh-LEX-in)

Keflet, Keflex, Keftab

A cephalosporin antibiotic used to treat infections caused by certain bacteria.

Precautions

DO NOT USE if you are allergic to any cephalosporin or penicillin.

BEFORE USING THIS MEDICINE, tell your healthcare provider if you are allergic to cephalosporins or penicillins; are pregnant or breastfeeding; or if you are taking, will be taking or stop taking any prescription or nonprescription medicine; or if you have any other medical conditions.

Side Effects

Every medicine can cause side effects, but many people have no, or minor, side effects. Tell your healthcare provider if any of the following occurs: skin rash; hives; itching; joint/muscle pain or swelling; fever; difficulty breathing; fluid retention; numbness; chills; nausea; vomiting; severe diarrhea; or unusual bleeding or bruising.

Guidelines for Use

USE EXACTLY AS PRESCRIBED.

May cause stomach upset; take with food or milk.

Take at even intervals around the clock as prescribed.

If a dose is missed, take it as soon as possible. If several hours have passed or if it is nearing time for the next dose, do not double the dose to catch up, unless advised by your healthcare provider. If more than one dose is missed, contact your healthcare provider.

Continue use until all the prescribed medicine has been taken. Failure to take all of the medicine may prevent complete elimination of bacteria, causing the infection to return.

Diabetes-May interfere with urine tests for glucose and may give false test results.

Cephalothin Sodium

(seff-AY-low-thin SO-dee-uhm)

Keflin

A cephalosporin antibiotic used to treat a variety of infections.

Side Effects

Every medicine can cause side effects, but many people have no, or minor, side effects. Tell your healthcare provider if any of the following occurs: nausea; vomiting; diarrhea; loss of appetite; taste distortion; inflammation of the tongue; abdominal pain; gas; heartburn; stomach cramps; upset stomach; headache; dizziness; lethargy; fatigue; abnormal skin sensations; excessive sweating; flushing; irritation at the injection site; fever; difficulty breathing; vaginal discharge; mouth sores; loss of sleep; sleepiness; nervousness; insomnia; hyperactivity; confusion.

Patient Information

Tell your healthcare provider if you have experienced allergic reactions to any cephalosporins, penicillins or their relatives.

Tell your healthcare provider of nausea, vomiting or diarrhea, especially if the diarrhea is severe or contains blood, mucus or pus.

Tell your healthcare provider if you are breastfeeding.

A false-positive reaction for urine glucose may occur with the nonspecific urine test. Use an enzyme-based test.

Cephapirin Sodium

(SEFF-uh-PIE-rin SO-dee-uhm)

Cefadyl

A cephalosporin antibiotic used to treat a variety of infections.

Side Effects

Every medicine can cause side effects, but many people have no, or minor, side effects. Tell your healthcare provider if any of the following occurs: nausea; vomiting; diarrhea; loss of appetite; taste distortion; inflammation of the tongue; abdominal pain; gas; heartburn; stomach cramps; upset stomach; headache; dizziness; lethargy; fatigue; abnormal skin sensations; excessive sweating; flushing; irritation at the injection site; fever; difficulty breathing; vaginal discharge; mouth sores; loss of sleep; sleepiness; nervousness; insomnia; hyperactivity; confusion.

Patient Information

Tell your healthcare provider if you have experienced allergic reactions to any cephalosporins, penicillins or their relatives.

Tell your healthcare provider of nausea, vomiting or diarrhea, especially if the diarrhea is severe or contains blood, mucus or pus.

Tell your healthcare provider if you are breastfeeding.

A false-positive reaction for urine glucose may occur with the nonspecific urine test. Use an enzyme-based test.

Cephradine

(SEFF-ruh-deen)

Velosef

A cephalosporin antibiotic used to treat infections caused by certain bacteria.

Precautions

DO NOT USE if you are allergic to any cephalosporin or penicillin.

BEFORE USING THIS MEDICINE, tell your healthcare provider if you are pregnant or breastfeeding; or if you are taking, will be taking or stop taking any prescription or nonprescription medicine; or if you have any other medical conditions.

Side Effects

Every medicine can cause side effects, but many people have no, or minor, side effects. Tell your healthcare provider if any of the following occurs: skin rash; hives; itching; joint/muscle pain or swelling; fever; difficulty breathing; fluid retention; numbness; chills; nausea; vomiting; severe diarrhea; or unusual bleeding or bruising.

Guidelines for Use

USE EXACTLY AS PRESCRIBED.

May cause stomach upset; take with food or milk.

Take at even intervals around the clock as prescribed.

If a dose is missed, take it as soon as possible. If several hours have passed or if it is nearing time for the next dose, do not double the dose to catch up, unless advised by your healthcare provider. If more than one dose is missed, contact your healthcare provider.

Continue use until all the prescribed medicine has been taken. Failure to take all of the medicine may prevent complete elimination of bacteria, causing the infection to return.

Diabetes-May interfere with urine tests for glucose and may give false test results.

Suspension-Shake well before using. Store in the refrigerator. Do not freeze. Discard after 14 days.

Charcoal, Activated

(CHAR-kole)

Actidose-Aqua, Actidose with Sorbitol, Charcoaid, Liqui-Char, SuperChar

Used to treat poisoning and medicine overdoses caused by swallowing.

Precautions

DO NOT USE if there is an overdose of cyanide, mineral acids, iron, alcohol and alkalies. DO NOT give to a semiconscious or unconscious patient.

Side Effects

Every medicine can cause side effects, but many people have no, or minor, side effects. Tell your healthcare provider if any of the following occurs: constipation; diarrhea; black stools; vomiting.

Guidelines for Use

USE EXACTLY AS PRESCRIBED.

Contact your healthcare provider or poison control center for all poisoning or suspected poisoning.

Give only to conscious (alert) persons.

If ipecac syrup also is given, give the ipecac first; give activated charcoal after vomiting occurs.

Do not mix charcoal with milk, ice cream or sherbet since they will decrease the effectiveness of the activated charcoal.

Keep in closed container.

Chloral Hydrate

(KLOR-uhl HIGH-drate)

Aquachloral Supprettes

This medicine causes drowsiness to aid in falling asleep. It generally is used to treat insomnia for a short period of time (1 to 2 weeks).

Precautions

DO NOT USE if you are allergic to this medicine.

BEFORE USING THIS MEDICINE, tell your healthcare provider if you are pregnant or breastfeeding; or if you are taking, will be taking or stop taking any prescription or nonprescription medicine; if you have any other medical conditions; or if you are allergic to tartrazine.

Side Effects

Every medicine can cause side effects, but many people have no, or minor, side effects. Tell your healthcare provider if any of the following occurs: stomach upset; diarrhea; vomiting; constipation; confusion; excitement; nightmares; drowsiness; dizziness; headache; incoordination; decreased mobility; incoherence; rash; hives; redness; unpleasant taste in mouth; sleepwalking.

Guidelines for Use

USE EXACTLY AS PRESCRIBED.

May cause drowsiness or dizziness. Use caution while driving or performing other tasks requiring mental alertness.

Dilute syrup in a half glass of water, ginger ale or fruit juice.

Avoid alcohol and other medicines that cause drowsiness (eg, pain relievers, sedatives, antihistamines).

May be habit-forming.

Do not discontinue this medicine abruptly, especially if you have a history of seizures. Withdrawal symptoms may occur when the medicine is stopped.

Contact your healthcare provider if visual changes, irregular heartbeats, chest pains, yellowing of skin or eyes, rash or unusual bleeding or bruising occurs.

Chlorambucil

(klor-AM-byoo-sill)

Leukeran

A medicine used to treat lymphomas, leukemia and Hodgkin's disease. It may occasionally be prescribed for other reasons.

Precautions

DO NOT USE if you are allergic to this medicine or to any other nitrogen mustard medicine or if you are breastfeeding. Not recommended for use in children.

BEFORE USING THIS MEDICINE, tell your healthcare provider if you are pregnant or breastfeeding; if you are taking, will be taking or stop taking any prescription or nonprescription medicine; or if you have any other medical condition.

Side Effects

Every medicine can cause side effects, but many people have no, or minor, side effects. Tell your healthcare provider if any of the following occurs: unusual skin sensitivity; hair loss; discoloration (eg, yellowing of skin); rash; nausea; vomiting; diarrhea; mouth sores; cessation of menstruation; tremors; confusion; agitation; incoordination; fever; breathing problems; abnormal sensations.

Guidelines for Use

USE EXACTLY AS PRESCRIBED.

Notify your healthcare provider of unusual bleeding or bruising, black tarry stools, nausea, vomiting, weight loss, fever, chills, sore throat, cough, shortness of breath, seizures, lack of menstrual flow, unusual lumps or masses, flank or stomach pain, joint pain, sores in mouth or on the lips, yellow discoloration of the skin or eyes or skin rash.

Contraceptive (birth control) measures are recommended during therapy for both men and women.

If a dose is missed, take it as soon as possible. If several hours have passed or if it is nearing time for the next dose, do not double the dose to catch up, unless advised by your healthcare provider. If more than one dose is missed, contact your healthcare provider.

Be careful to avoid injury, use a soft toothbrush and avoid medication that contains aspirin.

While taking this medicine, blood studies will be necessary every 1 to 2 weeks. Be sure to keep appointments.

This medicine may impair your body's ability to fight infection. Notify your healthcare provider if any signs of infection occur, including fever, sore throat, rashes or chills.

Chloramphenicol Oral

(KLOR-am-FEN-ih-kahl)

Chloromycetin

A medicine used to treat a variety of infections, acute infections of typhoid fever, and to treat infections in cystic fibrosis patients. It is intended only when less dangerous medicines have been ineffective or not recommended.

Precautions

DO NOT USE if you are allergic to this medicine.

BEFORE USING THIS MEDICINE, tell your healthcare provider if you are pregnant or breastfeeding; or if you are taking, will be taking or stop taking any prescription or nonprescription medicine; or if you have any other medical conditions.

Side Effects

Every medicine can cause side effects, but many people have no, or minor, side effects. Tell your healthcare provider if any of the following occurs: irritation; burning; stinging; itching; eye lid swelling or redness; secondary infection; blood abnormalities; headache; confusion; depression; diarrhea; nausea; vomiting; fever; rash; sore throat; hives; unusual bleeding or bruising; fatigue; changes in vision; difficulty breathing.

Guidelines for Use

USE EXACTLY AS PRESCRIBED.

Take on an empty stomach 1 hour before or 2 hours after a meal. Take with food if stomach upset occurs.

If a dose is missed, take it as soon as possible. If several hours have passed or if it is nearing time for the next dose, do not double the dose to "catch up," unless advised to do so by your healthcare provider. If more than one dose is missed, contact your healthcare provider.

Usually taken every 6 hours around the clock.

Continue to use until all of the prescribed medicine is used. Failure to take all of the medicine may prevent complete elimination of bacteria, causing the infection to return.

Report any of the following symptoms to your healthcare provider: bleeding, fever, sore throat, itching, nausea, vomiting, diarrhea, bruising, vision problems, numbness or weakness of hands or feet.

This drug is not to be used to treat minor infections (eg, colds, flu). Never try to self-treat infections or self-prescribe antibiotics.

Store below 86° F. Protect from moisture.

Chloramphenicol Otic

(KLOR-am-FEN-ih-kahl)

Chloromycetin Otic

A medicine used to treat certain bacterial infections of the outer ear.

Precautions

DO NOT USE if you are allergic to this medicine.

BEFORE USING THIS MEDICINE, tell your healthcare provider if you are pregnant or breastfeeding; or if you are taking, will be taking or stop taking any prescription or nonprescription medicine; or if you have any other medical conditions.

Side Effects

Every medicine can cause side effects, but many people have no, or minor, side effects. Tell your healthcare provider if any of the following occurs: local irritation; itching; burning; redness; and rash.

Guidelines for Use

USE EXACTLY AS PRESCRIBED.

If burning or itching occurs or persists after use, contact your healthcare provider.

To properly administer ear drops, the following steps should be taken: Avoid touching the dropper to the ear. Hold the container in the hand for a few minutes to warm it if it has been refrigerated. Lie on your side or tilit the affected ear up to administer the medicine. Administer the prescribed number of drops. Keep the ear tilted for about 2 minutes. To assist the drops in running into the external ear canal, hold the earlobe up and back in adults and down and back in children.

Chloramphenicol Ophthalmic

(KLOR-ăm-FEN-ih-kahl)

AK Chlor, Chloroptic, Chloroptic SOP

Precautions

DO NOT USE if you are allergic to this medicine.

BEFORE USING THIS MEDICINE, tell your healthcare provider if you are pregnant or breastfeeding; or if you are taking, will be taking or stop taking any prescription or nonprescription medicine; or if you have any other medical conditions.

Side Effects

Every medicine can cause side effects, but many people have no, or minor, side effects. Tell your healthcare provider if any of the following occurs: burning; stinging; itching; irritation; redness; dryness; widening of the pupils; watering of the eyes; blurred vision; headache; allergic reactions (itching, rash, hives, fever, chills).

Guidelines for Use

USE EXACTLY AS PRESCRIBED.

May cause temporary blurring of vision or stinging following administration.

Avoid contact between the dispensing container and the eye.

Contact your doctor if stinging, burning or itching becomes pronounced or if redness, irritation, swelling, decreasing vision or pain persists or worsens.

Avoid contact between the dispensing container and the eye.

Chloramphenicol Topical

(KLOR-am-FEN-ih-kahl)

A topical medicine used to treat susceptible bacteria and to prevent infections after minor skin lacerations or abrasions.

Precautions

DO NOT USE if you are allergic to this medicine.

BEFORE USING THIS MEDICINE, tell your healthcare provider if you are pregnant or breastfeeding; or if you are taking, will be taking or stop taking any prescription or nonprescription medicine; or if you have any other medical conditions.

Side Effects

Every medicine can cause side effects, but many people have no, or minor, side effects. Tell your healthcare provider if any of the following occurs: rash; itching; burning; redness; swelling.

Guidelines for Use

USE EXACTLY AS PRESCRIBED.

Apply a small amount of the medicine in a thin layer on the affected area 1 to 5 times daily. Cover the area with a loose gauze if desired.

Clean the affected area prior to applying the medicine.

Deeper skin infections may require oral or injectable antibiotic therapy in addition to the topical medicine.

Do not use in or near the eyes.

If rash or irritation develops or worsens where the antibiotic is applied, contact your healthcare provider.

Chlordiazepoxide

(klor-DIE-aze-ee-POX-ide)

Libritabs, *Librium*, *Mitran*, *Reposans-10*

A benzodiazepine medicine generally used to treat anxiety. It may occasionally be prescribed for other reasons.

Precautions

DO NOT USE if you are allergic to this medicine or its relatives or are breastfeeding.

BEFORE USING THIS MEDICINE, tell your healthcare provider if you are pregnant, or if you are taking, will be taking or stop taking any prescription or nonprescription medicine; or if you have any other medical conditions.

Side Effects

Every medicine can cause side effects, but many people have no, or minor, side effects. Tell your healthcare provider if any of the following occurs: stomach upset; constipation; diarrhea; change in appetite; vomiting; confusion; depression; nervousness; memory loss; drowsiness; fatigue; dizziness; crying; disorientation; dreams; headache; changes in heart rate; pounding in the chest; itching; rash; hair growth; yellowing of skin or eyes; visual/hearing disturbances; slurred speech; loss of bladder function; change in sex drive; urine retention; menstrual problems; dry mouth; fever; difficult breathing; swelling; excessive sweating; joint pain; weight gain or loss; dehydration; fainting.

Guidelines for Use

USE EXACTLY AS PRESCRIBED.

May be taken with food or water if stomach upset occurs.

If a dose is missed, take it as soon as possible. If several hours have passed or if it is nearing time for the next dose, do not double the dose to catch up, unless advised by your healthcare provider. If more than one dose is missed, contact your healthcare provider.

This medication can be addictive if used in large doses or for a long time. Discuss overuse with your healthcare provider.

May cause drowsiness. Use caution while driving or performing other tasks requiring mental alertness, coordination and dexterity. Avoid alcohol and other medications that cause drowsiness while taking this medication.

Excitement, stimulation and acute rage have been reported. If these symptoms occur, tell your healthcare provider.

Patients on long-term or high-dosage therapy may have withdrawal symptoms if therapy is suddenly stopped. Do not stop therapy abruptly or change dosage without asking your healthcare provider.

Chlordiazepoxide/Amitriptyline

(klor-DIE-aze-ee-POX-ide/am-ee-TRIP-tih-leen)

Limbitrol DS 10–25

A combination medicine used to treat moderate to severe depression associated with moderate to severe anxiety.

Precautions

DO NOT USE if you are allergic to benzodiazepines or tricyclic antidepressants or while you are using a monoamine oxidase inhibitor (MAOI).

BEFORE USING THIS MEDICINE, tell your healthcare provider if you are pregnant or breastfeeding; if you are taking, will be taking or stop taking any prescription or nonprescription medicine; or if you have any other medical conditions.

Side Effects

Every medicine can cause side effects, but many people have no, or minor, side effects. Tell your healthcare provider if any of the following occurs: indigestion; constipation; diarrhea; nausea; gas; change in appetite; vomiting; confusion; anxiety; disturbed concentration; depression; behavior changes; memory loss; drowsiness; fatigue; dizziness; feeling of whirling motion; exaggerated sense of well-being; restlessness; hallucinations; speech problems; disorientation; sleep disturbances; incoordination; vivid or abnormal dreams; headache; weakness; unsteadiness; hives; itching; rash; visual disturbances; speech problems; hearing disturbances; nasal congestion; nosebleeds; slurred speech; loss of voice; yawning; incontinence; changes in sex drive; sexual dysfunction in males; urine retention; menstrual problems; dry mouth; difficulty swallowing; hiccups; fever; sore throat; cough; ankle and facial swelling; breast enlargement; breast pain; swelling of the testicles; fluid retention; excessive perspiration; joint pain; weight changes; fainting; sensitivity to light.

Guidelines for Use

USE EXACTLY AS PRESCRIBED.

May be taken with food or water if stomach upset occurs.

If a dose is missed, take it as soon as possible. If several hours have passed or if it is nearing time for the next dose, do not double the dose to catch up, unless advised by your healthcare provider. If more than one dose is missed, contact your healthcare provider.

Avoid alcohol and medicines that cause drowsiness (eg, pain relievers, sedatives, barbiturates).

This medicine may cause drowsiness or blurred vision. Use caution while driving or performing other tasks requiring mental alertness, coordination and dexterity.

Notify your healthcare provider if dry mouth, blurred vision, increased heart rate, impaired coordination, difficult urination, excessive sedation or seizures occur.

May cause sensitivity to sunlight. Avoid prolonged exposure to the sun. Use sunscreen and wear protective clothing until tolerance is determined.

This medicine may be addictive if used in large doses or for a long time. Do not exceed prescribed dose. Discuss overuse with your healthcare provider.

Patients on long-term or high dosage therapy may experience withdrawal symptoms on abrupt cessation of therapy. Do not discontinue therapy abruptly or change dosage except on advice of your healthcare provider.

Store at room temperature.

Chlorhexidine Gluconate

(klor-HEX-ih-deen GLUE-koe-nate)

Dyna-Hex, Exidine, Hibiclens, Hibistat, Peridex

An oral rinse that kills bacteria in the mouth and treats inflammation of the gums; skin/wound cleanser.

Precautions

DO NOT USE if you are allergic to this medicine.

BEFORE USING THIS MEDICINE, tell your healthcare provider if you are pregnant or breastfeeding; or if you are taking, will be taking or stop taking any prescription or nonprescription medicine; or if you have any other medical conditions.

Side Effects

Every medicine can cause side effects, but many people have no, or minor, side effects. Tell your healthcare provider if any of the following occurs: staining of teeth, dental work and the tongue; increase in plaque formation; altered taste perception; minor peeling of the oral mucosa (especially in children); inflammation of salivary glands; stomach upset or nausea (if swallowed).

Guidelines for Use

USE EXACTLY AS PRESCRIBED.

Begin therapy after a thorough cleaning of teeth by a dentist or dental hygienist. Dental checkups every 6 months are necessary.

Use twice daily as an oral rinse for 30 seconds, morning and evening, after brushing the teeth.

Staining of the teeth may occur. Stain can be removed by usual professional techniques.

Taste changes may occur during use.

Do not swallow the medicine. Expectorate (spit out) after rinsing.

Chloroquine

(KLOR-oh-kwin)

Aralen

A medicine used to prevent and treat acute attacks of malaria caused by certain strains of parasites. It may occasionally be prescribed for other reasons.

Precautions

DO NOT USE if you are allergic to this medicine or have visual changes.

BEFORE USING THIS MEDICINE, tell your healthcare provider if you are pregnant or breastfeeding; or if you are using, will be using or stop using any prescription or nonprescription medicine; or if you have any other medical conditions.

Side Effects

Every medicine can cause side effects, but many people have no, or minor, side effects. Tell your healthcare provider if any of the following occurs: visual disturbances; blurred vision; difficulty focusing; foggy vision; night blindness; nausea; vomiting; diarrhea; stomach upset or cramps; appetite loss; rash; itching; pigment changes; ringing in the ears; hearing loss; headache; muscle weakness; abnormal sensations; mental changes; faintness; seizures (rare).

Guidelines for Use

USE EXACTLY AS PRESCRIBED.

May cause stomach upset. Take with food.

Dose and length of therapy depend on the patient's age and situation being treated. Take the medicine specifically as prescribed for the full course of therapy.

Report any change in vision, ringing in the ears or hearing impairment to your healthcare provider immediately.

Overdosage can be especially severe and is extremely dangerous in children. Keep this medicine in a child-proof container and out of the reach of children.

May cause rash, nausea, vomiting, stomach pain, diarrhea, appetite loss or muscle weakness. Notify your healthcare provider if these persist or become bothersome.

Irreversible damage to the retina of the eye, usually with long-term, high-dose use, has been reported. When long-term use is expected, eye exams should occur every 3 to 6 months. Notify your healthcare provider immediately if there is any blurring or change in vision. Retinal changes and visual disturbances may continue even after stopping therapy.

Deafness may occur with long-term use.

Drinking alcohol may increase the risk of upset stomach or liver damage.

Occasionally, certain strains of malaria will become resistant to this medicine. Discuss your travel plans carefully with your healthcare provider.

Chlorotrianisene

(klor-oh-try-AN-ih-seen)

Tace

A hormone used to treat or prevent a variety of conditions due to menopause (hot flashes, vaginal tissue breakdown), to treat breast engorgement immediately after childbirth, for estrogen replacement therapy, to treat advanced cancer of the prostate gland in men and to relieve the symptoms of breast cancer in selected men and women, or those with metastatic disease. It may occasionally be prescribed for other reasons.

Precautions

DO NOT USE if you are allergic to this medicine or are pregnant.

BEFORE USING THIS MEDICINE, tell your healthcare provider if you are breastfeeding; or if you are taking, will be taking or stop taking any prescription or nonprescription medicine; or if you have any other medical conditions.

Side Effects

Every medicine can cause side effects, but many people have no, or minor, side effects. Tell your healthcare provider if any of the following occurs: change in menstrual flow; vaginal bleeding at abnormal times; vaginal infection; unusual vaginal secretions; painful menstruation; nausea; vomiting; stomach cramps; bloating; diarrhea; headache; migraine; dizziness; fainting; depression; weakness; seizures; unusual body movements; loss of scalp hair; excessive hair growth; oversensitivity to sunlight or tanning lamps; itching; rash; hives; skin discoloration including yellowing of the skin; intolerance to contact lenses; weight gain or loss; breast tenderness and enlargement; breast milk secretion; pain in groin or calves; chest pain; shortness of breath; vision problems; abnormal blood glucose; fluid retention; high blood pressure; change in sex drive.

Guidelines for Use

USE EXACTLY AS PRESCRIBED.

If a dose is missed, take it as soon as possible. If several hours have passed or if it is nearing time for the next dose, do not double the dose to catch up, unless advised by your doctor. If more than one dose is missed, contact your healthcare provider.

Diabetes — This drug may cause abnormal blood glucose.

May cause sensitivity to sunlight. Avoid prolonged exposure to the sun. Use sunscreens and wear protective clothing until tolerance is determined.

Chlorpheniramine Maleate Oral

(klor-fen-AIR-uh-meen MAL-ee-ate)

Aller-Chlor, Clo-Amine, Chlor-Trimeton, Chlorate, Chlorspan-12, Chlortab-4, Chlortab-8, Pfeiffer's Allergy, Phenetron, Telachlor, Teldrin, Chlor-Tripolon, Chlor-Tripolon Repetabs

A medicine used to relieve symptoms associated with seasonal and year-round allergic runny nose; allergic conjunctivitis (watering, itching eyes); hives (mild and uncomplicated); and rash, insect bites and stings where there is mild to moderate itching and no complications.

Precautions

DO NOT USE if you are allergic to this medicine or if you are using a monoamine oxidase inhibitor.

BEFORE USING THIS MEDICINE, tell your healthcare provider if you are pregnant or breastfeeding; or if you are taking, will be taking or stop taking any prescription or nonprescription medicine; or if you have any other medical conditions.

Side Effects

Every medicine can cause side effects, but many people have no, or minor, side effects. Tell your healthcare provider if any of the following occurs: stomach ache; constipation; appetite changes; nausea; vomiting; diarrhea; drowsiness; dizziness; mental confusion; decreased coordination; fatigue; headache; sleeplessness; sleepiness; pounding in the chest; dry nose, throat and mouth; thickening of mucus in the respiratory tract; wheezing; nasal stuffiness; sensitivity to light; difficult urination; urine retention; sore throat; ringing in the ears; blurred and double vision; rash; hives; excessive perspiration; chills.

Guidelines for Use

USE EXACTLY AS PRESCRIBED.

May cause stomach upset; take with food.

May cause drowsiness or dizziness. Use caution while driving or performing tasks requiring mental alertness, coordination and dexterity.

Avoid alcohol and medicines that cause drowsiness.

May cause dry mouth.

Use alone when sneezing and runny nose exist, but nasal congestion is slight.

When nasal congestion accompanies sneezing and runny nose, an oral decongestant may be added.

Elderly patients are more likely to experience dizziness, sedation, decreased coordination, mental confusion and fainting when they take antihistamines.

May produce unexpected excitation, restlessness, irritability and insomnia in rare instances. This is most likely to occur in children and elderly patients.

Do not take for several days before allergy skin testing.

Chlorpromazine Hydrochloride

(klor-PRO-muh-zeen HIGH-droe-KLOR-ide)

Ormazine, Thorazine

A medicine used to control nausea and vomiting. It also is used to improve concentration and self-control in patients with psychotic behavior. It may occasionally be prescribed for other purposes.

Precautions

DO NOT USE if you are allergic to this medicine or its relatives. Laboratory tests may be needed.

BEFORE USING THIS MEDICINE, tell your healthcare provider if you are pregnant or breastfeeding; or if you are taking, will be taking or stop taking any prescription or nonprescription medicine; if you have any other medical conditions; or if you are allergic to tartrazine.

Side Effects

Every medicine can cause side effects, but many people have no, or minor, side effects. Tell your healthcare provider if any of the following occurs: tremors; drooling; shuffling gait; restlessness; muscle spasms; aching or numbness; sore throat; fever; unusual bleeding or bruising; skin rash; weakness; impaired vision; dark-colored urine; pale stools; yellowing of skin or eyes; drowsiness.

Guidelines for Use

USE EXACTLY AS PRESCRIBED.

Take this medicine routinely as directed; it controls illness symptoms and is not habit-forming.

If a dose is missed, take it as soon as possible. If several hours have passed or if it is nearing time for the next dose, do not double the dose to catch up, unless advised by your healthcare provider. If more than one dose is missed, contact your healthcare provider.

Improvement may not be seen for several weeks.

May cause drowsiness. Use caution while driving or performing other tasks requiring mental alertness. Avoid alcohol and medicines that cause drowsiness.

May cause sunlight sensitivity. Avoid long exposure to the sun. Use sunscreens and protective clothing until tolerance is known.

If dizziness or fainting occurs (more common during first week of therapy), avoid sudden changes in posture.

This medicine may increase risk of heat-stroke.

Capsule-Do not crush or chew. Swallow whole.

Suppository-Remove the foil wrapper. Avoid excessive handling of the suppository; it melts at body temperature. Insert completely into the rectum with gentle pressure, pointed end first.

Liquid Concentrate-May be added to 2 ounces of liquid such as tomato or fruit juice, simple or orange syrup, carbonated beverages, coffee, tea or water. Also may be put into some foods such as soup or pudding. Slight yellowing of solution is acceptable. Discard if significant discoloration occurs.

Lab tests may be needed. Be sure to keep appointments.

Chlorpropamide

(klor-PRO-puh-mide)

Diabinese

An oral antidiabetic medicine that lowers blood sugar. It is used only in patients with non-insulin-dependent diabetes mellitus (Type II) who cannot manage blood sugar levels by diet and exercise alone.

Precautions

DO NOT USE if you have an allergy to this medicine or sulfa drugs.

BEFORE USING THIS MEDICINE, tell your healthcare provider if you are pregnant or breastfeeding; or if you are taking, will be taking or stop taking any prescription or nonprescription medicine; or if you have any other medical conditions.

Side Effects

Every medicine can cause side effects, but many people have no, or minor, side effects. Tell your healthcare provider if any of the following occurs: nausea; vomiting; heartburn; diarrhea; fever; sore throat; rash; itching; weakness; unusual bruising or bleeding.

Guidelines for Use

USE EXACTLY AS PRESCRIBED.

Take 30 minutes before a meal. Take with food if nausea or stomach upset occurs.

Avoid alcohol, which can cause flushing, weakness, dizziness, a tingling sensation and headache.

Monitor blood sugar levels daily. Notify your healthcare provider if low blood sugar develops (eg, fatigue, nausea, confusion, agitation, excessive hunger, profuse sweating, numbness or tingling of lips, tongue or extremities) or if excessive thirst or urination, or other symptoms of high blood sugar levels occur (glucose or ketones in the urine or blood).

Proper diet and exercise are important.

To prevent low blood sugar: 1. Know the symptoms of low blood sugar. 2. Keep track of your blood sugar levels. 3. Keep a source of quick-acting sugar with you at all times. 4. Maintain an adequate diet. 5. Know how diet and exercise affect your blood sugar level. Acute illness (eg, physical trauma, infection, fever, surgery) may require the temporary administration of insulin.

Chlorthalidone

(klor-THAL-ih-dohn)

Hygroton, Thalitone

A diuretic (water pill) that decreases excess water in the body and increases urine flow. This medicine is used to treat high blood pressure and edema (excess fluid) due to a variety of causes.

Precautions

DO NOT USE if you are allergic to this medicine or its relatives; oral diabetic medicines; sulfa antibiotics; or if you have severe kidney disease or loss of kidney function.

BEFORE USING THIS MEDICINE, tell your healthcare provider if you are pregnant or breastfeeding; or if you are taking, will be taking or stop taking any prescription or nonprescription medicine; or if you have any other medical conditions.

Side Effects

Every medicine can cause side effects, but many people have no, or minor, side effects. Tell your healthcare provider if any of the following occurs: thirst; irregular heartbeat; confusion; mood changes; nausea; vomiting; unusual tiredness; weakness; weak pulse; muscle cramps; appetite loss; stomach upset; bloating; diarrhea; constipation; dizziness; lightheadedness; headache; tingling of toes and fingers; blurred vision; nervousness; insomnia; chest pain; sun sensitivity; rash; hives; itching; dry skin; yellowing of skin or eyes; unusual bruising; difficulty breathing; blood sugar imbalance; muscle cramps; joint pain; fever; chills; weight loss; nose bleeds; gout attack.

Guidelines for Use

USE EXACTLY AS PRESCRIBED.

Increases urination; to avoid disruption of sleep at night, take early in the day usually as a single dose.

May cause stomach upset. May be taken with food or milk.

May cause loss of potassium. If signs of potassium loss occur (eg, weakness, cramps, nausea, dizziness), contact your healthcare provider. Ask about foods high in potassium.

Diabetes — May increase blood sugar levels.

Dizziness or lightheadedness may occur if you stand up too fast from lying or sitting. Get up slowly, and notify your healthcare provider.

Sensitivity to sunlight may occur. Use sunscreen and wear protective clothing until tolerance is determined.

Your healthcare provider may want to periodically check your blood to ensure that your medicine is working properly.

This information is advisory only; it does not contain all information about this medicine. If you have any questions about your medicine, ask your healthcare provider.

Chlorzoxazone

(klor-ZOX-uh-zone)

Paraflex, Parafon Forte DSC Tablets, Remular-S

A medicine used to relieve muscle discomfort due to strain and sprain.

Precautions

DO NOT USE if you are allergic to this medicine or its relatives or if you are breastfeeding.

BEFORE USING THIS MEDICINE, tell your healthcare provider if you are pregnant or breastfeeding; or if you are taking, will be taking or stop taking any prescription or nonprescription medicine; or if you have any other medical conditions.

Side Effects

Every medicine can cause side effects, but many people have no, or minor, side effects. Tell your healthcare provider if any of the following occurs: stomach upset; vomiting; drowsiness; fatigue; dizziness; itching; rash; yellowing of skin or eyes; lightheadedness; difficulty breathing.

Guidelines for Use

USE EXACTLY AS PRESCRIBED.

May be taken with food or water if stomach upset occurs.

If a dose is missed, take it as soon as possible. If several hours have passed or if it is nearing time for the next dose, do not double the dose to catch up unless advised by your healthcare provider. If more than one dose is missed, contact your healthcare provider.

May cause drowsiness or dizziness. Use caution while driving or performing other tasks requiring mental alertness, coordination and dexterity. Avoid alcohol and other medication that cause drowsiness while taking this medication (eg, sleeping pills, tranquilizers, antihistamines).

Patients on long-term or high-dosage therapy may have withdrawal symptoms if therapy is suddenly stopped. Do not stop therapy abruptly or change dosage without asking your healthcare provider.

May discolor the urine orange or purple-red.

Cholestyramine

(koe-less-TIE-ruh-meen)

Questran, Questran Light

A medicine used to lower the level of cholesterol in the blood and to relieve itching associated with partial biliary obstruction. It may occasionally be prescribed for other reasons.

Precautions

DO NOT USE if you are allergic to this medicine.

BEFORE USING THIS MEDICINE, tell your healthcare provider if you are pregnant or breastfeeding; constipated; or if you are taking, will be taking or stop taking any prescription or nonprescription medicines; or have any other medical conditions.

Side Effects

Every medicine can cause side effects, but many people have no, or minor, side effects. Tell your healthcare provider if any of the following occurs: unusual bleeding; constipation; gas; nausea; heartburn.

Guidelines for Use

USE EXACTLY AS PRESCRIBED.

Take before meals.

Mix with liquid (water or noncarbonated drinks), very liquid soups or cereals, or with pulpy fruits (applesauce or crushed pineapple). Do not take the dry powder. Mix the contents of one powder packet or one level scoopful with 2 to 6 fl oz water or noncarbonated beverage.

May interfere with the effects of other medicines if taken at the same time. Generally take other medicines either 1 hour before or 4 to 6 hours after this medicine.

Most effective when used with a diet that decreases the intake of cholesterol and saturated fats.

Cimetidine

(sigh-MET-ih-deen)

Tagamet, Tagamet HB

An anti-ulcer medicine used to treat stomach and duodenal (upper small intestine) ulcers; hypersecretory (increased acid secretion) conditions (eg, Zollinger-Ellison syndrome); heartburn and gastroesophageal reflux disease (GERD), or the bubbling of stomach contents into the food pipe, which causes heartburn. It may occasionally be prescribed for other reasons.

Precautions

DO NOT USE if you are allergic to this medicine, nizatidine, ranitidine or famotidine.

BEFORE USING THIS MEDICINE, tell your healthcare provider if you are pregnant or breastfeeding; or if you are taking, will be taking or stop taking any prescription or nonprescription medicine; or if you have any other medical conditions.

Side Effects

Every medicine can cause side effects, but many people have no, or minor, side effects. Tell your healthcare provider if any of the following occurs: headache; nausea; diarrhea; dizziness; joint pain; behavioral changes; rash; itching; unusual bleeding or bruising; sore throat; difficult breathing; shortness of breath; fever; sleep disturbances; sexual difficulties; drowsiness; breast lumps (males and females).

Guidelines for Use

USE EXACTLY AS PRESCRIBED.

Take without regard to meals. Take with plenty of fluids.

Over—the—counter (non-prescription) tablets—Do not take this medicine on a daily basis for longer than 2 weeks unless instructed to do so by your healthcare provider.

Do not take directly with antacids; separate doses by at least an hour.

If a dose is missed, take it as soon as possible. If several hours have passed or if it is nearing time for the next dose, do not double the dose to catch up, unless advised by your healthcare provider. If more than one dose is missed, contact your healthcare provider.

It may be necessary to make significant lifestyle changes to assist in the treatment and prevention of ulcers and other digestive problems that can include stress-reduction programs, exercise and dietary changes.

Notify your healthcare provider if there are any symptoms that suggest a bleeding ulcer, such as black, tarry stools or coffee-ground vomit.

Never self-diagnose or self-treat ulcers with this or any other medicine.

Ciprofloxacin Ophthalmic

(sip-ROW-FLOX-uh-sin)

Ciloxan

A medicine that is used to treat superficial eye infections caused by susceptible bacteria.

Precautions

DO NOT USE if you are allergic to this medicine or its relatives.

BEFORE USING THIS MEDICINE, tell your healthcare provider if you are pregnant or breastfeeding; or if you are taking, will be taking or stop taking any prescription or nonprescription medicine; or if you have any other medical conditions.

Side Effects

Every medicine can cause side effects, but many people have no, or minor, side effects. Tell your healthcare provider if any of the following occurs: irritation; burning; stinging; itching; lid swelling; redness; lid crusting; crystals/scales; bad taste in mouth; secondary infection.

Guidelines for Use

USE EXACTLY AS PRESCRIBED.

May cause temporary blurring of vision or stinging following administration.

Contact your healthcare provider if stinging, burning or itching becomes pronounced or if redness, irritation, swelling, decreasing vision or pain persists or worsens.

Avoid contact between the dispensing container and the eye or any other surface.

Discontinue if skin rash or other sign of allergic reaction occurs.

Protect from light.

Ciprofloxacin Systemic

(sip-ROW-FLOX-uh-sin)

Cipro, Cipro IV

A quinolone antibiotic medicine used to treat infections caused by certain bacteria.

Precautions

DO NOT USE if you are allergic to this medicine or any of its relatives.

BEFORE USING THIS MEDICINE, tell your healthcare provider if you are pregnant or breastfeeding; or if you are taking, will be taking or stop taking any prescription or nonprescription medicine; or if you have any other medical conditions.

Side Effects

Every medicine can cause side effects, but many people have no, or minor, side effects. Tell your healthcare provider if any of the following occurs: severe nausea; diarrhea; rash; hives; itching; difficult breathing; wheezing; dizziness; headache.

Guidelines for Use

USE EXACTLY AS PRESCRIBED.

May be taken without regard to meals, but preferably 2 hours after a meal.

Drink plenty of liquids.

Do not take antacids, sucralfate (*Carafate*), or iron or zinc-containing products within 4 hours before or 2 hours after using this medicine.

If a dose is missed, take it as soon as possible. If several hours have passed or if it is nearing time for the next dose, do not double the dose to catch up, unless advised by your healthcare provider. If more than one dose is missed, contact your healthcare provider.

Continue use until all the prescribed medicine has been taken. Failure to take all of the medicine may prevent complete elimination of bacteria, causing the infection to return. Do not stop therapy without asking your healthcare provider.

May cause dizziness or lightheadedness. Use caution when driving or performing other tasks requiring mental alertness.

May cause sensitivity to sunlight. Avoid prolonged exposure to the sun. Use sunscreens and wear protective clothing until tolerance is determined.

Cisapride

(SIS-uh-PRIDE)

Propulsid

A medicine used for the treatment of nighttime heartburn due to gastroesophageal reflux disease.

Precautions

DO NOT USE if you are allergic to this medicine; if you have stomach or intestinal bleeding or blockage; intestinal perforation; or are taking any of the following medicines: ketoconazole (*Nizoral*)), itraconazole (*Sporanox*), miconazole IV (*Monistat*), fluconazole (*Diflucan*), troleandomycin (*TAO*), erythromycin or clarithromycin (*Biaxin*).

Rare cases of serious heart problems (abnormal heart rhythms) have been reported in patients taking this medicine. Most of these patients already had heart problems and were taking other medicines. If you are concerned about this issue, contact your healthcare provider.

BEFORE USING THIS MEDICINE, tell your healthcare provider if you are pregnant or breastfeeding; or if you are taking, will be taking or stop taking any prescription or nonprescription medicine; or if you have any other medical conditions.

Side Effects

Every medicine can cause side effects, but many people have no, or minor, side effects. Tell your healthcare provider if any of the following occurs: headache; diarrhea; nausea; constipation; gas; upset stomach; vomiting; dehydration; stuffy nose; sinus infection; coughing; viral or upper respiratory infection; chest pain; urinary tract infection; sleeplessness; anxiety; depression; nervousness; rash; itching; muscle/joint pain; abnormal vision; vaginal infection; dizziness; back pain.

Guidelines for Use

USE EXACTLY AS PRESCRIBED.

Suspension — Shake well before use.

Take this medicine 4 times daily, at least 15 minutes before meals and at bedtime.

If symptoms do not improve, contact your healthcare provider.

If a dose is missed, take it as soon as possible. If several hours have passed or if it is nearing time for the next dose, do not double the dose to "catch up," unless advised by your healthcare provider. If more than one dose is missed, contact your healthcare provider.

This medicine can cause some other medicines (eg, tranquilizers) and alcohol to have increased sedative or drowsiness effects. Use caution while driving or performing other tasks requiring alertness, coordination or physical dexterity.

Exams will be required. Be sure to keep appointments.

Store at room temperature. Tablets — Store at away from light and moisture.

Clarithromycin

(kluh-RITH-row-MY-sin)

Biaxin

An antibiotic used to treat infections caused by certain bacteria.

Precautions

DO NOT USE if you are allergic to this medicine or to erythromycin or if you are taking astemizole or terfenadine or have electrolyte disturbances.

BEFORE USING THIS MEDICINE, tell your healthcare provider if you are pregnant or breastfeeding; or if you are taking, will be taking or stop taking any prescription or nonprescription medicine; or if you have any other medical conditions.

Side Effects

Every medicine can cause side effects, but many people have no, or minor, side effects. Tell your healthcare provider if any of the following occurs: abdominal pain; diarrhea; gas; headache; nausea; rash; altered taste; vomiting; indigestion; unusual tiredness; yellowing of skin and eyes; itching; dark urine; pale stools.

Guidelines for Use

USE EXACTLY AS PRESCRIBED.

May be taken with or without food or milk.

Suspension-Shake well before using.

Take the 2 daily doses at evenly spaced intervals throughout the day, preferably every 12 hours.

If a dose is missed, take it as soon as possible. If several hours have passed or if it is nearing time for the next dose, do not double the dose to catch up, unless advised by your healthcare provider. If more than one dose is missed, contact your healthcare provider.

Continue use until all the prescribed medicine has been taken. Failure to take all of the medicine may prevent complete elimination of bacteria, causing the infection to return.

If diarrhea or stomach pain occurs, contact your healthcare provider immediately. This could be a symptom of a severe side effect (pseudomembranous colitis) requiring immediate medical attention.

Store at room temperature; do not refrigerate.

Use within 14 days. Discard any unused medication.

Follow each dose with liquids (preferably 6 to 8 ounces).

Clemastine Fumarate

(KLEM-ass-teen FEW-muh-rate)

Tavist, Tavist-1

A medicine (antihistamine) used for relief of seasonal allergy symptoms and symptoms associated with some types of hives and skin rash with mild to moderate itching.

Precautions

DO NOT USE if you are allergic to this medicine.

BEFORE USING THIS MEDICINE, tell your healthcare provider if you are pregnant or breastfeeding; or if you are taking, will be taking or stop taking any prescription or nonprescription medicine; or if you have any other medical conditions.

Side Effects

Every medicine can cause side effects, but many people have no, or minor, side effects. Tell your healthcare provider if any of the following occurs: stomach ache; constipation; appetite changes; nausea; vomiting; diarrhea; drowsiness; dizziness; mental confusion; decreased coordination; fatigue; headache; sleeplessness; sleepiness; irregular heartbeat; pounding in the chest; dry nose, throat and mouth; thickening of mucus in respiratory tract; wheezing; nasal stuffiness; sensitivity to sunburn; difficult urination; urine retention; sore throat; ringing in the ears; blurred and double vision; rash; hives; itching; chills.

Guidelines for Use

USE EXACTLY AS PRESCRIBED.

May cause stomach upset; take with food.

May cause drowsiness or dizziness. Use caution while driving or performing tasks requiring alertness. Avoid alcohol and other sedatives, hypnotics, tranquilizers, etc.

Elderly patients are more likely to experience dizziness, sedation, decreased coordination, mental confusion and fainting when they take antihistamines.

Do not take for several days before allergy skin testing because of interference with test.

May produce tolerance if taken regularly for a long time. Loss of effectiveness with a particular antihistamine can be restored if an antihistamine from a different chemical class is substituted for several days. Such alternating may be necessary if antihistamine therapy is continued over several weeks or months.

May cause blurred vision, weakness, headache or nervousness. Tell your healthcare provider if they become severe.

If dry mouth occurs, it may be helpful to sip water, suck on ice chips or sugarless hard candy or chew sugarless gum.

Avoid prolonged exposure to sunlight or UV light; may increase the risk of sunburn.

Clindamycin Oral

(KLIN-duh-MY-sin)

Cleocin, Cleocin Pediatric

A medicine used to treat a variety of serious infections, especially in patients who are allergic to pencillin.

Precautions

DO NOT USE if you are allergic to this medicine or lincomycin.

BEFORE USING THIS MEDICINE, tell your healthcare provider if you are pregnant or breastfeeding; or if you are taking, will be taking or stop taking any prescription or nonprescription medicine; or if you have any other medical conditions.

Side Effects

Every medicine can cause side effects, but many people have no, or minor, side effects. Tell your healthcare provider if any of the following occurs: nausea; vomiting; diarrhea; skin rashes; itching; flushing; abdominal pain; loss of appetite; metallic or unpleasant taste in mouth; yellowing of skin or eyes; difficulty breathing.

Guidelines for Use

USE EXACTLY AS PRESCRIBED.

Capsules — Usually taken in 3–4 daily doses for 7–10 days.

If a dose is missed, take it as soon as possible. If several hours have passed or if it is nearing time for the next dose, do not double the dose to "catch up," unless advised by your healthcare provider. If more than one dose is missed, contact your healthcare provider.

May cause diarrhea; tell your healthcare provider if this occurs. This could be a symptom of a severe side effect (pseudomembranous colitis) requiring immediate medical attention.

Do not treat diarrhea without consulting your healthcare provider.

Take each dose with a full glass of water.

May be taken without regard to meals.

Complete full course of therapy.

Injection — Store IV bags (piggybacks) at room temperature or in the refrigerator. Discard unused solution after 16 days if stored at room temperature or after 32 days if stored in refrigerator.

Clindamycin Topical

(KLIN-duh-MY-sin)

Cleocin T

An antibiotic put on the skin to treat acne in patients over 12 years old.

Precautions

DO NOT USE if you have an allergy to this medicine or lincomycin, or have a history of antibiotic-related diarrhea or colitis.

BEFORE USING THIS MEDICINE, tell your healthcare provider if you have diarrhea, colitis; if you are pregnant or breastfeeding; if you are taking, will be taking or if you stop taking any prescription or nonprescription medicine; or if you have any other medical conditions.

Side Effects

Every medicine can cause side effects, but many people have no, or minor, side effects. Tell your healthcare provider if any of the following occurs: skin dryness and irritation; stinging; burning; redness; inflammation of hair follicles; oily skin; rash; itching; peeling; diarrhea; stomach pain.

Guidelines for Use

USE EXACTLY AS PRESCRIBED.

Lotion — Shake well before using.

For external use only.

Apply a thin layer of the gel or solution to the affected area twice daily after washing and drying the skin. Do not use more often than prescribed.

If a dose is missed, apply it as soon as possible. If several hours have passed, or if it is nearing time for the next dose, do not double the dose to "catch up," unless advised by your healthcare provider.

Avoid contact with eyes, nose, mouth or other mucous membranes and damaged skin. Burning or irritation may occur. If this occurs, bathe the area with large amounts of tap water for several minutes.

Apply cautiously in those patients with a history of skin allergies.

If diarrhea or stomach pain occurs, contact your doctor immediately. This could be a symptom of a severe side effect (pseudomembranous colitis) requiring immediate medical attention. Do not treat diarrhea without consulting your doctor.

Use with caution in the elderly. Older patients with severe illness may not tolerate diarrhea well. Watch for changes in bowel frequency.

Clindamycin Vaginal

(KLIN-duh-MY-sin)

Cleocin

A medicine used to treat certain vaginal bacterial infections.

Precautions

DO NOT USE if you have an allergy to this medicine or its relatives (benzyl alcohol, lincomycin) or have a history of antibiotic-related diarrhea or colitis.

BEFORE USING THIS MEDICINE, tell your healthcare provider if you are pregnant or breastfeeding; or if you are taking, will be taking or stop taking any prescription or nonprescription medicine; or if you have any other medical conditions.

Side Effects

Every medicine can cause side effects, but many people have no, or minor, side effects. Tell your healthcare provider if any of the following occurs: headache; local pain/itching; vaginal yeast infection; dizziness; rash; heartburn; vomiting; constipation; severe diarrhea.

Guidelines for Use

USE EXACTLY AS PRESCRIBED.

For vaginal use only. Wash hands after using.

Specific instructions for use are enclosed in each package.

Disposable applicators are provided with the medicine.

Use at bedtime. This will help retain the medicine in the vagina and reduce leaking.

Complete a full course of therapy. Keep using, even during the menstrual period.

If the medicine causes local burning, pain or itching, or if symptoms worsen, contact your healthcare provider.

Avoid sexual intercourse during treatment. This product contains mineral oil, which may weaken products such as condoms and diaphragms. Do not use such products within 72 hours following treatment with this medicine.

A sanitary napkin or mini-pad may be used to prevent staining of clothing due to seepage. Do not use tampons.

If infection returns, other factors may be involved. Factors that increase the risk of infection include AIDS, diabetes, chronic antibiotic therapy, pregnancy, corticosteroid use and birth control tablet use.

Avoid contact with eyes. If contact occurs, rinse eyes with large amounts of water.

Store at room temperature. Do not freeze.

Clofibrate

(kloe-FIH-brate)

Atromid-S

A medicine used to lower high levels of triglycerides and cholesterol. Used alone or in conjunction with other medicines and diet.

Precautions

DO NOT USE if you are allergic to this medicine or if you are pregnant or breast-feeding.

BEFORE USING THIS MEDICINE, tell your healthcare provider if you are taking, will be taking or stop taking any prescription or nonprescription medicine; or if you have any other medical conditions.

Side Effects

Every medicine can cause side effects, but many people have no, or minor, side effects. Tell your healthcare provider if any of the following occurs: stomach pain; nausea; vomiting; diarrhea; upset stomach or heartburn; gas; bloating; loose stools; weakness; drowsiness; dizziness; headache; chest pain; rash; itching; dry skin; hair loss; dry brittle hair; hives; weight gain; swelling (especially in the ankles or feet); decreased urination; painful urination; blood in urine; decreased sexual function; flu-like symptoms (muscle aches; soreness or cramps); mouth irritation; excessive thirst; susceptibility to infection, gallstones.

Guidelines for Use

USE EXACTLY AS PRESCRIBED.

Patient package insert is available.

If upset stomach occurs, take with food.

Most effective when used with a diet that will lower intake of cholesterol and saturated fats.

Notify your healthcare provider if any of the following occurs: chest pain; shortness of breath; irregular heartbeat; severe stomach pain with nausea and vomiting; fever and chills or sore throat; blood in the urine; unusually low urine output; swelling of the lower extremities; weight gain.

Clomiphene Citrate

(KLOE-mih-feen SIH-trate)

Clomid, Milophene, Serophene

An ovulation stimulant that is used to treat female infertility when the patient desires pregnancy, the sexual partner is fertile and potent, and the patient has normal liver function and normal estrogen levels. It may occasionally be prescribed for other reasons.

Precautions

DO NOT USE if you are allergic to this medicine, are pregnant, or have a history of liver disease. Multiple births are a risk. The risk of a multiple pregnancy is increased approximately 6 times when this medicine is given.

BEFORE USING THIS MEDICINE, tell your healthcare provider if you are breastfeeding; or if you are taking, will be taking or stop taking any prescription or nonprescription medicine; or if you have any other medical conditions.

Side Effects

Every medicine can cause side effects, but many people have no, or minor, side effects. Tell your healthcare provider if any of the following occurs: nausea; vomiting; headache; dizziness; lightheadedness; blurred vision; blurred spots or flashes of light; multiple pregnancy; hot flashes; stomach or pelvic pain; bloating; abnormal uterine bleeding; breast tenderness.

Guidelines for Use

USE EXACTLY AS PRESCRIBED.

Use caution while driving or performing tasks requiring mental alertness.

Blurring or other visual symptoms may occur. If visual symptoms occur, discontinue treatment and call your healthcare provider about a complete eye evaluation.

Multiple pregnancy is possible and poses potential hazards.

Properly timed intercourse is important for good results.

The likelihood of conception diminishes with each succeeding course of therapy. If pregnancy has not been achieved after three courses of treatment, further treatment is not recommended. Long-term cyclic therapy is not recommended.

Clomipramine Hydrochloride

(kloe-MIH-pruh-meen HIGH-droe-KLOR-ide)

Anafranil

A mood elevating medicine usually used for the treatment of obsessive-compulsive disorder. It may occasionally be prescribed for other reasons.

Precautions

DO NOT USE if you are allergic to this medicine or its relatives, or if you are using monoamine oxidase inhibitors (eg, *Nardil*, *Parnate*).

BEFORE USING THIS MEDICINE, tell your healthcare provider if you are pregnant or breastfeeding; or if you are taking, will be taking or stop taking any prescription or nonprescription medicine; or if you have any other medical conditions.

Side Effects

Every medicine can cause side effects, but many people have no, or minor, side effects. Tell your healthcare provider if any of the following occurs: dry mouth; blurred vision; increased heart rate; impaired coordination; difficult urination; excessive sedation; seizures.

Guidelines for Use

USE EXACTLY AS PRESCRIBED.

Take as directed with a full glass of water, with or without food.

If a dose is missed, take it as soon as possible. If several hours have passed or if it is nearing time for the next dose, do not double the dose to catch up, unless advised by your healthcare provider. If more than one dose is missed, contact your healthcare provider.

This medicine may not be effective for 2 to 3 weeks.

May cause drowsiness or blurred vision. Use caution while driving or performing other tasks requiring mental alertness.

Using this medicine with alcohol or other central nervous system depressants (eg, pain relievers, sedatives, antihistamines) may cause added drowsiness.

May cause sensitivity to sunlight. Avoid prolonged exposure to the sun. Use sunscreens and wear protective clothing until tolerance is determined.

Taking this medicine at bedtime may help reduce side effects (eg, daytime drowsiness). Discuss this possibility with your healthcare provider.

Clonazepam

(kloe-NAY-ze-pam)

Klonopin

A medicine that helps control epilepsy and seizures. It may occasionally be prescribed for other reasons.

Precautions

DO NOT USE if you are allergic to this medicine or its relatives.

BEFORE USING THIS MEDICINE, tell your healthcare provider if you are pregnant or breastfeeding; or if you are taking, will be taking or stop taking any prescription or nonprescription medicine; or if you have any other medical conditions.

Side Effects

Every medicine can cause side effects, but many people have no, or minor, side effects. Tell your healthcare provider if any of the following occurs: constipation; diarrhea; nausea; appetite changes; headache; confusion; depression; memory loss; mood changes; behavior changes (especially children); sleeplessness; tremor; feeling of whirling motion; severe weakness; incoordination; drowsiness; abnormal involuntary body movements; hallucinations; pounding in chest; difficult breathing; chest congestion; runny nose; excessive growth or loss of hair; blurred vision; double vision; glassy-eyed appearance; unusual eye movements; fever; loss of voice; increased salivation or dry mouth; coated tongue; changes in urination; fluid retention; difficulty speaking; sore gums; swollen lymph nodes; weight changes; increased sex drive; incontinence of urine or feces; muscle pain or weakness; dehydration.

Guidelines for Use

USE EXACTLY AS PRESCRIBED.

May cause stomach upset. Take with food.

If the medication does not seem to be working as well after taking it for a few weeks, check with your healthcare provider. Do not change the dose you are taking until you have checked with your healthcare provider.

If you stop taking this medication suddenly, you may experience withdrawal symptoms. Check with your healthcare provider before stopping this medication.

May cause drowsiness, dizziness or blurred vision. Use caution when driving or performing other tasks requiring mental alertness.

Using this medication with alcohol or other central nervous system depressants (eg, pain relievers, sedatives, antihistamines) may cause added drowsiness.

Carry identification indicating you are using this medication.

Clonidine Hydrochloride

(KLOE-nih-DEEN HIGH-droe-KLOR-ide)

Catapres, Catapres T.T.S.

A medicine used to lower high blood pressure. It may occasionally be prescribed for other reasons.

Precautions

DO NOT USE if you are allergic to this medicine.

BEFORE USING THIS MEDICINE, tell your healthcare provider if you are pregnant or breastfeeding; or if you are taking, will be taking or stop taking any prescription or nonprescription medicine; or if you have any other medical conditions.

Side Effects

Every medicine can cause side effects, but many people have no, or minor, side effects. Tell your healthcare provider if any of the following occurs: dry mouth; drowsiness; constipation; nausea; change in taste; dry throat; fatigue; headache; difficulty sleeping; rash; nervousness; dizziness (especially when arising from a seated or lying position); impotence; sexual difficulties; vision changes.

Guidelines for Use

USE EXACTLY AS PRESCRIBED.

Do not stop taking this medicine suddenly. If your healthcare provider discontinues this medicine, the dose must be reduced gradually over several days to avoid a rapid increase in blood pressure.

If a dose is missed, take it as soon as possible. If several hours have passed or if it is nearing time for the next dose, do not double the dose to catch up, unless advised by your healthcare provider. If more than one dose is missed, contact your healthcare provider.

Patients being treated for high blood pressure often feel tired and run down for a few weeks after beginning therapy. It takes time for the body to adjust. Continue taking your medication even though you may not feel quite normal. Check with your healthcare provider if symptoms cause concern.

Have your blood pressure checked regularly and keep regular appointments with your healthcare provider even if you feel well.

Most patients with high blood pressure do not feel sick.

Avoid alcohol while taking this medicine; it may cause excessive drowsiness.

Transdermal patch—Apply to hairless area of skin on upper arm or torso, once every 7 days. Use a different skin site from the previous application.

If the system loosens during the 7–day wearing, apply the adhesive overlay directly over the system to ensure good adhesion.

Therapeutic blood levels of this medicine from the transdermal patch are not reached for 2 to 3 days after initial application.

Clorazepate Dipotassium

(klor-AZE-uh-PATE DIE-poe-TASS-ee-uhm)

Gen-Xene, Tranxene, Tranxene-SD, Tranxene-SD Half Strength

A benzodiazepine medicine used to treat symptoms of anxiety and certain types of seizures.

Precautions

DO NOT USE if you are allergic to this medicine or its relatives, or are breastfeeding.

BEFORE USING THIS MEDICINE, tell your healthcare provider if you are pregnant; if you are taking, will be taking or stop taking any prescription or nonprescription medicine; or if you have any other medical conditions.

Side Effects

Every medicine can cause side effects, but many people have no, or minor, side effects. Tell your healthcare provider if any of the following occurs: stomach upset; constipation; diarrhea; change in appetite; vomiting; confusion; depression; nervousness; memory loss; drowsiness; fatigue; dizziness; crying; disorientation; vivid dreams; headache; seizures; changes in heart rate; pounding in the chest; itching; rash; hair growth; yellowing of skin or eyes; visual or hearing disturbances; slurred speech; loss of bladder function; change in sex drive; urine retention; menstrual problems; dry mouth; fever; tremors/uncontrollable muscle movement; difficult breathing; swelling; excessive perspiration; joint pain; weight gain or loss; dehydration; fainting.

Guidelines for Use

USE EXACTLY AS PRESCRIBED.

May be taken with food or water if stomach upset occurs.

If a dose is missed, take it as soon as possible. If several hours have passed or if it is nearing time for the next dose, do not double the dose to catch up, unless advised by your healthcare provider. If more than one dose is missed, contact your healthcare provider.

This medication can be addictive if used in large doses or for a long time. Discuss overuse with your healthcare provider.

May cause drowsiness. Use caution while driving or performing other tasks requiring mental alertness, coordination and dexterity. Avoid alcohol and other medications that cause drowsiness while taking this medication.

Patients on long-term or high-dosage therapy may have withdrawal symptoms if therapy is suddenly stopped.

Carry identification if this medication is being used to treat a seizure disorder.

Clotrimazole Oral

(kloe-TRIM-uh-zole)

Mycelex Troches

An antifungal lozenge that is used to treat oral thrush (mouth infection) in adults and children over 3 years of age. This medicine is also used to prevent oral thrush in patients undergoing chemotherapy, radiology or steroid therapy.

Precautions

DO NOT USE if you have an allergy to this medicine.

BEFORE USING THIS MEDICINE, tell your healthcare provider if you are pregnant or breastfeeding; or if you are taking, will be taking or stop taking any prescription or nonprescription medicine; or if you have any other medical conditions.

Side Effects

Every medicine can cause side effects, but many people have no, or minor, side effects. Tell your healthcare provider if any of the following occurs: nausea; vomiting; unpleasant taste or mouth sensations; itching.

Guidelines for Use

USE EXACTLY AS PRESCRIBED.

For oral use only.

Allow each troche (lozenge) to dissolve slowly in the mouth. Do not swallow whole.

Usual dose is one lozenge 5 times a day for 14 days to treat oral thrush.

To prevent oral thrush, use one lozenge 3 times daily for the duration of chemotherapy or until steroids are reduced to maintenance levels.

Continue to use until all of the prescribed medicine has been taken. Failure to take all of the prescribed medicine may prevent complete elimination of fungi, causing the infection to return.

If a dose is missed, use it as soon as possible. If several hours have passed or if it is nearing time for the next dose, do not double the dose to "catch up," unless advised by your healthcare provider. If more than one dose is missed, contact your healthcare provider.

Do not use for treating fungal infection other than in the mouth.

If condition persists or worsens or if irritation or itching occurs, discontinue use and notify your healthcare provider.

Store at room temperature; do not freeze.

Clotrimazole Topical

(kloe-TRIM-uh-zole)

Lotrimin AF, Lotrimin, Mycelex, Mycelex OTC

A topical antifungal used to treat tinea pedis (athlete's foot), tinea cruris (jock itch), tinea corporis (ringworm), tinea versicolor (pityriasis) and candidiasis (yeast) in adults and children over 12 years old.

Precautions

DO NOT USE if you are allergic to this medicine.

BEFORE USING THIS MEDICINE, tell your healthcare provider if you are pregnant or breastfeeding; or if you are taking, will be taking or stop taking any prescription or nonprescription medicine; or if you have any other medical conditions.

Side Effects

Every medicine can cause side effects, but many people have no, or minor, side effects. Tell your healthcare provider if any of the following occurs: redness; stinging; itching; burning; blistering; peeling; hives; swelling; oozing; signs of increased irritation.

Guidelines for Use

USE EXACTLY AS PRESCRIBED.

For external use only.

Shake solution well before using.

Gently massage into affected and surrounding skin areas twice daily, morning and evening.

Avoid contact with the eyes.

Apply after cleansing and thoroughly drying the affected area, unless directed otherwise by your healthcare provider.

If a dose is missed, apply it as soon as possible. If several hours have passed or if it is nearing time for the next dose, do not double the dose in order to "catch up," unless advised by your healthcare provider. If more than one dose is missed, contact your healthcare provider.

Do not use for treating fungal infection other than on the skin.

Continue to use until all of the prescribed medicine has been taken. Failure to take all of the prescribed medicine may prevent complete elimination of fungi, causing the infection to return. Contact your healthcare provider if there is no improvement after 4 weeks of treatment.

If condition persists or worsens, discontinue use and notify your doctor.

Store at room temperature.

Clotrimazole Vaginal

(kloe-TRIM-uh-zole)

Femcare, Gyne-Lotrimin, Gyne-Lotrimin Combination Pack, Mycelex-7, Mycelex-G, Mycelex Twin Pack

A medicine used to treat vaginal yeast infections and the itching related to these infections in females over 12 years of age.

Precautions

DO NOT USE if you are allergic to this medicine.

BEFORE USING THIS MEDICINE, tell your healthcare provider if you are pregnant or breastfeeding; or if you are taking, will be taking or stop taking any prescription or nonprescription medicine; or if you have any other medical conditions.

Side Effects

Every medicine can cause side effects, but many people have no, or minor, side effects. Tell your healthcare provider if any of the following occurs: local irritation; burning; itching; rash; stomach cramps; bloating; frequent urination; painful/difficult intercourse.

Guidelines for Use

USE EXACTLY AS PRESCRIBED.

Patient instructions for proper use are enclosed in each package.

Usual dose is one vaginal tablet or applicator full.

Insert high into the vagina, except during pregnancy, preferably at bedtime for 7 days.

Complete a full course of therapy. Keep using, even during the menstrual period.

If a dose is missed, contact your healthcare provider for instruction.

If the medicine causes burning or irritation, or if symptoms worsen, contact your healthcare provider.

Contact your healthcare provider immediately if you experience any of the following: fever (over 100°F); pain in lower back, abdomen or shoulders; vaginal discharge that smells bad; headaches; rash; hives.

Refrain from sexual intercourse during treatment since the infection can spread to your partner. Also, the base in this formulation may interact with (weaken) certain latex products such as condoms or diaphragms. Do not rely on condoms or diaphragms to prevent pregnancy or sexually transmitted diseases.

A sanitary napkin or mini-pad may be used to prevent staining of clothing due to seepage or leakage. Do not use a tampon.

If infection recurs within 2 months, other factors may be involved. Factors that increase the risk of infection include AIDS, diabetes, chronic antibiotic therapy, pregnancy, steroid use and oral contraceptive use.

For best results, follow instructions exactly; wear cotton underwear and loose clothing; dry vaginal area thoroughly after bathing; wipe away from the vagina after bowel movements or urination; do not douche; do not scratch area.

If your partner experiences penile itching, redness or discomfort, he should contact his healthcare provider and mention that you are using this medication.

Store at room temperature away from children.

Clozapine

(KLOE-zuh-peen)

Clozaril

An antipsychotic medicine that helps the brain modify behavior in schizophrenic patients who do not respond to other antipsychotic treatments.

Precautions

DO NOT USE if you are severely depressed, if you have a bone marrow disorder, glaucoma, prostatic enlargement, drink alcohol, or if you are breastfeeding. Safe use in children under the age of 16 has not been established.

BEFORE USING THIS MEDICINE, tell your healthcare provider if you are pregnant; or if you are taking, will be taking or stop taking any prescription or nonprescription medicine; or if you have any other medical conditions.

Side Effects

Every medicine can cause side effects, but many people have no, or minor, side effects. Tell your healthcare provider if any of the following occurs: tiredness; weakness; headache; fever; sore throat; nausea; vomiting; constipation; stomach pain; seizures; dizziness; headache; tremor; fainting; insomnia; nightmares; restlessness; confusion; increased heart rate; dry mouth; visual disturbances; increased salivation; urinary abnormalities.

Guidelines for Use

USE EXACTLY AS PRESCRIBED.

May cause drowsiness or dizziness. Use caution while driving or performing other tasks requiring alertness.

Orthostatic hypotension (dizziness or drowsiness when rising quickly from a seated or lying position) may occur. Avoid sudden changes in posture.

Tell your healthcare provider immediately if any of the following symptoms occurs: tiredness, weakness, fever, sore throat, signs of infection, flu-like symptoms or seizures.

Do not take any prescription or over-the-counter medicines without first consulting your healthcare provider.

Watch for signs of overdose or toxicity, such as altered states of consciousness, including drowsiness, delirium and coma, increased heart rate, increased blood pressure, difficulty breathing, and excessive salivation.

Regular blood and laboratory tests will be needed. Be sure to keep appointments.

Codeine

(KOE-deen)

A medicine used to relieve mild to moderate pain and to suppress cough.

Precautions

DO NOT USE if you are allergic to this medicine or have acute bronchial asthma.

BEFORE USING THIS MEDICINE, tell your healthcare provider if you are pregnant or breastfeeding; or if you are taking, will be taking or stop taking any prescription or nonprescription medicine; if you have any other medical conditions; or if you are allergic to sulfite preservatives.

Side Effects

Every medicine can cause side effects, but many people have no, or minor, side effects. Tell your healthcare provider if any of the following occurs: lightheadedness; dizziness; drowsiness; nausea; vomiting; abdominal pain; cramps; constipation; euphoria (exaggerated sense of well-being); anxiety; nervousness; depression; incoordination; weakness; headache; dizziness or lightheadedness that occurs when rising from a sitting or lying position; rash; itching; hives; decreased urination; blurred vision; shortness of breath.

Guidelines for Use

USE EXACTLY AS PRESCRIBED.

May cause nausea; take with food.

May cause constipation (long-term use). Stool softeners or fiber laxatives may be required if use is prolonged. Drink plenty of water.

May cause drowsiness, dizziness or blurred vision. Use caution while driving or performing other tasks requiring mental alertness, coordination and dexterity. Avoid alcohol and drowsiness-causing medicine.

Long-term use may lead to addiction. Early signs include medicine ineffectiveness.

This medicine works best if taken on a routine basis. Narcotics are more effective in preventing pain than in treating pain after it occurs.

Give the medicine ample time to work before determining if more is needed (at least 30 minutes to 1 hour for oral agents).

If a dose is missed, take it as soon as possible. If several hours have passed or if it is nearing time for the next dose, do not double the dose to catch up, unless advised by your healthcare provider. If more than one dose is missed, contact your healthcare provider.

Sometimes this medicine is given in combination with nonnarcotic pain relievers. Make sure your healthcare provider knows if you have had problems taking aspirin or acetaminophen in the past. Notify your healthcare provider if shortness of breath or difficulty breathing occurs.

Colchicine

(KOHL-chih-seen)

A medicine used to relieve the pain of acute gout attacks and to prevent acute attacks. It may occasionally be prescribed for other reasons.

Precautions

DO NOT USE if you are allergic to this medicine.

BEFORE USING THIS MEDICINE, tell your healthcare provider if you are pregnant or breastfeeding; or if you are taking, will be taking, or stop taking any prescription or nonprescription medicine; or if you have any other medical conditions.

Side Effects

Every medicine can cause side effects, but many people have no, or minor, side effects. Tell your healthcare provider if any of the following occurs: vomiting; nausea; diarrhea; stomach pain; tiredness; weakness; numbness; hair loss; rash; fever; sore throat; unusual bleeding or bruising; tingling in hands or feet; blood in urine; reduced urination.

Guidelines for Use

USE EXACTLY AS PRESCRIBED.

Acute gout attack--Start taking at the first sign of an attack.

Stop taking as soon as gout pain is relieved or at the first sign of stomach pain, nausea, vomiting or diarrhea (unless directed by your healthcare provider). If symptoms persist notify your healthcare provider.

Notify your healthcare provider if rash, sore throat, fever, unusual bleeding, bruising, tiredness, weakness, numbness or tingling occurs.

With long-term therapy, periodic blood studies will be performed. Be sure to keep appointments.

Colestipol Hydrochloride

(koe-LESS-tih-pole HIGH-droe-KLOR-ide)

Colestid

A medicine used to lower the level of cholesterol in the blood.

Precautions

DO NOT USE if you are allergic to this medicine or if you have obstruction of the gall bladder or bile duct.

BEFORE USING THIS MEDICINE, tell your healthcare provider if you are pregnant or breastfeeding; constipated; or if you are taking, will be taking or stop taking any prescription or nonprescription medicine; or if you have any other medical conditions.

Side Effects

Every medicine can cause side effects, but many people have no, or minor, side effects. Tell your healthcare provider if any of the following occurs: unusual bleeding; constipation; gas; nausea; vomiting; diarrhea; heartburn; loss of appetite; rash.

Guidelines for Use

USE EXACTLY AS PRESCRIBED.

Take before meals.

Granules-Mix with liquid (water or noncarbonated drinks), very liquid soups or cereals, or with pulpy fruits (applesauce or crushed pineapple). Do not take the dry powder.

May interfere with the effects of other medicines if taken at the same time. Generally take other medicines either 1 hour before or 4 to 6 hours after this medicine.

Most effective when used with a diet that decreases the intake of cholesterol and saturated fats.

If therapy is long-term, absorption of fat-soluble vitamins (A, D, E and K) may be impaired. Supplemental vitamins may be required.

Report any unusual bleeding to your healthcare provider.

Corticotropin

(core-tih-koe-TROE-pin)

ACTH, ACTH-40, ACTH-80, Acthar

A medicine that is used to treat increased calcium levels in blood associated with certain conditions (eg, cancer, inflammation of the thyroid gland, multiple sclerosis). It is also used to monitor the adrenal cortex.

Precautions

DO NOT USE if you are allergic to this medicine.

BEFORE USING THIS MEDICINE, tell your healthcare provider if you are pregnant or breastfeeding; or if you are taking, will be taking or stop taking any prescription or nonprescription medicine; or if you have any other medical conditions.

Side Effects

Every medicine can cause side effects, but many people have no, or minor, side effects. Tell your healthcare provider if any of the following occurs: sodium and fluid retention; potassium and calcium loss; nausea; vomiting, ulceration of esophagus; inflammation of the pancreas; peptic ulcer; vertigo (feeling of whirling motion); headache; euphoria; sleeplessness; mood swings; depression; seizures; high blood pressure; heart failure; impaired wound healing; increased sweating; freckling; thin, fragile skin; redness; acne; excessive body hair growth; rash; easy bruising; infection; menstrual irregularities; suppression of growth in children; cataracts; glaucoma; muscle weakness; loss of muscle mass; osteoporosis.

Guidelines for Use

USE EXACTLY AS PRESCRIBED.

May mask signs of infection. There may be decreased resistance and inability to localize infection.

Diabetes-Insulin or oral blood-sugar-lowering agent requirements may increase.

This medicine can increase blood pressure and potassium and calcium excretion and cause salt and water retention. A salt-restricted diet and potassium supplements may be necessary.

Avoid immunization with live vaccines (eg, smallpox) when receiving this medicine.

Cortisone Oral

(CORE-tih-sone)

Cortone Acetate

A hormone used as replacement therapy when the adrenal cortex gland is not functioning properly. It is also used for its anti-inflammatory action. It may be prescribed for other reasons.

Precautions

DO NOT USE if you are allergic to this medicine or its relatives.

BEFORE USING THIS MEDICINE, tell your healthcare provider if you are pregnant or breastfeeding; or if you are taking, will be taking or stop taking any prescription or nonprescription medicine; or if you have any other medical conditions.

Side Effects

Every medicine can cause side effects, but many people have no, or minor, side effects. Tell your healthcare provider if any of the following occurs: appearance of round, swollen moonface; fat deposits (eg, shoulders, midsection); nausea; vomiting; increased appetite; weight gain; peptic ulcer; local pain; rectal bleeding with enemas; seizures; dizziness; headache; behavior changes; sleeplessness; hiccups; fluid retention; low or high blood pressure; irregular heart rhythm; impaired wound healing; thinning of skin and layer of fat under the skin; excessive pigmentation of skin; acne; excessive body hair growth; rash; hives; loss of muscle mass; osteoporosis; bone fractures; menstrual irregularities; growth suppression in children; higher blood sugar levels.

Guidelines for Use

USE EXACTLY AS PRESCRIBED.

May cause stomach upset. Take with meals or snacks.

Take single daily or alternate day doses in the morning prior to 9 a.m. Take multiple doses at evenly spaced intervals throughout the day.

Patients on long-term therapy should carry identification.

High-dose or long-term therapy: DO NOT change or stop therapy unless directed by your healthcare provider. Sudden withdrawal of therapy may cause symptoms of fatigue, loss of appetite, nausea, vomiting, diarrhea, weight loss, weakness, dizziness and low blood sugar.

Diabetics may require increased doses of insulin or oral diabetes (hypoglycemic) medications.

Cosyntropin

(koe-sin-TROE-pin)

Cortrosyn

Used for the diagnostic testing of adrenocortical function.

Side Effects

Every medicine can cause side effects, but many people have no, or minor, side effects. Tell your healthcare provider if any of the following occurs: fluid retention; muscle weakness; stomach distention; increased sweating; thinning of the skin; flushing of the face; acne; convulsions; feeling of a whirling motion; headache; menstrual irregularities; growth suppression (children); excess hair growth; dizziness; nausea; vomiting; shock; skin reactions.

Patient Information

This medicine may mask signs of infection.

Avoid immunizations with live vaccines; consult your healthcare provider.

Diabetes--Requirements for insulin or oral hypoglycemia may increase.

Tell your healthcare provider if marked fluid retention; muscle weakness, abdominal pain, seizures or headache occur.

Cromolyn Sodium Inhalation

(KROE-moe-lin SO-dee-uhm)

Intal

A medicine used to prevent various types of asthma and decrease the severity of allergy attacks; to prevent or treat allergic rhinitis. It may occasionally be prescribed for other reasons.

Precautions

DO NOT USE if you are allergic to this medicine or its relatives. This medicine is not useful to treat acute asthma attacks.

BEFORE USING THIS MEDICINE, tell your healthcare provider if you are pregnant or breastfeeding; or if you are taking, will be taking or stop taking any prescription or nonprescription medicine; or if you have any other medical conditions.

Side Effects

Every medicine can cause side effects, but many people have no, or minor, side effects. Tell your healthcare provider if any of the following occurs: coughing; wheezing; dizziness; headache; rash; joint pain.

Guidelines for Use

USE EXACTLY AS PRESCRIBED.

Not for the treatment of an existing asthma attack. Start when an asthma attack is under control and you can breathe well.

Effectiveness depends on continuous use. Do not stop therapy suddenly except on the advice of your healthcare provider.

For inhalation only. Do not swallow capsule.

Notify your healthcare provider if coughing or wheezing occurs.

Prevent exercise-induced asthma - Give one of the daily doses 1 hour before beginning exercise.

If allergic rhinitis is seasonal, continue treatment through the season. If the allergic rhinitis is year-round, continuous use may be necessary. Use may decrease or eliminate the need for antihistamines or decongestants.

Cromolyn Sodium Nasal

Nasalcrom

A medicine used to prevent various types of asthma and decrease the severity of allergy attacks; to prevent or treat allergic rhinitis. It may occasionally be prescribed for other reasons.

Precautions

DO NOT USE if you are allergic to this medicine or its relatives. This medicine is not useful to treat acute asthma attacks.

BEFORE USING THIS MEDICINE, tell your healthcare provider if you are pregnant or breastfeeding; or if you are taking, will be taking or stop taking any prescription or nonprescription medicine; or if you have any other medical conditions.

Side Effects

Every medicine can cause side effects, but many people have no, or minor, side effects. Tell your healthcare provider if any of the following occurs: sneezing; nasal irritation; bad taste in mouth; nosebleeds.

Guidelines for Use

USE EXACTLY AS PRESCRIBED.

For inhalation only. Do not swallow capsule.

Not for the treatment of an existing asthma attack. Start when an asthma attack is under control and you can breathe well.

Effectiveness depends on continuous use. Do not stop therapy suddenly except on the advice of your healthcare provider.

Notify your healthcare provider if coughing or wheezing occurs.

Prevent exercise-induced asthma - Give one of the daily doses 1 hour before beginning exercise.

Blow your nose before using the nasal solution.

If allergic rhinitis is seasonal, continue treatment through the season. If the allergic rhinitis is year-round, continuous use may be necessary.

Use may decrease or eliminate the need for antihistamines or decongestants.

Nasal solution may cause mild nasal stinging or sneezing, but this rarely requires stopping therapy.

Cromolyn Sodium Ophthalmic

(KROE-moe-lin SO-dee-uhm)

Crolom

Eyedrops used to decrease allergy symptoms of the eye in adults and children over 4 years old. The medicine may sometimes be used with a corticosteroid eyedrop.

Precautions

DO NOT USE if you are allergic to this medicine or its relatives. Do not wear contact lenses while using this medicine.

BEFORE USING THIS MEDICINE, tell your healthcare provider if you are pregnant or breastfeeding; or if you are taking, will be taking or stop taking any prescription or nonprescription medicine; or if you have any other medical conditions.

Side Effects

Every medicine can cause side effects, but many people have no, or minor, side effects. Tell your healthcare provider if any of the following occurs: watery eyes; itchy eyes; dryness around the eye; puffy eyes; eye irritation; styes; continued stinging, burning or itching after use.

Guidelines for Use

USE EXACTLY AS PRESCRIBED.

Place 1–2 drops in the affected eye(s) 4–6 times daily at regular intervals. Do not exceed this dosage. Wait at least 5 minutes before using any other eye medications.

Effectiveness depends on continuous use. Consult your healthcare provider about stopping the medicine.

Brief stinging or burning of the eye may occur after administration. This is normal. Contact your healthcare provider if the symptom(s) continues.

Do not touch the dropper tip to any surface, including your eye, since this may contaminate the contents or cause damage to the eye.

Do not increase or decrease this medicine without your healthcare provider's approval.

If a dose is missed, instill it as soon as possible. If several hours have passed or if it is nearing time for the next dose, do not double the dose to "catch up," unless advised by your healthcare provider. If more than one dose is missed, contact your healthcare provider.

Soft contact lenses — Do not wear during treatment. Soft contact lens wear may be resumed within a few hours after stopping the drug.

Relief of symptoms (itching, tearing, redness and discharge) is usually seen within a few days, but can take up to 6 weeks.

Continue to use the medicine on a regular basis even after the symptoms are relieved in order to prevent the return of the symptoms.

Do not use if there are any signs of tampering with the product (eg, broken seal).

Keep out of reach of children.

Do not share this medicine with anyone else.

Store at room temperature with container tightly closed. Protect from light.

Cromolyn Sodium Oral

(KROE-moe-lin SO-dee-uhm)

Gastrocrom

A medicine used to relieve symptoms of mastocytosis

Precautions

DO NOT USE if you are allergic to this medicine or its relatives.

BEFORE USING THIS MEDICINE, tell your healthcare provider if you are pregnant or breastfeeding; or if you are taking, will be taking or stop taking any prescription or nonprescription medicine; or if you have any other medical conditions.

Side Effects

Every medicine can cause side effects, but many people have no, or minor, side effects. Tell your healthcare provider if any of the following occurs: headache; diarrhea.

Guidelines for Use

USE EXACTLY AS PRESCRIBED.

Effectiveness depends on continuous use. Do not stop therapy suddenly. Consult your healthcare provider about stopping the medicine.

Take at least 30 minutes before meals.

Do not mix with fruit juice, milk, or foods. Be sure to mix exactly as directed. Open capsules and pour contents into half a glass of hot water. Stir until dissolved. Add an equal quantity of cold water while stirring. Drink all of the liquid.

Oral capsules are NOT for inhalation.

Cyanocobalamin (Vitamin B_{12}) Injectable

(sigh-an-oh-koe-BAL-uh-min)

Crystamine, Cyanoject, Cyomin, Rubesol-1000, Rubramin PC

A medicine used to treat B12 deficiency due to malabsorption caused by a variety of conditions. It also is used to fill increased vitamin B12 requirements associated with pregnancy, thyrotoxicosis, hemolytic anemia, hemorrhage, malignancy and hepatic and renal disease.

Precautions

DO NOT USE if you are allergic to this medicine or to cobalt or to benzyl alcohol.

BEFORE USING THIS MEDICINE, tell your healthcare provider if you are pregnant or breastfeeding; or if you are taking, will be taking or stop taking any prescription or nonprescription medicine; or if you have any other medical conditions.

Side Effects

Every medicine can cause side effects, but many people have no, or minor, side effects. Tell your healthcare provider if any of the following occurs: itching; rash; pain at injection site; fluid retention and swelling; mild diarrhea; visual problems.

Guidelines for Use

USE EXACTLY AS PRESCRIBED.

Patients with pernicious anemia will require monthly injections of vitamin B_{12} for the rest of their lives. Failure to do so will result in return of the anemia and in development of severe and irreversible damage to the nerves of the spinal cord.

A well-balanced dietary intake is necessary; talk with your healthcare provider.

Do not take folic acid instead of vitamin B_{12} because folic acid may prevent anemia, but allow progression of nerve damage and mask anemia symptoms.

Periodic blood tests will be required to monitor response. Keep appointments.

Report any rash, itching, breathing problems or visual changes immediately to your healthcare provider.

Cyanocobalamin (Vitamin B_{12})

(sigh-an-oh-koe-BAL-uh-min)

Ener-B, Vitamin B_{12}

A medicine used to correct vitamin B_{12} deficiency, which causes certain forms of anemia and neurologic problems.

Precautions

DO NOT USE if you are allergic to this medicine or to cobalt.

BEFORE USING THIS MEDICINE, tell your healthcare provider if you are pregnant or breastfeeding; or if you are taking, will be taking or stop taking any prescription or nonprescription medicine; or if you have any other medical conditions.

Side Effects

Every medicine can cause side effects, but many people have no, or minor, side effects. Tell your healthcare provider if any of the following occurs: rash, itching or breathing difficulty may indicate allergic reaction.

Guidelines for Use

USE EXACTLY AS PRESCRIBED.

Recommended Dietary Allowances (RDAs)--2 mcg.

Take only as directed.

Dose needs to be individualized by your healthcare provider depending on severity of deficiency.

Vegetarians are especially prone to vitamin B_{12} deficiency and may require supplementation.

Cyclobenzaprine

(SIGH-kloe-BEN-zuh-preen)

Flexeril

A muscle relaxant used to relieve muscle discomfort due to strain, sprain or injury.

Precautions

DO NOT USE if you are allergic to this medicine; are taking monoamine oxidase inhibitors (phenelzine, tranylcypromine); or have porphyria.

BEFORE USING THIS MEDICINE, tell your healthcare provider if you are pregnant or breastfeeding; or if you are taking, will be taking or stop taking any prescription or nonprescription medicine; or if you have any other medical conditions. This medicine is not a substitute for rest or physical therapy needed for proper healing.

Side Effects

Every medicine can cause side effects, but many people have no, or minor, side effects. Tell your healthcare provider if any of the following occurs: dry mouth; difficult urination; constipation; headache; skin rash; yellowing of skin or eyes; fever; nasal congestion; rapid heart rate; palpitations (pounding in the chest); confusion.

Guidelines for Use

USE EXACTLY AS PRESCRIBED.

May cause stomach upset. Take with food.

Do not use a larger dose or use more often than prescribed. It is likely to cause drowsiness.

Use with extreme caution when driving or performing other tasks requiring mental alertness. Avoid alcohol and other medication that cause drowsiness (eg, narcotics, tranquilizers, antihistamines) during treatment.

Dizziness or lightheadedness may occur when arising quickly from a sitting or lying position. Avoid sudden changes in posture. Use caution when climbing stairs, etc.

This medicine makes an injury temporarily feel better. Do not rush your recovery. Lifting or exercising too soon may further damage muscles.

Cyclophosphamide

(sigh-kloe-FOSS-fuh-mide)

Cytoxan, Neosar

A medicine used to treat certain specific forms of cancer. It may occasionally be prescribed for other reasons.

Precautions

DO NOT USE if you are allergic to this medicine or to any other nitrogen mustard medicine or if you are breastfeeding, or if you have severe bone marrow suppression.

BEFORE USING THIS MEDICINE, tell your healthcare provider if you are pregnant or breastfeeding; if you are taking, will be taking or stop taking any prescription or nonprescription medicine; or if you have any other medical condition.

Side Effects

Every medicine can cause side effects, but many people have no, or minor, side effects. Tell your healthcare provider if any of the following occurs: hair loss; discoloration (eg, yellowing of skin); rash; nausea; vomiting; diarrhea; mouth sores; prolonged infertility; cessation of menstruation; tremors; confusion; agitation; incoordination; seizures; fever; difficulty breathing; blood in urine/stools; skin/nail pigment changes.

Guidelines for Use

USE EXACTLY AS PRESCRIBED.

Take on an empty stomach. If stomach upset is severe, take with food.

Notify your healthcare provider of unusual bleeding or bruising, black tarry stools, nausea, vomiting, weight loss, fever, chills, sore throat, cough, shortness of breath, seizures, lack of menstrual flow, unusual lumps or masses, flank or stomach pain, joint pain, sores in mouth or on the lips, yellow discoloration of the skin or eyes or skin rash.

Contraceptive (birth control) measures are recommended during therapy for both men and women.

This medicine may impair your ability to fight infection. Notify your healthcare provider of any signs of infection including fever, sore throat, rashes or chills.

May cause darkening of skin and fingernails. Contact your healthcare provider if these become pronounced.

Blood and urine tests should be conducted regularly to monitor and reduce medicine toxicity. Be sure to keep appointments.

Cycloserine

(sigh-kloe-SER-een)

Seromycin

A medicine used in combination with other medications to treat tuberculosis and certain types of urinary tract infections.

Precautions

DO NOT USE if you are allergic to the medicine or use alcohol excessively.

BEFORE USING THIS MEDICINE, tell your healthcare provider if you are pregnant or breastfeeding; or if you are taking, will be taking or stop taking any prescription or nonprescription medicine; or if you have any other medical conditions.

Side Effects

Every medicine can cause side effects, but many people have no, or minor, side effects. Tell your healthcare provider if any of the following occurs: nausea; vomiting; appetite loss; diarrhea; stomach pain; rash; itching; hives; dizziness; weakness; drowsiness; confusion; headache; numbness, pain or tingling in hands or feet; slurred speech; tremor; convulsions; partial paralysis; exaggerated reflexes; feeling of whirling motion; disorientation with memory loss; psychosis; irritability; aggression; suicidal thoughts.

Guidelines for Use

USE EXACTLY AS PRESCRIBED.

Take as directed. Avoid missing doses. Do not stop taking before consulting your healthcare provider.

If a dose is missed, take it as soon as possible. If several hours have passed or if it is nearing time for the next dose, do not double the dose to catch up, unless advised by your healthcare provider. If more than one dose is missed, contact your healthcare provider.

May cause drowsiness. Use caution while driving or performing other tasks requiring mental alertness, coordination and dexterity.

Avoid alcohol consumption. The risk of seizures is increased.

Notify your healthcare provider if skin rash, mental confusion, dizziness, headache or tremor occurs.

While taking this medicine, blood, kidney and liver studies will be necessary. Regular follow-up visits with your healthcare provider are important.

If you develop an allergic-type reaction or symptoms of toxicity (eg, convulsions, psychosis, depression, confusion, headache, tremor, feeling of a whirling motion, partial paralysis, slurred speech), discontinue the medicine and contact your healthcare provider. Toxicity is closely related to excessive blood levels.

Cyclosporine

(SIGH-kloe-spore-EEN)

Sandimmune, Neoral

A medicine used to prevent rejection of organ or tissue transplants. Used with corticosteroids. It also is used to treat transplant rejection in patients previously treated with other immunosuppressive agents. It occasionally may be prescribed for other reasons.

Precautions

DO NOT USE if you are allergic to this medicine or polyoxyethylated castor oil or if you are breastfeeding.

BEFORE USING THIS MEDICINE, tell your healthcare provider if you are pregnant; or if you are taking, will be taking or stop taking any prescription or nonprescription medicine; or if you have any other medical conditions.

Side Effects

Every medicine can cause side effects, but many people have no, or minor, side effects. Tell your healthcare provider if any of the following occurs: nausea; vomiting; stomach pain or discomfort; appetite loss; diarrhea; confusion; seizures; depression; tremors; headache; rash; itching; acne; unusual hair growth; brittle fingernails; flushing; night sweats; difficult urination; blood in urine; unusual growth of the gums; numbness or tingling in hands or feet; swelling of or lumps in the breast (male or female); swelling; fever; hearing loss; ringing in the ears; visual disturbance; signs of infection; muscle cramps or pain; hiccups; fever; sore throat; tiredness; frequent or cloudy urine.

Guidelines for Use

USE EXACTLY AS PRESCRIBED.

To improve the flavor, dilute with milk, chocolate milk or orange juice (preferably at room temperature).

Do not stop taking this medication unless advised to do so by your healthcare provider.

See your healthcare provider regularly to ensure that the medicine is working properly and that no serious side effects are developing.

Use a glass container when taking this medication.

Do not allow it to stand before drinking. Stir oral solution well and drink all at once. Rinse glass and drink again to ensure that the entire dose was taken.

Contact your healthcare provider if fever, sore throat, tiredness or unusual bleeding or bruising occurs.

Use mechanical contraceptive measures (eg, diaphragm, condom) during treatment. Do not use oral contraceptives.

While taking this medication, kidney and liver studies will be necessary.

Practice good oral hygiene and have regular dental checkups.

Cyproheptadine Hydrochloride

(sip-row-HEP-tuh-deen HIGH-droe-KLOR-ide)

Periactin

A medicine used for relief of allergy symptoms and symptoms associated with hives (mild and uncomplicated), some insect bites and stings and skin conditions with mild to moderate itching.

Precautions

DO NOT USE if you are allergic to this medicine or its relatives; are breastfeeding; or are taking monoamine oxidase inhibitors (MAOIs, eg, *Nardil*, *Parnate*).

BEFORE USING THIS MEDICINE, tell your healthcare provider if you are pregnant; or if you are taking, will be taking or stop taking any prescription or nonprescription medicine; or if you have any other medical conditions.

Side Effects

Every medicine can cause side effects, but many people have no, or minor, side effects. Tell your healthcare provider if any of the following occurs: drowsiness; dizziness; dry mouth; stomach upset; constipation; blurred vision; difficult urination; confusion; fainting; irregular heartbeat.

Guidelines for Use

USE EXACTLY AS PRESCRIBED.

Take with food.

This drug may cause drowsiness or dizziness. Use caution while driving or performing tasks requiring mental alertness, coordination or physical dexterity. Avoid alcohol and drowsiness-causing medicines.

May be used when sneezing and runny nose exist but nasal congestion is slight. When more severe nasal congestion occurs with sneezing and runny nose, an oral or topical decongestant also may be used.

Use with caution in the presence of liver disease.

Do not take for several days before allergy skin testing.

Cysteamine Bitartrate

(sis-tea-UH mean by- TAR-trate)

Cystagon

A urinary tract product used to manage nephropathic cystinosis (a rare, serious kidney disease) in children and adults. This disease may cause kidney failure, other organ damage or growth reduction.

Precautions

DO NOT USE if you are allergic to this medicine or to penicillamine (eg, *Cuprimine*). Do not begin or continue use of this medicine if a skin rash is present; contact your healthcare provider.

BEFORE USING THIS MEDICINE, tell your healthcare provider if you are pregnant or breastfeeding; if you are taking; will be taking or stop taking any prescription or nonprescription medicine; or if you have any other medical conditions.

Side Effects

Every medicine can cause side effects, but many people have no, or minor, side effects. Tell your healthcare provider if any of the following occurs: vomiting; diarrhea; appetite loss; nausea; bad breath; rash; constipation; stomach ache; indigestion; fever; tiredness; headache; convulsions; seizures; incoordination; confusion; impaired hearing; dizziness; hives; nervousness; abnormal thinking; emotions or dreams; dehydration; flushing; lightheadedness.

Guidelines for Use

USE EXACTLY AS PRESCRIBED.

Take in four divided doses about 6 hours apart, or as directed.

Young children may not be able to swallow the capsules. Contents of the capsules should be sprinkled over food or mixed in formula for children under 6 years of age.

Older patients should follow their healthcare provider's instructions with regard to food.

Do not increase or decrease this medicine without your healthcare provider's approval.

If a dose is missed, take it as soon as possible. If several hours have passed or if it is within 2 hours of the next dose, do not double the dose to "catch up," unless advised by your healthcare provider. If more than one dose is missed, contact your healthcare provider.

Contact your healthcare provider if any of the following occurs: rash, fever, seizures, weakness, tiredness, drowsiness, incoordination, difficluty breathing, strange behavior, unusual thinking or emotions, depression, nausea, diarrhea, vomitiing, appetite loss, abdominal pain.

Dacarbazine

(da-CAR-buh-zeen)

DTIC-Dome

Used to treat metastatic malignant melanoma; it also is used in combination with other medicines to treat Hodgkin's disease.

Side Effects

Every medicine can cause side effects, but many people have no, or minor, side effects. Tell your healthcare provider if any of the following occurs: loss of appetite; nausea; vomiting; flu-like symptoms (fever, muscle aches, general body discomfort); hair loss; facial flushing; abnormal skin sensations (facial).

Guidelines for Use

USE EXACTLY AS PRESCRIBED.

May cause sensitivity to sunlight. Avoid prolonged exposure to the sun and other ultraviolet light. Use sunscreens and wear protective clothing until tolerance is determined.

Dalteparin Sodium

(dal-TEH-puh-rin SO-dee-uhm)

Fragmin

This medicine is a blood thinner used to prevent deep vein thrombosis (or blood clots) in adults after abdominal surgery.

Precautions

DO NOT USE if you are allergic to this medicine, heparin or pork products; or if you are prone to heavy bleeding.

BEFORE USING THIS MEDICINE, tell your healthcare provider if you are pregnant or breastfeeding; if you are taking, will be taking or stop taking any prescription or nonprescription medicine; or if you have any other medical conditions.

Side Effects

Every medicine can cause side effects, but many people have no, or minor, side effects. Tell your healthcare provider if any of the following occurs: heavy or unusual bleeding/bruising or pain at the injection site.

Guidelines for Use

USE EXACTLY AS PRESCRIBED.

This medicine should be given once daily, with the first dose given 1-2 hours before surgery. Treatment may continue for 5-10 days.

Use proper technique; inject under the skin, NOT into muscle.

If a dose is missed, take it as soon as possible. If more than 12 hours have passed, do not double the dose to "catch up." If more than one dose is missed, contact your healthcare provider.

Contact your healthcare provider if you experience: bleeding, bruising, dizziness, lightheadedness, itching, rash, fever, swelling or difficulty breathing.

Do not use or substitute other blood thinners without first checking with your healthcare provider.

Lab tests may be required to monitor therapy. Be sure to keep appointments.

Injections are given around the navel, upper thigh or buttocks. The injection site will be changed daily.

Store at room temperature.

Danazol

(DAN-uh-ZOLE)

Danocrine

A medicine used to treat pain and infertility caused by endometriosis; to treat fibrocystic breast disease; to treat hereditary angioedema (swelling of the abdominal organs and tissue, extremities, face and airway). It may occasionally be prescribed for other reasons.

Precautions

DO NOT USE if you are allergic to this medicine, or if you are pregnant or breast-feeding.

BEFORE USING THIS MEDICINE, tell your healthcare provider if you are taking, will be taking or stop taking any prescription or nonprescription medicine; or if you have any other medical conditions.

Side Effects

Every medicine can cause side effects, but many people have no, or minor, side effects. Tell your healthcare provider if any of the following occurs: acne; fluid retention; mild abnormal growth of fine body hair; oily skin or hair; weight gain; flushing; sweating; vaginitis (itching, dryness, burning and vaginal bleeding); nervousness; dizziness; headache; sleep disorders; fatigue; tremor; prickling or burning sensation in extremities; visual disturbances; anxiety; depression; appetite changes; chills; fever; hair loss; yellowing of the skin or eyes; muscle cramps or spasms; joint lock-up or swelling; pain in back, neck or legs; blood in urine; change in sex drive; pelvic pain; carpal tunnel syndrome; nasal congestion; decreased breast size; deepening of voice; stomach upset; nausea; vomiting; constipation.

Guidelines for Use

USE EXACTLY AS PRESCRIBED.

Schedule regular visits with your healthcare provider to make sure the medicine is working effectively.

It is common for women taking this medicine to have no, or irregular, menstrual periods. After stopping the medication, menstrual periods should return within 90 days.

Tell your healthcare provider if masculinizing effects occur (eg, abnormal growth of facial or fine body hair, deepening of the voice, acne, decrease in breast size).

Use a nonhormonal birth control method (eg, condom, diaphragm) during therapy. Discontinue use if pregnancy is suspected.

Diabetes — Insulin requirements may increase. Abnormal glucose (sugar) tolerance tests may be seen. Monitor urine and blood sugar levels.

Males (especially teenagers) receiving this medicine should have their semen checked every 3 to 4 months.

Fluid retention caused by this medicine may aggravate epilepsy, migraine, heart or kidney disease.

Report any rash or yellowing of skin or eyes immediately to your healthcare provider.

Dantrolene Sodium Injectable

(dan-troe-LEEN SO-dee-uhm)

Dantrium

A medicine used to treat malignant hyperthermia (life-threatening rapid rises in body temperature resulting from the use of an anesthetic). It also is used after malignant hyperthermia has occurred during an operation to prevent a recurrence.

Precautions

DO NOT USE if patient is allergic to this medicine or is breastfeeding.

BEFORE RECEIVING THIS MEDICINE, tell your healthcare provider if you are pregnant; or if you are taking any prescription medicine; or if you have any other medical conditions.

Side Effects

Every medicine can cause side effects, but many people have no, or minor, side effects. Tell your healthcare provider if any of the following occurs: shortness of breath; hives; pain over a vein; redness of the skin.

Guidelines for Use

USE EXACTLY AS PRESCRIBED.

May decrease the grip strength and increase weakness of leg muscles, especially walking down stairs.

May cause drowsiness, dizziness or lightheadedness. Avoid alcohol and medicines that can cause drowsiness, dizziness or lightheadedness.

Use caution while eating because choking and difficulty swallowing can occur after the medicine is administered.

Notify your healthcare provider if skin rash, itching, bloody or black tarry stools, or yellowish discoloration of the skin or eyes occurs.

Dantrolene Sodium Oral

(dan-troe-LEEN SO-dee-uhm)

Dantrium

A medicine used to treat muscle spasms due to certain nerve disorders (eg, cerebral palsy, multiple sclerosis, spinal cord injury or stroke). It also is given before an operation to prevent malignant hyperthermia (life-threatening rapid rises in body temperature resulting from the use of an anesthetic) or after an operation to prevent a recurrence. It occasionally may be prescribed for other reasons.

Precautions

DO NOT USE if you are allergic to this medicine or are breastfeeding.

BEFORE USING THIS MEDICINE, tell your healthcare provider if you are pregnant; or if you are taking, will be taking or stop taking any prescription or nonprescription medicine; or if you have any other medical conditions.

Side Effects

Every medicine can cause side effects, but many people have no, or minor, side effects. Tell your healthcare provider if any of the following occurs: increased frequency of urination; blood in urine; loss of urine control; difficulty with urination; frequent urination at night; diarrhea; nausea; constipation; bleeding; loss of appetite; taste alterations; difficulty swallowing; upset stomach; abdominal cramps; yellowing of skin and eyes; drowsiness; dizziness; difficulty with sleep; depression; confusion; nervousness; weakness; tiredness; vision problems; double vision; headache; swelling, pain and tenderness over a vein; chest pain; unusual hair growth; rash; itching; sweating; general feeling of ill health; sore muscles; backache; chills and fever; feeling of suffocation; excessive tearing.

Guidelines for Use

USE EXACTLY AS PRESCRIBED.

If no apparent benefit is observed after 45 days of treatment, the medicine should be stopped.

May cause drowsiness, dizziness or lightheadedness. Use caution when driving or performing other tasks requiring mental alertness, coordination and dexterity. Avoid alcohol and medicines that can cause drowsiness, dizziness or lightheadedness.

Use caution while eating because choking and difficulty swallowing can occur after the medicine is administered.

May cause sensitivity to sunlight. Avoid prolonged exposure to the sun. Use sunscreen and wear protective clothing until tolerance is determined.

May cause weakness, malaise, fatigue, nausea and diarrhea. Notify your healthcare provider if these effects persist.

Notify your healthcare provider if skin rash, itching, bloody or black tarry stools, or yellowish discoloration of the skin or eyes occurs.

Desipramine Hydrochloride

(dess-IPP-ruh-meen HIGH-droe-KLOR-ide)

Norpramin, Pertofrane

A mood elevating medicine usually used for the relief of depression. It occasionally may prescribe it for other reasons.

Precautions

DO NOT USE if you are allergic to this medicine or its relatives, or if you are using monoamine oxidase inhibitors (eg, Nardil, Parnate).

BEFORE USING THIS MEDICINE, tell your healthcare provider if you are pregnant or breastfeeding; or if you are taking, will be taking or stop taking any prescription or nonprescription medicine; or if you have any other medical conditions.

Side Effects

Every medicine can cause side effects, but many people have no, or minor, side effects. Tell your healthcare provider if any of the following occurs: dry mouth; blurred vision; increased heart rate; impaired coordination; difficult urination; excessive sedation; seizures.

Guidelines for Use

USE EXACTLY AS PRESCRIBED.

Take as directed with a full glass of water, with or without food.

If a dose is missed, take it as soon as possible. If several hours have passed or if it is nearing time for the next dose, do not double the dose to catch up, unless advised by your healthcare provider. If more than one dose is missed, contact your healthcare provider.

This medicine may not be effective for 2 to 3 weeks.

Using this medicine with alcohol or other central nervous system depressants (eg, pain relievers, sedatives, antihistamines) may cause added drowsiness.

May cause drowsiness or blurred vision. Use caution while driving or performing other tasks requiring mental alertness.

May cause sensitivity to sunlight. Avoid prolonged exposure to the sun. Use sunscreens and wear protective clothing until tolerance is determined.

Taking this medicine at bedtime may help reduce side effects (eg, daytime drowsiness). Discuss this possibility with your doctor.

Symptoms of nausea, headache or fatigue may develop after abruptly stopping long-term use.

Desmopressin Acetate

(DESS-moe-PRESS-in ASS-uh-TATE)

DDAVP

A medicine used to treat primary nocturnal bed wetting, central cranial diabetes insipidus, certain types of hemophilia A and von Willebrand's disease (Type I), during surgery and postoperatively. It occasionally may be prescribed for other reasons.

Precautions

DO NOT USE if you are allergic to this medicine.

BEFORE USING THIS MEDICINE, tell your healthcare provider if you are pregnant or breastfeeding; or if you are taking, will be taking or stop taking any prescription or nonprescription medicine; or if you have any other medical conditions.

Side Effects

Every medicine can cause side effects, but many people have no, or minor, side effects. Tell your healthcare provider if any of the following occurs: headache; runny nose; nausea; mild abdominal cramps, vulval pain; facial flushing; nosebleed; sore throat; cough. Injection only: local flushing, swelling, burning pain.

Guidelines for Use

USE EXACTLY AS PRESCRIBED.

Patient instructions provided with the intranasal product. Be sure to review the instructions with your healthcare provider.

Be sure to follow any instructions you have been given by your healthcare provider regarding fluid intake.

If used for bleeding disorder (eg, hemophilia A) and bleeding is not controlled, contact your healthcare provider.

Notify your healthcare provider if headache, shortness of breath, heartburn, nausea, abdominal cramps or vulval pain occurs.

Storage--Refrigerate. Nasal solution may be stored for 3 weeks at room temperature.

Desmopressin

(DESS-moe-PRESS-in)

Stimate

A medicine used to treat some forms of hemophilia A and von Willebrand's disease (Type I). It occasionally may be prescribed for other reasons.

Precautions

DO NOT USE if you are allergic to this medicine.

BEFORE USING THIS MEDICINE, tell your healthcare provider if you are pregnant or breastfeeding; or if you are taking, will be taking or stop taking any prescription or nonprescription medicine; or if you have any other medical conditions.

Side Effects

Every medicine can cause side effects, but many people have no, or minor, side effects. Tell your healthcare provider if any of the following occurs: drowsiness; dizziness; itchy or light-sensitive eyes; sleeplessness; chills; warm feeling; pain; chest pain; pounding in the chest; upset stomach; fluid retention; vomiting; agitation; inflammation of the penis.

Guidelines for Use

USE EXACTLY AS PRESCRIBED.

Patient instructions provided with the intranasal product. Be sure to review the instructions with your healthcare provider.

Be sure to follow any instructions you have been given by your healthcare provider.

If bleeding is not controlled, contact your healthcare provider.

Notify your healthcare provider if headache, shortness of breath, heartburn, nausea, abdominal cramps or vulval pain occurs.

Storage--Refrigerate. Nasal solution may be stored for 3 weeks at room temperature.

The bottle accurately delivers 25 doses; discard any solution remaining after 25 doses. Do not transfer the remaining solution to another bottle.

May cause sensitivity to bright lights. This may be minimized by wearisng sunglasses.

Dexamethasone Ophthalmic

(DEX-uh-METH-uh-sone)

AK-Dex, Decadron Phosphate, Maxidex Ointment

An anti-inflammatory agent for the eye. It works by inhibiting the inflammatory response of tissues to mechanical, chemical or allergy-causing agents.

Precautions

DO NOT USE if you are allergic to this medicine.

BEFORE USING THIS MEDICINE, tell your healthcare provider if you are pregnant or breastfeeding; or if you are taking, will be taking or stop taking any prescription or nonprescription medicine; or if you have any other medical conditions.

Side Effects

Every medicine can cause side effects, but many people have no, or minor, side effects. Tell your healthcare provider if any of the following occurs: visual defects; temporary stinging or burning; muscle weakness.

Guidelines for Use

USE EXACTLY AS PRESCRIBED.

Do not stop using this medicine without consulting your doctor.

May cause sensitivity to light. This may be reduced by wearing sunglasses.

Notify your doctor if improvement is not seen after 7 or 8 days, if condition worsens, or if pain, itching or swelling occurs.

Some of these products may contain sulfite preservatives, which can cause allergic reactions in certain individuals. Check package label when available or consult your healthcare provider.

Dexamethasone

(DEX-uh-METH-sone)

Decadron, Dexone, Hexadrol, Aeroseb-Dex, Decaspray

A hormone used as replacement therapy when the adrenal cortex is not functioning properly. It is also used for its anti-inflammatory action. It occasionally may be prescribe for a variety of other uses.

Precautions

DO NOT USE if you have an allergy to this medicine or its relatives.

BEFORE USING THIS MEDICINE, tell your healthcare provider if you are pregnant or breastfeeding; or if you are taking, will be taking or stop taking any prescription or nonprescription medicine; or if you have any other medical conditions.

Side Effects

Every medicine can cause side effects, but many people have no, or minor, side effects. Tell your healthcare provider if any of the following occurs: appearance of round, swollen moonface; fat deposits (eg, shoulders, midsection); nausea; vomiting; increased appetite; weight gain; peptic ulcer; rectal bleeding with the enema dose form; seizures; dizziness; headache; behavior changes; sleeplessness; hiccups; fluid retention; low or high blood pressure; irregular heart rhythm; impaired wound healing; thinning of skin and layer of fat under the skin; excessive pigmentation of skin; acne; excessive body hair growth; rash; hives; loss of muscle mass; osteoporosis; bone fractures; menstrual irregularities; growth suppression in children; higher blood sugar levels.

Guidelines for Use

USE EXACTLY AS PRESCRIBED.

Oral: May cause stomach upset. Take with meals or snacks.

Take single daily or alternate day doses in the morning prior to 9 a.m. Take multiple doses at evenly spaced intervals throughout the day.

Patients on long-term therapy should carry identification.

Notify your healthcare provider if any of the above side effects occur.

High dose or long-term therapy: DO NOT change or stop therapy unless directed by your doctor. Sudden withdrawal of therapy may cause symptoms of fatigue, loss of appetite, nausea, vomiting, diarrhea, weight loss, weakness, dizziness and low blood sugar.

Diabetes — May require increased doses of insulin or oral diabetes (hypoglycemic) medications.

Cream: Apply in a light film; rub in gently.

Aerosol: Shake well and spray on affected area holding container about 3 to 6 inches away. Spray for about 2 seconds to cover an area the size of your hand. Take care not to inhale the vapors. If you are spraying your face or near your face, cover your eyes.

Dextroamphetamine Sulfate

(DEX-troe-am-FET-uh-meen SULL-fate)

Dexedrine, Ferndex, Oxydess II, Spancap No. 1

A medicine that is used to treat narcolepsy, attention deficit disorder in children and as a short-term addition in a weight reduction program.

Precautions

DO NOT USE if you are allergic to this medicine; if you have drug abuse tendencies or an irritable or excitable personality; or if you have a thyroid condition, heart disease or glaucoma.

BEFORE USING THIS MEDICINE, tell your healthcare provider if you are pregnant or breastfeeding; or if you are taking, will be taking or stop taking any prescription or nonprescription medicines; or if you have any other medical conditions.

Side Effects

Every medicine can cause side effects, but many people have no, or minor, side effects. Tell your healthcare provider if any of the following occurs: diarrhea; constipation; nausea; stomach cramps; psychological problems; headache; anxiety; tension; nervousness; dizziness; depression (between doses or after stopping); inability to sleep; excessive restlessness; irritability; pounding in the chest; rash; flushing; sweating; hives; fever; muscle tremor or twitching; sexual problems; fatigue between doses or after stopping; weight loss (children); stunted growth (children); rapid breathing/panting.

Guidelines for Use

USE EXACTLY AS PRESCRIBED.

Take early in the day to avoid nighttime sleep loss.

This medicine may impair your ability to drive or perform other tasks requiring alertness, coordination, and physical dexterity.

May mask extreme fatigue and cause dizziness.

May cause nervousness, restlessness, sleeplessness, dizziness and digestive tract disturbances. Tell your healthcare provider if these effects become pronounced.

Attention deficit disorder in children--Your doctor may occasionally interrupt therapy to determine if there is a recurrence of symptoms.

Weight control--Appropriate lifestyle changes (eg, diet and exercise) should be made while on therapy. Use beyond 8 to 12 weeks is not encouraged.

Elixir--Contains alcohol.

Sustained release capsule--Do not crush or chew.

Dextromethorphan

(DEX-troe-meth-OR-fan)

Children's Hold, Delsym, Hold DM, Pertussin CS, Robitussin Cough Calmers, Robitussin Pediatric, Scot-Tussin DM Cough Chasers, St. Joseph Cough Suppressant, Sucrets Cough Control, Suppress, Trocal

Used to relieve or suppress nonproductive cough (no mucous production) or cough due to colds or allergy.

Precautions

DO NOT USE if you are allergic to this medicine.

BEFORE USING THIS MEDICINE, tell your healthcare provider if you are pregnant or breastfeeding; or if you are taking, will be taking or stop taking any prescription or nonprescription medicine; or if you have any other medical conditions.

Side Effects

Every medicine can cause side effects, but many people have no, or minor, side effects. Tell your healthcare provider if any of the following occurs: constipation; nausea; stomach upset; mild dizziness; itching; nasal congestion; difficulty breathing; drowsiness; rash.

Guidelines for Use

USE EXACTLY AS PRESCRIBED.

Do not exceed recommended dose.

Do not take for persistent or chronic cough, such as occurs with smoking, asthma or emphysema or where cough is accompanied by excessive secretions, except under supervision of your healthcare provider.

If cough continues beyond 7 to 10 days or is accompanied by a fever, consult your healthcare provider.

Diazepam

(DIE-aze-uh-pam)

Valium, Valrelease, Zetran

A benzodiazepine medicine generally used to treat anxiety.

Precautions

DO NOT USE if you are allergic to this medicine or its relatives, or if you are breastfeeding.

BEFORE USING THIS MEDICINE, tell your healthcare provider if you are pregnant; or if you are taking, will be taking or stop taking any prescription or nonprescription medicine; or if you have any other medical conditions.

Side Effects

Every medicine can cause side effects, but many people have no, or minor, side effects. Tell your healthcare provider if any of the following occurs: stomach upset; constipation; diarrhea; appetite change; vomiting; confusion; depression; nervousness; memory loss; drowsiness; fatigue; dizziness; crying; vivid dreams; headache; seizures; itching; rash; hair growth; yellowing of skin or eyes; visual or hearing disturbances; slurred speech; change in bladder function; change in sex drive; menstrual problems; dry mouth; fever; tremors/uncontrollable muscle movement; difficult breathing; swelling; excessive perspiration; joint pain; weight gain or loss; fainting.

Guidelines for Use

USE EXACTLY AS PRESCRIBED.

May be taken with food or water if stomach upset occurs.

If a dose is missed, take it as soon as possible. If several hours have passed or it is nearing time for the next dose, do not double the dose to catch up, unless advised by your healthcare provider. If more than one dose is missed, contact your healthcare provider.

May cause drowsiness. Use caution while driving or performing other tasks requiring mental alertness, coordination and dexterity. Avoid alcohol and other medication that cause drowsiness while taking this medication (eg, sleeping pills, antihistamines).

If excitement, stimulation or acute rage occurs tell your healthcare provider.

Patients on long-term or high dosage therapy may have withdrawal symptoms if therapy is suddenly stopped.

Do not stop therapy abruptly or change dosage without asking your healthcare provider.

Carry identification if this medicine is used for seizures.

Diazoxide Oral

(DIE-aze-OX-ide)

Proglycem

A medicine used in the management of hypoglycemia (low blood sugar) due to hyperinsulinism.

Precautions

DO NOT USE if you are allergic to this medicine or any other thiazide or if you have low blood sugar (other than due to hyperinsulinism).

BEFORE USING THIS MEDICINE, tell your healthcare provider if you are pregnant or breastfeeding; or if you are taking, will be taking, or stop taking any prescription or nonprescription medicine; or if you have any other medical conditions.

Side Effects

Every medicine can cause side effects, but many people have no, or minor, side effects. Tell your healthcare provider if any of the following occurs: fluid retention; loss of appetite; nausea; vomiting; abdominal pain; diarrhea; temporary loss of taste; pounding in the chest; chest pain; decreased urination; blood in the urine; headache; weakness; general body discomfort; anxiety; dizziness; sleeplessness; abnormal sensations; blurred vision; double vision; excessive tearing; abnormal hairiness; skin rash; itching; herpes; loss of scalp hair; gout; excessive/spontaneous flow of breast milk; enlargement or lump in breast; fever.

Guidelines for Use

USE EXACTLY AS PRESCRIBED.

Follow all dietary instructions.

If a dose is missed, take it as soon as possible. If several hours have passed or if it is nearing time for the next dose, do not double the dose to catch up, unless advised by your healthcare provider. If more than one dose is missed, contact your healthcare provider.

Monitor urine regularly for glucose and ketones. Report any abnormalities to your healthcare provider.

Promptly report increased urinary frequency, increased thirst, fruity breath odor.

Suspension--Protect from light.

Diclofenac Ophthalmic

(die-KLOE-fen-ak)

Voltaren

A medicine used for the relief of redness, soreness and irritation after cataract surgery. It occasionally may be prescribed for other reasons.

Precautions

DO NOT USE if you are allergic to this medicine or its relatives, or if you wear soft contact lenses.

BEFORE USING THIS MEDICINE, tell your healthcare provider if you are pregnant or breastfeeding; or if you are taking, will be taking or stop taking any prescription or nonprescription medicine; or if you have other medical conditions.

Side Effects

Every medicine can cause side effects, but many people have no, or minor, side effects. Tell your healthcare provider if any of the following occurs: temporary burning or stinging; irritation; redness/burning (contact lens wearers); inflammation of outer membrane of eye; eye allergy; nausea; vomiting.

Guidelines for Use

USE EXACTLY AS PRESCRIBED.

For use in the eye.

Contact your healthcare provider if you have experienced bleeding tendencies, are on medicines that prolong bleeding time (eg, blood thinners).

Tell your healthcare provider if you have herpes simplex of the eye.

Mild burning or stinging after instillation is no cause for alarm unless symptoms persist or worsen.

Diclofenac Oral

(die-KLOE-fen-ak)

Voltaren

A nonsteroidal anti-inflammatory medicine (NSAID) generally used to treat osteoarthritis (degenerative joint disease) and rheumatoid arthritis. It occasionally may be prescribed for other reasons.

Precautions

DO NOT USE if you are allergic to this medicine or its relatives, aspirin or iodides.

BEFORE USING THIS MEDICINE, tell your healthcare provider if you are pregnant or breastfeeding; use alcohol chronically; are prone to fluid retention; or if you are taking, will be taking or stop taking any prescription or nonprescription medicines; or have any other medical conditions.

Side Effects

Every medicine can cause side effects, but many people have no, or minor, side effects. Tell your healthcare provider if any of the following occurs: allergic reaction (eg, rash, itching, fever); changes in vision; weight gain; fluid retention; stomach problems (eg, nausea, vomiting, diarrhea, pain); black stools; constipation; persistent headache; dizziness; nervousness; weakness; ringing in the ears; taste changes; unusual bruising or bleeding.

Guidelines for Use

USE EXACTLY AS PRESCRIBED.

Avoid aspirin and alcoholic beverages.

If stomach upset occurs, take with food, milk or antacids. If stomach pain continues, tell your healthcare provider.

If a dose is missed, take it as soon as possible. If several hours have passed or if it is nearing time for the next dose, do not double the dose to catch up, unless advised by your healthcare provider. If more than one dose is missed, contact your healthcare provider.

May cause drowsiness or dizziness. Observe caution while driving or performing other tasks requiring mental alertness, coordination and dexterity.

May cause sensitivity to sunlight. Avoid prolonged exposure to the sun. Use sunscreens and wear protective clothing until tolerance is determined.

Diclofenac Potassium

(die-KLOE-fen-ak)

Cataflam

A nonsteroidal anti-inflammatory medicine (NSAID) used for the relief of mild pain; arthritis, ankylosing spondylitis; and menstrual cramps.

Precautions

DO NOT USE if you are allergic to this medicine, aspirin or any other nonsteroidal anti-inflammatory medicine.

BEFORE USING THIS MEDICINE, tell your healthcare provider if you are pregnant or breastfeeding; use alcohol chronically; are prone to fluid retention; or if you are taking, will be taking or stop taking any prescription or nonprescription medicine; or if you have any other medical conditions.

Side Effects

Every medicine can cause side effects, but many people have no, or minor, side effects. Tell your healthcare provider if any of the following occurs: abdominal pain or cramps; headache; abdominal swelling; diarrhea; indigestion; nausea; constipation; fluid retention (edema); gas; dizziness; rash; itching; ringing in the ears; swelling of eyelids, lips, or throat; difficulty breathing.

Guidelines for Use

USE EXACTLY AS PRESCRIBED.

If stomach upset occurs, take with food or milk or antacids. If stomach pain continues, call your healthcare provider. If a dose is missed, take it as soon as possible. If several hours have passed or if it is nearing time for the next dose, do not double the dose to catch up, unless advised by your healthcare provider. If more than one dose is missed, contact your healthcare provider.

May cause drowsiness or dizziness. Observe caution while driving or performing other tasks requiring mental alertness, coordination and dexterity.

May cause sensitivity to sunlight. Avoid prolonged exposure to the sun. Use sunscreens and wear protective clothing until tolerance is determined.

Avoid the use of aspirin and alcoholic beverages while taking this medicine.

Dicloxacillin Sodium

(DIE-klox-uh-SILL-in SO-dee-uhm)

Dycill, Dynapen, Pathocil

A penicillin antibiotic used to treat infections caused by certain bacteria.

Precautions

DO NOT USE if you are allergic to any cephalosporin or penicillin.

BEFORE USING THIS MEDICINE, tell your healthcare provider if you are pregnant or breastfeeding; or if you are taking, will be taking or stop taking any prescription or nonprescription medicine; or if you have any other medical conditions.

Side Effects

Every medicine can cause side effects, but many people have no, or minor, side effects. Tell your healthcare provider if any of the following occurs: itching; rash; hives; severe diarrhea; shortness of breath; wheezing; dizziness; black tongue; nausea; vomiting; swollen joints; or any unusual bleeding or bruising; sore throat; fever.

Guidelines for Use

USE EXACTLY AS PRESCRIBED.

Take on an empty stomach approximately 30 minutes to one hour before meals or two hours after a meal.

Take at even intervals, preferably around the clock.

If a dose is missed, take it as soon as possible. If several hours have passed or if it is nearing time for the next dose, do not double the dose to "catch up," unless advised by your healthcare provider. If more than one dose is missed, contact your healthcare provider.

Continue until all the prescribed medicine has been taken. Failure to take a full course of therapy may cause a relapse of the infection.

Suspension: Store in the refrigerator. Do not freeze. Shake well before using.

Dicyclomine Hydrochloride

(die-SIGH-kloe-meen HIGH-droe-KLOR-ide)

Antispas, Bemote, Bentyl, Byclomine, Dibent, Neoquess, Spasmoject

A medicine used to treat certain stomach and intestinal disorders.

Precautions

DO NOT USE if you are allergic to this medicine or to the dye tartrazine. This medicine may cause excitement, agitation, drowsiness and other mental reactions in the elderly.

BEFORE USING THIS MEDICINE, tell your healthcare provider if you are pregnant or breastfeeding; or if you are taking, will be taking or stop taking any prescription or nonprescription medicine; or if you have any other medical conditions.

Side Effects

Every medicine can cause side effects, but many people have no, or minor, side effects. Tell your healthcare provider if any of the following occurs: excitement; tremors; hallucinations; delirium; uncoordinated walking; seizures; headache; nervousness; drowsiness; dizziness; inability to sleep; pounding in the chest; difficult breathing; nasal congestion; itching; rash; flushing; decreased sweating; difficult urination; eye pain; muscle weakness or loss of muscle function; dry mouth; altered taste perception; difficulty swallowing; urine retention; impotence; blurred vision; sensitivity to light; reduced breast milk production and flow; thirst; fever; widening pupils.

Guidelines for Use

USE EXACTLY AS PRESCRIBED.

Take 30 minutes before meals.

May cause drowsiness. Use caution when driving or performing other tasks requiring mental alertness or coordination.

May cause dry mouth, difficulty in urination, constipation or increased sensitivity to light, skin rash, flushing or eye pain. Notify your healthcare provider if these effects persist or become severe.

These products may cause drying of the eyes. Contact lens wearers should use appropriate lubricating solution while taking this medicine.

May cause sensitivity to bright lights. This may be minimized by wearing sunglasses.

Didanosine (ddI; dideoxyinosine)

(die-DAN-oh-SEEN)

Videx

A medicine used for the treatment of advanced HIV infection.

Precautions

DO NOT USE if you are allergic to this medicine or if you are breastfeeding. Children should have an eye examination every six months or if a change in vision occurs.

BEFORE USING THIS MEDICINE, tell your healthcare provider if you are pregnant; or if you are taking, will be taking or stop taking any prescription or nonprescription medicine; or if you have any other medical conditions.

Side Effects

Every medicine can cause side effects, but many people have no, or minor, side effects. Tell your healthcare provider if any of the following occurs: Adults: diarrhea; nausea; vomiting; stomach pain; appetite loss; weight loss; indigestion; gas; constipation; headache; numbness; tingling or pain in the feet or hands; weakness; sleeplessness; seizures; confusion; nervousness; dizziness; infection; fluid retention; muscle pain; mouth swelling; arthritis (pain or swelling in the joints); taste changes; dry mouth; hair loss; cough; rash.

Children: appetite changes; weight loss; stomach pain; constipation; diarrhea; nausea; vomiting; bloody stools; black vomit; dizziness; lethargy; nervousness; headache; sleeplessness; poor coordination; weakness; seizures; cough; difficulty breathing; runny nose; congestion; sweating; rash; itching; redness; hair loss; flu-like symptoms; chills; fever; sore throat; numbness or tingling in hands/feet; joint/muscle pain; ear/hearing problems; sensitivity to light; dry mouth; mouth sores; nosebleed; vision problems; frequent urination.

Guidelines for Use

USE EXACTLY AS PRESCRIBED.

This medicine is not a cure for HIV infection. You may still acquire illnesses associated with AIDS or ARC (AIDS-Related Complex). Tell your healthcare provider if any significant change in your health occurs.

Take this medicine on an empty stomach.

This medicine does NOT reduce the risk of transmitting HIV to others through sexual contact or blood contamination.

Alcohol and certain medicines may increase the toxic effects of this medicine. Check with your healthcare provider before use.

Pediatric oral solution--Shake well before using. Store in refrigerator.

Oral solution--Open packet carefully and pour contents into 4 ounces of water (only); stir until completely dissolved (2 to 3 minutes); drink entire solution.

Diethylpropion Hydrochloride

(die-ETH-uhl-PRO-pee-ahn HIGH-droe-KLOR-ide)

Tenuate, Tenuate Dospan, Tepanil, Tepanil Ten-Tab

For short-term use (8 to 12 weeks) as part of an overall diet plan to reduce weight. It occasionally may be prescribed for other reasons.

Precautions

DO NOT USE if you are allergic to this medicine.

BEFORE USING THIS MEDICINE, tell your healthcare provider if you are pregnant or breastfeeding; or if you are taking, will be taking or stop taking any prescription or nonprescription medicine; or if you have any other medical conditions.

Side Effects

Every medicine can cause side effects, but many people have no, or minor, side effects. Tell your healthcare provider if any of the following occurs: nausea; vomiting; constipation; stomach cramps; diarrhea; restlessness; tremor; nervousness; anxiety; tension; confusion; sleeplessness; fainting; overstimulation; weakness; headache; pounding in the chest; chest pain; hair loss; flushing; chills; sweating; hives; dry mouth; unpleasant taste; muscle aches; menstrual changes; sexual problems; blurred vision; eye irritation; rapid breathing/panting; rash; fever; dizziness.

Guidelines for Use

USE EXACTLY AS PRESCRIBED.

Appetite suppressants are not a substitute for proper dieting. Make lifestyle changes (eg, diet and exercise) while on therapy to avoid continued use of these products.

Take one hour before meals.

May cause sleeplessness. Avoid taking this medicine late in the day.

Avoid alcohol.

May produce dizziness or blurred vision. Use caution while driving or performing other tasks requiring mental alertness, coordination and dexterity.

May cause dry mouth and constipation. Tell your healthcare provider if these become pronounced or if pounding in the chest, nervousness or dizziness occurs.

Use of this medicine to improve athletic skills, mental alertness or to stay awake is dangerous and illegal.

Never share medicine with others.

Sustained release--Do not crush or chew.

Diethylstilbestrol (DES)

(die-ETH-uhl-still-BESS-trahl)

A hormone used to treat advanced cancer of the prostate gland in men.

Precautions

DO NOT USE if you are allergic to this medicine, or if you have breast cancer or other forms of cancer, have blood clots or are a woman.

BEFORE USING THIS MEDICINE, tell your healthcare provider if you are taking, will be taking or stop taking any prescription or nonprescription medicine; or if you have any other medical conditions.

Side Effects

Every medicine can cause side effects, but many people have no, or minor, side effects. Tell your healthcare provider if any of the following occurs: nausea; vomiting; stomach cramps; bloating; diarrhea; headache; migraine; dizziness; fainting; depression; weakness; seizures; unusual body movements; loss of scalp hair; excessive hair growth; oversensitivity to sunlight or tanning lamps; itching; rash; hives; skin discoloration including yellowing of the skin; intolerance to contact lenses; weight gain or loss; breast tenderness and enlargement; breast milk secretion; pain in groin or calves; chest pain; shortness of breath; vision problems; fluid retention; change in sex drive.

Guidelines for Use

USE EXACTLY AS PRESCRIBED.

If a dose is missed, take it as soon as possible. If several hours have passed or if it is nearing time for the next dose, do not double the dose to catch up, unless advised by your doctor. If more than one dose is missed, contact your healthcare provider.

May cause sensitivity to sunlight. Avoid prolonged exposure to the sun. Use sunscreens and wear protective clothing until tolerance is determined.

Those who wear contact lenses may notice a change in their vision. Lens wear may not be possible.

Lab test will be required to monitor treatment. Be sure to keep appointments.

Diabetic patients should be prepared to monitor their blood sugar levels more frequently. Loss of glucose may occur.

Store at room temperature. Protect from light.

Diflunisal

(die-FLOO-nih-sal)

Dolobid

An aspirin-related medicine used to relieve mild to moderate pain and inflammation and to treat osteoarthritis (degenerative joint disease) and rheumatoid arthritis. It occasionally may be prescribe for other reasons.

Precautions

DO NOT USE if you are allergic to this medicine or its relatives, aspirin or iodides.

BEFORE USING THIS MEDICINE, tell your healthcare provider if you are pregnant or breastfeeding; use alcohol chronically; are prone to fluid retention; or if you are taking, will be taking or stop taking any prescription or nonprescription medicines; or have any other medical conditions.

Side Effects

Every medicine can cause side effects, but many people have no, or minor, side effects. Tell your healthcare provider if any of the following occurs: allergic reaction (eg, rash, itching, fever); changes in vision; weight gain; fluid retention; stomach problems (eg, nausea, vomiting, diarrhea, pain); black stools; constipation; persistent headache; dizziness; nervousness; weakness; ringing in the ears; taste changes; unusual bruising or bleeding.

Guidelines for Use

USE EXACTLY AS PRESCRIBED.

Avoid aspirin and alcoholic beverages.

If stomach upset occurs, take with food, milk or antacids. If stomach pain continues, tell your healthcare provider.

If a dose is missed, take it as soon as possible. If several hours have passed or if it is nearing time for the next dose, do not double the dose to catch up, unless advised by your healthcare provider. If more than one dose is missed, contact your healthcare provider.

May cause drowsiness or dizziness. Observe caution while driving or performing other tasks requiring mental alertness, coordination and dexterity.

May cause sensitivity to sunlight. Avoid prolonged exposure to the sun. Use sunscreens and wear protective clothing until tolerance is determined.

Digitoxin

(dih-juh-TOX-in)

Crystodigin

A heart medicine that improves the heart's pumping action in congestive heart failure and helps the heart rhythm when the heart is beating too fast or too irregularly to function normally.

Precautions

DO NOT USE if you are allergic to this medicine or experience some type of irregular heartbeat.

BEFORE USING THIS MEDICINE, tell your healthcare provider if you are pregnant or breastfeeding; or if you are taking, will be taking or stop taking any prescription or nonprescription medicine; or if you have any other medical conditions.

Side Effects

Every medicine can cause side effects, but many people have no, or minor, side effects. Tell your healthcare provider if any of the following occurs: loss of appetite; lower stomach pain; nausea; vomiting; diarrhea; unusual tiredness or weakness; irregular heartbeat; drowsiness; depression; headache; blurred or yellow vision; skin rash; itching or hives.

Guidelines for Use

USE EXACTLY AS PRESCRIBED.

This medicine must be taken consistently, generally at the same time of day, usually in the morning.

It can be taken without regard to meals.

Do not stop taking medication without first checking with your healthcare provider.

It is important to keep regular appointments with your healthcare provider, to make sure this medicine is working properly.

Avoid nonprescription antacids, cough, cold, allergy and diet medicines unless you ask your healthcare provider.

Digoxin

(dih-JOX-in)

Lanoxicaps, Lanoxin

A heart medicine that improves the heart's pumping action in congestive heart failure and helps the heart rhythm when the heart is beating too fast or too irregularly to function normally.

Precautions

DO NOT USE if you are allergic to this medicine, have taken too much of this medicine or experience some type of irregular heartbeat.

BEFORE USING THIS MEDICINE, tell your healthcare provider if you are pregnant or breastfeeding; or if you are taking, will be taking or stop taking any prescription or nonprescription medicine; or if you have any other medical conditions.

Side Effects

Every medicine can cause side effects, but many people have no, or minor, side effects. Tell your healthcare provider if any of the following occurs: loss of appetite; lower stomach pain; nausea; vomiting; diarrhea; unusual tiredness or weakness; irregular heartbeat; drowsiness; depression; headache; blurred or yellow vision; skin rash; itching or hives.

Guidelines for Use

USE EXACTLY AS PRESCRIBED.

This medicine must be taken consistently, generally at the same time of day, usually in the morning.

It can be taken without regard to meals.

Do not stop taking medication without first checking with your healthcare provider.

It is important to keep regular appointments with your healthcare provider, to make sure this medicine is working properly.

Avoid nonprescription antacids, cough, cold, allergy and diet medicines unless you ask your healthcare provider.

Dihydroergotamine Mesylate

(DIE-high-droe-err-GOT-uh-meen MEH-sih-LATE)

D.H.E. 45

A medicine used to abort or prevent vascular headaches such as migraine, migraine variant and cluster headaches.

Precautions

DO NOT USE if you are allergic to this medicine, are pregnant or may become pregnant, or are breastfeeding.

BEFORE USING THIS MEDICINE, tell your healthcare provider if you are taking, will be taking or stop taking any prescription or nonprescription medicine; or if you have any other medical conditions.

Side Effects

Every medicine can cause side effects, but many people have no, or minor, side effects. Tell your healthcare provider if any of the following occurs: nausea; vomiting; numbness and tingling of fingers and toes; muscle pain in the extremities; weakness in the legs; chest pain; fluid retention; itching; irritation at the injection site.

Guidelines for Use

USE EXACTLY AS PRESCRIBED.

Start therapy at the first sign of attack. Do NOT exceed the maximum dose or prescribed duration of therapy.

Avoid alcohol, smoking and exposure to cold. These can aggravate migraine headaches.

Notify your healthcare provider if any of the following occurs: irregular heart beat, chest pain, nausea, vomiting, numbness or tingling of fingers or toes or pain or weakness of extremities, itching or swelling.

Diltiazem Hydrochloride

(dill-TIE-uh-zem HIGH-droe-KLOR-ide)

Cardizem, Cardizem CD, Cardizem SR, Dilacor XR

A calcium channel blocker medicine that is used to treat high blood pressure and chronic stable angina in adults. It may be used alone or in combination with other blood pressure products. It occasionally may be prescribed for other reasons.

Precautions

DO NOT USE if you are allergic to this medicine.

BEFORE USING THIS MEDICINE, tell your healthcare provider if you are pregnant or breastfeeding; or if you are taking, will be taking or stop taking any prescription or nonprescription medicine; or if you have any other medical conditions.

Side Effects

Every medicine can cause side effects, but many people have no, or minor, side effects. Tell your healthcare provider if any of the following occurs: increased frequency/severity of angina; shortness of breath; swelling of hands and feet; dizziness or light headedness; headache; sore throat; running nose; increased cough; flu-like symptoms; muscle, back, joint and stomach pain; diarrhea; vomiting; sinus discomfort; weakness; indigestion; flushing; ringing in the ears; abnormal dreams; constipation; nausea; symptoms of a drug allergy (eg, itching, rash, hives, difficult breathing); gum enlargement; unusual bruising or bleeding.

Guidelines for Use

USE EXACTLY AS PRESCRIBED.

Take this medicine in the morning on an empty stomach.

Do not open, crush or chew capsules; they should be swallowed whole.

If a dose is missed, take it as soon as possible. If several hours have passed or if it is nearing time for the next dose, do not double the dose to "catch up," unless advised by your healthcare provider. If more than one dose is missed, contact your healthcare provider.

Do not suddenly stop taking this medicine as this may cause serious health problems. This can be minimized if the medicine is tapered slowly by your healthcare provider.

It is important to brush and floss your teeth and see your dentist regularly.

Contact your healthcare provider if any of the following occurs: irregular heartbeat, difficulty breathing, swelling of hands or feet, pronounced dizziness, constipation, nausea or rash.

Low blood pressure may occur (usually as dizziness or lightheadedness). Tell your healthcare provider if this occurs, especially from a lying or sitting position. Use caution while driving or performing other tasks requiring mental alertness.

Lab tests may be required. Be sure to keep appointments.

Store at room temperature.

Keep out of the reach of children.

Dimenhydrinate

(die-men-HIGH-drih-nate)

Calm-X, Dimetabs, Dommanate, Dramamine, Dramanate, Dramoject, Dymenate, Hydrate, Nico-Vert, Triptone, Vertab, Wehamine

A medicine used to treat nausea, vomiting, motion sickness and vertigo (feeling of whirling motion).

Precautions

DO NOT USE if you are allergic to this medicine.

BEFORE USING THIS MEDICINE, tell your healthcare provider if you are pregnant or breastfeeding; or if you are taking, will be taking or stop taking any prescription or nonprescription medicine; or if you have any other medical conditions.

Side Effects

Every medicine can cause side effects, but many people have no, or minor, side effects. Tell your healthcare provider if any of the following occurs: nausea; vomiting; constipation; diarrhea; drowsiness (common); nervousness; insomnia (especially in children); difficult urination; rash; blurred vision; dry mouth; difficult breathing.

Guidelines for Use

USE EXACTLY AS PRESCRIBED.

For motion sickness, the first dose should be taken 30 minutes before exposure to motion.

Avoid alcohol and other depressants (eg, sleeping pills, tranquilizers, narcotic pain relievers, antihistamines).

May cause drowsiness or blurred vision. Use caution while driving or performing other tasks requiring mental alertness or coordination.

May cause dry mouth.

Diphenhydramine Hydrochloride

(die-fen-HIGH-druh-meen HIGH-droe-KLOR-ide)

AllerMax, Banophen, Belix, Benadryl, Benahist, Ben-Allergin-50, Benoject, Benylin Cough, Bydramine Cough, Compoz Nightime Sleep Aid, Diphen Cough, Diphenacen-50, Genahist, Gen-D-phen, Hydramine, Hydramyn, Hyrexin-50, Maximum Strength Sleepinal, Maximum Strength Unisom SleepGels, Nidryl, Nytol, Phendry, Sleep-Eze 3, Sleepwell 2–nite, Sominex, Tusstat, Twilite, UniBent Cough, Wehdryl

A medicine used for several different problems including relief of allergy symptoms, hives (mild and uncomplicated), some insect bites/stings, skin rash with mild to moderate itching, cough, motion sickness and Parkinson's disease.

Precautions

DO NOT USE if you are allergic to this medicine or its relatives; are breastfeeding; or are taking monoamine oxidase inhibitors (MAOIs).

BEFORE USING THIS MEDICINE, tell your healthcare provider if you are pregnant; or if you are taking, will be taking or stop taking any prescription or nonprescription medicine; or if you have any other medical conditions.

Side Effects

Every medicine can cause side effects, but many people have no, or minor, side effects. Tell your healthcare provider if any of the following occurs: drowsiness; dizziness; dry mouth; stomach upset; constipation; blurred vision; rash; hives; difficult breathing; difficult urination; confusion; fainting; irregular heart beat.

Guidelines for Use

USE EXACTLY AS PRESCRIBED.

Take with food.

Avoid alcohol and drowsiness-causing medicines (eg, tranquilizers, some pain medicine).

Use caution while driving or performing tasks requiring mental alertness and coordination.

Children and the elderly may be more likely to experience side effects, and paradoxical reactions such as excitement, irritability and sleeplessness.

Motion sickness — The first dose should be taken 30 minutes before exposure to motion.

Do not take for several days before allergy skin testing.

Orthostatic hypotension (dizziness or lightheadedness when rising quickly from a seated or lying position) may occur. Avoid sudden changes in posture.

Diphenoxylate Hydrochloride/Atropine Sulfate

(die-fen-OX-ih-late HIGH-droe-KLOR-ide/AT-troe-peen SULL-fate)

Diphenatol Hydrochloride, Lonox, Lo-Trol, Lomanate, Lomotil

A medicine used to relieve diarrhea.

Precautions

DO NOT USE if you are allergic to this medicine; for diarrhea associated with antibiotic therapy; if you have jaundice (yellowing of the skin or eyes); in children under two years of age. Safety and effectiveness in children under 12 have not been established. Use with caution, especially in children with Down's syndrome.

BEFORE USING THIS MEDICINE, tell your healthcare provider if you are pregnant or breastfeeding; or if you are taking, will be taking or stop taking any prescription or nonprescription medicine; or if you have any other medical conditions.

Side Effects

Every medicine can cause side effects, but many people have no, or minor, side effects. Tell your healthcare provider if any of the following occurs: nausea; vomiting; stomach ache; appetite loss; constipation; dizziness; drowsiness; restlessness; difficulty sleeping; confusion; hallucinations; headache; dry skin; flushing; redness; hives; itching; fever; blurred vision; burning eyes; dry mouth; difficulty urinating; difficulty breathing; irregular heartbeat; swelling of the gums.

Guidelines for Use

USE EXACTLY AS PRESCRIBED.

Do not take more than the prescribed dose.

Avoid alcohol and other sedatives that may cause drowsiness.

May cause drowsiness or dizziness. Use caution when driving or performing other tasks requiring mental alertness or physical coordination.

May cause dry mouth.

Keep out of reach of children since accidental overdosage may result in severe, even fatal, breathing problems.

Notify your healthcare provider if diarrhea persists or if fever, palpitations or abdominal distention occurs.

This medicine can be habit forming. If you have been taking large doses and suddenly stop taking the medication, symptoms of withdrawal may occur. These symptoms include muscle cramps, stomach cramps, unusual sweating, nausea, vomiting and shaking or trembling.

Practice good oral hygiene and have regular dental checkups.

Solution: Shake well before using.

Dipyridamole

(DIE-pih-RID-uh-mole)

Persantine, Persantine IV

An antiplatelet agent normally given with oral coumarin anticoagulants (eg, warfarin) to prevent blood clots after heart surgery in patients over 12 years of age. It occasionally may be prescribed for other reasons.

Precautions

DO NOT USE if you are allergic to this medicine.

BEFORE USING THIS MEDICINE, tell your healthcare provider if you are pregnant or breastfeeding; or if you are taking, will be taking or stop taking any prescription (especially adenosine) or nonprescription medicine; or if you have any other medical conditions.

Side Effects

Every medicine can cause side effects, but many people have no, or minor, side effects. Tell your healthcare provider if any of the following occurs: stomach ache; nausea; vomiting; diarrhea; headache; rash; itching; flushing; dizziness; lightheadedness; fainting.

Guidelines for Use

USE EXACTLY AS PRESCRIBED.

Take without regard to food.

Do not stop taking this medicine except on your healthcare provider's advice.

If using this medicine in combination with coumarin anticoagulants (eg, warfarin), do not take aspirin unless directed by your heathcare provider.

Do not change from one brand of this drug to another without consulting your pharmacist or healthcare provider. Products manufactured by different companies may not be equally effective.

If a dose is missed, take it as soon as possible. If several hours have passed or if it is nearing time for the next dose, do not double the dose to catch up, unless advised by your healthcare provider. If more than one dose is missed, contact your healthcare provider.

Low blood pressure — This medicine may cause lightheadedness in people with low blood pressure. Be cautious when rising from a sitting or lying position.

Dirithromycin

(die-RITH-row-MY-sin)

Dynabac

An antibiotic to treat mild to moderate respiratory and skin infections in persons over 12 years of age.

Precautions

DO NOT USE if you are allergic to this medication or to erythromycin or other similar antibiotics.

BEFORE USING THIS MEDICINE, tell your healthcare provider if you are pregnant or breastfeeding; if you are taking, will be taking or stop taking any prescription or nonprescription medicine; or if you have any other medical conditions.

Side Effects

Every medicine can cause side effects, but many people have no, or minor, side effects. Tell your healthcare provider if any of the following occurs: stomach pain; nausea; diarrhea; vomiting; indigestion; gas; headache; weakness; dizziness; sleeplessness; cough; difficulty breathing; hives; rash; itching.

Guidelines for Use

USE EXACTLY AS PRESCRIBED.

Take once a day with food or within 1 hour of having eaten.

Do not cut, chew or crush the tablets.

Continue use until all of the prescribed medicine has been taken (usually 7-14 days). Failure to take all of the medicine may prevent complete elimination of bacteria, causing the infection to return.

If a dose is missed, take it as soon as possible. If several hours have passed or if it is nearing time for the next dose, do not double the dose to "catch up," unless advised by your healthcare provider. If more than one dose is missed, contact your healthcare provider.

Contact your healthcare provider if skin rash, hives, itching, difficulty breathing, nausea, vomiting, severe stomach pain or diarrhea occurs.

Store at room temperature.

Disopyramide

(DIE-so-PIR-uh-mide)

Norpace, Norpace CR

A heart medicine (antiarrhythmic) used to correct or prevent various types of irregular heartbeats and heart rhythm disturbances. May occasionally be prescribed for other reasons.

Precautions

DO NOT USE if you are allergic to this medicine or have sinus syndrome.

BEFORE USING THIS MEDICINE, tell your healthcare provider if you are pregnant or breastfeeding; or if you are taking, will be taking or stop taking any prescription or nonprescription medicine; or if you have any other medical conditions.

Side Effects

Every medicine can cause side effects, but many people have no, or minor, side effects. Tell your healthcare provider if any of the following occurs: sweating; chills; tremors; constipation; nausea; vomiting; gas; loss of appetite; diarrhea; headache; depression; dizziness; tiredness; weakness; sleeplessness; chest pain; pounding in the chest; rash; itching; urinary frequency/urgency; painful urination; shortness of breath; weight gain; blurred vision; impotence; dry mouth, nose and throat; aches and pain.

Guidelines for Use

USE EXACTLY AS PRESCRIBED.

Do not discontinue medication unless instructed by your healthcare provider.

Low blood glucose (sugar) levels may occur. Contact your healthcare provider if symptoms develop.

Take this medication at evenly spaced intervals around the clock.

Timed release--Do not crush or chew.

Disulfiram

(die-SULL-fih-ram)

Antabuse

A medicine used in the management of selected alcoholics who wish to remain in a state of enforced sobriety.

Precautions

DO NOT USE if you have heart disease, psychosis or are allergic to this medicine, rubber or to thiuram derivatives used in pesticides. Do not use if you recently received metronidazole (*Flagyl*), paraldehyde or with alcohol or alcohol-containing products. This medicine plus alcohol, even in small amounts, produces flushing, throbbing in the head and neck, throbbing headaches, fainting, nausea, severe vomiting, sweating, thirst, chest pain, pounding in the chest, difficulty breathing, weakness, feeling of whirling motion, blurred vision and confusion. Severe reactions may include collapse, irregular heart rhythm, heart attack, acute congestive heart failure, unconsciousness, convulsions and death. The severity of the attack is proportional to the amounts of alcohol ingested with the medicine.

BEFORE USING THIS MEDICINE, tell your healthcare provider if you are pregnant or breastfeeding; if you are taking, will be taking or stop taking any prescription or nonprescription medicine; or if you have any other medical conditions.

Side Effects

Every medicine can cause side effects, but many people have no, or minor, side effects. Tell your healthcare provider if any of the following occurs: drowsiness; fatigue; headache; restlessness; psychotic reaction; changes in vision or color perception; abnormal sensations; rash; acne; metallic or garlic-like aftertaste; impotence.

Guidelines for Use

USE EXACTLY AS PRESCRIBED.

Ethylene dibromide (a fumigant and additive in anti-knock gasoline) and its vapors may be harmful to patients receiving this medicine; avoid exposure.

Never use in intoxicated individuals or without an individual's knowledge. Patient's relatives should be instructed accordingly.

Do not take for at least 12 hours after drinking alcohol. A reaction may occur for up to 2 weeks after the medicine has been stopped.

If a dose is missed, take it as soon as possible. If several hours have passed or if it is nearing time for the next dose, do not double the dose in order to catch up, unless advised to do so by your healthcare provider. If more than one dose is missed, contact your healthcare provider.

Avoid alcohol in all forms, including: alcoholic beverages, including beer and wine, vinegars, many liquid medications (including prescription and nonprescription), some sauces, aftershave lotions, colognes, liniments, etc. Reactions with alcohol can have a severe effect on the heart and breathing. Always read product labels or ask your pharmacist about the alcohol content of all liquid medications before choosing one.

Tablets can be crushed or mixed with liquid.

May cause drowsiness. Use caution while driving or performing other tasks requiring alertness.

Always carry identification indicating that you are taking this medicine. Include the phone numbers of your healthcare provider and the medical facility that should be contacted in case of a reaction.

Docusate

(DOCK-you-sate)

Colace, DC Softgels, Dialose, Diocto, Diocto-K, Dioeze, Disonate, DOK, DOS Softgels, Doxinate, DSS, Kasof, Modane Soft, Perestan, Pro-Cal-Sof, Pro-Sof, Regulax SS, Regutol, Sulfalax Calcium, Surfak Liquigels

Used for the short-term prevention and treatment of constipation. It also is used to soften the stool in patients who should not strain at the stool (eg, patients who have hernias, severe high blood pressure or heart disease, women who have just had babies and people who have had recent rectal surgery).

Precautions

DO NOT USE if you are allergic to this medicine; if you have appendicitis symptoms (eg, nausea, vomiting, stomach pain); intestinal obstruction; stool impaction; or with mineral oil.

BEFORE USING THIS MEDICINE, tell your healthcare provider if you are pregnant or breastfeeding; or if you are taking, will be taking or stop taking any prescription or nonprescription medicine; or if you have any other medical conditions.

Side Effects

Every medicine can cause side effects, but many people have no, or minor, side effects. Tell your healthcare provider if any of the following occurs: rash; nausea; vomiting; stomach ache; bowel cramping; diarrhea.

Guidelines for Use

USE EXACTLY AS PRESCRIBED.

Take with a full glass of water or juice.

Laxative use is only a temporary measure. When normal bowel habits return, stop use of these products.

Do not use for more than one week except on the advice of your healthcare provider.

Do not use in the presence of abdominal pain, nausea or vomiting.

Notify your healthcare provider if unrelieved constipation or rectal bleeding occurs.

Liquid--Put in milk, fruit juice or infant formula to mask taste.

Effects occur in 24 to 72 hours.

Dornase Alfa

(DOR-nace AL-fuh)

Pulmozyme

A medicine used in cystic fibrosis patients to reduce the frequency of severe respiratory infections and to improve lung function.

Precautions

DO NOT USE if you are allergic to this medicine or any part of it.

BEFORE USING THIS MEDICINE, tell your healthcare provider if you are pregnant or breastfeeding; or if you are taking, will be taking or stop taking any prescription or nonprescription medicine; or if you have any other medical conditions.

Side Effects

Every medicine can cause side effects, but many people have no, or minor, side effects. Tell your healthcare provider if any of the following occurs: chest pain; throat inflammation; voice changes; rash; inflammation of the eye.

Guidelines for Use

USE EXACTLY AS PRESCRIBED.

This medicine must be stored in the refrigerator and should not be exposed to room temperature for longer than a total time of 24 hours.

Once opened, the entire ampule must be used or discarded.

The solution should be discarded if it is cloudy or discolored.

Protect from strong light.

Patients should be instructed in the proper maintenance of the nebulizer and compressor system. Talk to your healthcare provider for instructions.

Do not dilute or mix other drugs in the nebulizer.

If a dose is missed, take it as soon as possible. If several hours have passed or if it is nearing time for the next dose, do not double the dose to catch up, unless advised by your healthcare provider. If more than one dose is missed, contact your healthcare provider.

Dorzolamide Hydrochloride

(dore-ZOLE-uh-mide HIGH-droe-KLOR-ide)

Trusopt

Eyedrops used to lower fluid pressure in the eye (intraocular pressure) in adults with ocular hypertension or open-angle glaucoma.

Precautions

DO NOT USE if you are allergic to this medication, its relatives (eg, sulfa drugs) or any of its ingredients. Soft contact lenses should not be worn during treatment with this medicine.

BEFORE USING THIS MEDICATION, tell your healthcare provider if you are pregnant or breastfeeding; if you are taking, will be taking or stop taking any prescription or nonprescription medicine; or if you have any other medical conditions.

Side Effects

Every medicine can cause side effects, but many people have no, or minor, side effects. Tell your healthcare provider if any of the following occurs: burning, stinging or discomfort after use; bitter taste after use; redness; itching; discharge; tearing; blurred vision; dryness; light sensitivity; skin or eyelid reactions; yellowing of the skin or eyes.

Guidelines for Use

USE EXACTLY AS PRESCRIBED.

Place one drop in the affected eye(s) 3 times daily. Wait 10 minutes before using any other eye medications.

Brief stinging or burning of the eye may occur after administration. This is normal. Contact your healthcare provider if the symptom(s) continues.

Do not touch the dropper tip to any surface, including your eye, since this may contaminate the contents or cause damage to the eye.

Do not increase or decrease this medicine without your healthcare provider's approval. If a dose is missed, take it as soon as possible. If several hours have passed or if it is within 2 hours of the next dose, do not double the dose to "catch up," unless advised by your healthcare provider. If more than one dose is missed, contact your healthcare provider.

Soft contact lenses-Do not wear during treatment.

Discontinue this medicine immediately and contact your healthcare provider if any of the following occurs: redness, itching, discharge, tearing, swelling of the eyelid or any other signs of an infection.

This medicine may cause a sensitivity to bright light. Protect your eyes and wear sunglasses.

Notify your healthcare provider that you are taking this medication if you receive an eye injury or undergo eye surgery; this medication may need to be changed.

Store at room temperature.

Doxazosin Mesylate

(DOX-uh-ZOE-sin MEH-suh-late)

Cardura

A medicine used to lower high blood pressure. It also is used to treat benign prostatic hyperplasia (BPH), or swelling of the prostate in older men. It occasionally may be prescribed for other reasons.

Precautions

DO NOT USE if you are allergic to this medicine or similar medicine such as prazosin or terazosin.

BEFORE USING THIS MEDICINE, tell your healthcare provider if you are pregnant or breastfeeding; or if you are taking, will be taking or stop taking any prescription or nonprescription medicine; or if you have any other medical conditions.

Side Effects

Every medicine can cause side effects, but many people have no, or minor, side effects. Tell your healthcare provider if any of the following occurs: pounding in the chest; nausea; diarrhea; constipation; shortness of breath; muscle pain; blurred vision; visual problems; drowsiness/fatigue; nervousness; headache; lightheadedness; dizziness (especially when arising from a seated or lying position); swelling; feeling of whirling motion; indigestion; gas; dry mouth; ringing in the ears; nosebleed; urinary problems; weight gain; skin rash; itching.

Guidelines for Use

USE EXACTLY AS PRESCRIBED.

If a dose is missed, take it as soon as possible. If several hours have passed or it is nearing time for the next dose, do not double the dose to "catch up," unless advised by your healthcare provider. If more than one dose is missed, contact your healthcare provider.

Take the first dose at bedtime in order to reduce the risk of dizziness, which may occur early in therapy.

Dizziness or lightheadedness may occur if you stand up too fast from a lying or sitting position. If this occurs, get up slowly and avoid sudden changes in posture.

If dizziness, lightheadedness or palpitations are bothersome, contact your doctor. A dose adjustment may be needed.

Patients being treated for high blood pressure often feel tired and run down for a few weeks after beginning therapy. It takes time for the body to adjust to lowered blood pressure. Continue taking your medicine even though you may not feel quite normal.

Check with your healthcare provider during this time regarding any new symptoms that occur to ensure that they are a normal consequence of changes in blood pressure.

May cause drowsiness, dizziness, lightheadedness or blurred vision. Use caution when driving or performing other tasks requiring mental alertness, coordination and dexterity.

Do not take nonprescription decongestants, weight loss products, cold, sinus or allergy medications without first consulting your healthcare provider.

May cause sodium and water retention when used alone to treat high blood pressure. Report any unusual swelling or weight gain to your healthcare provider.

Keep regular appointments with your healthcare provider.

Doxepin Hydrochloride

(DOX-uh-pin HIGH-droe-KLOR-ide)

Adapin, Sinequan, Sinequan Concentrate, Zonalon

A mood elevating medicine usually used for the relief of depression. It may occasionally be prescribed for other reasons.

Precautions

DO NOT USE if you are allergic to this medicine or its relatives or if you are using monoamine oxidase inhibitors (MAOIs); if you have glaucoma; or if you have difficulty urinating.

BEFORE USING THIS MEDICINE, tell your healthcare provider if you are pregnant or breastfeeding; or if you are taking, will be taking, or stop taking any prescription or nonprescription medicine; or if you have any other medical conditions.

Side Effects

Every medicine can cause side effects, but many people have no, or minor, side effects. Tell your healthcare provider if any of the following occurs: dry mouth; blurred vision; difficult urination; seizures; drowsiness; confusion; hallucinations; numbness; tremors; fever; constipation.

Guidelines for Use

USE EXACTLY AS PRESCRIBED.

Take as directed with a full glass of water, with or without food.

Oral concentrate: Mix with 4 oz of water, milk or fruit juice. Do not mix with carbonated beverages or prepare and store in bulk.

If a dose is missed, take it as soon as possible. If several hours have passed or if it is nearing time for the next dose, do not double the dose to "catch up," unless advised by your healthcare provider. If more than one dose is missed, contact your healthcare provider.

This medicine may not be effective for 2 to 3 weeks.

May increase or decrease blood sugar levels in diabetics.

May cause drowsiness or blurred vision. Use caution while driving or performing other tasks requiring mental alertness.

Using this medicine with alcohol or other central nervous system depressants (eg, pain relievers, sedatives, antihistamines) may cause added drowsiness.

May cause sensitivity to sunlight. Avoid prolonged exposure to the sun. Use sunscreens and wear protective clothing until tolerance is determined.

Taking this medicine at bedtime may help reduce side effects (eg, daytime drowsiness). Discuss this possibility with your healthcare provider.

Symptoms of nausea, headache or fatigue may develop after abruptly stopping long-term use.

Lab tests may be required to monitor therapy; keep appointments.

Store at room temperature. Protect from light.

Doxorubicin Hydrochloride (ADR)

(DOX-oh-RUE-bih-sin HIGH-droe-KLOR-ide)

Adriamycin PFS, Adriamycin RDF, Rubex

Used to produce regression in a variety of cancers.

Side Effects

Every medicine can cause side effects, but many people have no, or minor, side effects. Tell your healthcare provider if any of the following occurs: severe nausea and vomiting; hair loss; changes in nailbeds; streaking of the skin along injection site; fever; chills; hives; mouth sores; anal bleeding; appetite loss; diarrhea; flushing; rash; difficulty breathing.

Patient Information

Urine will be a red color for 1 to 2 days after administration.

Doxycycline

(DOX-ee-SIGH-kleen)

Doryx, Doxy 100, Doxy 200, Doxy-Caps, Doxychel Hyclate, Monodox, Vibramycin, Vibramycin IV, Vibra-Tabs

An anti-infection medicine used to treat a wide variety of infections caused by certain bacteria. It also is used as a preventative treatment of certain types of malaria in short-term travelers.

Precautions

DO NOT USE if you are allergic to this medicine or its relatives, if you are pregnant, in children under 8 years of age or if it is out of date.

BEFORE USING THIS MEDICINE, tell your healthcare provider if you are breastfeeding; or if you are taking, will be taking or stop taking any prescription medicine; or if you have any other medical conditions.

Side Effects

Every medicine can cause side effects, but many people have no, or minor, side effects. Tell your healthcare provider if any of the following occurs: headache; vomiting; nausea; diarrhea; vaginal infections; visual disturbances.

Guidelines for Use

USE EXACTLY AS PRESCRIBED.

May be taken without regard to meals.

Avoid taking at the same time with antacids, laxatives, dairy products or iron-containing products. Generally allow 2 to 3 hours before or after taking this medicine.

May be stored at cool room temperatures.

If a dose is missed, take it as soon as possible. If several hours have passed of if it is nearing time for the next dose, do not double the dose to "catch up," unless advised by your healthcare provider. If more than one dose is missed, contact your healthcare provider.

Continue to take until all the prescribed medicine is gone. Failure to take all of the medicine may prevent complete elimination of bacteria, causing the infection to return.

May cause a sensitivity to sunlight. Avoid prolonged exposure to the sun and other ultraviolet light. Use sunscreens and wear protective clothing until tolerance is determined.

Do not use outdated medicine since it may be highly toxic.

Dronabinol

(droe-NAB-ih-nahl)

Marinol

A medicine used to treat nausea and vomiting associated with chemotherapy or to stimulate appetite in some cases.

Precautions

DO NOT USE if you are are allergic to this medicine, marijuana or sesame oil.

BEFORE USING THIS MEDICINE, tell your healthcare provider if you are pregnant; or if you are taking, will be taking or stop taking any prescription or nonprescription medicines; or have any other medical conditions.

Side Effects

Every medicine can cause side effects, but many people have no, or minor, side effects. Tell your healthcare provider if any of the following occurs: nausea; loss of appetite; drowsiness; heightened awareness; dizziness or lightheadedness when rising from a sitting or lying position; anxiety; difficulty concentrating; irritability; unsteadiness; depression; weakness; hallucinations; memory loss; confusion; nightmares; increased heart rate; pounding in the chest; flushing; dry mouth; numbness or tingling in the hands and feet; visual problems (distortions).

Guidelines for Use

USE EXACTLY AS PRESCRIBED.

Avoid alcohol and barbiturates.

Use medicines that cause drowsiness (eg, antianxiety agents, narcotic pain relievers) with caution.

May cause dizziness or drowsiness. Do not drive or perform tasks requiring mental alertness.

Possible changes in mood and other behavioral effects are possible with this medicine. Do not panic in the event of such manifestations.

Remain under the supervision of a responsible adult.

This medicine is highly abusable. Use caution.

Orthostatic hypotension (dizziness or lightheadedness when rising from a seated or lying position) may occur. Avoid sudden changes in posture.

Econazole Nitrate

(ee-CON-uh-zole NYE-trate)

Spectazole

A medicine used to treat athlete's foot, jock itch, ringworm, tinea versicolor (pityriasis) and skin candidiasis infections.

Precautions

DO NOT USE if you have an allergy to this medicine.

BEFORE USING THIS MEDICINE, tell your healthcare provider if you are pregnant or breastfeeding; or if you are taking, will be taking or stop taking any prescription or nonprescription medicine; or if you have any other medical conditions.

Side Effects

Every medicine can cause side effects, but many people have no, or minor, side effects. Tell your healthcare provider if any of the following occurs: *At application site* — burning; itching; stinging; redness; dryness; local irritation.

Guidelines for Use

USE EXACTLY AS PRESCRIBED.

For external use only. Avoid contact with the eyes, nose, mouth or other mucous membranes.

Use only as directed. Cleanse and dry the area to be treated before application.

Avoid inhalation.

Apply with caution to blistered or raw skin, oozing skin or skin over a deep puncture wound.

Avoid the use of air-tight dressings unless directed by your healthcare provider.

Use this medication for the full treatment time, even if the symptoms improve.

For athlete's foot, wear well-fitted, ventilated shoes and change socks at least once a day.

Allergic reactions may occur. If the condition being treated worsens or irritation, burning, redness, swelling or stinging persists, discontinue use and contact your healthcare provider.

Enalapril Maleate

(EH-NAL-uh-prill-MAL-ee-ate)

Vasotec

An angiotensin converting enzyme (ACE) inhibitor medicine generally used to lower high blood pressure or treat heart failure.

Precautions

DO NOT USE if you are allergic to this medicine or if you are pregnant.

BEFORE USING THIS MEDICINE, tell your healthcare provider if you are breastfeeding; or if you are taking, will be taking or stop taking any prescription or nonprescription medicine; or if you have any other medical conditions.

Side Effects

Every medicine can cause side effects, but many people have no, or minor, side effects. Tell your healthcare provider if any of the following occurs: stomach pain; vomiting; diarrhea; constipation; appetite loss; depression; headache; dizziness; nervousness; sleeping difficulties; fatigue; dizziness/lightheadedness when rising quickly from a sitting or lying position; shortness of breath; cough; nasal congestion; bronchitis; sinus inflammation; rash; sweating; flushing; yellowing of skin or eyes; muscle cramps; weight loss; taste loss; dry mouth; decreased sex drive; back, joint and shoulder pain; urination changes; fever; vision disturbances; numbness/tingling of hands or feet.

Guidelines for Use

USE EXACTLY AS PRESCRIBED.

May be taken without regard to meals.

Patients starting treatment for high blood pressure may at first feel tired. It takes time for the body to adjust. Continue taking medication and check with your healthcare provider.

If a dose is missed, take it as soon as possible. If several hours have passed or if it is nearing time for the next dose, do not double the dose to "catch up," unless advised by your healthcare provider. If more than one dose is missed, contact your healthcare provider.

Do not interrupt or stop medication without consulting your healthcare provider.

Do not use salt substitutes without telling your healthcare provider.

A persistent, dry, nonproductive cough may occur; tell your healthcare provider. Recovery is rapid when the medicine is stopped.

Dizziness, fainting or lightheadedness is most likely after the first dose or in the first days of therapy; avoid sudden changes in posture.

If fainting occurs, discontinue medicine until talking to your healthcare provider.

Enalapril with Hydrochlorothiazide

(EH-NAL-uh-prill MAL-ee-ate with high-droe-klor-oh-THIGH-uh-zide)

Hydrochlorothiazide w/Enalapril Tablets, Vaseretic 10-25 Tablets

A combination medicine used to treat high blood pressure.

Precautions

DO NOT USE if you have an allergy to this medicine, oral diabetic or sulfa medicines, or are pregnant.

BEFORE USING THIS MEDICINE, tell your healthcare provider if you are pregnant or breastfeeding; or if you are taking, will be taking or stop taking any prescription or nonprescription medicine; or if you have any other medical conditions.

Side Effects

Every medicine can cause side effects, but many people have no, or minor, side effects. Tell your healthcare provider if any of the following occurs: dry mouth; thirst; irregular heartbeat; confusion/mood changes; nausea; vomiting; fatigue; weakness; appetite loss; bloating; diarrhea; constipation; lightheadedness; headache; tingling of toes/fingers; vision changes; depression; nervousness; sleeplessness; fall in blood pressure upon standing that may cause dizziness, fainting and blurred vision; chest pain; sun sensitivity; rash; hives; itching; dry skin; flushing; unusual bruising; cough; sinus congestion; sore throat; difficulty breathing; frequent urination; impotence; reduced sex drive; muscle cramps; joint pain; fever; chills; weight loss; nosebleeds; gout.

Guidelines for Use

USE EXACTLY AS PRESCRIBED.

If upset stomach occurs, take with food or milk.

Increases urination; take early in the day when possible.

Patients treated for high blood pressure may feel tired for a few weeks after starting therapy. It takes time for the body to adjust. Continue taking your medicine even if you may not feel normal.

If a dose is missed, take as soon as possible. If several hours have passed or if it is nearing time for the next dose, do not double the dose to "catch up," unless advised by your healthcare provider. If more than one dose is missed, contact your healthcare provider.

Tell your healthcare provider immediately, if any of the following occurs: weakness, muscle cramps, dizziness, nausea, unusual swelling of the face/neck, lightheadedness/faintness upon standing, sore throat, chest pain, or a dry and persistent cough.

Do not use salt substitutes unless advised by your healthcare provider.

Enoxacin

(en-OX-uh-SIN)

Penetrex

A quinolone antibiotic medicine used to treat infections caused by certain bacteria.

Precautions

DO NOT USE if you are allergic to this medicine or any of its relatives.

BEFORE USING THIS MEDICINE, tell your healthcare provider if you are pregnant or breastfeeding; or if you are taking, will be taking or stop taking any prescription or nonprescription medicine; or if you have any other medical conditions.

Side Effects

Every medicine can cause side effects, but many people have no, or minor, side effects. Tell your healthcare provider if any of the following occurs: severe nausea and vomiting; diarrhea; rash; hives; itching; difficulty breathing; wheezing; dizziness; headache; insomnia; nervousness.

Guidelines for Use

USE EXACTLY AS PRESCRIBED.

May be taken without regard to meals, but preferably 2 hours after a meal.

Drink plenty of liquids.

Do not take antacids, sucralfate (*Carafate*), or iron or zinc-containing products within 4 hours before or 2 hours after using this medicine.

If a dose is missed, take it as soon as possible. If several hours have passed or if it is nearing time for the next dose, do not double the dose to "catch up," unless advised by your healthcare provider. If more than one dose is missed, contact your healthcare provider.

Continue use until all the prescribed medicine has been taken. Failure to take all of the medicine may prevent complete elimination of bacteria, causing the infection to return.

Dose and duration of therapy depends on the condition being treated and its severity.

Do not stop therapy without asking your healthcare provider.

May cause dizziness or lightheadedness. Use caution when driving or performing other tasks requiring mental alertness.

May cause sensitivity to sunlight. Avoid prolonged exposure to the sun. Use sunscreens and wear protective clothing until tolerance is determined.

Enoxaparin Sodium Injection

(eh-NOX-uh-par-in SO-dee-uhm)

Lovenox

This medicine is an anticoagulant or "blood thinner" used in adults to prevent deep vein thrombosis (or blood clots) after hip and knee replacement surgery.

Precautions

DO NOT USE if you are allergic to this medicine, heparin or pork products; or if you are prone to heavy bleeding.

BEFORE USING THIS MEDICINE, tell your healthcare provider if you are pregnant or breastfeeding; if you are taking, will be taking or stop taking any prescription or nonprescription medicine; or if you have any other medical conditions.

Side Effects

Every medicine can cause side effects, but many people have no, or minor, side effects. Tell your healthcare provider if any of the following occurs: heavy or unusual bleeding or bruising; pain, redness, bruising or hardness at the injection site; fever; nausea; swelling, possibly in the arms and legs; confusion.

Guidelines for Use

USE EXACTLY AS PRESCRIBED.

This medicine should be used twice daily, with the first dose given right after surgery. Treatment usually lasts 7–10 days, but may continue for up to 14 days.

Use proper technique; inject under the skin, NOT into muscle.

If a dose is missed, take it as soon as possible. If more than 6 hours have passed, do not double the dose to "catch up." If more than one dose is missed, contact your healthcare provider.

Contact your healthcare provider if you experience bleeding, bruising, dizziness, lightheadedness, itching, rash or difficulty breathing.

Do not use or substitute other blood thinners without first checking with your healthcare provider.

Lab tests may be required to monitor therapy. Be sure to keep appointments.

Store at or below room temperature. Do not freeze.

Ephedrine

(eh-FED-rin)

Kondon's, Pretz-D, Vicks Vatronol

A decongestant used to treat nasal stuffiness due to the common cold, sinusitis, hay fever and other allergies. It also is used to relieve air block and pressure pain during air travel. It may occasionally be prescribed for other reasons.

Precautions

DO NOT USE if you have an allergy to this medicine.

BEFORE USING THIS MEDICINE, tell your healthcare provider if you are pregnant or breastfeeding; or if you are taking, will be taking or stop taking any prescription or nonprescription medicine; if you have any other medical conditions; or if you are allergic to sulfite preservatives.

Side Effects

Every medicine can cause side effects, but many people have no, or minor, side effects. Tell your healthcare provider if any of the following occurs: nausea; vomiting; appetite loss; anxiety; restlessness; tremors; headache; dizziness; drowsiness; sleeplessness; hallucinations; convulsions; depression; pounding in the chest; sweating; pallor; difficulty breathing; chest pain; tearing; eye irritation; sensitivity of eyes to light; urinary retention; painful urination; burning; stinging; sneezing; dryness of nose; local irritation; rebound congestion.

Guidelines for Use

USE EXACTLY AS PRESCRIBED.

Do not exceed recommended dosage and do not use longer than 3 to 5 days.

Stinging, burning or drying of the nose may occur.

Too much use may cause certain side effects (nervousness, dizziness or sleeplessness) that are more likely in the elderly and children.

Long-term, high-dose therapy may be habit-forming.

Rebound congestion may occur after the dose wears off.

Stop using the medicine gradually; stop using the medicine in one nostril, then both nostrils.

An oral decongestant may be substituted.

Epinephrine Hydrochloride

(epp-ih-NEFF-rin)

Adrenalin Chloride, AsthmaNefrin, Bronitin, Bronkaid Mist, Epifrin, Epinal, Epinephrine Pediatric, Eppy/N, Glaucon, MicroNefrin, Nephron, Primatene Mist, Racepinephrine, S-2, SusPhrine, Vaponefrin

A medicine used to treat various heart conditions, Adams-Stokes syndrome, syncope due to heart block or carotid sinus hypersensitivity, symptomatic relief of serum sickness, urticaria and angioedema, nasal congestion due to the common cold, sinusitis, hay fever and other allergies. It also is used to relieve air block and pressure pain during air travel, to relieve eustachian tube congestion, and to treat bronchial asthma. Ophthalmic solution: used to treat open-angle glaucoma. It may occasionally be prescribed for other reasons.

Precautions

DO NOT USE if you have an allergy to this medicine.

BEFORE USING THIS MEDICINE, tell your healthcare provider if you are pregnant or breastfeeding; or if you are taking, will be taking or stop taking any prescription or nonprescription medicine; if you have any other medical conditions; or if you are allergic to sulfite preservatives.

Side Effects

Every medicine can cause side effects, but many people have no, or minor, side effects. Tell your healthcare provider if any of the following occurs: nausea; vomiting; appetite loss; anxiety; restlessness; tremors; headache; dizziness; drowsiness; sleeplessness; hallucinations; convulsions; depression; pounding in the chest; sweating; pallor; difficulty breathing; chest pain; tearing; eye irritation; sensitivity of eyes to light; urinary retention; painful urination; nasal burning, stinging, dryness; sneezing; local irritation; rebound congestion.

Guidelines for Use

USE EXACTLY AS PRESCRIBED.

Topical decongestant: Do not take more than the recommended dosage and do not use longer than 3 to 5 days. Stinging, burning or drying of the nose may occur. Long-term, high-dose therapy may be habit-forming. Rebound congestion may occur after the dose wears off. Excessive use may cause certain side effects (nervousness, dizziness or sleeplessness) that are more likely in the elderly and children. Stop using the medicine gradually; stop using the medicine in one nostril, then both nostrils. An oral decongestant may be substituted.

Ophthalmic solution: Tell your healthcare provider if you experience prolonged blurred vision, headache, palpitations, tremors, sweating and fainting. Use caution while driving or performing other hazardous tasks. Stinging of the eyes will occur on instillation. Do not wear soft contact lenses during therapy; discoloration of lenses may result.

Inhalation: Tell your healthcare provider if no relief from your symptoms occurs, or if you experience dizziness or chest pain.

Injection: Tell your healthcare provider if you experience lightheadedness, fainting, pounding in the chest, weakness or chest pain.

Epoetin Alfa

(EH-poe-EH-TIN AL-fuh)

Epogen, Procrit

Used for treatment of anemia associated with chronic renal failure (CRF); treatment of anemia related to AZT therapy in HIV-infected patients; treatment of anemia in cancer patients on chemotherapy. It may occasionally be prescribed for other reasons.

Precautions

DO NOT USE if you are allergic to mammalian cell-derived products or to human albumin or with uncontrolled high blood pressure.

BEFORE USING THIS MEDICINE, tell your healthcare provider if you are pregnant or breastfeeding; or if you are taking, will be taking or stop taking any prescription or nonprescription medicine; or if you have any other medical conditions.

Side Effects

Every medicine can cause side effects, but many people have no, or minor, side effects. Tell your healthcare provider if any of the following occurs: *CRF-treated patients*--headache; joint pain; nausea; swelling of the extremities; fatigue; diarrhea; vomiting; chest pain; reaction at the injection site; weakness; dizziness. *Zidovudine-treated patients*--fever; fatigue; headache; cough; diarrhea; rash; nausea; congestion; shortness of breath; weakness; skin reaction at the injection site; dizziness. *Cancer patients*--fever; diarrhea; nausea; vomiting; swelling of the extremities; weakness; fatigue; shortness of breath; abnormal skin sensations; upper respiratory infection. *All*--seizures (rarely); skin rash, itching.

Guidelines for Use

USE EXACTLY AS PRESCRIBED.

Follow dietary guidelines given to you by your healthcare provider.

Home dialysis patients--Follow your healthcare provider's instructions carefully.

Ask your healthcare provider for information on signs and symptoms that indicate an allergic reaction.

Talk to your healthcare provider concerning the need for an iron supplement.

Patient information is available with the product.

Periodic blood counts are required to monitor response to this product.

Keep lab appointments.

Ergoloid Mesylates

(err-GO-loyd MEH-suh-lates)

Gerimal, Hydergine, Hydergine LC, Niloric

A medicine used to treat age-related decrease in mental ability, including decreased alertness, short-term memory loss, decreased self-care and sociability or age-related changes in mood in people over 60.

Precautions

DO NOT USE if you have an allergy to this medicine.

BEFORE USING THIS MEDICINE, tell your healthcare provider if you are pregnant or breastfeeding; or if you are taking, will be taking or stop taking any prescription or nonprescription medicine; or if you have any other medical conditions.

Side Effects

Every medicine can cause side effects, but many people have no, or minor, side effects. Tell your healthcare provider if any of the following occurs: irritation under the tongue (sublingual tablets); nausea; stomach upset.

Guidelines for Use

USE EXACTLY AS PRESCRIBED.

May cause nausea and stomach upset during start of treatment.

If a dose is missed, take it as soon as possible. If several hours have passed or if it is nearing time for the next dose, do not double the dose to "catch up," unless advised by your healthcare provider. If more than one dose is missed, contact your healthcare provider.

Results may not be apparent for 3 to 4 weeks. Do not stop therapy or change the dose without consulting your healthcare provider.

Treatment for up to 6 months may be necessary in order to determine maximum effectiveness.

Sublingual tablets--Allow to dissolve under your tongue. Do not chew, crush or swallow.

Erythromycin Ophthalmic

(eh-RITH-row-MY-sin)

Ilotycin Ophthalmic

A medicine used to treat superficial eye infections caused by susceptible bacteria and to prevent eye infection in newborns.

Precautions

DO NOT USE if you are allergic to this medicine; do not use with astemizole (*Hismanal*) or terfenadine (*Seldane*).

BEFORE USING THIS MEDICINE, tell your healthcare provider if you are pregnant or breastfeeding; or if you are taking, will be taking or stop taking any prescription or nonprescription medicine; or if you have any other medical conditions.

Side Effects

Every medicine can cause side effects, but many people have no, or minor, side effects. Tell your healthcare provider if any of the following occurs: irritation; burning; stinging; itching; lid swelling; redness.

Guidelines for Use

USE EXACTLY AS PRESCRIBED.

May cause temporary blurring of vision or stinging following administration.

Contact your healthcare provider if stinging, burning or itching becomes pronounced or if redness, irritation, swelling, decreasing vision or pain persists or worsens.

Avoid contact between the dispensing container and the eye.

Protect from light.

Erythromycin Systemic

(eh-RITH-row-MY-sin)

Ane-mycin, Del-Mycin, Eramycin, Erygel, E-Base, E-Mycin, EryPed, Erythrocin Stearate, Ery-Tab, Eryc, PCE Dispertab, Robimycin

An anti-infection medicine used to treat infections caused by certain bacteria.

Precautions

DO NOT USE if you are allergic to this medicine or its relatives; do not use with astemizole (*Hismanal*) or terfenadine (*Seldane*).

BEFORE USING THIS MEDICINE, tell your healthcare provider if you are pregnant or breastfeeding; or if you are taking, will be taking or stop taking any prescription or nonprescription medicine; or if you have any other medical conditions.

Side Effects

Every medicine can cause side effects, but many people have no, or minor, side effects. Tell your healthcare provider if any of the following occurs: vomiting; diarrhea; stomach cramps; unusual tiredness; severe abdominal pain; yellowing of skin or eyes; rash; itching; hives; dark urine; or pale stools.

Guidelines for Use

USE EXACTLY AS PRESCRIBED.

Take on an empty stomach, 1 hour before or 2 hours after meals.

If stomach upset occurs, take with food.

Take each dose with an adequate amount of fluid (preferably 6 to 8 ounces).

Take at evenly spaced intervals throughout the day, preferably around the clock.

If a dose is missed, take it as soon as possible. If several hours have passed or if it is nearing time for the next dose, do not double the dose to "catch up," unless advised by your healthcare provider. If more than one dose is missed, contact your healthcare provider.

Continue use until all the prescribed medicine has been taken. Failure to take all of the medicine may prevent complete elimination of bacteria, causing the infection to return.

Erythromycin Topical

(eh-RITH-row-MY-sin)

Akne-mycin, A/TIS, Del-Mycin, Erycette, Eryderm 2, Erygel, Erymax, Ery-Sol, Erythra-Derm, Staticin, Theramycin, T-Stat

A topical antibiotic used to treat acne and minor skin infections.

Precautions

DO NOT USE if you are allergic to this medicine.

BEFORE USING THIS MEDICINE, tell your healthcare provider if you are pregnant or breastfeeding; or if you are taking, will be taking or stop taking any prescription or nonprescription medicine; or if you have any other medical conditions.

Side Effects

Every medicine can cause side effects, but many people have no, or minor, side effects. Tell your healthcare provider if any of the following occurs: flushing; redness; sloughing, burning or tenderness in treated area; dryness; itching; oily skin; eye irritation.

Guidelines for Use

USE EXACTLY AS PRESCRIBED.

For external use only.

Keep away from eyes, nose, mouth and other mucous membranes.

Apply to the affected area in the morning and evening (unless advised to do otherwise by your healthcare provider).

Before applying medicine, wash the area with soap and warm water, rinse well and pat dry.

Apply with an applicator or the fingertips. Wash hands after application.

If excessive irritation or dryness occurs, discontinue use and consult with your healthcare provider.

Keep out of reach of children.

Store at room temperature. Keep tightly closed. Keep away from heat and open flames.

Erythromycin Ethylsuccinate/Sulfisoxazole

(eh-RITH-row-MY-sin ETH-il-SUX-i-nate/sul-fih-SOX-uh-zole)

Eryzole Granules, Pediazole

A medicine used in children to treat middle ear infections caused by susceptible strains of *Haemophilus influenzae*.

Precautions

DO NOT USE if you are allergic to this medicine or its relatives or sulfonamides. Do not use with terfenadine (*Seldane*) or astemizole (*Hismanal*).

BEFORE USING THIS MEDICINE, tell your healthcare provider if you are pregnant or breastfeeding; or if you are taking, will be taking or stop taking any prescription or nonprescription medicine; or if you have any other medical conditions. Use is not recommended for infants less than two months of age.

Side Effects

Every medicine can cause side effects, but many people have no, or minor, side effects. Tell your healthcare provider if any of the following occurs: stomach cramps; appetite loss; nausea; vomiting; diarrhea; headache; sleeplessness; vertigo (feeling of whirling motion); rash; itching; hives; hair loss; sensitivity to light; yellowing of skin or eyes; temporary hearing loss; fever; chills.

Guidelines for Use

USE EXACTLY AS PRESCRIBED.

Shake well before using.

Doses should be equally divided into 4 daily doses and administered for 10 days.

Take with meals or on an empty stomach.

Take with a full glass of water.

Refrigerate after reconstitution. Discard unused portion in 14 days.

Avoid prolonged exposure to the sun. Use sunscreens and wear protective clothing until tolerance is determined.

May cause nausea, vomiting, diarrhea, pale stools, unusual tiredness or stomach cramps. Contact your healthcare provider if effects persist.

Estradiol Oral

(ESS-truh-DIE-ole)

Estrace

Female hormones. This medicine has a variety of uses including various treatment of symptoms of menopause, replacement therapy, osteoporosis (loss of bone cells with aging) and some cancers.

Precautions

DO NOT USE if you are allergic to estrogens, are pregnant, or have abnormal undiagnosed vaginal bleeding.

BEFORE USING THIS MEDICINE, tell your healthcare provider if you are pregnant or breastfeeding; a cigarette smoker; or if you are taking, will be taking or stop taking any prescription or nonprescription medicine; or if you have any other medical conditions.

Side Effects

Every medicine can cause side effects, but many people have no, or minor, side effects. Tell your healthcare provider if any of the following occurs: pain in the groin or calves; sharp chest pain or sudden shortness of breath; abnormal vaginal bleeding; breast lumps; sudden severe headache; dizziness or fainting; vision or speech problems; weakness or numbness in an arm or leg; severe abdominal pain; yellowing of the skin or eyes; severe depression.

Guidelines for Use

USE EXACTLY AS PRESCRIBED.

Diabetes-Blood sugar changes may occur. Monitor urine or blood sugar closely and report changes to your healthcare provider.

Have regular physical exams.

Tell your healthcare provider if you miss a menstrual period or suspect pregnancy.

Avoid prolonged exposure to the sun and other ultraviolet light sources (e.g., tanning beds). Use sunscreens and wear protective clothing until tolerance is determined.

Report contact lens intolerance.

If a dose is missed, take it as soon as possible. If several hours have passed or if it is nearing time for the next dose, do not double the dose to "catch up," unless advised by your healthcare provider. If more than one dose is missed, contact your healthcare provider.

Estradiol Transdermal

(ESS-truh-DIE-ole)

Estraderm Transdermal

A female hormone (estrogen) in a special skin patch. It is used primarily to prevent numerous vascular symptoms associated with menopause, atrophic vaginitis and osteoporosis, although it has a variety of other uses.

Precautions

DO NOT USE if you are allergic to estrogens, pregnant or have abnormal undiagnosed vaginal bleeding.

BEFORE USING THIS MEDICINE, tell your healthcare provider if you are pregnant or breastfeeding; a cigarette smoker; or if you are taking, will be taking or stop taking any prescription or nonprescription medicine; or if you have any other medical conditions.

Side Effects

Every medicine can cause side effects, but many people have no, or minor, side effects. Tell your healthcare provider if any of the following occurs: pain in the groin or calves; sharp chest pain or sudden shortness of breath; abnormal vaginal bleeding; breast lumps; sudden severe headache; dizziness or fainting; vision or speech problems; weakness or numbness in an arm or leg; severe abdominal pain; yellowing of the skin or eyes; severe depression.

Guidelines for Use

USE EXACTLY AS PRESCRIBED.

Place adhesive side on a clean, dry area of the trunk, preferably the abdomen, NOT the breasts.

Rotate the application site with an interval of at least 1 week between applications to one site.

The area should not be oily, damaged or irritated. Avoid the waistline.

Apply immediately after opening and removing the protective liner.

Press firmly in place with palm of hand for 10 seconds. Make sure there is good contact, especially around edges.

If the system should fall off, reapply. If necessary, apply a new system.

In either case, continue original treatment schedule.

Diabetes-Blood sugar changes may occur. Monitor urine or blood sugar closely and report changes to your healthcare provider if he/she advises.

Tell your healthcare provider if you miss a menstrual period or suspect pregnancy.

Have regular physical exams.

Avoid prolonged exposure to the sun and other ultraviolet light sources (eg, tanning beds). Use sunscreens and wear protective clothing until sun tolerance is determined.

Estradiol Vaginal

(ESS-truh-DIE-ole)

Estrace Vaginal Cream

A female hormone primarily used to treat vaginal breakdown and dryness associated with declining ovarian function and menopause.

Precautions

DO NOT USE if you are pregnant or if you have an allergy to estrogens, or have abnormal undiagnosed vaginal bleeding.

BEFORE USING THIS MEDICINE, tell your healthcare provider if you are pregnant or breastfeeding; a cigarette smoker; or if you are taking, will be taking or stop taking any prescription or nonprescription medicine; or if you have any other medical conditions.

Side Effects

Every medicine can cause side effects, but many people have no, or minor, side effects. Tell your healthcare provider if any of the following occurs: pain in the groin or calves; sharp chest pain or sudden shortness of breath; abnormal vaginal bleeding; breast lumps; sudden severe headache; dizziness/fainting; vision or speech disturbance; weakness or numbness in an arm or leg; severe abdominal pain; yellowing of the skin or eyes; severe depression.

Guidelines for Use

USE EXACTLY AS PRESCRIBED.

Insert high into the vagina with the applicator provided.

Tell your healthcare provider if you miss a menstrual period or suspect pregnancy.

May cause sensitivity to light. Avoid prolonged exposure to the sun and other ultraviolet light. Use sunscreens and wear protective clothing until tolerance is determined.

Diabetes-Monitor urine or blood sugar closely and report changes to your healthcare provider if he/she advises.

Have regular physical exams.

Estramustine Phosphate Sodium

(ESS-truh-muss-TEEN FOSS-fate SO-dee-uhm)

Emcyt

A medicine used with other anti-cancer medicines for the treatment of advanced, inoperable cancer of the prostate.

Precautions

DO NOT USE if you are allergic to this medicine or nitrogen mustard or if you have a clotting disorder.

BEFORE USING THIS MEDICINE, tell your healthcare provider if you are taking, will be taking or stop taking any prescription or nonprescription medicine; or if you have any other medical conditions.

Side Effects

Every medicine can cause side effects, but many people have no, or minor, side effects. Tell your healthcare provider if any of the following occurs: pain, redness or swelling over a vein; fluid retention; difficulty breathing; leg cramps; upper respiratory discharge; hoarseness; nausea; vomiting; diarrhea; loss of appetite; gas; burning throat; thirst; minor stomach upset; rash; itching; dry skin; peeling skin of fingertips; easy bruising; flushing; thinning hair; feeling of indifference; drowsiness; sleeplessness; headache; anxiety; chest pain; tearing of eyes; breast tenderness; mild to moderate breast enlargement; black or tarry stools.

Guidelines for Use

USE EXACTLY AS PRESCRIBED.

Because of the possibility of birth defects, contraceptive measures are recommended during therapy.

Take three to four times daily with water at least 1 hour before or 2 hours after meals.

This medicine may lower your body's ability to fight infection. Tell your healthcare provider of any signs of infection including fever, sore throat, rashes or chills.

If a dose is missed, take as soon as possible. If several hours have passed or if it is nearing time for the next dose, do not double the dose to "catch up," unless advised by your healthcare provider. If more than one dose is missed, contact your healthcare provider.

Diabetes-Be prepared to monitor blood sugar more often to track loss of glucose control.

Milk, milk products and calcium-rich foods or medicine (eg, calcium-containing antacids) must not be taken simultaneously with this medicine.

Consult your healthcare provider periodically for evaluation of blood pressure.

Storage--Refrigerate. Capsules may be left out of the refrigerator for 24 to 48 hours without affecting potency.

Estrogens, Conjugated

(ESS-truh-janz, KAHN-juh-gay-tuhd)

Premarin, Premarin IV

A medicine used to control abnormal uterine bleeding due to hormonal imbalance.

Precautions

DO NOT USE if you have an allergy to this medicine, are pregnant or have undiagnosed vaginal bleeding.

BEFORE USING THIS MEDICINE, tell your healthcare provider if you are pregnant or breastfeeding; are taking, will be taking or stop taking any prescription or nonprescription medicine; or if you have any other medical conditions.

Side Effects

Every medicine can cause side effects, but many people have no, or minor, side effects. Tell your healthcare provider if any of the following occurs: breakthrough bleeding; spotting; change in menstrual flow; premenstrual-like symptoms; nausea; vomiting; abdominal cramps; bloating; yellowing of the skin or eyes; scalp hair loss; excess hair; headache; migraine; dizziness; mental depression; convulsions; pain at injection site; postinjection redness; weight changes; swelling; changes in sex drive; breast tenderness, enlargement or secretion.

Guidelines for Use

USE EXACTLY AS PRESCRIBED.

Contact your healthcare provider if any of the following occurs: pain in the groin or calves; sharp chest pain or sudden shortness of breath; abnormal vaginal bleeding; missed menstrual period or suspected pregnancy; lumps in the breast; sudden severe headache, dizziness or fainting; vision or speech disturbance; weakness or numbness in an arm or leg; severe abdominal pain; yellowing of the skin or eyes; severe depression.

Diabetes--Glucose tolerance may be decreased; monitor urine, sugar or serum glucose closely and report abnormalities to your healthcare provider.

Estropipate Oral

(ESS-troe-PIH-pate)

Ogen, Ortho-Est

Female hormones. This medicine has a variety of uses including treatment of various symptoms of menopause, replacement therapy, osteoporosis (loss of bone cells with aging) and some cancers.

Precautions

DO NOT USE if you are allergic to estrogens, are pregnant or have abnormal undiagnosed vaginal bleeding.

BEFORE USING THIS MEDICINE, tell your healthcare provider if you are pregnant or breastfeeding; a cigarette smoker; or if you are taking, will be taking or stop taking any prescription or nonprescription medicine; or if you have any other medical conditions.

Side Effects

Every medicine can cause side effects, but many people have no, or minor, side effects. Tell your healthcare provider if any of the following occurs: pain in the groin or calves; sharp chest pain or sudden shortness of breath; abnormal vaginal bleeding; breast lumps; sudden severe headache; dizziness or fainting; vision or speech problems; weakness or numbness in an arm or leg; severe abdominal pain; yellowing of the skin or eyes; severe depression.

Guidelines for Use

USE EXACTLY AS PRESCRIBED.

Diabetes-Blood sugar changes may occur. Monitor urine or blood sugar closely and report changes to your healthcare provider if he/she advises.

Have regular physical exams.

Tell your healthcare provider if you miss a menstrual period or suspect pregnancy.

Avoid prolonged exposure to the sun and other ultraviolet light sources (eg, tanning beds). Use sunscreens and wear protective clothing until sun tolerance is determined.

Report contact lens intolerance.

If a dose is missed, take it as soon as possible. If it is nearing time for the next dose, do not double the dose to "catch up," unless advised by your healthcare provider. If more than one dose is missed, contact your healthcare provider.

Estropipate Vaginal

(ESS-troe-PIH-pate)

Ogen

Used for treatment of atrophic vaginitis and kraurosis vulvae associated with menopause.

Precautions

DO NOT USE if you are allergic to this medicine.

BEFORE USING THIS MEDICINE, tell your healthcare provider if you are pregnant or breastfeeding; or if you are taking, will be taking or stop taking any prescription or nonprescription medicine; or if you have any other medical conditions.

Side Effects

Every medicine can cause side effects, but many people have no, or minor, side effects. Tell your healthcare provider if any of the following occurs: breakthrough bleeding; spotting; change in menstrual flow; menstrual irregularities; nausea; vomiting; abdominal cramps; bloating; scalp hair loss; excess hairiness; rash; itching; intolerance to contact lenses; headache; migraine; dizziness; mental depression; convulsions; increase or decrease in weight; swelling of the extremities; changes in sex drive; breast swelling.

Guidelines for Use

USE EXACTLY AS PRESCRIBED.

Package insert is available with this medicine.

Insert high into the vagina with the applicator.

Diabetes: Glucose tolerance may be decreased; monitor urine sugar or serum glucose closely and report abnormalities to your healthcare provider.

Ethacrynate and Ethacrynic Acid

(eth-uh-KRIN-ate and eth-uh-KRIN-ik acid)

Edecrin Tablets

This medicine is used to treat serious fluid accumulation (edema) due to a variety of causes.

Precautions

DO NOT USE if you are allergic to this medicine or its relatives; oral diabetic medicines; sulfa antibiotics; or if you have severe kidney disease or loss of kidney function.

BEFORE USING THIS MEDICINE, tell your healthcare provider if you are pregnant or breastfeeding; or if you are taking, will be taking or stop taking any prescription or nonprescription medicine; or if you have any other medical conditions.

Side Effects

Every medicine can cause side effects, but many people have no, or minor, side effects. Tell your healthcare provider if any of the following occurs: thirst; irregular heartbeat; mental confusion and mood changes; nausea; vomiting; unusual tiredness; weakness; weak pulse; muscle cramps; appetite loss; stomach upset; bloating; diarrhea; constipation; dizziness; lightheadedness; headache; tingling of toes and fingers; blurred vision; nervousness; insomnia; chest pain; ringing in the ears; hearing loss (reversible); sun sensitivity; rash; hives; itching; dry skin; yellow skin or eyes; unusual bruising; difficulty breathing; blood sugar imbalance; muscle cramps; joint pain; fever; chills; weight loss; nosebleeds; gout attack.

Guidelines for Use

USE EXACTLY AS PRESCRIBED.

Increases urination, therefore to avoid disruption of sleep at night take early in the day usually as a single dose.

May cause stomach upset. May be taken with food or milk. May cause loss of potassium.

If signs of potassium loss occur (eg, weakness, cramps, nausea, dizziness), contact your healthcare provider. Ask about foods high in potassium.

Diabetes-May increase blood sugar levels.

May cause gout attacks.

Call your healthcare provider if sudden joint pain occurs.

Dizziness or lightheadedness may occur during therapy; avoid sudden changes in posture.

Sensitivity to sunlight may occur. Use sunscreen and wear protective clothing until tolerance is determined.

Your healthcare provider may want to periodically check your blood to ensure that your medicine is working properly.

Ethchlorvynol

(eth-klor-VIH-nahl)

Placidyl Capsules

This medicine causes drowsiness to aid in falling asleep. It generally is used to treat insomnia for a short period of time (1 to 2 weeks).

Precautions

DO NOT USE if you are allergic to this medicine or to tartrazine.

BEFORE USING THIS MEDICINE, tell your healthcare provider if you are pregnant or breastfeeding; or if you are taking, will be taking or stop taking any prescription or nonprescription medicine; or if you have any other medical conditions.

Side Effects

Every medicine can cause side effects, but many people have no, or minor, side effects. Tell your healthcare provider if any of the following occurs: stomach upset; diarrhea; vomiting; constipation; confusion; excitement; nightmares; drowsiness; dizziness; headache; incoordination; decreased mobility; incoherence; rash; hives; redness; unpleasant taste in mouth.

Guidelines for Use

USE EXACTLY AS PRESCRIBED.

May cause drowsiness or dizziness. Use caution while driving or performing other tasks requiring mental alertness.

Symptoms of giddiness, incoordination and stomach upset may be reduced if medication is taken with food.

Take capsules with a full glass of water or fruit juice. Swallow capsules whole. Do not chew.

Avoid alcohol and other medicines that cause drowsiness (eg, pain relievers, sedatives, antihistamines).

There is a risk of oversedation, morning hangover (grogginess in the morning), dizziness and confusion.

Dose may need to be reduced. May be habit-forming.

Do not discontinue the medicine abruptly, especially if you have a history of seizures. Withdrawal symptoms may occur when the medicine is stopped.

Contact your healthcare provider if visual changes, irregular heartbeats, chest pains, yellowing of skin or eyes, rash or unusual bleeding or bruising occurs.

Ethosuximide

(ETH-oh-SUX-ih-mide)

Zarontin

A medicine used to control absence (petit mal) seizures.

Precautions

DO NOT USE if you are allergic to this medicine or other succinimides.

BEFORE USING THIS MEDICINE, tell your healthcare provider if you are pregnant or breastfeeding; or if you are taking, will be taking or stop taking any prescription or nonprescription medicine; or if you have any other medical conditions.

Side Effects

Every medicine can cause side effects, but many people have no, or minor, side effects. Tell your healthcare provider if any of the following occurs: nausea; vomiting; stomach discomfort; loss of appetite; diarrhea; constipation; abdominal pain; hiccups; drowsiness; dizziness; mood changes; headache; nervousness; exaggerated sense of well being; dream-like feeling; hyperactivity; confusion; fatigue; impaired coordination; sleep disturbances; depression; unusual bleeding or bruising; hives; increased growth and darkening of fine body hair; hair loss; joint pain; fever; sore throat; blurred vision; eyes sensitive to light; urinary frequency; blood in urine; muscle weakness; swelling of tongue and gums; swelling around the eyes.

Guidelines for Use

USE EXACTLY AS PRESCRIBED.

If stomach upset occurs, take with food or milk.

Do not change the dose or stop taking this medication without consulting your healthcare provider.

Abrupt withdrawal may cause seizures.

If a dose is missed, take it as soon as possible. If several hours have passed or if it is nearing time for the next dose, do not double the dose to "catch up," unless advised by your healthcare provider. If more than one dose is missed, contact your healthcare provider.

Keep scheduled appointments with your healthcare provider and carry Medic Alert identification listing your medical condition and medicine.

Avoid alcoholic beverages.

May cause drowsiness, dizziness, or blurred vision. Use caution while driving or performing other tasks requiring mental alertness, coordination and dexterity.

Notify your healthcare provider if any of the following occurs: skin rash, joint pain, unexplained fever, sore throat, unusual bleeding or bruising, drowsiness, dizziness, blurred vision, pregnancy, seizures, depression, aggressiveness.

Etidronate Disodium

(eh-TIH-DROE-nate die-SO-dee-uhm)

Didronel

A medicine used to treat Paget's disease of the bone. It also is used for the prevention and treatment of abnormal bone formation due to spinal injury or following total hip replacement. It may occasionally be prescribed for other reasons.

Precautions

DO NOT USE if you are allergic to this medicine.

BEFORE USING THIS MEDICINE, tell your healthcare provider if you are pregnant or breastfeeding; or if you are taking, will be taking or stop taking any prescription or nonprescription medicines; or have any other medical conditions.

Side Effects

Every medicine can cause side effects, but many people have no, or minor, side effects. Tell your healthcare provider if any of the following occurs: diarrhea; nausea; metallic, altered or loss of taste (temporary); increased or recurrent pain at pagetic sites (Paget's Disease); rash; hives; difficulty breathing; fever.

Guidelines for Use

USE EXACTLY AS PRESCRIBED.

To maximize absorption take on an empty stomach 2 hours before meals.

Avoid vitamins with mineral supplements or antacids high in metals (eg, calcium, iron, magnesium or aluminum).

Etodolac

(EE-toe-DOE-lak)

Lodine

A nonsteroidal anti-inflammatory medicine (NSAID) used to relieve mild to moderate pain and inflammation and to treat osteoarthritis (degenerative joint disease). It may occasionally be prescribed for other reasons.

Precautions

DO NOT USE if you are allergic to this medicine or its relatives, aspirin or iodides.

BEFORE USING THIS MEDICINE, tell your healthcare provider if you are pregnant or breastfeeding; use alcohol chronically; are prone to fluid retention; or if you are taking, will be taking or stop taking any prescription or nonprescription medicines; or have any other medical conditions.

Side Effects

Every medicine can cause side effects, but many people have no, or minor, side effects. Tell your healthcare provider if any of the following occurs: allergic reaction (eg, rash, itching, fever); changes in vision; weight gain; fluid retention; stomach problems (eg, nausea, vomiting, diarrhea, pain); black stools; constipation; persistent headache; dizziness; nervousness; weakness; ringing in the ears; taste changes; unusual bruising or bleeding.

Guidelines for Use

USE EXACTLY AS PRESCRIBED.

Avoid aspirin and alcoholic beverages.

If stomach upset occurs, take with food, milk or antacids. If stomach pain continues, tell your healthcare provider.

If a dose is missed, take it as soon as possible. If several hours have passed or if it is nearing time for the next dose, do not double the dose to "catch up," unless advised by your healthcare provider. If more than one dose is missed, contact your healthcare provider.

May cause drowsiness or dizziness. Observe caution while driving or performing other tasks requiring mental alertness, coordination and dexterity.

May cause sensitivity to sunlight. Avoid prolonged exposure to the sun. Use sunscreens and wear protective clothing until tolerance is determined.

Etoposide

(EH-toe-POE-side)

VePesid

An anticancer medicine.

Precautions

DO NOT USE if you are allergic to this medicine.

BEFORE USING THIS MEDICINE, tell your healthcare provider if you are pregnant or breastfeeding; or if you are taking, will be taking or stop taking any prescription or nonprescription medicine; or if you have any other medical conditions.

Side Effects

Every medicine can cause side effects, but many people have no, or minor, side effects. Tell your healthcare provider if any of the following occurs: nausea; vomiting; appetite loss; diarrhea; stomach ache; hair loss.

Guidelines for Use

USE EXACTLY AS PRESCRIBED.

If a dose is missed, take it as soon as possible. If several hours have passed or if it is nearing time for the next dose, do not double the dose to "catch up," unless advised by your healthcare provider. If more than one dose is missed, contact your healthcare provider.

This medicine may lower your body's ability to fight infection. Notify your healthcare provider if fever, sore throat, rashes or chills occur.

Also contact your healthcare provider if rapid heartbeat or difficulty breathing occurs.

Practice effective birth control measures during therapy.

Famciclovir

(fam-SIC-clo-ver)

Famvir

This medicine is used to treat acute herpes zoster (shingles) in adults with healthy immune systems.

Precautions

DO NOT USE if you are allergic to this medicine or to acyclovir (*Zovirax*).

BEFORE USING THIS MEDICINE, tell your healthcare provider if you are pregnant or breastfeeding; if you are taking, will be taking or stop taking any prescription or nonprescription medicine; or if you have any other medical conditions.

Side Effects

Every medicine can cause side effects, but many people have no, or minor, side effects. Tell your healthcare provider if any of the following occurs: fatigue; fever; pain; chills; stiffness; nausea; diarrhea; vomiting; constipation; loss of appetite; abdominal pain; back pain; joint pain; headache; dizziness; abnormal skin sensations; drowsiness; sore throat; sinus discomfort; itching; weakness.

Guidelines for Use

USE EXACTLY AS PRESCRIBED.

It is important to start treatment as soon as possible after the first sign of shingles. This medicine is most effective when started within 48 hours of the onset of the rash. It may not work after 72 hours of onset.

This medicine may be taken with or without food.

The usual dose of this medicine is 1 g (2 capsules) 3 times daily for 7 days. Elderly patients may take a smaller dose.

Continue taking until all of the prescribed medicine has been used, even if the rash or other symptoms have disappeared. Failure to take all of the medicine may prevent complete elimination of the virus.

If a dose is missed, take it as soon as possible. If several hours have passed or if it is nearing time for the next dose, do not double the dose to "catch up," unless advised by your healthcare provider. If more than one dose is missed, contact your healthcare provider.

This medicine is not recommended for use if you are infected by the HIV virus or have had a bone marrow transplant or kidney transplant.

Store at room temperature.

Famotidine

(fuh-MOE-tih-deen)

Pepcid, Pepcid AC

An anti-ulcer medicine used to treat stomach and duodenal (first part of small intestine) ulcers, hypersecretory (increased acid secretion) conditions (eg, Zollinger-Ellison syndrome) and gastroesophageal reflux (bubbling of stomach contents into the esophagus, which causes heartburn).

Precautions

DO NOT USE if you are allergic to this medicine.

BEFORE USING THIS MEDICINE, tell your healthcare provider if you have kidney or liver disease; are pregnant or breastfeeding; if you are taking, will be taking or stop taking any prescription or nonprescription medicines; or have any other medical conditions.

Side Effects

Every medicine can cause side effects, but many people have no, or minor, side effects. Tell your healthcare provider if any of the following occurs: nausea; vomiting; diarrhea; dizziness; rash; itching; unusual bleeding or bruising; fever; difficulty breathing; shortness of breath; sleep disturbances; joint pain; behavioral changes; headache; constipation.

Guidelines for Use

USE EXACTLY AS PRESCRIBED.

Suspension — Shake well before taking. Store below 86 degrees F; do not freeze. Discard unused portion after 30 days.

AC Tablets — Take 1 tablet with water, as needed, but do not exceed 2 tablets in 24 hours.

To prevent symptoms caused by eating or drinking certain foods or beverages, take 1 tablet before eating.

Do not take this medicine for longer than 2 weeks unless instructed to do so by your healthcare provider.

If a dose is missed, take it as soon as possible. If several hours have passed or if it is nearing time for the next dose, do not double the dose to "catch up," unless advised by your healthcare provider. If more than one dose is missed, contact your healthcare provider.

Never self-diagnose or self-treat ulcers with this or any other medicine.

It may be necessary to make significant lifestyle changes to assist in the treatment and prevention of ulcers and other digestive problems that can include stress-reduction programs, exercise and dietary changes.

Notify your healthcare provider if there are any symptoms that suggest a bleeding ulcer, such as black, tarry stools or coffee-ground vomit.

Felbamate

(FELL-buh-MATE)

Felbatol

An antiepileptic and anticonvulsant used in the treatment of partial seizures in adults with epilepsy and in the treatment of Lennox-Gastaut syndrome in children. This medicine should be used ONLY as secondary therapy in patients with severe refractory epilepsy who do not respond to other anticonvulsant medications.

Precautions

DO NOT USE if you are allergic to this medicine, its relatives or other carbamates; if you have liver disease/injury; or if you have a blood disease. This medicine should be used only when the risk of bone marrow failure and liver failure is deemed acceptable.

BEFORE USING THIS MEDICINE, tell your healthcare provider if you are pregnant or breastfeeding; or if you are taking, will be taking or stop taking any prescription or nonprescription medicine; or if you have any other medical conditions.

Side Effects

Every medicine can cause side effects, but many people have no, or minor, side effects. Tell your healthcare provider if any of the following occurs: appetite loss; indigestion; vomiting; nausea; constipation; diarrhea; stomach pain/bloating; anxiety; tremor; sleep disorders; dizziness; incoordination; chest pain; pounding in chest; fast heartbeat; headache; fever; fluid retention/swelling; urinary problems; unusual bleeding (women); dry mouth; altered taste; impaired vision; hiccoughs; abnormal skin sensations; confusion; unstable emotions; mood swings (mostly in children); abnormal thinking; congestion; sore throat; cough; middle ear infection; general body discomfort; pain; weakness; bleeding; bruising; acne; rash; itching; hives; yellowing of skin; weight changes.

Guidelines for Use

USE EXACTLY AS PRESCRIBED.

Shake well before use.

Take without regard to food.

Do not stop or adjust the dose unless directed.

If a dose is missed, take it as soon as possible. If several hours have passed or if it is nearing time for the next dose, do not double the dose to "catch up," unless advised by your healthcare provider. If more than one dose is missed, contact your healthcare provider.

Notify your healthcare provider immediately of fever, yellowing of the skin or eyes, appetite loss, abdominal pain or bloating, weakness, sore throat, unusual bleeding/bruising, rash, dark urine.

Lab tests will be needed to monitor therapy. Be sure to keep appointments.

May cause sensitivity to sunlight. Avoid long exposure to the sun and other ultraviolet light. Use sunscreen and wear protective clothing.

Store this medicine in a tightly closed container at room temperature away from excessive heat, direct sunlight or moisture.

Felodipine

(feh-LOW-dih-peen)

Plendil

A calcium channel blocker medicine that is used to treat high blood pressure. It may occasionally be prescribed for other reasons.

Precautions

DO NOT USE if you are allergic to this medicine.

BEFORE USING THIS MEDICINE, tell your healthcare provider if you are pregnant or breastfeeding; or if you are taking, will be taking or stop taking any prescription or nonprescription medicine; or if you have any other medical conditions.

Side Effects

Every medicine can cause side effects, but many people have no, or minor, side effects. Tell your healthcare provider if any of the following occurs: irregular heartbeat; increased frequency/severity of angina; shortness of breath; swelling of hands and feet; dizziness; constipation; nausea; low blood pressure (dizziness lightheadedness); or symptoms of a drug allergy (eg, itching, rash, hives, difficult breathing); swollen or enlarged gums; unusual bleeding or bruising.

Guidelines for Use

USE EXACTLY AS PRESCRIBED.

Swallow whole; do not crush or chew.

If a dose is missed, take it as soon as possible. If several hours have passed or if it is nearing time for the next dose, do not double the dose to "catch up," unless advised by your healthcare provider. If more than one dose is missed, contact your healthcare provider.

It is important to brush and floss your teeth and see your dentist regularly.

Do not suddenly stop taking this medicine as this may cause serious chest pains. This can be minimized if the medicine is tapered slowly by your healthcare provider.

Fenfluramine Hydrochloride

(fen-FLURE-uh-meen HIGH-droe-KLOR-ide)

Pondimin

A medicine that reduces appetite by suppressing the hunger center of the brain.

Precautions

DO NOT USE if you are pregnant; allergic to this medicine; or if you have a history of drug abuse.

BEFORE USING THIS MEDICINE, tell your healthcare provider if you are breastfeeding; or if you are taking, will be taking or stop taking any prescription or nonprescription medicine; or if you have any other medical conditions.

Side Effects

Every medicine can cause side effects, but many people have no, or minor, side effects. Tell your healthcare provider if any of the following occurs: nausea; vomiting; constipation; stomach cramps; diarrhea; restlessness; tremor; nervousness; anxiety; tension; confusion; insomnia; fainting; excitement; weakness; headache; aggressiveness; pounding in the chest; rapid pulse; irregular heart beats; chest pain; hair loss; flushing; chills; sweating; hives; rash; burning sensation; fever; muscle aches or pain; menstrual changes; sexual problems; dizziness; blurred vision; eye irritation; rapid breathing.

Guidelines for Use

USE EXACTLY AS PRESCRIBED.

Appetite suppressants are not substitutes for proper dieting. It is important to make lifestyle changes (eg, diet and exercise) while on therapy.

Take on an empty stomach.

May cause insomnia.

Avoid taking this medicine late in the day.

Avoid the use of alcohol.

May produce dizziness or blurred vision. Use caution while driving or performing other tasks requiring mental alertness.

Use of this medicine to improve athletic skills, mental alertness or to stay awake is dangerous and illegal.

Never share medicines with others.

Interrupted courses of therapy supervised by your healthcare provider may be useful in the treatment of obesity.

Fenoprofen Calcium

(FEN-oh-PRO-fen KAL-see-uhm)

Nalfon

A nonsteroidal anti-inflammatory medicine (NSAID) used to relieve mild to moderate pain and inflammation and to treat osteoarthritis (degenerative joint disease) and rheumatoid arthritis. It may occasionally be prescribed for other reasons.

Precautions

DO NOT USE if you are allergic to this medicine or its relatives, aspirin or iodides.

BEFORE USING THIS MEDICINE, tell your healthcare provider if you are pregnant or breastfeeding; use alcohol chronically; are prone to fluid retention; or if you are taking, will be taking or stop taking any prescription or nonprescription medicine; or if you have any other medical conditions.

Side Effects

Every medicine can cause side effects, but many people have no, or minor, side effects. Tell your healthcare provider if any of the following occurs: allergic reaction (eg, rash, itching, fever); changes in vision; weight gain; fluid retention; stomach problems (eg, nausea, vomiting, diarrhea, pain); black stools; constipation; persistent headache; dizziness; nervousness; weakness; ringing in the ears; taste changes; unusual bruising or bleeding.

Guidelines for Use

USE EXACTLY AS PRESCRIBED.

If stomach upset occurs, take with food, milk or antacids. If stomach pain continues, tell your healthcare provider.

Avoid aspirin and alcoholic beverages.

If a dose is missed, take it as soon as possible. If several hours have passed or if it is nearing time for the next dose, do not double the dose to "catch up," unless advised by your healthcare provider. If more than one dose is missed, contact your healthcare provider.

This medicine may cause drowsiness or dizziness. Use caution while driving or performing other tasks requiring mental alertness, coordination and dexterity.

May cause sensitivity to sunlight. Avoid prolonged exposure to the sun. Use sunscreen and wear protective clothing until tolerance is determined.

Fentanyl Citrate

(FEN-tuh-nill SIH-trate)

Fentanyl Citrate Oral Transmucosal, Fentanyl Oralet

This medicine is a narcotic analgesic used as an anesthetic premedication and also for sedation prior to a diagnostic or therapeutic procedure.

Precautions

DO NOT USE if you are allergic to this medicine. Do not use in children who weigh less than 33 pounds or to treat serious or chronic pain. The medicine should not be used if you have taken monoamine oxidase (MAO) inhibitors (eg, *Parnate*) within 14 days. Not for use at home or anywhere outside a hospital.

Side Effects

Every medicine can cause side effects, but many people have no, or minor, side effects. Tell your healthcare provider if any of the following occurs: shortness of breath; headache; flushing; paleness; nausea; vomiting; apathy; dizziness; fainting; exaggerated sense of well-being; abnormal skin sensations; itching; rash; vision changes.

Guidelines for Use

USE EXACTLY AS PRESCRIBED.

This medicine should only be used in a hospital.

Doses should be individualized.

Destroy unconsumed portions of the lozenge, consistent with state and federal regulations.

The medicine should be given 20 to 40 minutes before the desired effect is needed; the lozenge should be taken by sucking on it until it is gone (10 to 20 minutes).

Fentanyl Transdermal System

(FEN-tuh-nill)

Duragesic-25, Duragesic-50, Duragesic-75, Duragesic-100

A narcotic pain reliever used for chronic pain.

Precautions

DO NOT USE , if you are allergic to this medicine or its relatives.

BEFORE USING THIS MEDICINE, tell your healthcare provider if you are pregnant or breastfeeding; or if you are taking, will be taking or stop taking any prescription or nonprescription medicine; or if you have any other medical conditions. Long-term, regular use of narcotic pain relievers may lead to dependence and physical tolerance. Withdrawal symptoms may occur when therapy is stopped.

Side Effects

Every medicine can cause side effects, but many people have no, or minor, side effects. Tell your healthcare provider if any of the following occurs: lightheadedness; dizziness; drowsiness; nausea; vomiting; sweating; abdominal pain; constipation; diarrhea; urine retention; appetite loss; indigestion; excitability; vision problems; difficult breathing; headache; dry mouth; confusion; weakness; nervousness; itching.

Guidelines for Use

USE EXACTLY AS PRESCRIBED.

May cause drowsiness, dizziness or blurred vision. Use caution while driving or performing other tasks requiring mental alertness, judgment and coordination.

Avoid alcohol and other medicines that cause drowsiness (eg, sleeping pills, antihistamines).

May cause nausea, vomiting or constipation. Constipation may be avoided by using a stool softener or fiber laxative.

Keep all used and unused systems out of the reach of children.

This patch should be applied to a dry, nonirritated section of skin on the chest or back. Clip (don't shave) any hair at the application site, and clean the area with clear water only and then dry. Apply the patch immediately upon removal from the sealed package. Press firmly in place with the palm of the hand for 10 to 20 seconds, ensuring that all the edges are in contact with the skin.

Used systems should be flushed down the toilet immediately upon removal.

If the gel from the medicine reservoir accidentally comes in contact with the skin, the area should be washed with clear water.

Ferrous Salts

(FER-uhs salts)

Femiron, Feosol, Feratab, Fergon, Fer-In-Sol, Fer-Iron, Fero-Gradumet Filmtab, Ferospace, Ferra-TD, Ferralet, Ferralet Slow Release, Ferralyn Lanacaps, Ferrous Sulfate, Fumasorb, Fumerin, Hemocyte, Ircon, Mol-Iron, Nephro-Fer, Simron, Slow-FE, Span-FF

Used to prevent or treat iron deficiency anemia.

Precautions

DO NOT USE if you are allergic to iron; have inflammation of the small intestine; non-iron deficiency anemias or blood disorders; peptic ulcers; or ulcerative colitis.

BEFORE USING THIS MEDICINE, tell your healthcare provider if you are pregnant or breastfeeding; or if you are taking, will be taking or stop taking any prescription or nonprescription medicine; or if you have any other medical conditions.

Side Effects

Every medicine can cause side effects, but many people have no, or minor, side effects. Tell your healthcare provider if any of the following occurs: stomach ache; appetite loss; constipation; diarrhea; staining of teeth; iron overdose--unexplained tiredness, nausea, vomiting, abdominal pain, black, tarry stools, dehydration.

Guidelines for Use

USE EXACTLY AS PRESCRIBED.

Take after meals or with food if stomach upset occurs.

Avoid taking antacids, tetracycline or fluoroquinolones at the same time; allow 1 to 2 hours between.

Liquid iron preparations may be put in water or juice. Drink through a straw to prevent staining of teeth.

Medication may cause black stools, constipation or diarrhea.

Sustained release — Do not crush or chew.

Recommended Dietary Allowances (RDA): Adult males—10 mg; Adult females—15 mg; Pregnancy—30 mg; Breastfeeding—15 mg. Common sources of iron — Meat, eggs, vegetables and fortified enriched cereals.

In a true iron deficiency state, iron doses are higher than the RDA. Discuss the desired dose and duration of therapy with your healthcare provider if you are iron deficient.

Filgrastim

(fill-GRAH-stim)

Neupogen

Used to decrease the incidence of infection in patients with certain cancers receiving anti-cancer medicines associated with a significant incidence of severe low white blood cell count with fever. It also is used to reduce the duration of low white blood cell count in patients with malignancies undergoing chemotherapy followed by marrow transplantation; used to reduce the incidence and duration of symptoms of low white blood cell count in patients with certain types of neutropenia. It may occasionally be prescribed for other reasons.

Precautions

DO NOT USE if you are allergic to this medicine.

BEFORE USING THIS MEDICINE, tell your healthcare provider if you are pregnant or breastfeeding; or if you are taking, will be taking or stop taking any prescription or nonprescription medicine; or if you have any other medical conditions.

Side Effects

Every medicine can cause side effects, but many people have no, or minor, side effects. Tell your healthcare provider if any of the following occurs: *Patients receiving myelosuppressive chemotherapy*—nausea/vomiting; skeletal pain; hair loss; diarrhea; fever; fatigue; appetite loss; difficulty breathing; headache; cough; skin rash; chest pain; general weakness; sore throat; constipation; pain. *Bone marrow transplant patients*—rash; mouth irritation; nausea; vomiting; neck/mouth swelling. *Patients with severe chronic neutropenia*—mild to moderate bone pain; nosebleeds; injection site reaction; rash; joint pain; abdominal pain/swelling.

Guidelines for Use

USE EXACTLY AS PRESCRIBED.

Home care patients—Carefully follow your healthcare provider's instructions in regards to the proper disposal, and reuse of needles, syringes and medicine. Always use the puncture-resistant container supplied by your healthcare provider for disposal of used syringes and needles. Follow the directions for the safe disposal of the full container.

Bone pain is the most common side effect and can be usually controlled with non-narcotic pain relievers.

Periodic lab tests need to be performed to monitor your response to the medicine. Keep appointments.

Finasteride

(fih-NASS-teer-IDE)

Proscar

A medicine to treat nonmalignant prostate gland enlargement.

Precautions

DO NOT USE if you are allergic to this medicine; not intended for use in women. A woman who is pregnant or who may become pregnant should not handle crushed tablets because of the danger of absorption.

BEFORE USING THIS MEDICINE, tell your healthcare provider if you are taking, will be taking or stop taking any prescription or nonprescription medicine; or if you have any other medical conditions.

Side Effects

Every medicine can cause side effects, but many people have no, or minor, side effects. Tell your healthcare provider if any of the following occurs: impotence; decreased sex drive; decreased ejaculate.

Guidelines for Use

USE EXACTLY AS PRESCRIBED.

If a dose is missed, take it as soon as possible. If several hours have passed or if it is nearing time for the next dose, do not double the dose to "catch up," unless advised by your healthcare provider. If more than one dose is missed, contact your healthcare provider.

Although early improvement may be seen, at least 6 to 12 months of therapy may be necessary to assess response.

It is important to keep regular appointments with your healthcare provider for assessment and laboratory tests.

Women generally should avoid contact with this medicine.

Flavoxate

(flay-voke-sate)

Urispas

A medicine used for the relief of painful urination, frequency, urgency, nighttime urination, incontinence and pain associated with urinary tract disorders. It is not a definitive treatment but is compatible with other urinary tract medicines.

Precautions

DO NOT USE if you are allergic to this medicine.

BEFORE USING THIS MEDICINE, tell your healthcare provider if you are pregnant or breastfeeding; or if you are taking, will be taking or stop taking any prescription or nonprescription medicine; or if you have any other medical conditions.

Side Effects

Every medicine can cause side effects, but many people have no, or minor, side effects. Tell your healthcare provider if any of the following occurs: nausea; vomiting; nervousness; vertigo (feeling of whirling motion); headache; drowsiness; confusion; dry mouth; high fever; painful or difficult urination; increased heart rate; pounding in the chest; vision problems (eg, blurred vision); hives; rash; skin disorders.

Guidelines for Use

USE EXACTLY AS PRESCRIBED.

May cause drowsiness or blurred vision. Use caution while driving or performing other tasks requiring alertness, coordination or physical dexterity.

May cause dry mouth, hives and rash. If these or other side effects persist or worsen, contact your healthcare provider.

Flecainide Acetate

(fleh-CANE-ide ASS-uh-TATE)

Tambocor

A heart medicine (antiarrhythmic) used for various types of irregular heartbeats that lead to life-threatening heart rhythm disturbances.

Precautions

DO NOT USE if you are allergic to this medicine.

BEFORE USING THIS MEDICINE, tell your healthcare provider if you are pregnant or breastfeeding; or if you are taking, will be taking or stop taking any prescription or nonprescription medicine; or if you have any other medical conditions.

Side Effects

Every medicine can cause side effects, but many people have no, or minor, side effects. Tell your healthcare provider if any of the following occurs: nausea; vomiting; constipation; indigestion; appetite loss; diarrhea; dizziness; numbness and tingling of toes and fingers; tremor; headache; depression; sleeplessness; fatigue; weakness; incoordination; anxiety; new or worsened heart rhythm disturbances; heart rate changes; chest pain; pounding in the chest; rash; flushing; sweating; fluid retention; vision problems; ringing in the ears; difficulty breathing; fever; fainting.

Guidelines for Use

USE EXACTLY AS PRESCRIBED.

Serious heartbeat disturbances can result from missing any doses and serious side effects can result from increasing or decreasing doses without supervision.

Blood tests for medicine levels may be required to monitor your therapy; keep appointments.

Floxuridine

(flox-YUR-ih-deen)

FDUR

Used for the treatment of inoperable liver cancer.

Side Effects

Every medicine can cause side effects, but many people have no, or minor, side effects. Tell your healthcare provider if any of the following occurs: diarrhea; loss of appetite; nausea; vomiting; cramps; bleeding; loss of hair; nail changes including loss of nails; dry skin; splitting of the skin; flushing or increased skin pigmentation; general body discomfort; weakness; headache; lethargy; disorientation; confusion; fever; chest pain; mouth sores; black or bloody stools; rash; difficulty breathing; vision changes; drowsiness; pain or bleeding at the injection site; nosebleeds.

Patient Information

Contraceptive (birth control) measures are recommended for men and women during therapy.

Tell your healthcare provider if chills, nausea, vomiting, unusual bleeding or bruising, yellowing of the skin or eyes, abdominal pain, flank or joint pain or swelling of feet or legs occur.

Drink plenty of liquids while on this therapy.

May cause diarrhea, fever and weakness. Tell your healthcare provider if these become pronounced.

Fluconazole

(flew-KOE-nuh-zole)

Diflucan

An antifungal medicine used to treat certain yeast infections of the mouth and throat, the urinary tract, peritonium (lining of the abdomen and pelvis) and pneumonia. It may occasionally be prescribed for other reasons.

Precautions

DO NOT USE if you have an allergy to this medicine.

BEFORE USING THIS MEDICINE, tell your healthcare provider if you are pregnant or breastfeeding; or if you are taking, will be taking or stop taking any prescription or nonprescription medicine; or if you have any other medical conditions.

Side Effects

Every medicine can cause side effects, but many people have no, or minor, side effects. Tell your healthcare provider if any of the following occurs: nausea; vomiting; stomach ache; diarrhea; headache; rash.

Guidelines for Use

USE EXACTLY AS PRESCRIBED.

Take this medicine until it is all gone, or as directed by your healthcare provider.

If a dose is missed, take it as soon as possible. If several hours have passed or if it is nearing time for the next dose, do not double the dose to "catch up," unless advised by your healthcare provider. If more than one dose is missed, contact your healthcare provider.

Flucytosine

(flew-SITE-oh-seen)

Ancobon, 5–FC, 5–Fluorocytosine

A medicine used to treat serious fungal infections.

Precautions

DO NOT USE if you are allergic to this medicine.

BEFORE USING THIS MEDICINE, tell your healthcare provider if you are pregnant or breastfeeding; or if you are taking, will be taking or stop taking any prescription or nonprescription medicine; or if you have any other medical conditions.

Side Effects

Every medicine can cause side effects, but many people have no, or minor, side effects. Tell your healthcare provider if any of the following occurs: chest pain; difficulty breathing; rash; itching; hives; sensitivity to sunlight; nausea; vomiting; abdominal pain; diarrhea; loss of appetite; dry mouth; yellowing of the skin or eyes; incoordination; hearing loss; headache; abnormal skin sensations; tremors; rigid muscles; fever; feeling of a whirling motion; confusion; hallucinations; mental disturbances; sedation.

Guidelines for Use

USE EXACTLY AS PRESCRIBED.

May cause nausea and vomiting. Reduce or avoid by taking the capsules a few at a time over a 15-minute period. Tell your healthcare provider if symptoms become severe.

If a dose is missed, take it as soon as possible. If several hours have passed or if it is nearing time for the next dose, do not double the dose to "catch up," unless advised by your healthcare provider. If more than one dose is missed, contact your healthcare provider.

Medicine may cause drowsiness and feeling of whirling motion. Use caution while driving or performing other tasks requiring mental alertness, coordination or dexterity.

May cause sensitivity to sunlight. Avoid prolonged exposure to the sun. Use sunscreen and wear protective clothing until tolerance is determined.

Fludrocortisone Acetate

(flew-droe-CORE-tih-sone ASS-uh-TATE)

Florinef Acetate

A medicine that helps the kidney save sodium by increasing potassium and hydrogen loss in the urine. It treats lack of steroids from the adrenal cortex and excessive salt loss. It may occasionally be prescribed for other reasons.

Precautions

DO NOT USE if you are having glucose tolerance tests done or if you have an infection.

BEFORE USING THIS MEDICINE, tell your healthcare provider if you are pregnant or breastfeeding; or if you are taking, will be taking or stop taking any prescription or nonprescription medicine; or if you have any other medical conditions.

Side Effects

Every medicine can cause side effects, but many people have no, or minor, side effects. Tell your healthcare provider if any of the following occurs: fluid retention; joint pain; muscle weakness; headache; dizziness; unusual weight gain.

Guidelines for Use

USE EXACTLY AS PRESCRIBED.

Call your healthcare provider if dizziness, severe headaches, joint pain, extreme weakness, swelling of feet or lower legs, or unusual weight gain occurs.

If a dose is missed, take it as soon as possible. If several hours have passed or if it is nearing time for the next dose, do not double the dose to "catch up," unless advised by your healthcare provider. If more than one dose is missed, contact your healthcare provider.

Do not stop taking suddenly.

Lab tests may be needed to determine sodium and potassium levels in the blood. When fluid retention occurs, your healthcare provider may recommend a low-sodium diet.

Flunisolide

(flew-NIH-sole-ide)

AeroBid, AeroBid-M, Nasalide

A medicine used to treat allergy symptoms (eg, itching, runny nose, nasal congestion and sneezing) in patients over 6 years of age.

Precautions

DO NOT USE if you are allergic to this medicine or its ingredients, have nasal infections or herpes infections near the eye.

BEFORE USING THIS MEDICINE, tell your healthcare provider if you are pregnant or breastfeeding; or if you are taking, will be taking or stop taking any prescription or nonprescription medicines; or if you have any other medical conditions.

Side Effects

Every medicine can cause side effects, but many people have no, or minor, side effects. Tell your healthcare provider if any of the following occurs: sneezing; nasal irritation, burning, drying or stinging; nosebleed; blood in mucus; headache; stuffy nose; watery eyes; sore throat; nausea; vomiting; loss of smell or taste.

Guidelines for Use

USE EXACTLY AS PRESCRIBED.

Read and follow additional patient instructions carefully.

Do not exceed recommended dosage. Usual adult dose is 2 sprays per nostril twice a day (max. 8 sprays per nostril per day); children, 1 spray per nostril 3 times a day or 2 sprays per nostril twice a day (max. 4 sprays per nostril).

Effects are not immediate; benefit usually occurs in a few days.

Clear nasal passages prior to use by blowing the nose and using a saline solution if secretions are thick. If nasal passages are blocked, use a decongestant 15 minutes before using to ensure adequate penetration of the spray.

May be used alone, or with an antihistamine or decongestant.

Symptoms due to allergies (watering, itching eyes) are not significantly relieved by this medicine.

Use with caution if sores or injuries occur in the nasal passages (eg, frequent nosebleed). This medicine may prevent or slow proper healing.

Infection of the nose and throat has been linked with long-term use. Such infection may require stopping this medicine.

If symptoms do not improve within 3 weeks, contact your healthcare provider.

After the desired effect is obtained, reduce the maintenance dose to the smallest amount necessary to control the symptoms.

Report any unusual fever, joint/muscle pain, weakness, sneezing, nasal irritation, depression or fluid retention to your healthcare provider.

Avoid exposure to chickenpox, measles or other infections; if exposed, contact your healthcare provider immediately.

Exams may be necessary. Be sure to keep appointments.

Store at room temperature.

Fluorouracil (5-Fluorouracil; 5-FU)

(FLURE-oh-YUR-uh-sill)

Adrucil, Efudex, Fluoroplex

An anticancer medicine. A topical medicine used for precancerous skin growths and superficial basal cell carcinomas. It may occasionally be prescribed for other reasons.

Precautions

DO NOT USE if you are allergic to this medicine.

BEFORE USING THIS MEDICINE, tell your healthcare provider if you are pregnant or breastfeeding; or if you are taking, will be taking or stop taking any prescription or nonprescription medicine; or if you have any other medical conditions.

Side Effects

Every medicine can cause side effects, but many people have no, or minor, side effects. Tell your healthcare provider if any of the following occurs: diarrhea; temporary hair loss; fever; sore throat; chills; nausea; vomiting; unusual bleeding or bruising; black, tarry stools; darkened or bloody urine; yellowing of skin or eyes; mouth sores; flank or joint pain; swelling of feet or legs.

Guidelines for Use

USE EXACTLY AS PRESCRIBED.

Drink plenty of liquids.

Practice effective birth control measures during therapy.

If a dose is missed, take it as soon as possible. If several hours have passed or if it is nearing time for the next dose, do not double the dose to "catch up," unless advised by your healthcare provider. If more than one dose is missed, contact your healthcare provider.

Wash hands immediately after applying.

Use caution near eyes, nose and mouth.

Reaction in the treated area may be unsightly during and sometimes after therapy.

Avoid airtight bandages.

Fluoxetine Hydrochloride

(flew-OX-uh-teen HIGH-droe-KLOR-ide)

Prozac

An antidepressant and mood elevating agent used to relieve mental depression and to treat Obsessive-Compulsive Disorder (OCD) in adults. It may occasionally be prescribed for other reasons.

Precautions

DO NOT USE if you are allergic to this medicine or use monoamine oxidase inhibitors (eg, phenelzine, tranylcypromine).

BEFORE USING THIS MEDICINE, tell your healthcare provider if you are pregnant or breastfeeding; or if you are taking, will be taking or stop taking any prescription or non-prescription medicine; or have other medical conditions.

Side Effects

Every medicine can cause side effects, but many people have no, or minor, side effects. Tell your healthcare provider if any of the following occurs: rash; hives; anxiety; appetite changes; weight loss; headache; sleep disorders; tremor; dizziness; nausea; diarrhea; stomach ache; dry mouth; indigestion; sweating; sore throat; vomiting; constipation; gas; dark, bloody stools/vomit; lightheadedness; weakness; agitation; abnormal dreams/thinking; memory loss; twitching; confusion; pounding in chest; chest pain; nasal congestion; sinus infection; difficult breathing; yawning; cough; acne; itching; painful menstruation; sexual desire/ability changes; frequent urination; fever; general body pain; vision changes; taste changes; ringing in ears; chills; fluid retention; swollen lymph nodes.

Guidelines for Use

USE EXACTLY AS PRESCRIBED.

May be administered without regard to food.

If a dose is missed, take it as soon as possible. If several hours have passed or if it is nearing time for the next dose, do not double the dose to "catch up," unless advised by your healthcare provider. If more than one dose is missed, contact your healthcare provider.

Improvement may not be seen for several days to a few weeks.

May cause drowsiness, dizziness or impaired judgment. Use caution while driving or performing other tasks requiring alertness.

Avoid using alcohol or other depressants (eg, pain relievers, antihistamines) that may cause drowsiness and other side effects.

Diabetes — Monitor blood glucose levels daily.

Do not use with MAOIs (monoamine oxidase inhibitors) or within 14 days of discontinuing treatment with an MAOI. After stopping this medication, wait at least 5 weeks before starting an MAOI.

May cause sleeplessness if taken in evening. Take single doses in morning. Take twice daily doses in the morning and at noon.

Store in a dry place at room temperature.

Fluphenazine

(flew-FEN-uh-zeen)

Permitil, Prolixin, Prolixin Decanoate, Prolixin Enanthate

A neuroleptic or major tranquilizer generally used to improve concentration and self-control in patients with psychotic behavior.

Precautions

DO NOT USE if you are allergic to this medicine or its relatives. Laboratory tests may be needed including eye exams, blood counts and kidney and liver tests.

BEFORE USING THIS MEDICINE, tell your healthcare provider if you are pregnant or breastfeeding; or if you are taking, will be taking or stop taking any prescription or nonprescription medicine; if you have any other medical conditions; or if you are allergic to tartrazine.

Side Effects

Every medicine can cause side effects, but many people have no, or minor, side effects. Tell your healthcare provider if any of the following occurs: tremors; drooling; shuffling gait; restlessness; muscle spasms; aching or numbness; sore throat; fever; unusual bleeding or bruising; skin rash; weakness; impaired vision; dark-colored urine; pale stools; yellowing of skin or eyes.

Guidelines for Use

USE EXACTLY AS PRESCRIBED.

Take routinely as directed; it controls illness symptoms and is not habit-forming.

Improvement may not be seen for several weeks.

May cause drowsiness. Use caution while driving or performing other tasks requiring mental alertness.

Avoid alcohol and medicines that cause drowsiness (eg, sleeping pills, antihistamines).

May cause sunlight sensitivity. Avoid long exposure to the sun. Use sunscreens and protective clothing until tolerance is known.

May discolor the urine pink or reddish brown. This is not harmful.

If dizziness or fainting occurs, avoid sudden changes in posture and use caution when climbing stairs, etc (more common during first week of therapy).

Caution in hot weather: May increase risk of heat-stroke.

Flurazepam Hydrochloride

(flure-AZE-uh-pam HIGH-droe-KLOR-ide)

Dalmane

A benzodiazepine medicine that is a sleeping pill to treat insomnia for a short period of time (1 to 2 weeks). Long-term use generally is not recommended.

Precautions

DO NOT USE if you are allergic to this medicine or its relatives; or if you are pregnant.

BEFORE USING THIS MEDICINE, tell your healthcare provider if you are pregnant or breastfeeding; or if you are taking, will be taking or stop taking any prescription or nonprescription medicine; or if you have any other medical conditions.

Side Effects

Every medicine can cause side effects, but many people have no, or minor, side effects. Tell your healthcare provider if any of the following occurs: vision changes; irregular heartbeat; headache; chest pain; yellowing of skin or eyes; rash; unusual bleeding or bruising; vomiting; heartburn; diarrhea; constipation; appetite loss; nervousness; irritability; memory loss; sleeplessness; ringing in the ears; sore throat; joint pain.

Guidelines for Use

USE EXACTLY AS PRESCRIBED.

Do not exceed prescribed dosage.

Take with a full glass of water.

Use caution while driving or performing other tasks requiring mental alertness, coordination and dexterity.

May cause morning drowsiness, unusual tiredness in the morning or daytime sleepiness after using these medications for sleep. The elderly are particularly sensitive to these effects.

Avoid alcohol and other medications that cause drowsiness (eg, pain relievers, sedatives, antihistamines).

Nighttime sleep may be disturbed for 1 or 2 nights following stopping of the medication.

May be habit-forming.

Do not discontinue medicine abruptly, especially if you have a history of seizures, regardless of other antiseizure medications you may be taking.

Long-term use may result in dependence. Withdrawal symptoms may occur when the medication is stopped.

Flurbiprofen Ophthalmic

(FLURE-bih-PRO-fen)

Ocufen

A medicine that is used to prevent pupil constriction during surgery. It may occasionally be prescribed for other reasons.

Precautions

DO NOT USE if you are allergic to this medicine.

BEFORE USING THIS MEDICINE, tell your healthcare provider if you are pregnant or breastfeeding; or if you are taking, will be taking or stop taking any prescription or nonprescription medicine; or if you have any other medical conditions.

Side Effects

Every medicine can cause side effects, but many people have no, or minor, side effects. Tell your healthcare provider if any of the following occurs: temporary burning or stinging; irritation; redness; itching; sensitivity to light; increased bleeding during eye surgery.

Guidelines for Use

USE EXACTLY AS PRESCRIBED.

Surgery-One drop should be placed into the eye every half hour, beginning 2 hours before surgery (total of 4 drops).

Contact your healthcare provider if you have bleeding problems, are on medicine that prolongs bleeding time (eg, blood thinners), or have an active case or a history of herpes simplex infection of the eye. This medicine may delay wound healing.

Flurbiprofen Oral

(FLURE-bih-PRO-fen)

Ansaid

A nonsteroidal anti-inflammatory medicine (NSAID) generally used to treat osteoarthritis (degenerative joint disease) and rheumatoid arthritis. It may occasionally be prescribed for other reasons.

Precautions

DO NOT USE if you are allergic to this medicine or its relatives, aspirin or iodides.

BEFORE USING THIS MEDICINE, tell your healthcare provider if you are pregnant or breastfeeding; use alcohol chronically; are prone to fluid retention; or if you are taking, will be taking or stop taking any prescription or nonprescription medicines; or have any other medical conditions.

Side Effects

Every medicine can cause side effects, but many people have no, or minor, side effects. Tell your healthcare provider if any of the following occurs: allergic reaction (eg, rash, itching, fever); changes in vision; weight gain; fluid retention; stomach problems (eg, nausea, vomiting, diarrhea, pain); black stools; constipation; persistent headache; dizziness; nervousness; weakness; ringing in the ears; taste changes; unusual bruising or bleeding.

Guidelines for Use

USE EXACTLY AS PRESCRIBED.

Avoid aspirin and alcoholic beverages.

If stomach upset occurs, take with food, milk or antacids. If stomach pain continues, tell your healthcare provider.

If a dose is missed, take it as soon as possible. If several hours have passed or if it is nearing time for the next dose, do not double the dose to "catch up," unless advised by your healthcare provider. If more than one dose is missed, contact your healthcare provider.

May cause drowsiness or dizziness. Observe caution while driving or performing other tasks requiring mental alertness, coordination and dexterity.

May cause sensitivity to sunlight. Avoid prolonged exposure to the sun. Use sunscreens and wear protective clothing until tolerance is determined.

Flutamide

(FLEW-tuh-mide)

Eulexin

A medicine used in combination with other anti-cancer medicines to treat recurrent, inoperable prostate cancer.

Precautions

DO NOT USE if you are allergic to this medicine or if you are a woman.

BEFORE USING THIS MEDICINE, tell your healthcare provider if you are taking, will be taking or stop taking any prescription or nonprescription medicine; or if you have any other medical conditions.

Side Effects

Every medicine can cause side effects, but many people have no, or minor, side effects. Tell your healthcare provider if any of the following occurs: hot flashes; loss of sex drive; impotence; stomach upset; loss of appetite; diarrhea; nausea; vomiting; breast enlargement; swelling; itching; fluid retention; drowsiness; confusion; depression; anxiety; nervousness; rash; muscle cramps; swelling of hands or feet; discolored urine; anemia; unusual bleeding or bruising.

Guidelines for Use

USE EXACTLY AS PRESCRIBED.

DO NOT stop taking this medicine, or change the dose, without talking with your healthcare provider.

Usual dose is 2 capsules 3 times daily, 8 hours apart. Take on an empty stomach with a full glass of water. However, if stomach upset occurs, take with food.

Be sure to take this medicine in combination with your LHRH agonist analog (eg, Lupron) for the proper treatment.

If a dose is missed, take it as soon as possible. If several hours have passed, or if it is nearing time for the next dose, do not double the dose to "catch up," unless advised by your healthcare provider. If more than one dose is missed, contact your healthcare provider.

Report itching, dark urine, appetite loss, yellowing of skin or eyes, stomach pain/tenderness or flu-like symptoms to your healthcare provider immediately.

Lab tests will be required to monitor treatment. Be sure to keep appointments.

Store at room temperature away from moisture.

Fluvastatin

(FLEW-vah-stat-in)

Lescol

A medicine used to lower the level of cholesterol in the blood. It may occasionally be prescribed for other reasons.

Precautions

DO NOT USE if you are allergic to this medicine; if you are pregnant or if you are breastfeeding.

BEFORE USING THIS MEDICINE, tell your healthcare provider if you are taking, will be taking or stop taking any prescription or nonprescription medicine; or if you have any other medical conditions.

Side Effects

Every medicine can cause side effects, but many people have no, or minor, side effects. Tell your healthcare provider if any of the following occurs: back pain; indigestion; diarrhea; stomach pain; headache; cold- or flu-like symptoms; nausea; constipation; rash; muscle cramps.

Guidelines for Use

USE EXACTLY AS PRESCRIBED.

Take once daily at bedtime; may take with or without food.

If a dose is missed, take it as soon as possible. If several hours have passed or if it is nearing time for the next dose, do not double the dose to "catch up," unless advised by your healthcare provider. If more than one dose is missed, contact your healthcare provider.

If you are also taking cholestyramine, take this medicine at least 2 hours after taking cholestyramine.

Regular blood and laboratory tests may be necessary to make sure your medicine is working; be sure to keep appointments.

Tell your healthcare provider immediately of any unexplained muscle pain, tenderness or weakness, especially if accompanied by fever or general body discomfort.

Exercise and a diet that reduces the intake of cholesterol and saturated fats should accompany the use of this medicine.

Fluvoxamine Maleate

(flu-VOX-uh-meen MAL-ee-ate)

Luvox

An antidepressant and mood elevating agent used to treat obsessive-compulsive disorder (OCD) in patients over 18 years of age.

Precautions

DO NOT USE if you are allergic to this medicine, or are using monoamine oxidase inhibitors (MAOIs, eg *Nardil*), terfenadine (*Seldane*) or astemizole (*Hismanal*).

BEFORE USING THIS MEDICINE, tell your healthcare provider if you are pregnant or breastfeeding; if you are taking, will be taking or stop taking any prescription or nonprescription medicine; or if you have any other medical conditions. This medicine may not be as effective if you are a smoker.

Side Effects

Every medicine can cause side effects, but many people have no, or minor, side effects. Tell your healthcare provider if any of the following occurs: sleeplessness; nausea; drowsiness; dry mouth; tremor; changes in sexual desire or ability; sweating; taste changes; vomiting; constipation; indigestion; diarrhea; stomach pain; appetite changes; gas; headache; memory loss; indifference; incoordination; anxiety; dizziness; flushing; depression; chest pain; pounding in the chest; rapid heartbeat; lightheadedness; runny nose; congestion; difficulty breathing; cough; hives; itching; rash; unusual bruising; frequent urination; painful menstruation; general body discomfort; fluid retention; weight change; ear pain; muscle spasms; weakness; vision impairment; difficulty swallowing; seizures.

Guidelines for Use

USE EXACTLY AS PRESCRIBED.

Take in one or two doses without regard to food, but do not chew tablet.

If a single dose is prescribed, take it at bedtime; of two doses are prescribed, take the larger dose at bedtime.

Do not use if you are taking monoamine oxidase inhibitors (MAOIs) or within 14 days of stopping treatment with an MAOI. After stopping treatment with this medicine, wait 2 weeks before taking an MAOI.

If a dose is missed, take it as soon as possible. If several hours have passed or if it is nearing time for the next dose, do not double the dose to "catch up," unless advised by your healthcare provider. If more than one dose is missed, contact your healthcare provider.

Avoid alcohol and smoking while using this drug.

This medicine may cause drowsiness, dizziness or impaired judgement. Use caution while driving or performing other tasks requiring alertness, coordination or physical dexterity.

If rash, hives, other signs of an allergic reaction or seizures develop, contact your healthcare provider.

Foscarnet Sodium (Phosphonoformic Acid)

(foss-CAR-net SO-dee-uhm)

Foscavir

An antiviral medicine used to treat, not cure, cytomegaloviris (CMV) retinitis in AIDS patients.

Precautions

DO NOT USE if you are allergic to this medicine. Lab tests (eg, eye exams, blood tests) may be required during therapy.

BEFORE USING THIS MEDICINE, tell your healthcare provider if you are pregnant or breastfeeding; or if you are taking, will be taking or stop taking any prescription or nonprescription medicine; or if you have any other medical conditions.

Side Effects

Every medicine can cause side effects, but many people have no, or minor, side effects. Tell your healthcare provider if any of the following occurs: nausea; vomiting; diarrhea; stomach pain; dark or bloody stool; bloody vomit; headache; dizziness; aggressive behavior; hallucinations; chest pain; difficulty breathing; coughing up blood; rash; sweating; painful or difficult urination; excessive urination; general body discomfort; back pain; chills; fever; seizures; abnormal vision; leg cramps; difficulty swallowing.

Guidelines for Use

USE EXACTLY AS PRESCRIBED.

Drink plenty of fluids during therapy.

Do not exceed recommended dosage, frequency or rate of infusion.

Lab tests may be required during therapy. Be sure to keep appointments.

Fosinopril Sodium

(FAH-sin-oh-PRILL SO-dee-uhm)

Monopril

An angiotensin converting enzyme (ACE) inhibitor medicine generally used to lower high blood pressure.

Precautions

DO NOT USE if you are allergic to this medicine or if you are pregnant.

BEFORE USING THIS MEDICINE, tell your healthcare provider if you are breastfeeding; or if you are taking, will be taking or stop taking any prescription or nonprescription medicine; or if you have any other medical conditions.

Side Effects

Every medicine can cause side effects, but many people have no, or minor, side effects. Tell your healthcare provider if any of the following occurs: stomach pain; vomiting; diarrhea; constipation; appetite loss; depression; headache; dizziness; nervousness; sleeping difficulties; fatigue; rapid or irregular heartbeat; dizziness/lightheadedness when rising quickly from a sitting or lying position; shortness of breath; cough; nasal congestion; bronchitis; sinus inflammation; rash; sweating; flushing; yellowing of skin or eyes; muscle cramps; weight loss; taste loss; dry mouth; decreased sex drive; back, joint and shoulder pain; urination changes; fever; vision disturbances; numbness/tingling of hands or feet.

Guidelines for Use

USE EXACTLY AS PRESCRIBED.

May be taken without regard to meals.

Patients starting treatment for high blood pressure may at first feel tired. It takes time for the body to adjust. Continue taking your medication and check with your healthcare provider.

If a dose is missed, take it as soon as possible. If several hours have passed or if it is nearing time for the next dose, do not double the dose to "catch up," unless advised by your healthcare provider. If more than one dose is missed, contact your healthcare provider.

Do not interrupt or stop medication without consulting your healthcare provider.

Do not use salt substitutes without telling your healthcare provider.

A persistent, dry, nonproductive cough may occur. Tell your healthcare provider. Recovery is rapid when the medicine is stopped.

Dizziness, fainting or lightheadedness is most likely after the first dose or in the first days of therapy; avoid sudden changes in posture. If fainting occurs, discontinue medicine until talking to your healthcare provider.

Furosemide

(fyu-ROH-se-mide)

Lasix

A diuretic (water pill) that decreases excess water in the body and increases urine flow. This medicine is used to treat high blood pressure; edema (excess fluid) due to a variety of causes.

Precautions

DO NOT USE if you are allergic to this medicine or its relatives; oral diabetic medicines; sulfa antibiotics; or if you have severe kidney disease or loss of kidney function.

BEFORE USING THIS MEDICINE, tell your healthcare provider if you are pregnant or breastfeeding; or if you are taking, will be taking or stop taking any prescription or nonprescription medicine; or if you have any other medical conditions.

Side Effects

Every medicine can cause side effects, but many people have no, or minor, side effects. Tell your healthcare provider if any of the following occurs: thirst; irregular heartbeat; confusion; mood changes; nausea; vomiting; unusual tiredness; weakness; weak pulse; muscle cramps; appetite loss; stomach upset; bloating; diarrhea; constipation; dizziness; lightheadedness; headache; tingling of toes and fingers; blurred vision; nervousness; insomnia; chest pain; ringing in the ears; hearing loss (reversible); sun sensitivity; rash; hives; itching; dry skin; yellow skin or eyes; unusual bruising; difficult breathing; blood sugar imbalance; muscle cramps; joint pain; fever; chills; weight loss; nosebleeds; gout attack.

Guidelines for Use

USE EXACTLY AS PRESCRIBED.

Increases urination, therefore to avoid disruption of sleep at night take early in the day usually as a single dose.

May cause stomach upset. May be taken with food or milk.

May cause loss of potassium. If signs of potassium loss occur (weakness, cramps, nausea, dizziness, etc), contact your healthcare provider. Ask about foods high in potassium.

Diabetes-May increase blood sugar levels.

Dizziness or lightheadedness may occur if you stand up too fast from lying or sitting. Get up slowly, and notify healthcare provider.

Sensitivity to sunlight may occur. Use sunscreen and wear protective clothing until tolerance is determined.

Your healthcare provider may want to periodically check your blood to ensure that your medicine is working properly.

Gabapentin

(GAB-uh-PEN-tin)

Neurontin

A medicine used as part of overall therapy in the treatment of partial seizures in adults with epilepsy.

Precautions

DO NOT USE if you are allergic to this medicine.

BEFORE USING THIS MEDICINE, tell your healthcare provider if you are pregnant or breastfeeding; or if you are taking, will be taking or stop taking any prescription or nonprescription medicine; or if you have any other medical conditions.

Side Effects

Every medicine can cause side effects, but many people have no, or minor, side effects. Tell your healthcare provider if any of the following occurs: weakness; fatigue; dizziness; incoordination; tremor; weight gain; back pain; upset stomach; dry mouth or throat; constipation; fluid retention; general body discomfort; appetite loss; gas; bruising; dizziness; abnormal skin sensations; feelings of anxiety or hostility; pneumonia; abnormal vision; rapid eye movement; speech problems; memory loss; depression; abnormal thoughts; impotence; increased motor function (hyperactivity); drowsiness; inflammation of the gums.

Guidelines for Use

USE EXACTLY AS PRESCRIBED.

May cause drowsiness or dizziness. Use caution when driving or performing other tasks requiring mental alertness or physical activity.

May be taken with or without food.

Do not take with antacids. If stomach upset occurs, consult your healthcare provider.

If a dose is missed, take it as soon as possible. If several hours have passed or if it is nearing time for the next dose, do not double the dose to catch up, unless advised by your healthcare provider. If more than one dose is missed, contact your healthcare provider.

Store at room temperature.

Do not stop taking this medicine without the advice of the doctor.

Practice good oral hygiene and have regular dental checkups.

Ganciclovir Sodium

(gan-SIGH-kloe-VIHR SO-dee-uhm)

Cytovene

An antiviral drug used to treat cytomegalovirus (CMV) retinitis (inflammation of the retina) in patients over 13 years of age with immunocompromised (weakened) immune systems, including patients with the acquired immunodeficiency syndrome (AIDS). Safety and effectiveness of this medicine have not been established for treating any signs of CMV disease other than maintenance treatment of CMV retinitis.

Precautions

DO NOT USE if you are allergic to this medicine or to acyclovir. This medicine may reduce your body's ability to fight infections. It is important that you keep appointments to monitor blood counts.

BEFORE USING THIS MEDICINE, tell your healthcare provider if you are pregnant or breastfeeding; or if you are taking, will be taking or stop taking any prescription or nonprescription medicine (especially zidovudine, *Retrovir*; didanosine, *Videx*); or if you have any other medical conditions.

Side Effects

Every medicine can cause side effects, but many people have no, or minor, side effects. Tell your healthcare provider if any of the following occurs: nausea; vomiting; diarrhea; indigestion; stomach pain; appetite loss; gas; headache; weakness; rash; itching; abnormal skin sensations; sweating; fever; chills; general body pain; fertility problems; kidney or liver problems; phlebitis; pneumonia.

Guidelines for Use

USE EXACTLY AS PRESCRIBED.

Take with food.

Do not open or crush capsules.

Do not alter or exceed recommended dose unless instructed.

If a dose is missed, take it as soon as possible. If several hours have passed or if it is nearing time for the next dose, do not double the dose to catch up, unless advised by your doctor. If more than one dose is missed, contact your healthcare provider.

Avoid contact with skin or nasal tissues. If contact occurs, wash skin with soap and water; rinse eyes thoroughly with plain water.

This medicine is not a cure for CMV retinitis, and you may continue to experience effects of retinitis during or following treatment.

Lab tests and eye exams will be required. Be sure to keep appointments.

Contraceptive (birth control) use is recommended for men and women during therapy. Men should use barrier contraception during and for at least 90 days after taking this medicine.

Refer to package literature for reconstitution, stability, storage and disposal information.

Gemfibrozil

(gem-FIE-broe-ZILL)

Lopid

A medicine that lowers blood levels of triglycerides and cholesterol. It occasionally may be prescribed for other reasons.

Precautions

DO NOT USE if you are allergic to this medicine.

BEFORE USING THIS MEDICINE, tell your healthcare provder if you are pregnant or breastfeeding; or if you are taking, will be taking or stop taking any prescription or nonprescription medicine; or if you have any other medical conditions.

Side Effects

Every medicine can cause side effects, but many people have no, or minor, side effects. Tell your healthcare provider if any of the following occurs: abdominal pain, diarrhea, constipation; nausea; vomiting; headache; dizziness; fatigue; itching; sore throat; fever; chills; muscle ache; taste changes; tingling in hands/feet.

Guidelines for Use

USE EXACTLY AS PRESCRIBED.

Take this drug 30 minutes before morning and evening meals.

Most effective when used with a diet that reduces the intake of cholesterol and saturated fats.

May cause dizziness or blurred vision. Use caution when driving or performing other tasks requiring mental alertness.

Diabetes — This medicine may cause an increase in blood sugar. Carefully monitor blood sugar levels.

It is important to keep regular appointments with your healthcare provider.

Gentamicin

(JEN-tuh-MY-sin)

Garamycin, Genoptic, Genoptic S.O.P., Gentacidin, Gentak, G-myticin

A medicine that is used to treat surface eye infections.

Precautions

DO NOT USE if you are allergic to this medicine or its relatives.

BEFORE USING THIS MEDICINE, tell your healthcare provider if you are pregnant or breastfeeding; or if you are taking, will be taking or stop taking any prescription or nonprescription medicine; or if you have any other medical conditions.

Side Effects

Every medicine can cause side effects, but many people have no, or minor, side effects. Tell your healthcare provider if any of the following occurs: headache; itching; burning; irritation; stinging; lid swelling; redness; pupil dilation; watering; blurred vision; lid crusting; crystals/scales.

Guidelines for Use

USE EXACTLY AS PRESCRIBED.

Avoid contact between the dispensing container and the eye.

May cause temporary blurring of vision or stinging following administration.

Contact your healthcare provider if stinging, burning or itching becomes pronounced or if redness, irritation, swelling, decreasing vision or pain persists or worsens.

Glimepiride

(GLIE-meh-pie-ride)

Amaryl

An oral antidiabetic medicine (sulfonylurea) used to lower blood sugar in adult patients with type II (non-insulin dependent) diabetes whose high blood sugar cannot be controlled by diet and exercise alone. It is also used in combination with insulin for type II diabetics whose high blood sugar cannot be controlled by diet, exercise and glimepiride together.

Precautions

DO NOT USE if you are allergic to this medicine or other sulfonylureas or have diabetic ketoacidosis or insulin-dependent diabetes mellitus.

BEFORE USING THIS MEDICINE, tell your healthcare provider if you are pregnant or breastfeeding; or if you are taking, will be taking or stop taking any prescription or nonprescription medicine; or if you have any other medical conditions.

Side Effects

Every medicine can cause side effects, but many people have no, or minor, side effects. Tell your healthcare provider if any of the following occurs: low blood sugar; dizziness; weakness; headache; nausea.

Guidelines for Use

USE EXACTLY AS PRESCRIBED.

Each patient, especially elderly, debilitated or malnourished patients, or patients with kidney or liver problems, may require a different dosing regimen.

Usual starting dose — 1–2 mg tablet taken with breakfast or the first main meal of the day. Usual maintenance dose — 1–4 mg once daily with the maximum recommended dose of 8 mg once daily. Combination therapy dose — 8 mg daily taken with the first main meal of the day.

Combination therapy with insulin is used in patients with secondary failure to oral sulfonylureas.

If a dose is missed, take it as soon as possible. If several hours have passed or if it is nearing time for the next dose, do not double the dose to "catch up," unless advised by your healthcare provider. If more than one dose is missed, contact your healthcare provider.

Do not change the dose or discontinue therapy unless advised to do so by your healthcare provider.

It is very important that you follow the diet and exercise program prescribed by your healthcare provider, otherwise this medicine may not be as effective.

To prevent low blood sugar: 1. Know the symptoms of low blood sugar. 2. Keep track of your blood sugar levels. 3. Keep a source of quick-acting sugar with you at all times. 4. Maintain an adequate diet. 5. Know how diet and exercise affect your blood sugar level. Acute illness (eg, physical trauma, infection, fever, surgery) may require the temporary administration of insulin.

Contact your healthcare provider if you notice any loss of effectiveness.

If you are planning to become pregnant, contact your healthcare provider as other drug therapy may be required.

Lab tests will be required; be sure to keep appointments.

Store at room temperature in a tightly-closed container with a secure cap.

Glipizide

(GLIP-ih-zide)

Glucotrol

An oral antidiabetic medicine that lowers blood sugar. It is used only in patients with non-insulin-dependent diabetes mellitus (Type II) who cannot manage blood sugar levels by diet and exercise alone.

Precautions

DO NOT USE if you have an allergy to this medicine or sulfa drugs.

BEFORE USING THIS MEDICINE, tell your healthcare provider if you are pregnant or breastfeeding; or if you are taking, will be taking or stop taking any prescription or nonprescription medicine; or if you have any other medical conditions.

Side Effects

Every medicine can cause side effects, but many people have no, or minor, side effects. Tell your healthcare provider if any of the following occurs: nausea; vomiting; heartburn; diarrhea; fever; sore throat; rash; itching; weakness; unusual bruising or bleeding.

Guidelines for Use

USE EXACTLY AS PRESCRIBED.

Take 30 minutes before a meal.

Take with food if nausea or stomach upset occurs.

Avoid alcohol, which can cause flushing, weakness, dizziness, a tingling sensation and headache.

Monitor blood sugar levels daily. Notify the doctor if low blood sugar develops (eg, fatigue, nausea, confusion, agitation, excessive hunger, profuse sweating, numbness or tingling of lips, tongue or extremities), or if excessive thirst or urination, or other symptoms of high blood sugar levels occur (glucose or ketones in the urine or blood).

Proper diet and exercise are important.

To prevent low blood sugar: 1. Know the symptoms of low blood sugar. 2. Keep track of your blood sugar levels. 3. Keep a source of quick-acting sugar with you at all times. 4. Maintain an adequate diet. 5. Know how diet and exercise affect your blood sugar level. Acute illness (eg, physical trauma, infection, fever, surgery) may require the temporary administration of insulin.

Glucagon

(GLUE-kuh-gahn)

A hormone used to treat low blood sugar levels and unconscious diabetics. It is also used in the x-ray examination of the stomach, small intestine and colon. It occasionally may be prescribed for other reasons.

Precautions

DO NOT USE if you are allergic to this medicine.

BEFORE USING THIS MEDICINE, tell your healthcare provider if you are pregnant or breastfeeding; or if you are taking, will be taking or stop taking any prescription or nonprescription medicine; or if you have any other medical conditions.

If used for emergency treatment of low blood sugar levels, notify your healthcare provider so adjustments in insulin dose and dietary factors can be made. In addition, patients should be given food after they become conscious. Self monitor blood glucose frequently so that blood sugar levels are not allowed to get too low.

Side Effects

Every medicine can cause side effects, but many people have no, or minor, side effects. Tell your healthcare provider if any of the following occurs: nausea; vomiting; rash; respiratory distress; low blood pressure (dizziness, lightheadedness).

Guidelines for Use

USE EXACTLY AS PRESCRIBED.

All patients with diabetes should have a glucagon emergency kit.

Low blood sugar (conscious patient)-Consume fast-acting sugars (eg, *B-D Glucose Tablets*, *Glutose*).

Low blood sugar (unconscious patient)-This medicine is the treatment of choice.

Instruct friends, co-workers and family members of patients with diabetes how to administer glucagon.

The glucagon emergency kit has a diluting fluid in a unit (one) dose syringe. This diluting fluid is injected into a vial of the glucagon crystals. The vial is then shaken and the contents brought back into the syringe. The glucagon crystals now in the diluting fluid are given either intravenously, intramuscularly or under the skin.

Use glucagon immediately after it has been mixed with the diluting fluid because the medicine is stable for only a short time.

Orthostatic hypotension (lightheadedness and dizziness when rising from a seated or lying position) may occur. Avoid sudden changes in posture.

Glutethimide

(glue-TETH-ih-mide)

Doriden

This medicine causes drowsiness to aid in falling asleep. It generally is used to treat insomnia for a short period of time (1 to 2 weeks).

Precautions

DO NOT USE if you are allergic to this medicine.

BEFORE USING THIS MEDICINE, tell your healthcare provider if you are pregnant or breastfeeding; or if you are taking, will be taking or stop taking any prescription or nonprescription medicine; or if you have any other medical conditions.

Side Effects

Every medicine can cause side effects, but many people have no, or minor, side effects. Tell your healthcare provider if any of the following occurs: stomach upset; diarrhea; vomiting; constipation; confusion; excitement; nightmares; drowsiness; dizziness; headache; incoordination; decreased mobility; incoherence; rash; hives; redness; unpleasant taste in mouth.

Guidelines for Use

USE EXACTLY AS PRESCRIBED.

May cause drowsiness or dizziness. Use caution while driving or performing other tasks requiring mental alertness.

Avoid alcohol and other medicines that cause drowsiness (eg, pain relievers, sedatives, antihistamines).

There is a risk of oversedation, morning hangover (grogginess in the morning), dizziness and confusion. Dose may need to be reduced.

May be habit forming.

Do not discontinue this medicine abruptly, especially if you have a history of seizures, regardless of other antiseizure medications you may be taking.

Withdrawal symptoms may occur when the medicine is stopped.

Contact your doctor if rash occurs.

Glyburide

(glie-BYOO-ride)

DiaBeta, Glynase PresTab, Micronase

An oral antidiabetic medicine that lowers blood sugar. It is used only in patients with non-insulin-dependent diabetes mellitus (Type II) who cannot manage blood sugar levels by diet and exercise alone.

Precautions

DO NOT USE if you have an allergy to this medicine or to sulfa drugs.

BEFORE USING THIS MEDICINE, tell your healthcare provider if you are pregnant or breastfeeding; or if you are taking, will be taking or stop taking any prescription or nonprescription medicine; or if you have any other medical conditions.

Side Effects

Every medicine can cause side effects, but many people have no, or minor, side effects. Tell your healthcare provider if any of the following occurs: nausea; vomiting; heartburn; diarrhea; fever; sore throat; rash; itching; weakness; unusual bruising or bleeding.

Guidelines for Use

USE EXACTLY AS PRESCRIBED.

Take 30 minutes before a meal.

Take with food if nausea or stomach upset occurs.

Avoid alcohol, which can cause flushing, weakness, dizziness, a tingling sensation and headache.

Monitor blood sugar levels daily. Notify your healthcare provider if low blood sugar develops (eg, fatigue, nausea, confusion, agitation, excessive hunger, profuse sweating, numbness or tingling of lips, tongue or extremities) or if excessive thirst or urination, or other symptoms of high blood sugar levels occur (glucose or ketones in the urine or blood).

Proper diet and exercise are important.

To prevent low blood sugar: 1. Know the symptoms of low blood sugar. 2. Keep track of your blood sugar levels. 3. Keep a source of quick-acting sugar with you at all times. 4. Maintain an adequate diet. 5. Know how diet and exercise affect your blood sugar level. Acute illness (eg, physical trauma, infection, fever, surgery) may require the temporary administration of insulin.

Glycerin Oral

(GLIH-suh-rin)

Osmoglyn

Used to stop attacks of glaucoma. It also is used before and after eye surgery where reduction of the eye pressure is needed. It occasionally may be prescribed for other reasons.

Precautions

DO NOT USE if you are allergic to this medicine or dehydrated.

Side Effects

Every medicine can cause side effects, but many people have no, or minor, side effects. Tell your healthcare provider if any of the following occurs: nausea; vomiting; headache; confusion; disorientation; thirst.

Glycerin Rectal

(GLIH-suh-rin)

Fleet Babylax, Sani-Supp

This medicine is used for the short-term treatment of constipation, and to treat constipation in infants and children.

Precautions

DO NOT USE if you are allergic to this product; have appendicitis symptoms (eg, nausea, vomiting, abdominal pain); intestinal obstruction; stool impaction.

BEFORE USING THIS MEDICINE, tell your healthcare provider if you are pregnant or breastfeeding; or if you are taking, will be taking or stop taking any prescription or nonprescription medicine; or if you have any other medical conditions.

Side Effects

Every medicine can cause side effects, but many people have no, or minor, side effects. Tell your healthcare provider if any of the following occurs: pounding in the chest; bowel cramping; muscle cramps or pain; irritation or bleeding in the rectal area.

Guidelines for Use

USE EXACTLY AS PRESCRIBED.

Laxative use is only a temporary measure. Stop use when normal bowel habits return.

Do not use in the presence of abdominal pain, nausea or vomiting.

Tell your healthcare provider if unrelieved constipation, rectal bleeding or symptoms of electrolyte imbalance (eg, muscle cramps or pain, weakness, dizziness) occurs.

Effects usually occur in 30 minutes.

Insert one suppository high in the rectum and retain for 15 minutes. It does not need to melt to produce laxative action. Use the correct size suppository on infants and children.

Store at room temperature. Protect from moisture.

Glycopyrrolate Injection

(glie-koe-PIE-row-late)

Robinul

A medicine used before surgery to reduce oral, stomach and intestinal secretions and to prevent the side effects of other medicines on the heart.

Precautions

DO NOT USE if you are allergic to this medicine or any other anticholinergic medicines.

BEFORE USING THIS MEDICINE, tell your healthcare provider if you are pregnant or breastfeeding; or if you are taking, will be taking or stop taking any prescription or nonprescription medicine; or if you have any other medical conditions.

Side Effects

Every medicine can cause side effects, but many people have no, or minor, side effects. Tell your healthcare provider if any of the following occurs: nausea; vomiting; bloating; heartburn; constipation; confusion; excitement; restlessness; tremors; headache; nervousness; drowsiness; dizziness; inability to sleep; pounding in the chest; rapid heart rate; nasal congestion; rash; itching; flushing; decreased sweating; eye pain; fever; weakness; dry mouth; altered taste perception; difficult swallowing; urine retention; difficult urination; impotence; blurred vision; sensitivity to light; reduced breast milk production and flow; thirst.

Guidelines for Use

USE EXACTLY AS PRESCRIBED.

Given 30 to 60 minutes before surgery.

May cause sensitivity to bright lights. This may be minimized by wearing sunglasses.

Glycopyrrolate Tablets

(glie-koe-PIE-row-late)

Robinul, Robinul Forte

A medicine used in the treatment of stomach and intestinal disorders (eg, ulcers, cramping, diarrhea).

Precautions

DO NOT USE if you are allergic to this medicine or any other anticholinergic medicine.

BEFORE USING THIS MEDICINE, tell your healthcare provider if you are pregnant or breastfeeding; or if you are taking, will be taking or stop taking any prescription or nonprescription medicine; or if you have any other medical conditions.

Side Effects

Every medicine can cause side effects, but many people have no, or minor, side effects. Tell your healthcare provider if any of the following occurs: nausea; vomiting; bloating; heartburn; constipation; confusion; restlessness; headache; nervousness; drowsiness; dizziness; inability to sleep; pounding in the chest; rapid heart rate; difficulty breathing; nasal congestion; rash; itching; flushing; decreased sweating; dry mouth; altered taste perception; urine retention; difficult urination; impotence; blurred vision; visual sensitivity to light; reduced breast milk production and flow; thirst.

Guidelines for Use

USE EXACTLY AS PRESCRIBED.

Take 30 to 60 minutes before meals.

May cause drowsiness or blurred vision. Use caution when driving or performing other tasks requiring alertness.

Notify your healthcare provider if skin rash or visual problems occur.

May cause difficulty in urination, constipation or increased sensitivity to light. Tell your doctor if these effects persist or become severe.

If a dose is missed, take it as soon as possible. If several hours have passed or if it is nearing time for the next dose, do not double the dose to "catch up," unless advised by your healthcare provider. If more than one dose is missed, contact your healthcare provider.

This medicine can reduce sweating. When exposed to hot weather, this can cause heat prostration, fever and heatstroke.

Diarrhea can be an early symptom of incomplete intestinal obstruction. Check with your healthcare provider before taking anything for diarrhea while using this medicine.

Contact lens use — Can cause drying of the eyes. Contact lens wearers should use an appropriate lubricant.

Gold Sodium Thiomalate

(gold SO-dee-uhm thigh-oh-MAL-ate)

Myochrysine, Aurolate

Used to treat active adult and juvenile rheumatoid arthritis that are not adequately controlled by other therapies. It occasionally may be prescribed for other reasons.

Precautions

DO NOT USE if you are allergic to this medicine (eg, gold) or if you are pregnant.

BEFORE USING THIS MEDICINE, tell your healthcare provider if you are breastfeeding; or if you are taking, will be taking or stop taking any prescription or nonprescription medicine; or if you have any other medical conditions.

Side Effects

Every medicine can cause side effects, but many people have no, or minor, side effects. Tell your healthcare provider if any of the following occurs: indigestion; nausea; vomiting; diarrhea; constipation; stomach cramps; loss of appetite; gas; bloody or black stools; confusion; hallucinations; dizziness; fainting; fever; weakness; cough; shortness of breath; rash; itching; hives; swelling; yellowing of the skin and eyes; flushing; redness; light sensitivity; sweating; easy bruising; blood in urine; sore mouth or throat; swollen gums or tongue; nosebleeds; metallic taste; hair loss; loss of fingernails.

Guidelines for Use

USE EXACTLY AS PRESCRIBED.

Joint aches may occur a day or two after injection. They usually subside after the first few injections. These reactions are usually mild, but occasionally may be so severe that treatment is stopped.

Tell your healthcare provider if rash, sore mouth, indigestion, metallic taste, easy bruising or nosebleeds or itching occurs.

A gray-to-blue discoloration of your skin may occur, especially on exposed areas. Minimize exposure to sunlight or artificial ultraviolet light (tanning booths).

Observe good oral hygiene during therapy.

Regular follow-up with your healthcare provider is needed to monitor for side effects.

Goserelin Acetate

(GO-suh-REH-lin ASS-uh-TATE)

Zoladex

A medicine used for the treatment of advanced prostate cancer. It also is used for the treatment of endometriosis.

Precautions

DO NOT USE if you are allergic to this medicine or if you are pregnant or breast-feeding.

BEFORE USING THIS MEDICINE, tell your healthcare provider if you are taking, will be taking or stop taking any prescription or nonprescription medicine; or if you have any other medical conditions.

Side Effects

Every medicine can cause side effects, but many people have no, or minor, side effects. Tell your healthcare provider if any of the following occurs: Men—hot flashes; sexual dysfunction; decreased erections; edema or swelling; rash; loss of appetite; dizziness; sleeplessness; nausea; depression; application site reaction. Women—hot flashes; vaginitis; headache; changes in sexual urge; emotional swings; depression; sweating; acne; changes in breast size; edema or swelling; painful intercourse; sleeplessness; nausea; facial hair growth; application site reaction.

Guidelines for Use

USE EXACTLY AS PRESCRIBED.

Menstruation should stop with effective doses of this medicine. Tell your healthcare provider if regular menstruation persists.

If you miss one or more successive doses, you may experience breakthrough bleeding.

After therapy is discontinued, there may be a delay in the return of your menstrual periods.

Tell your healthcare provider if pregnancy occurs during this treatment.

To prevent pregnancy, use a nonhormonal method of contraception during treatment.

The implant is injected under the skin of the abdominal (belly) wall every 28 days. Be sure to keep appointments for replacement of the implant.

This medicine may cause hot flashes, headache, vaginal dryness, emotional changes, change in sex drive, depression, sweating and change in breast size.

Treatment induces a hypoestrogenic state that results in a loss of bone mineral density over the course of treatment, some of which may not be reversible.

Griseofulvin

(griss-ee-oh-FULL-vin)

Fulvicin U/F, Fulvicin P/G, Grifulvin V, Grisactin, Grisactin Ultra, Gris-PEG

A medicine used to treat ringworm (fungal) infections of the hair, skin and nails.

Precautions

DO NOT USE if you are allergic to this medicine or if you are pregnant.

BEFORE USING THIS MEDICINE, tell your healthcare provider if you are pregnant or breastfeeding; or if you are taking, will be taking or stop taking any prescription or nonprescription medicine; or if you have any other medical conditions.

Side Effects

Every medicine can cause side effects, but many people have no, or minor, side effects. Tell your healthcare provider if any of the following occurs: nausea; vomiting; diarrhea; stomach ache; headache; fatigue; dizziness; confusion; inability to sleep; impaired coordination; rash; hives; itching; fever; sore throat; oral thrush; tingling and numbness in hands and feet.

Guidelines for Use

USE EXACTLY AS PRESCRIBED.

Beneficial effects may not be apparent for weeks or months. Take the complete course of therapy.

May cause dizziness. Use caution while driving or performing other tasks requiring mental alertness, coordination or dexterity.

Good hygiene must be observed during treatment to help control infection and prevent reinfection.

Topical antifungal therapy may accompany oral therapy. Topical therapy is especially useful in athlete's foot (tinea pedis) and jock itch (tinea cruris).

If a dose is missed, take it as soon as possible. If several hours have passed or if it is nearing time for the next dose, do not double the dose to "catch up," unless advised by your healthcare provider. If more than one dose is missed, contact your healthcare provider.

This medicine may cause sensitivity to sunlight. Avoid prolonged exposure to the sun. Use sunscreen and wear protective clothing until tolerance is determined.

Tell your healthcare provider if fever, sore throat or skin rash occurs.

Oral suspension: shake well before using.

Guaifenesin

(GWHY-fen-ah-sin)

Amonidrin, Anti-Tuss, Breonesin, Diabetic Tussin EX, Fenesin, Gee-Gee, Genatuss, GG-Cen, Glyate, Glycotuss, Glytuss, GuiaCough CF, GuiaCough PE, Guiatuss, Halotussin, Humibid L.A., Humibid Sprinkle, Hytuss, Malotuss, Mytussin, Naldecon Senior EX, Pneumomist, Robitussin, Scot-Tussin Expectorant, Uni-tussin

Used for the symptomatic relief of respiratory conditions characterized by dry, nonproductive cough and the presence of mucous in the respiratory tract.

Precautions

DO NOT USE if you are allergic to this medicine.

BEFORE USING THIS MEDICINE, tell your healthcare provider if you are pregnant or breastfeeding; or if you are taking, will be taking or stop taking any prescription or nonprescription medicine; or if you have any other medical conditions.

Side Effects

Every medicine can cause side effects, but many people have no, or minor, side effects. Tell your healthcare provider if any of the following occurs: nausea; vomiting; dizziness; headache; rash.

Guidelines for Use

USE EXACTLY AS PRESCRIBED.

Do not take these products for persistent or chronic cough such as occurs with smoking, asthma, chronic bronchitis or emphysema, or when cough is accompanied by excessive phlegm, unless directed by your healthcare provider.

A persistent cough may be a sign of a serious condition. If cough persists for more than one week, tends to recur, or is accompanied by fever, rash or persistent headache, talk to your healthcare provider.

Drink a glass of water or other fluid with each dose. A well-hydrated body (due to fluid intake) is responsible for thinning respiratory tract mucus, and may be as valuable or more so than the expectorant itself.

Guanabenz Acetate

(GWAHN-uh-benz ASS-uh-TATE)

Wytensin

A medicine used to treat high blood pressure. This medicine frequently is used with other medicines to lower blood pressure.

Precautions

DO NOT USE if you are allergic to this medicine. DO NOT stop taking this medicine without consulting your healthcare provider. Sudden withdrawal of treatment may result in high blood pressure, rapid pulse, irregular heartbeat, nervousness and anxiety.

BEFORE USING THIS MEDICINE, tell your healthcare provider if you are pregnant or breastfeeding; or if you are taking, will be taking or stop taking any prescription or nonprescription medicine; or if you have any other medical conditions.

Side Effects

Every medicine can cause side effects, but many people have no, or minor, side effects. Tell your healthcare provider if any of the following occurs: nausea; vomiting; stomach ache; diarrhea; constipation; depression; sleep disturbances; dizziness; weakness; headache; nervousness; drowsiness; chest pain; pounding in the chest; shortness of breath; nasal congestion; fluid retention; dry mouth; unsteady walk; muscle aches (arms and legs); problems with sexual function; breast enlargement (men); taste disturbance; urinary frequency; blurred vision; rash; itching.

Guidelines for Use

USE EXACTLY AS PRESCRIBED.

Patients being treated for high blood pressure often feel tired and run down for a few weeks after beginning therapy. It takes time for the body to adjust to lowered blood pressure. Continue taking your medication even though you may not feel quite normal. Check with your healthcare provider during this time regarding any new symptoms that occur to ensure that these new feelings are normal consequence of changes in blood pressure.

If a dose is missed, take it as soon as possible. If several hours have passed or if it is nearing time for the next dose, do not double the dose to "catch up," unless advised by your healthcare provider. If more than one dose is missed, contact your healthcare provider.

Dizziness or lightheadedness may occur if you stand up too fast from a lying or sitting position. If this occurs, get up slowly and avoid sudden changes in posture.

This medicine may cause drowsiness or dizziness. Use caution while driving or performing other tasks requiring mental alertness, coordination or physical dexterity.

Guanadrel Sulfate

(GWAHN-uh-drell SULL-fate)

Hylorel

A medicine used to treat high blood pressure, alone or in conjunction with other high blood pressure medications.

Precautions

DO NOT USE if you are allergic to this medicine or with, or within one week of taking, monoamine oxidase inhibitors (MAOIs).

BEFORE USING THIS MEDICINE, tell your healthcare provider if you are pregnant or breastfeeding; or if you are taking, will be taking or stop taking any prescription or nonprescription medicine; or if you have any other medical conditions.

Side Effects

Every medicine can cause side effects, but many people have no, or minor, side effects. Tell your healthcare provider if any of the following occurs: severe diarrhea; gas pain; indigestion; nausea; vomiting; decreased appetite; constipation; headache; sleep disturbances; confusion; fatigue; faintness; drowsiness; depression; chest pain; pounding in the chest; dizziness or lightheadedness upon standing; shortness of breath at rest or during exercise; cough; ankle swelling; weight gain or excess fluid retention; decreased sexual ability; leg cramps and aches; muscle pain; dry mouth; increased urination; inflamed tongue; visual disturbances; tingling or numbness in hands or feet.

Guidelines for Use

USE EXACTLY AS PRESCRIBED.

Patients being treated for high blood pressure often feel tired and run down for a few weeks after beginning therapy. It takes time for the body to adjust to lowered blood pressure. Continue taking your medication even though you may not feel quite normal. Do not stop therapy or change dose unless advised by your doctor.

If a dose is missed, take it as soon as possible. If several hours have passed or it is nearing time for the next dose, do not double the dose to "catch up," unless advised by your healthcare provider. If more than one dose is missed, contact your healthcare provider.

This medicine may cause drowsiness or dizziness. Use caution while driving or performing other tasks requiring mental alertness, coordination and dexterity.

Dizziness is common. Sit or lie down immediately at the onset of dizziness or weakness to prevent fainting.

Avoid sudden or prolonged standing or exercise.

Excess heat or fevers can worsen the dizziness.

Guanethidine Monosulfate

(gwahn-ETH-ih-deen MAH-no-SULL-fate)

Ismelin

A medicine used to lower high blood pressure. It occasionally may be prescribed for other reasons.

Precautions

DO NOT USE if you are allergic to this medicine, are breastfeeding or if you are taking a monoamine oxidase inhibitor.

Orthostatic hypotension: Dizziness or lightheadedness frequently can occur when rising quickly from a sitting or lying position. If you feel faint, it is important to lie down at the first signs of dizziness or weakness. Avoid sudden or prolonged standing or exercise while taking this medicine. Get out of bed slowly, sit for a few minutes before standing, then stand for a few minutes before walking. Hot weather, fever and alcohol may worsen the problem. If dizziness is persistent or bothersome, contact your healthcare provider.

BEFORE USING THIS MEDICINE, tell your healthcare provider if you are pregnant; or if you are taking, will be taking or stop taking any prescription or nonprescription medicine; or if you have any other medical conditions.

Side Effects

Every medicine can cause side effects, but many people have no, or minor, side effects. Tell your healthcare provider if any of the following occurs: dizziness, weakness and fainting (orthostatic hypotension); diarrhea; nausea; vomiting; depression; chest pain or numbness; nasal congestion; difficult or painful breathing; asthma; scalp hair loss; sexual problems; muscle tremors or aches; dry mouth; fluid retention (edema); increased urination; loss of bladder control; weight gain; blurred vision.

Guidelines for Use

USE EXACTLY AS PRESCRIBED.

Patients being treated for high blood pressure often feel tired and run down for a few weeks after beginning therapy. It takes time for the body to adjust to lowered blood pressure. Continue taking your medication even though you may not feel quite normal.

This medicine may cause drowsiness or dizziness. Use caution while driving or performing other tasks requiring mental alertness, coördination and dexterity.

Do not discontinue this medicine unless instructed to do so by your healthcare provider.

Take on a regular daily schedule; do not exceed recommended dose.

Contact your healthcare provider if you experience severe diarrhea, frequent dizziness or fainting.

Avoid alcohol while taking this medicine.

Orthostatic hypotension (dizziness or lightheadedness when rising quickly from a seated or lying position) may occur. Avoid sudden changes in posture.

Guanfacine Hydrochloride

(GWAHN-fay-seen HIGH-droe-KLOR-ide)

Tenex

A medicine to treat high blood pressure. It may occasionally be prescribed for other reasons.

Precautions

DO NOT USE if you are allergic to this medicine.

BEFORE USING THIS MEDICINE, tell your healthcare provider if you are pregnant or breastfeeding; or if you are taking, will be taking or stop taking any prescription or nonprescription medicine; or if you have any other medical conditions.

Side Effects

Every medicine can cause side effects, but many people have no, or minor, side effects. Tell your healthcare provider if any of the following occurs: dry mouth; sleepiness or insomnia; dizziness; headache; impotence; constipation; weakness; fatigue; confusion; runny nose.

Guidelines for Use

USE EXACTLY AS PRESCRIBED.

Take daily dose at bedtime to decrease daytime sedation unless advised by your healthcare provider.

May produce drowsiness or dizziness. Use caution while driving or performing other tasks requiring mental alertness, especially in the first weeks of therapy.

Avoid alcohol and other depressants.

Take this medication daily as directed.

Have your blood pressure checked regularly and keep appointments with your healthcare provider even if you feel well. Most patients with high blood pressure do not feel sick.

Patients being treated for high blood pressure often feel tired and run down for a few weeks after beginning therapy. It takes time for the body to adjust to lowered blood pressure. Continue taking your medication even though you may not feel quite normal.

Do not discontinue taking this medicine without consulting your healthcare provider.

Haloperidol

(HAL-oh-pehr-i-dahl)

Haldol

A neuroleptic or major tranquilizer generally used to improve concentration and self-control in patients with psychotic behavior.

Precautions

DO NOT USE if you are allergic to this medicine, its relatives or tartrazine. Laboratory tests may be needed including eye exams, blood counts and kidney and liver tests.

BEFORE USING THIS MEDICINE, tell your healthcare provider if you are pregnant or breastfeeding; or if you are taking, will be taking or stop taking any prescription or nonprescription medicine; or if you have any other medical conditions.

Side Effects

Every medicine can cause side effects, but many people have no, or minor, side effects. Tell your healthcare provider if any of the following occurs: tremors; drooling; shuffling gait; restlessness; muscle spasms; aching or numbness; sore throat; fever; unusual bleeding or bruising; skin rash; weakness; impaired vision; dark-colored urine; pale stools; jaundice.

Guidelines for Use

USE EXACTLY AS PRESCRIBED.

Take routinely as directed; it controls illness symptoms and is not habit-forming. Improvement may not be seen for several weeks.

If a dose is missed, take it as soon as possible. If several hours have passed or if it is nearing time for the next dose, do not double the dose to "catch up," unless advised by your healthcare provider. If more than one dose is missed, contact your healthcare provider.

May cause drowsiness. Use caution while driving or performing other tasks requiring mental alertness.

Avoid alcohol and medicines that cause drowsiness (eg, sleeping pills, antihistamines).

May cause sunlight sensitivity. Avoid long exposure to the sun. Use sunscreens and protective clothing until tolerance is known.

May discolor the urine pink or reddish brown. This is not harmful.

If dizziness or fainting occurs, avoid sudden changes in posture and use caution when climbing stairs, etc (more common during first week of therapy).

Use with caution in hot weather; may increase risk of heatstroke.

Heparin

(HEP-uh-rin)

Heparin Sodium, Heparin Sodium Lock Flush, Hep-Lock, Hep-Lock U/P, Liquaemin Sodium

An injectable anticoagulant medicine that prevents blood clots from forming. It will not dissolve already-formed blood clots, but will prevent them from becoming larger. Generally used to prevent blood-clotting complications of surgery and to reduce the risk of heart attack or stroke. It may occasionally be prescribed for other reasons.

Precautions

DO NOT USE by intramuscular injection; if you are allergic to this medicine; or have a bleeding disorder (eg, hemophilia).

BEFORE USING THIS MEDICINE, tell your healthcare provider if you are pregnant or breastfeeding; or if you are taking, will be taking or stop taking any prescription or nonprescription medicine; or if you have any other medical conditions.

Side Effects

Every medicine can cause side effects, but many people have no, or minor, side effects. Tell your healthcare provider if any of the following occurs: difficult breathing; hives; itching; irritation; hair loss; unusual bleeding or bruising; chills; fever; painful sustained erection; nausea; vomiting; stomach pain; tarry stools; chest pain; increased blood pressure; runny nose; mild pain; redness/bruising at injection site; tearing; joint pain; headaches; abnormal blood counts; shock; swelling; osteoporosis (long-term use).

Guidelines for Use

USE EXACTLY AS PRESCRIBED.

Avoid intramuscular (IM) use.

Usually given by healthcare provider as an injection.

Report any bleeding (eg, nose bleeds or bleeding gums) or bruising, itching, chills, fever, or difficulty breathing immediately to your healthcare provider.

This medicine is derived from animal tissue; use with caution if there is a history of allergies.

Avoid alcohol while using this medicine.

Laboratory tests are required to make sure the therapy is working properly. Be sure to keep appointments

Store at room temperature.

Hydralazine Hydrochloride

(high-DRAL-uh-zeen HIGH-droe-KLOR-ide)

Apresoline

A medicine that lowers high blood pressure by relaxing and widening blood vessels.

Precautions

DO NOT USE if you are allergic to any part of this medicine.

BEFORE USING THIS MEDICINE, tell your healthcare provider if you are pregnant or breastfeeding; or if you are taking, will be taking or stop taking any prescription or nonprescription medicine; or if you have any other medical conditions; or allergy to tartrazine.

Side Effects

Every medicine can cause side effects, but many people have no, or minor, side effects. Tell your healthcare provider if any of the following occurs: nausea; vomiting; diarrhea; constipation; headache; tiredness; lightheadedness; depression; anxiety; disorientation; chest pain; increased heartbeat; breathing difficulty; rash; flushing; yellowing of skin and/or eyes; hives; easy bruising and bleeding; joint pain; fever; muscle aches; hoarseness; lymph node swelling; difficult urination; decreased sexual ability; numbness or tingling of hands or feet; chills; fluid retention.

Guidelines for Use

USE EXACTLY AS PRESCRIBED.

Take with meals.

If a dose is missed, take it as soon as possible. If several hours have passed or if it is nearing time for the next dose, do not double the dose to "catch up," unless advised by your healthcare provider. If more than one dose is missed, contact your healthcare provider.

Patients being treated for high blood pressure often feel tired and run down for a few weeks after beginning therapy. It takes time for the body to adjust to lowered blood pressure. Continue taking your medicine even though you may not feel quite normal. Take this medicine daily as directed, have your blood pressure checked regularly and keep your appointment with your healthcare provider even if you feel well. Most patients with high blood pressure do not feel sick.

Notify your healthcare provider of unusual prolonged tiredness, muscle or joint aching, chest pain, fever, numbness or tingling of hands or feet, rash.

Dizziness or lightheadedness may occur if you stand up too fast from sitting or lying. Get up slowly and notify your healthcare provider.

Hydrochlorothiazide (HCTZ)

(high-droe-klor-oh-THIGH-uh-zide)

Esidrix, Ezide, Hydro-Par, HydroDIURIL, Oretic

A diuretic (water pill) for use in adults to decrease excess water in the body and to increase urine flow. This medicine is also used to treat high blood pressure and edema (excess fluid) due to a variety of causes. It may be prescribed for other reasons.

Precautions

DO NOT USE if you are allergic to this medicine or its relatives, oral diabetic medicines, sulfa antibiotics; if you have kidney disease (inability to urinate); or if you are in the second or third trimester of pregnancy.

BEFORE USING THIS MEDICINE, tell your healthcare provider if you are pregnant or breastfeeding; or if you are taking, will be taking or stop taking any prescription or nonprescription medicine; if you have any other medical conditions; or are allergic to tartrazine.

Side Effects

Every medicine can cause side effects, but many people have no, or minor, side effects. Tell your healthcare provider if any of the following occurs: thirst; confusion; mood changes; nausea; vomiting; tiredness; weakness; muscle cramps; appetite loss; stomach upset; bloating; diarrhea; constipation; dizziness; lightheadedness; headache; tingling of toes/fingers; blurred vision; nervousness; sleeplessness; chest pain; sun sensitivity; rash; hives; itching; dry skin; yellowing of skin or eyes; unusual bruising; difficult breathing; blood sugar imbalance; muscle cramps; joint pain; fever; chills; weight loss; nose bleeds; gout attack; swelling of the lower legs; back or leg pain; cough; stuffy nose; sore throat.

Guidelines for Use

USE EXACTLY AS PRESCRIBED.

Do not adjust the dosage without consulting your healthcare provider.

Increases urination; therefore, to avoid disruption of sleep at night, take early in the day, usually as a single dose.

If a dose is missed, take it as soon as possible. If several hours have passed or if it is nearing time for the next dose, do not double the dose to "catch up," unless advised by your healthcare provider. If more than one dose is missed, contact your healthcare provider.

May cause stomach upset. If upset occurs, it may be taken with food or milk.

If signs of potassium loss occur (weakness, cramps, nausea, dizziness), contact your healthcare provider. Ask about foods high in potassium. Do not use salt substitutes containing potassium without consulting your healthcare provider.

Diabetes — May increase blood sugar levels.

Contact your healthcare provider if sudden, significant joint pain occurs.

Dizziness or lightheadedness may occur if you stand up too fast from a lying or sitting position. Get up slowly, and notify your healthcare provider.

Sensitivity to sunlight may occur. Use sunscreen and wear protective clothing until tolerance is determined.

Do not use alcohol while taking this medicine.

Lab test may be required. Be sure to keep appointments.

Store at room temperature in a tightly sealed container away from light.

Hydrochlorothiazide/Triamterene (HCTZ/Triamterene)

(high-droe-klor-oh-THIGH-uh-zide/try-AM-tur-een)

Dyazide, Maxzide, Maxzide-25MG

Combination of two diuretics (water pills) used to treat fluid accumulation (edema) and lower blood pressure. Contains a potassium-sparing diuretic to minimize potassium loss from the body.

Precautions

DO NOT USE if you are allergic to this medicine or its relatives.

BEFORE USING THIS MEDICINE, tell your healthcare provider if you are pregnant or breastfeeding; or if you are taking, will be taking or stop taking any prescription or nonprescription medicine; or if you have any other medical conditions.

Side Effects

Every medicine can cause side effects, but many people have no, or minor, side effects. Tell your healthcare provider if any of the following occurs: weakness; cramps; nausea; dizziness; fever; sore throat; mouth sores; unusual bleeding or bruising; gout; increased blood sugar levels.

Guidelines for Use

USE EXACTLY AS PRESCRIBED.

May cause stomach upset. May be taken with food or milk.

Avoid prolonged exposure to sunlight. Photosensitivity (sensitivity to sunlight) may occur. Take protective measures (eg, sunscreens, protective clothing) against exposure to sunlight or other ultraviolet light.

If a dose is missed, take it as soon as possible. If several hours have passed or if it is nearing time for the next dose, do not double the dose to "catch up," unless advised by your doctor. If more than one dose is missed, contact your healthcare provider.

Patients being treated for high blood pressure often feel tired and run down for a few weeks after beginning therapy. It takes time for the body to adjust to lowered blood pressure. Continue taking your medication and check with your healthcare provider.

Diuretics are usually given as a single daily dose in the morning.

Hydrocodone Bitartrate/Acetaminophen

(HIGH-droe-KOE-dohn by-TAR-trate/ass-ett-ah-MEE-noe-fen)

Amacodone, Anexsia, Anodynos DHC, Bancap-HC, Co-Gesic, Dolacet, Duocet, Duradyne DHC, HY-PHEN, Hydrocet, Hydrogesic, Lorcet-HD, Lortab, Margesic H, Norcet, Stagesic, T-Gesic, Vicodin ES, Vicodin, Zydone

A medicine used to relieve moderate to severe pain.

Precautions

DO NOT USE if you are allergic to this medicine.

BEFORE USING THIS MEDICINE, tell your healthcare provider if you are pregnant or breastfeeding; or if you are taking, will be taking or stop taking any prescription or nonprescription medicine; or if you have any other medical conditions.

Side Effects

Every medicine can cause side effects, but many people have no, or minor, side effects. Tell your healthcare provider if any of the following occurs: drowsiness; dizziness; blurred vision; nausea; vomiting; constipation; difficulty breathing; rash; yellowing of the skin.

Guidelines for Use

USE EXACTLY AS PRESCRIBED.

May cause nausea. Take with food.

May cause drowsiness, dizziness or blurred vision. Use caution while driving or performing other tasks requiring mental alertness.

Avoid alcohol and other sedative or drowsiness-causing substances.

Long-term use may lead to addiction. An early sign of this is medicine ineffectiveness. Dependence is not an issue in terminal illness pain where patient comfort is more important.

May cause constipation with long-term use. Use stool softener or fiber laxative.

Narcotics are more effective in preventing pain than in treating pain after it occurs.

Significant overdosage requires emergency treatment.

Hydrocortisone Anorectal

(HIGH-droe-CORE-tih-sone)

Analpram-HC, Anucort, Anucort-HC, Anumed HC Suppositories, Anusol-HC, Cort-Dome High Potency, Hemorrhoidal HC, Pramoxine HC, Proctofoam-HC, Rectacort

A medicine used for the relief of discomfort associated with hemorrhoids (piles) or itching or irritation.

Precautions

DO NOT USE if you are allergic to this medicine.

BEFORE USING THIS MEDICINE, tell your healthcare provider if you are pregnant or breastfeeding.

Side Effects

Every medicine can cause side effects, but many people have no, or minor, side effects. Tell your healthcare provider if any of the following occurs: bleeding; protrusion; seepage.

Guidelines for Use

USE EXACTLY AS PRESCRIBED.

For external use only.

Avoid contact with eyes.

Tell your healthcare provider if symptoms do not improve in 7 days, or if bleeding, protrusion or seepage occurs.

Maintain normal bowel movements by proper diet, adequate fluid intake and regular exercise.

Avoid excessive laxative use. Stool softeners or bulk laxatives may be useful as an aid to the therapy.

Hydrocortisone Systemic

(HIGH-droe-CORE-tih-sone)

A-hydroCort, Cortef, Hydrocortone, Solu-Cortef

A hormone used as replacement therapy when the adrenal cortex gland is not functioning properly. It is also used for its anti-inflammatory action. It may occasionally be prescribed for other reasons.

Precautions

DO NOT USE if you are allergic to this medicine or its relatives.

BEFORE USING THIS MEDICINE, tell your healthcare provider if you are pregnant or breastfeeding; or if you are taking, will be taking or stop taking any prescription or nonprescription medicine; or if you have any other medical conditions.

Side Effects

Every medicine can cause side effects, but many people have no, or minor, side effects. Tell your healthcare provider if any of the following occurs: appearance of a round, swollen moonface; fat deposits (eg, shoulders, midsection); nausea; vomiting; increased appetite; weight gain; peptic ulcer; local pain; rectal bleeding with enemas; seizures; dizziness; headache; behavior changes; sleeplessness; hiccups; fluid retention; low or high blood pressure; irregular heart rhythm; impaired wound healing; thinning of skin and layer of fat under the skin; excessive pigmentation of skin; acne; excessive body hair growth; rash; hives; loss of muscle mass; osteoporosis; bone fractures; menstrual irregularities; growth suppression in children; higher blood sugar levels.

Guidelines for Use

USE EXACTLY AS PRESCRIBED.

May cause stomach upset. Take with meals or snacks.

Take single daily or alternate day doses in the morning prior to 9 a.m.

Take multiple doses at evenly spaced intervals throughout the day.

Patients on long-term therapy with this medicine should carry identification.

Notify your healthcare provider if any of the above side effects occurs.

High-dose or long-term therapy: DO NOT change or stop therapy unless directed by your healthcare provider. Sudden withdrawal of therapy may cause symptoms of fatigue, loss of appetite, nausea, vomiting, diarrhea, weight loss, weakness, dizziness and low blood sugar.

Diabetes—May require increased doses of insulin or oral diabetes medications.

Hydrocortisone Topical

(HIGH-droe-CORE-tih-sone)

CaldeCort, Cortef Feminine Itch, Cortaid with Aloe, Corticaine, Extra Strength Gynecort 10, Gynecort-5, Lanacort 5, Lanacort 10, Proctocort, U-Cort, Westcort

A topical anti-inflammatory agent used to treat rash or skin irritation.

Precautions

DO NOT USE near eyes or eyelids or if you have an allergy to this medicine.

BEFORE USING THIS MEDICINE, tell your healthcare provider if you are pregnant or breastfeeding; or if you are taking, will be taking or stop taking any prescription or nonprescription medicine; or if you have any other medical conditions.

Side Effects

Every medicine can cause side effects, but many people have no, or minor, side effects. Tell your healthcare provider if any of the following occurs: burning; itching; irritation; redness; dryness; acne; streaks in skin; stinging and cracking; elevated blood sugar; cataracts and glaucoma (prolonged use near eyes); numbness of fingers.

Guidelines for Use

USE EXACTLY AS PRESCRIBED.

Apply sparingly as a thin film. Rub in lightly.

Wash or soak the affected area before application as this may increase medicine penetration.

Avoid contact with the eyes.

Avoid prolonged use, especially near the eyes, on the face, on genital and rectal areas, and in skin folds.

Do not use tight-fitting diapers or plastic pants on children being treated in the diaper area.

Do not wrap the treated area with bandages or tight-fitting clothing unless specifically directed by your healthcare provider.

Skin infections may worsen. It may be necessary to stop the corticosteroid and treat the infection.

Skin wasting may occur in 3 to 4 weeks.

Do not mix these products with other products. Allergic reactions may occur.

If the condition being treated gets worse or irritation, burning, redness, swelling or stinging persists, do not reapply the medicine. Contact your healthcare provider.

Alcohol-containing preparations may cause drying, burning or irritation of open lesions.

Hydromorphone Hydrochloride

(HIGH-droe-MORE-phone HIGH-droe-KLOR-ide)

Dilaudid, Dilaudid HP

A narcotic pain reliever used for moderate to severe pain.

Precautions

DO NOT USE if you are allergic to this medicine or its relatives.

BEFORE USING THIS MEDICINE, tell your healthcare provider if you are pregnant or breastfeeding; or if you are taking, will be taking or stop taking any prescription or nonprescription medicine; or if you have any other medical conditions. Long term, regular use of narcotic pain relievers may lead to dependence and physical tolerance. Withdrawal symptoms may occur when therapy is stopped. Some products may contain sulfite preservatives that can cause allergic reactions in some people. Ask your pharmacist.

Side Effects

Every medicine can cause side effects, but many people have no, or minor, side effects. Tell your healthcare provider if any of the following occurs: lightheadedness; dizziness; drowsiness; nausea; vomiting; sweating; abdominal pain; cramps; constipation; diarrhea; urine retention; appetite loss; indigestion; gas; excitability; vision problems; difficult breathing.

Guidelines for Use

USE EXACTLY AS PRESCRIBED.

Take with food if stomach upset occurs.

May cause drowsiness, dizziness or blurred vision. Use caution while driving or performing other tasks requiring mental alertness, judgment and coordination.

Avoid alcohol and other medicines that cause drowsiness (eg, sleeping pills, antihistamines).

May cause nausea, vomiting or constipation. Constipation may be avoided by using a stool softener or fiber laxative.

This medicine works best if taken regularly. It is more effective in preventing pain than in treating pain after it occurs.

Give the medicine ample time to work before taking more (approximately 30 minutes to 1 hour).

If a dose is missed, take it as soon as possible. If several hours have passed or if it is nearing time for the next dose, do not double the dose to "catch up," unless advised by your healthcare provider. If more than one dose is missed, contact your healthcare provider.

Suppository: If you do not know the correct way to insert a suppository, ask your healthcare provider.

Hydroxychloroquine Sulfate

(high-drox-ee-KLOR-oh-kwin SULL-fate)

Plaquenil Sulfate

A medicine used to treat acute or chronic rheumatoid arthritis. It also is used for the treatment of acute attacks of malaria and lupus erythematosus.

Precautions

DO NOT USE if you are allergic to this medicine or if you are pregnant.

Lab tests — Lab tests may be required during treatment with this medicine. Tests may include eye exams, blood counts and knee and ankle reflex testing.

BEFORE USING THIS MEDICINE, tell your healthcare provider if you are breastfeeding; or if you are taking, will be taking or stop taking any prescription or nonprescription medicine; or if you have any other medical conditions.

Side Effects

Every medicine can cause side effects, but many people have no, or minor, side effects. Tell your healthcare provider if any of the following occurs: appetite loss; vomiting; nausea; diarrhea; abdominal cramps; irritability; nervousness; nightmares; unusual behavior; headache; weakness; dizziness; vertigo (feeling of whirling motion); convulsions; incoordination; visual difficulties/disturbances; blurred vision; missing or blacked-out areas in the visual field; light flashes and streaks; sensitivity to light; hives; bleaching of hair; hair loss; itching; changes in pigmentation; muscle weakness; ringing in the ears; hearing loss; weight loss.

Guidelines for Use

USE EXACTLY AS PRESCRIBED.

Do not exceed prescribed dosage. Damage to the eyes may occur if dosage is exceeded.

If you experience any change in vision, hearing loss or ringing in the ears, contact your healthcare provider.

May cause stomach upset. Take with food or milk.

Periodic blood counts should be taken if therapy is prolonged.

Avoid long-term therapy in children.

If favorable results do not occur within six months, talk to your healthcare provider about discontinuing use.

Hydroxyurea

(high-DROX-ee-you-REE-uh)

Hydrea

A medicine used to treat certain types of skin cancer (melanoma, primary squamous cell carcinoma), resistant chronic myelocytic leukemia and inoperable ovarian cancer.

Precautions

DO NOT USE if you are allergic to this medicine.

BEFORE USING THIS MEDICINE, tell your healthcare provider if you are pregnant or breastfeeding; or if you are taking, will be taking or stop taking any prescription or nonprescription medicine; or if you have any other medical conditions.

Side Effects

Every medicine can cause side effects, but many people have no, or minor, side effects. Tell your healthcare provider if any of the following occurs: fever; drowsiness; chills; headache; appetite loss; diarrhea; constipation; stomach pain; nausea; vomiting; dizziness; hair loss; itching; redness; rash; sweating; allergic reaction; inflammation of mucous membranes; difficult urination; hallucinations; seizures.

Guidelines for Use

USE EXACTLY AS PRESCRIBED.

This medicine is usually taken as a single dose every day or every third day. Use a calendar or some other device to help ensure that no doses are missed.

If a dose is missed, take it as soon as possible. If more than half the time between doses has passed, do not take unless advised to do so by your healthcare provider. If more than one dose is missed, contact your healthcare provider.

Contraceptive measures (birth control) are recommended during therapy. Notify your healthcare provider immediately if you become pregnant.

Notify your healthcare provider if fever, chills, sore throat, nausea, vomiting, loss of appetite, diarrhea, sores in mouth and on the lips, unusual bleeding or bruising occurs.

May cause drowsiness, constipation, redness of face, skin rash, itching and loss of hair. Notify your healthcare provider if these become pronounced or bothersome.

This medicine may cause drowsiness or dizziness. Use caution while driving or performing other tasks requiring mental alertness, coordination or dexterity.

Hydroxyzine Hydrochloride

(high-DROX-ih-zeen HIGH-droe-KLOR-ide)

Anxanil, Atarax, Atarax 100, E-Vista, Hydroxacen, Hyzine-50, Quiess, Vistacon, Vistaject-25, Vistaject-50, Vistaquel 50, Vistaril, Vistazine 50

An antihistamine and agent used to relieve nervousness and anxiety. Decreases anxiety by suppressing activity in the anxiety centers in the brain. This medicine also is used as an anti-allergy, bronchodilator, analgesic, antispasmodic and antiemetic.

Precautions

DO NOT USE if you are allergic to this medicine, or if you are pregnant or breast-feeding.

BEFORE USING THIS MEDICINE, tell your healthcare provider if you are taking, will be taking or stop taking any prescription or nonprescription medicine; or if you have any other medical conditions.

Side Effects

Every medicine can cause side effects, but many people have no, or minor, side effects. Tell your healthcare provider if any of the following occurs: tremor; seizures; drowsiness; dizziness; wheezing; difficulty breathing; chest tightness; involuntary movements; dry mouth.

Guidelines for Use

USE EXACTLY AS PRESCRIBED.

If a dose is missed, take it as soon as possible. If several hours have passed or if it is nearing time for the next dose, do not double the dose to catch up, unless advised by your healthcare provider. If more than one dose is missed, contact your healthcare provider.

May cause drowsiness. Use caution while driving or performing other tasks requiring alertness.

Avoid alcohol or depressant medicines while taking this medicine.

Discontinue medicine at first appearance of wheezing, breathing difficulty or chest tightness. Tell your healthcare provider immediately.

Suspension: Shake well before using.

Ibuprofen

(eye-BYOO-pro-fen)

Aches-N-Pain, Advil, Excedrin IB, Genpril, Haltran, Ibu-Tab, Ibuprin, Medipren, Midol IB, Motrin, Motrin IB, Nuprin, Pedia-Profen, Rufen, Saleto-200, Trendar

A nonsteroidal anti-inflammatory medicine (NSAID) used to relieve mild to moderate pain and inflammation, to reduce fever and to treat osteoarthritis (degenerative joint disease), rheumatoid arthritis, and symptoms of PMS and dysmenorrhea (cramps). It may occasionally be prescribed for other reasons.

Precautions

DO NOT USE if you are allergic to this medicine or its relatives, aspirin or iodides.

BEFORE USING THIS MEDICINE, tell your healthcare provider if you are pregnant or breastfeeding; use alcohol chronically; are prone to fluid retention; or if you are taking, will be taking or stop taking any prescription or nonprescription medicines; or have any other medical conditions.

Side Effects

Every medicine can cause side effects, but many people have no, or minor, side effects. Tell your healthcare provider if any of the following occurs: allergic reaction (eg, rash, itching, fever); changes in vision; weight gain; fluid retention; stomach problems (eg, nausea, vomiting, diarrhea, pain); black stools; constipation; persistent headache; dizziness; nervousness; weakness; ringing in the ears; taste changes; unusual bruising or bleeding.

Guidelines for Use

USE EXACTLY AS PRESCRIBED.

Avoid aspirin and alcoholic beverages.

If stomach upset occurs, take with food, milk or antacids. If stomach pain continues, tell your healthcare provider.

If a dose is missed, take it as soon as possible. If several hours have passed or if it is nearing time for the next dose, do not double the dose to "catch up," unless advised by your healthcare provider. If more than one dose is missed, contact your healthcare provider.

May cause drowsiness or dizziness. Use caution while driving or performing other tasks requiring mental alertness, coordination and dexterity.

May cause sensitivity to sunlight. Avoid prolonged exposure to the sun. Use sunscreens and wear protective clothing until tolerance is determined.

Idarubicin Hydrochloride

(eye-DUH-RUE-bih-sin HIGH-droe-KLOR-ide)

Idamycin

Used in combination with other medicines to treat acute myeloid leukemia.

Precautions

DO NOT USE if you are pregnant.

Side Effects

Every medicine can cause side effects, but many people have no, or minor, side effects. Tell your healthcare provider if any of the following occurs: nausea; vomiting; hair loss; abdominal cramps; diarrhea; fever; headache; unusual bleeding or bruising; rash; difficulty breathing; chest pain; irritation at the injection site.

Idoxuridine (IDU)

(EYE-dox-YOU-rih-deen)

Herplex

A medicine used to treat herpes simplex keratitis (a viral infection of the cornea of the eye).

Precautions

DO NOT USE if you are allergic to this medicine.

BEFORE USING THIS MEDICINE, tell your healthcare provider if you are pregnant or breastfeeding; or if you are taking, will be taking or stop taking any prescription or nonprescription medicine; or if you have any other medical conditions.

Side Effects

Every medicine can cause side effects, but many people have no, or minor, side effects. Tell your healthcare provider if any of the following occurs: irritation; pain; itching; swelling of the eye or lids; increased tearing; sensitivity to bright light; clouding of vision.

Guidelines for Use

USE EXACTLY AS PRESCRIBED.

May cause sensitivity to bright lights. This may be minimized by wearing sunglasses.

Temporary burning or stinging may occur upon administration. This is not a cause for alarm.

If a dose is missed, use it as soon as possible. Do not double the dose to "catch up," unless advised by your healthcare provider. If several doses are missed, contact your healthcare provider.

Do not stop using the medicine unless instructed by your healthcare provider.

Use the full course of therapy.

Notify your healthcare provider if improvement is not seen after 14 days, if condition worsens, or if pain, itching or swelling of the eye occurs.

Recurrence may be seen if medication is not continued for 5 to 7 days after the lesion is apparently healed.

Storage--Store at room temperature and protect from light.

Do not mix with other medications.

Ifosfamide

(eye-FOSS-fuh-MIDE)

Ifex

Used in combination with other medicines to treat certain types of cancer.

Side Effects

Every medicine can cause side effects, but many people have no, or minor, side effects. Tell your healthcare provider if any of the following occurs: nausea; vomiting; loss of appetite; diarrhea; constipation; hair loss; sleepiness; confusion; severe depression; hallucinations; dizziness.

Patient Information

Tell your healthcare provider of unusual bleeding/bruising, fever, chills, sore throat, cough, shortness of breath, seizures, lack of menstrual flow, unusual lumps or masses, flank, stomach or joint pain, sores in mouth or on lips, yellow discoloration of skin or eyes.

Contraceptive (birth control) measures are recommended for men and women during therapy.

Imiglucerase

(eye-mih-GLU-cer-ace)

Cerozyme

An enzyme replacement used for the long-term treatment of patients with confirmed Type 1 Gaucher's disease.

Precautions

DO NOT USE if you are allergic to this medicine.

BEFORE USING THIS MEDICINE, tell your healthcare provider if you are pregnant or breastfeeding; or if you are taking, will be taking or stop taking any prescription or nonprescription medicine; or if you have any other medical conditions.

Side Effects

Every medicine can cause side effects, but many people have no, or minor, side effects. Tell your healthcare provider if any of the following occurs: headache; nausea; abdominal discomfort; dizziness; rash; itching; decreased urinary frequency.

Guidelines for Use

USE EXACTLY AS PRESCRIBED.

Careful monitoring and evaluation to determine if dosage should be changed should occur every 3 to 6 months.

Contact your healthcare provider if you have any signs of an allergic reaction.

Imipenem/Cilastatin IM

(ih-mih-PEN-em/SIGH-luh-STAT-in)

Primaxin IM

Used to treat infections caused by certain bacteria.

Precautions

DO NOT USE if you are allergic to this medicine or its relatives.

Side Effects

Every medicine can cause side effects, but many people have no, or minor, side effects. Tell your healthcare provider if any of the following occurs: irritation at the injection site; nausea; vomiting; diarrhea; difficulty breathing; rash; itching.

Guidelines for Use

USE EXACTLY AS PRESCRIBED.

If a dose is missed, inject it as soon as possible. If several hours have passed or if it is nearing time for the next dose, do not double the dose to catch up, unless advised to do so by your healthcare provider. If more than one dose is missed, contact your healthcare provider.

Continue use until all of the prescribed drug has been used, even if fever or other symptoms have disappeared. Failure to use a full course of therapy may prevent complete elimination of the bacteria, causing a relapse of the infection.

Imipenem/Cilastatin IV

(ih-mih-PEN-em/SIGH-luh-STAT-in)

Primaxin IV

Used to treat infections caused by certain bacteria.

Precautions

DO NOT USE if your are allergic to this medicine or its relatives.

Side Effects

Every medicine can cause side effects, but many people have no, or minor, side effects. Tell your healthcare provider if any of the following occurs: irritation at the injection site; nausea; vomiting; diarrhea; stomach ache; heartburn; mental confusion; dizziness; vertigo; seizures; headache; fever; pounding in the chest; difficulty breathing; itching; rash; hives; flushing; blue skin; sore throat; ringing in the ears; hearing loss; joint pain; muscle weakness.

Guidelines for Use

USE EXACTLY AS PRESCRIBED.

If a dose is missed, take it as soon as possible. If several hours have passed or if it is nearing time for the next dose, do not double the dose in order to catch up, unless advised to do so by your healthcare provider. If more than one dose is missed, contact your healthcare provider.

Continue use until all the prescribed drug has been used, even if fever or other symptoms have disappeared. Failure to use a full course of therapy may prevent complete elimination of the bacteria, causing a relapse of the infection.

Imipramine

(im-IPP-ruh-meen)

Imipramine Pamoate, Janimine, Tipramine, Tofranil, Tofranil-PM

A mood elevating medicine usually used for the relief of depression. It may occasionally be prescribed for other reasons.

Precautions

DO NOT USE if you are allergic to this medicine or its relatives, or if you are using monoamine oxidase inhibitors (eg, *Nardil, Parnate*).

BEFORE USING THIS MEDICINE, tell your healthcare provider if you are pregnant or breastfeeding; or if you are taking, will be taking or stop taking any prescription or nonprescription medicine; or if you have any other medical conditions.

Side Effects

Every medicine can cause side effects, but many people have no, or minor, side effects. Tell your healthcare provider if any of the following occurs: dry mouth; blurred vision; increased heart rate; impaired coordination; difficult urination; excessive sedation; seizures.

Guidelines for Use

USE EXACTLY AS PRESCRIBED.

Take as directed with a full glass of water, with or without food.

If a dose is missed, take it as soon as possible. If several hours have passed or if it is nearing time for the next dose, do not double the dose to catch up, unless advised by your healthcare provider. If more than one dose is missed, contact your healthcare provider.

This medicine may not be effective for 2 to 3 weeks.

Using this medicine with alcohol or other central nervous system depressants (eg, pain relievers, sedatives, antihistamines) may cause added drowsiness.

May cause drowsiness or blurred vision. Use caution while driving or performing other tasks requiring mental alertness.

May cause sensitivity to sunlight. Avoid prolonged exposure to the sun. Use sunscreens and wear protective clothing until tolerance is determined.

Taking this medicine at bedtime may help reduce side effects (eg, daytime drowsiness). Discuss this possibility with your healthcare provider.

Symptoms of nausea, headache or fatigue may develop after abruptly stopping long-term use.

Indapamide

(IN-DAP-uh-mide)

Lozol

A diuretic (water pill) that decreases excess water in the body and increases urine flow. This medicine is used to treat high blood pressure; edema (excess fluid) due to a variety of causes.

Precautions

DO NOT USE if you are allergic to this medicine or its relatives; oral diabetic medicines; sulfa antibiotics; or if you have severe kidney disease or loss of kidney function.

BEFORE USING THIS MEDICINE, tell your healthcare provider if you are pregnant or breastfeeding; or if you are taking, will be taking or stop taking any prescription or nonprescription medicine; or if you have any other medical conditions.

Side Effects

Every medicine can cause side effects, but many people have no, or minor, side effects. Tell your healthcare provider if any of the following occurs: thirst; irregular heartbeat; confusion; mood changes; nausea; vomiting; unusual tiredness; weakness; weak pulse; muscle cramps; appetite loss; stomach upset; bloating; diarrhea; constipation; dizziness; lightheadedness; headache; tingling of toes and fingers; blurred vision; nervousness; insomnia; chest pain; sun sensitivity; rash; hives; itching; dry skin; yellowing of skin or eyes; unusual bruising; difficult breathing; blood sugar imbalance; muscle cramps; joint pain; fever; chills; weight loss; nose bleeds; gout attack.

Guidelines for Use

USE EXACTLY AS PRESCRIBED.

Increases urination, therefore to avoid disruption of sleep at night take early in the day usually as a single dose.

May cause stomach upset. May be taken with food or milk.

May cause loss of potassium. If signs of potassium loss occur (weakness, cramps, nausea, dizziness, etc), contact your healthcare provider. Ask about foods high in potassium.

Diabetes — May increase blood sugar levels.

Dizziness or lightheadedness may occur if you stand up too fast from lying or sitting. Get up slowly, and notify your healthcare provider.

Sensitivity to sunlight may occur. Use sunscreen and wear protective clothing until tolerance is determined.

Your healthcare provider may want to periodically check your blood to ensure that your medicine is working properly.

Indinavir Sulfate

(in-DIN-ah-veer SULL-fate)

Crixivan

This medicine is used to treat HIV infection in adults. This medicine is not a cure for HIV and patients may continue to develop infections and other complications associated with HIV disease. This medicine has not been shown to reduce the incidence or frequency of these illnesses, nor reduce the risk of transmission of HIV to others. The long-term effects of indinavir are unknown at this time.

Precautions

DO NOT USE if you are allergic to this medicine.

BEFORE USING THIS MEDICINE, tell your healthcare provider if you are pregnant or breastfeeding; or if you are taking, will be taking or stop taking any prescription or nonprescription medicine; or if you have any other medical conditions.

Side Effects

Every medicine can cause side effects, but many people have no, or minor, side effects. Tell your healthcare provider if any of the following occurs: kidney stones; flank pain; blood in the urine; yellowing of the skin or eyes; dark urine; stomach pain; weakness; fatigue; general body discomfort; nausea; diarrhea; vomiting; acid regurgitation; appetite loss; headache; sleeplessness; dizziness; drowsiness; bad taste in mouth.

Guidelines for Use

USE EXACTLY AS PRESCRIBED.

Do not take this medicine at the same time as any of your other medications.

Take 800 mg (two capsules) by mouth every 8 hours with water 1 hour before or 2 hours after a meal. Do not take with food. However, it can be taken with liquids such as skim milk, juice, coffee or tea, or with a light meal (eg, dry toast with jelly, juice and coffee with skim milk and sugar, or with corn flakes, skim milk and sugar) if the medicine causes stomach discomfort. Meals high in fat, protein and calories reduce the absorption of this medicine.

Do not stop taking this medicine or change the dose unless directed by your healthcare provider.

Be sure to notify your healthcare provider of any other medications you are taking or will be taking.

If a dose is missed, take the next dose at the regularly scheduled time and do not double the dose to "catch up," unless advised by your healthcare provider. If more than one dose is missed, contact your healthcare provider.

Drink at least 1.5 liters (48 ounces) of liquid every 24 hours while taking this medicine.

Notify your healthcare provider if you have any liver problems. Your dosage may need to be adjusted.

Lab tests may be required. Be sure to keep appointments.

Store in the original tightly-closed container at room temperature (59°-86°F) away from moisture.

Keep the drying packet in the original bottle to protect the capsules from moisture damage. Do not throw it away until all of the medicine has been used.

Indomethacin

(in-doe-METH-uh-sin)

Indochron E-R, Indocin, Indocin IV, Indocin SR, Indocin Suppositories, Indocin Suspension, Indomethacin Capsules, Indomethacin Suppositories, Indomethacin Suspension, Indomethacin Sustained Release Capsules

A nonsteroidal anti-inflammatory medicine (NSAID) generally used to treat osteoarthritis (degenerative joint disease), rheumatoid arthritis and acute gout. Doctors occasionally may prescribe it for other reasons.

Precautions

DO NOT USE if you are allergic to this medicine or its relatives, aspirin or iodides.

BEFORE USING THIS MEDICINE, tell your healthcare provider if you are pregnant or breastfeeding; use alcohol chronically; are prone to fluid retention; or if you are taking, will be taking or stop taking any prescription or nonprescription medicines; or have any other medical conditions.

Side Effects

Every medicine can cause side effects, but many people have no, or minor, side effects. Tell your healthcare provider if any of the following occurs: allergic reaction (eg, rash, itching, fever); changes in vision; weight gain; fluid retention; stomach problems (eg, nausea, vomiting, diarrhea, pain); black stools; constipation; persistent headache; dizziness; nervousness; weakness; ringing in the ears; taste changes; unusual bruising or bleeding.

Guidelines for Use

USE EXACTLY AS PRESCRIBED.

Avoid aspirin and alcoholic beverages.

If stomach upset occurs, take with food, milk or antacids. If stomach pain continues, tell your healthcare provider.

If a dose is missed, take it as soon as possible. If several hours have passed or if it is nearing time for the next dose, do not double the dose to catch up, unless advised by your healthcare provider. If more than one dose is missed, contact your healthcare provider.

May cause drowsiness or dizziness. Observe caution while driving or performing other tasks requiring mental alertness, coordination and dexterity.

May cause sensitivity to sunlight. Avoid prolonged exposure to the sun. Use sunscreens and wear protective clothing until tolerance is determined.

Sustained release: swallow whole; do not crush or chew.

Suspension: shake well before using.

Suppository: If you do not know the correct way to use a suppository, ask your healthcare provider.

Influenza Virus Vaccine

(in-flew-EN-zuh virus vaccine)

Fluzone, Flu-Imune, Fluogen, Flu-Shield

For immunization against influenza virus.

Side Effects

Every medicine can cause side effects, but many people have no, or minor, side effects. Tell your healthcare provider if any of the following occurs: soreness at injection site; fever; general body discomfort; muscle aches.

Insulin

(IN-suh-lin)

Humulin 70/30, Humulin L, Humulin N, Humulin R, Humulin U, Iletin I Lente, Iletin I NPH, Iletin I Regular, Iletin II Lente (Pork), Iletin II NPH, Iletin II Regular, Iletin II Regular Concentrate, Insulatard NPH, Lente Ilentin I, Lente L, Novolin 70/30, Novolin 70/30 PenFill, Novolin L, Novolin N, Novolin N PenFill, Novolin R, Novolin R PenFill, NPH Iletin I, NPH-N, Regular Iletin I, Regular Insulin, Ultralente U, Velosulin Human

A hormone used to treat diabetes mellitus that is self-injected to lower blood sugar levels that cannot be controlled by diet, exercise or oral medicine.

Precautions

DO NOT USE if you are allergic to this medicine.

BEFORE USING THIS MEDICINE, tell your healthcare provider if you are pregnant or breastfeeding; or if you are taking, will be taking or stop taking any prescription or nonprescription medicine; or if you have any other medical conditions.

Side Effects

Every medicine can cause side effects, but many people have no, or minor, side effects. Tell your healthcare provider if any of the following occurs: visual changes; rash; itching or other allergic symptoms at injection site; infection that does not heal; increased thirst; increased urination; dry mouth; burning sensation in feet, legs or hands; pain in legs after exercise; and, especially, frequent episodes of very low or very high blood sugar levels. The main concern is dangerously low blood sugar levels (also called hypoglycemia; insulin shock).

Guidelines for Use

USE EXACTLY AS PRESCRIBED.

Rotate the sites of injection to prevent scarring.

Monitor urine for glucose and ketones as prescribed.

Blood glucose monitoring is essential to achieve normal blood sugar levels.

Patients with diabetes should wear an ID tag (eg, *Medic-Alert*) so appropriate treatment can be given if complications occur away from home. You should be taught self-management of diabetes by a trained health professional.

Have your eyes examined annually; see your dentist regularly to avoid tooth and gum disease.

Store the bottle you are using at room temperature. Store unopened bottles in refrigerator. Do not freeze.

Interferon alfa-2a

(IN-ter-FEER-ahn AL-fuh 2a)

Roferon-A

Used to treat hairy cell leukemia and AIDS-related Kaposi's sarcoma in selected patients age 18 and over. It may occasionally be prescribed for other reasons.

Side Effects

Every medicine can cause side effects, but many people have no, or minor, side effects. Tell your healthcare provider if any of the following occurs: fever; drowsiness; chills; tiredness; sore throat; joint and muscle aches/pain; headache; appetite loss; diarrhea; constipation; stomach pain; nausea; vomiting; gas; heartburn; dizziness; confusion; forgetfulness; incoordination; mood disorders; nervousness; sleep problems; anxiety; fatigue; weakness; general body discomfort; depression; abnormal thinking; feeling of whirling motion; chest pain; pounding in the chest; hemorrhage; painful or difficult breathing; coughing; hair loss; itching; redness; rash; dry skin; skin disorders; sweating; muscle twitching; back pain; weight loss; taste changes; fluid loss; thirst; dry, swollen mouth; pain; hot flashes; cold sores; nosebleed; numbness and tingling; sensitivity to light; double vision; ear and eye pain; painful or difficult urination; blood in urine; temporary impotence; speech problems.

Patient Information

Contraceptive (birth control) measures are recommended during therapy. Tell your healthcare provider immediately if you suspect pregnancy.

Flu-like symptoms (fever, drowsiness, chills, tiredness, sore throat, muscle aches, headache, joint pain) are common with this medicine. Tell your healthcare provider if they become pronounced.

May cause drowsiness or dizziness. Use caution while driving or performing other tasks requiring mental alertness, coordination and dexterity.

Tell your healthcare provider if hives, itching, tightness in the chest, wheezing or lightheadedness occurs.

Drink plenty of fluids, especially in the early stages of treatment.

Interferon alfa-2b

(IN-ter-FEER-ahn AL-fuh-2b)

Intron A

Used to treat hairy cell leukemia, genital or venereal warts, chronic hepatitis or AIDS-related Kaposi's sarcoma in selected patients age 18 and over. It may occasionally be prescribed for other reasons.

Precautions

DO NOT USE if you are allergic to this medicine.

Side Effects

Every medicine can cause side effects, but many people have no, or minor, side effects. Tell your healthcare provider if any of the following occurs: fever; drowsiness; chills; tiredness; sore throat; joint and muscle aches/pain; headache; appetite loss; diarrhea; constipation; stomach pain; nausea; vomiting; gas; heartburn; dizziness; confusion; nervousness; sleep problems; anxiety; fatigue; weakness; general body discomfort; depression; feeling of whirling motion; chest pain; pounding in the chest; hemorrhage; painful or difficult breathing; coughing; hair loss; itching; redness; rash; dry skin; skin disorders; sweating; muscle twitching; back pain; weight loss; taste changes; cold sores; numbness and tingling; sensitivity to light; double vision; ear and eye pain; temporary impotence; ringing in the ears.

Guidelines for Use

USE EXACTLY AS PRESCRIBED.

Contraceptive (birth control) measures are recommended during therapy.

Tell your healthcare provider immediately if you suspect pregnancy.

Flu-like symptoms (fever, drowsiness, chills, tiredness, sore throat, muscle aches, headache, joint pain) are common with this medicine. Tell your healthcare provider if they become pronounced.

May cause drowsiness or dizziness. Use caution while driving or performing other tasks requiring mental alertness, coordination and dexterity.

Tell your healthcare provider if hives, itching, tightness in the chest, wheezing or lightheadedness occurs.

Drink plenty of fluids, especially in the early stages of treatment.

May cause sensitivity to sunlight. Avoid prolonged exposure to the sun. Wear sunscreen and protective clothing until tolerance is determined.

Interferon alfa-n3

(IN-ter-FEER-ahn AL-fuh-n3)

Alferon N

Used to treat hairy cell leukemia and AIDS-related Kaposi's sarcoma in selected patients age 18 and over. It may occasionally be prescribed for other reasons.

Side Effects

Every medicine can cause side effects, but many people have no, or minor, side effects. Tell your healthcare provider if any of the following occurs: fever; drowsiness; chills; tiredness; sore throat; joint and muscle aches/pain; headache; appetite loss; diarrhea; constipation; stomach pain; nausea; vomiting; gas; heartburn; dizziness; confusion; forgetfulness; incoordination; mood disorders; nervousness; sleep problems; anxiety; fatigue; weakness; general body discomfort; depression; abnormal thinking; feeling of whirling motion; chest pain; pounding in the chest; hemorrhage; painful or difficult breathing; coughing; hair loss; itching; redness; rash; dry skin; skin disorders; sweating; muscle twitching; back pain; weight loss; taste changes; fluid loss; thirst; dry, swollen mouth; pain; hot flashes; cold sores; nosebleed; numbness and tingling; sensitivity to light; double vision; ear and eye pain; painful or difficult urination; blood in urine; temporary impotence; speech problems; runny nose.

Patient Information

Contraceptive (birth control) measures are recommended during therapy.

Tell your healthcare provider immediately if you suspect pregnancy.

Flu-like symptoms (fever, drowsiness, chills, tiredness, sore throat, muscle aches, headache, joint pain) are common with this medicine. Tell your doctor if they become pronounced.

May cause drowsiness or dizziness. Use caution while driving or performing other tasks requiring mental alertness, coordination and dexterity.

Tell your healthcare provider if hives, itching, tightness in the chest, wheezing or lightheadedness occurs.

Drink plenty of fluids, especially in the early stages of treatment.

Interferon Beta-1b (rIFN-B)

(IN-ter-FEER-ahn BAY-tuh-1b)

Betaseron

A medicine used to treat relapsing-remitting multiple sclerosis to reduce the frequency of clinical attacks.

Precautions

DO NOT USE if you are allergic to this medicine or if you are pregnant. Immediately tell your healthcare provider if you experience any depression or suicidal thoughts.

BEFORE USING THIS MEDICINE, tell your healthcare provider if you are breastfeeding; or if you are taking, will be taking or stop taking any prescription or nonprescription medicine; or if you have any other medical conditions.

Side Effects

Every medicine can cause side effects, but many people have no, or minor, side effects. Tell your healthcare provider if any of the following occurs: pain and tenderness at the injection site; headache; fever; flu-like symptoms; pain; weakness; chills; abdominal pain; general body discomfort; fluid retention; pelvic pain; cysts; migraine; pounding in the chest; high blood pressure; bleeding; diarrhea; constipation; vomiting; cramps; sinus infection; difficulty breathing; laryngitis; weight gain or loss; joint and muscle aches and pain; anxiety; depression; sleeplessness; confusion; slurred speech; convulsions; sweating; hair loss; menstrual problems; breast pain; frequent urination; fibrous breast cysts.

Guidelines for Use

USE EXACTLY AS PRESCRIBED.

Do not change your dosage or times when you receive the medicine without talking to your healthcare provider.

You should receive thorough instructions on storage of and mixing the medicine, self-injection technique and procedures. Your first self-administered injection should be given under the supervision of a healthcare professional. A patient information sheet is provided.

Do not re-use needles/syringes. Your pharmacist can provide you with a puncture-resistant container for safe disposal of used syringes and needles along with instructions for safe disposal of container.

If you become pregnant or plan to become pregnant, talk to your healthcare provider immediately. Spontaneous abortions have occurred during this therapy.

May cause sunlight sensitivity. Avoid long exposure to the sun or sunlamps. Use sunscreens and protective clothing as needed.

Keep appointments with your healthcare provider. Lab tests will be required.

Interferon gamma-1b

(IN-ter-FEER-ahn GAM-uh-1b)

Actimmune

Used to reduce the frequency and severity of serious infections associated with chronic granulomatous disease.

Side Effects

Every medicine can cause side effects, but many people have no, or minor, side effects. Tell your healthcare provider if any of the following occurs: fever; headache; rash; chills; irritation at the injection site; fatigue; diarrhea; vomiting; nausea; abdominal pain; weight loss; muscle pain; loss of appetite; depression; joint pain; back pain.

Patient Information

If home use is prescribed, your healthcare provider will provide you with a puncture-resistant container for the disposal of used syringes and needles.

Carefully follow your healthcare provider's instructions on the safe disposal of used syringes and needles. Never reuse syringes or needles.

Your healthcare provider will provide you with a patient information sheet. Be sure to review all information with your healthcare provider.

The most common adverse reactions are flu-like symptoms such as fever, chills, headache, muscle pain and fatigue. Some of these symptoms may be minimized by bedtime administration.

Acetaminophen (*Tylenol*) may be used to prevent or partially treat the fever and headache.

Iodine Antiseptic

(EYE-uh-dine)

Iodine Tincture, Strong Iodine (Lugol's Solution)

Topical medicine used against bacteria, fungi, viruses, protozoa and yeasts. Also is used to disinfect the skin before surgery.

Precautions

DO NOT USE if you are allergic to this medicine.

BEFORE USING THIS MEDICINE, tell your healthcare provider if you are pregnant or breastfeeding; or if you are taking, will be taking or stop taking any prescription or nonprescription medicine; of if you have any other medical conditions.

Every medicine can cause side effects, but many people have no, or minor, side effects. Tell your healthcare provider if skin irritation occurs.

Guidelines for Use

USE EXACTLY AS PRESCRIBED.

For external use only.

Avoid contact with the eyes.

May stain skin and clothes.

Iodine Expectorant

(EYE-uh-dine)

Pima, SSKI

A medicine used for the treatment of lung disease where mucus complicates the conditions (emphysema, bronchial asthma, chronic bronchitis). It also is used as adjunctive treatment in respiratory conditions such as cystic fibrosis, chronic sinusitis and after surgery to help prevent lung collapse.

Precautions

DO NOT USE if you are allergic to this medicine.

BEFORE USING THIS MEDICINE, tell your healthcare provider if you are pregnant or breastfeeding; or if you are taking, will be taking or stop taking any prescription or nonprescription medicine; of if you have any other medical conditions.

Side Effects

Every medicine can cause side effects, but many people have no, or minor, side effects. Tell your healthcare provider if any of the following occurs: nausea; vomiting; diarrhea; stomach pain; bleeding; mental confusion; headache; numbness; fatigue; acne; rash; hives; skin and mucous membrane bleeding; joint pain; swelling of neck or throat; metallic taste; sore or burning mouth or throat; increased salivation; runny nose; sneezing; eyelid swelling; tingling; pain or weakness in hands or feet; weakness or heaviness of legs; fever; difficulty breathing; black or tar-like stools.

Guidelines for Use

USE EXACTLY AS PRESCRIBED.

Do not take this medicine for persistent or chronic cough such as occurs with smoking, asthma, chronic bronchitis or emphysema, or when cough is accompanied by excessive phlegm, unless directed by your healthcare provider.

A persistent cough may be a sign of a serious condition. If cough persists for more than one week, tends to recur, or is accompanied by fever, rash or persistent headache, talk to your healthcare provider.

Drink a glass of water or other fluid with each dose.

Stop if stomach pain, rash, nausea, vomiting, bloating or a metallic taste occurs.

Iodine (Thyroid Agent)

(EYE-uh-dine)

Strong Iodine (Lugol's Solution), Thyro-Block

Used with an antithyroid medicine in hyperthyroid patients prior to thyroid surgery or to treat an overactive thyroid gland. It also is used to block the thyroid gland during a radiation emergency (eg, radioactive fallout). It may occasionally be prescribed for other reasons.

Precautions

DO NOT USE if you are allergic to this medicine.

BEFORE USING THIS MEDICINE, tell your healthcare provider if you are pregnant or breastfeeding; or if you are taking, will be taking or stop taking any prescription or nonprescription medicine; or if you have any other medical conditions.

Side Effects

Every medicine can cause side effects, but many people have no, or minor, side effects. Tell your healthcare provider if any of the following occurs: metallic taste; burning mouth and throat; sore gums; upset stomach; diarrhea; vomiting; symptoms of a head cold; shortness of breath; runny nose; rash; acne; fever; joint pain; swelling of parts of the face and body; inflammation of the eye (with watering); bloating; nervous irritability; irritation at the injection site.

Guidelines for Use

USE EXACTLY AS PRESCRIBED.

Strong iodine solutions--Dilute with water or fruit juice to improve taste.

Thyroid surgery--Oral iodine-containing products are usually given for 10 days prior to surgery.

Discontinue use and tell your doctor if any of the following occurs: fever, skin rash, metallic taste, swelling of the throat, burning of the mouth and throat, sore gums, head cold symptoms, severe stomach distress.

Recommended Dietary Allowances (RDA)--Adults: 150 mcg.

Ipecac Syrup

(IPP-uh-kak)

Available as generic only

Used to treat overdoses and certain poisoning caused by swallowing.

Precautions

DO NOT USE if you are pregnant or breastfeeding; if poisoning is by corrosives (eg, alkalies, strong acid), petroleum distillates or strychnine. DO NOT give to a semiconscious or unconscious patient.

BEFORE USING THIS MEDICINE, tell your healthcare provider if you are pregnant or breastfeeding; or if you are taking, will be taking or stop taking any prescription or nonprescription medicine; of if you have any other medical conditions.

Side Effects

Every medicine can cause side effects, but many people have no, or minor, side effects. Tell your healthcare provider if any of the following occurs: diarrhea; drowsiness; stomach ache.

Guidelines for Use

USE EXACTLY AS PRESCRIBED.

Give only to conscious (alert) persons.

Give with plenty of water.

Do not exceed recommended dosage.

Do not take with milk or carbonated drinks (eg, soda).

Always consult your doctor or poison control center in cases of accidental ingestion.

Ipecac syrup may not work on an empty stomach.

Have the patient sit upright with head forward before administering dose. Children--(1 to 12 years)--15 ml (1 tbsp) followed by 1 to 2 glasses of water. Adults--15 to 30 ml (1 to 2 tbsp) followed by 3 to 4 glasses of water. Repeat the dosage once if vomiting does not occur within 20 minutes. If vomiting does not occur within 30 minutes after the second dose, contact your healthcare provider or poison control center. If vomiting does not occur after taking ipecac syrup, or if excessive doses are used, it may be absorbed into the body and cause problems with the heart. Contact your healthcare provider.

Ipratropium Bromide

(IH-pruh-TROE-pee-uhm BROE-mide)

Atrovent

A medicine that widens the passageways in the lungs and is used to treat various breathing problems.

Precautions

DO NOT USE if you are allergic to atropine or any of its relatives.

BEFORE USING THIS MEDICINE, tell your healthcare provider if you are pregnant or breastfeeding; or if you are taking, will be taking or stop taking any prescription or nonprescription medicine; or if you have any other medical conditions.

Side Effects

Every medicine can cause side effects, but many people have no, or minor, side effects. Tell your healthcare provider if any of the following occurs: nervousness; dizziness; headaches; nausea; abdominal discomfort; blurred vision; dry mouth and throat; cough; drowsiness; palpitations (pounding in chest); rash.

Guidelines for Use

USE EXACTLY AS PRESCRIBED.

Not for the treatment of acute episodes of bronchospasm where rapid response is required.

Temporary blurring of vision may occur if the medicine is sprayed in the eye. Use of a nebulizer with a mouthpiece, rather than a face mask, may be preferable to reduce the liklihood of the solution reaching the eyes. Solution can be mixed in the nebulizer with albuterol if used within one hour of mixing together.

Protect from sunlight. Store unused vials in the foil pouch.

Store at room temperature.

Avoid excessive humidity.

The total daily dose should not exceed 12 inhalations/24 hours.

Isoetharine

(EYE-so-ETH-uh-reen)

Arm-a-Med Isoetharine Hydrochloride, Bronkosol

A medicine that makes breathing easier by widening breathing passages of the lung and by removing (expectorating) mucus and other debris that cause congestion in the lungs. May be used to treat asthma, bronchitis or emphysema.

Precautions

DO NOT USE if you are allergic to this medicine or have heart rhythm disturbances associated with a rapid heart rate.

BEFORE USING THIS MEDICINE, tell your healthcare provider if you are pregnant or breastfeeding; or if you are taking, will be taking or stop taking any prescription or nonprescription medicine; or if you have any other medical conditions.

Side Effects

Every medicine can cause side effects, but many people have no, or minor, side effects. Tell your healthcare provider if any of the following occurs: nausea; vomiting; loss of appetite; heartburn; nervousness; restlessness; dizziness; lightheadedness; headache; anxiety; tension; tremor; drowsiness; weakness; sleeplessness; chest pain; pounding in chest (palpitations); breathing problems; coughing; flushing; sweating; hives; muscle cramps; unusual or bad taste in mouth; drying or irritation of mouth; excitement.

Guidelines for Use

USE EXACTLY AS PRESCRIBED.

Shake well before use.

Tell your healthcare provider if palpitations, chest pain, muscle tremors, dizziness, headache, flushing or difficult urination occurs, or if breathing difficulty or nervousness persists.

Patient instructions are available with products.

Do not exceed recommended dosage. Excessive use may lead to side effects or loss of effectiveness.

Do not stop or adjust the dose except on the recommendation of your healthcare provider.

Administer pressurized inhalation during the second half of breath intake.

Solution for inhalation: This medicine is usually delivered over 15–20 minutes and does not need to be repeated more often than every 4 hours. However, more frequent administration may be necessary in severe cases.

Aerosol: The average adult dose is 1–2 inhalations (puffs).

If more than one inhalation per dose is necessary, wait at least one full minute between doses. If you do not get the usual relief from your normal dose, do not increase your dose, but call your healthcare provider immediately.

If a dose is missed, inhale it as soon as possible. If several hours have passed or if it is nearing time for the next dose, do not double the dose to "catch up," unless advised by your healthcare provider. If more than one dose is missed, contact your healthcare provider.

Do not use epinephrine or other inhaled bronchodilators while using this medicine.

Storage: Do not use if solution is discolored or cloudy. Protect from heat and light.

Isometheptene/Dichloralphenazone/Acetaminophen

(eye-so-meth-EPP-teen/die-klor-uhl-FEN-uh-zone/ASS-et-ah-MEE-noe-fen)

Isocom, Isopap, Midchlor, Midrin, Migratine

A medicine used for treatment of migraine.

Precautions

DO NOT USE if you are allergic to these medicines.

BEFORE USING THIS MEDICINE, tell your healthcare provider if you are pregnant or breastfeeding; or if you are taking, will be taking or stop taking any prescription or nonprescription medicine; or if you have any other medical conditions such as high blood pressure, heart disease, glaucoma, kidney or liver problems.

Side Effects

Every medicine can cause side effects, but many people have no, or minor, side effects. Tell your healthcare provider if any of the following occurs: irregular heartbeat; nausea; vomiting; dizziness; skin rash; yellowing of skin or eyes.

Guidelines for Use

USE EXACTLY AS PRESCRIBED.

Start therapy at first sign of attack. Do NOT exceed maximum dose.

Isoniazid

(eye-so-NYE-uh-zid)

Laniazid, Nydrazid

Used to prevent and treat tuberculosis. It may occasionally be prescribed for other reasons.

Precautions

DO NOT USE if you have liver problems or if you are allergic to this medicine. Severe and sometimes fatal hepatitis may occur or develop after taking this medicine. The risk of developing hepatitis increases with age and frequent use of alcohol. Report any of the following signs of hepatitis to your healthcare provider: fatigue, weakness, general body discomfort, appetite loss, nausea, vomiting, yellowing of skin/eyes.

BEFORE USING THIS MEDICINE, tell your healthcare provider if you are pregnant or breastfeeding; or if you are taking, will be taking or stop taking any prescription or nonprescription medicine; or if you have any other medical conditions.

Side Effects

Every medicine can cause side effects, but many people have no, or minor, side effects. Tell your healthcare provider if any of the following occurs: nausea; vomiting; appetite loss; diarrhea; stomach pain; dizziness; unusual tiredness; weakness; drowsiness; confusion; rash; itching; hives; muscle pain or arthritis; headache; vision problems; fever; numbness, pain or tingling in hands or feet; general body discomfort; yellowing of the eyes or skin; breast enlargement; increased blood sugar; joint pain; irritation at injection site.

Guidelines for Use

USE EXACTLY AS PRESCRIBED.

Take on an empty stomach, at least 1 hour before or 2 hours after meals. If stomach upset occurs, take with food.

Take as directed.

Minimize alcohol use. Alcohol increases risk of hepatitis.

Do not stop taking before talking with your healthcare provider.

Avoid missing doses, however, if a dose is missed, take it as soon as possible. If several hours have passed or it is nearing time for the next dose, do not double the dose to "catch up," unless advised to do so by your healthcare provider. If more than one dose is missed, contact your healthcare provider.

Vitamin B6 deficiency is sometimes seen during treatment with this medicine. Talk to your healthcare provider to determine if vitamin B6 supplements are required.

To avoid a possible interaction, avoid tyramine-containing foods (cheese/dairy products, beef or chicken liver, fish, meats prepared with tenderizer; fermented sausages, game meat, caviar, dried fish, avocado, yeast extracts, bananas, figs, raisins, soy sauce, fava beans, chocolate, caffeine-containing beverages) and foods containing histamine (skipjack, tuna, sauerkraut juice, yeast extract).

Contact your healthcare provider if any of the following occurs: fever, rash, appetite loss, nausea, vomiting, yellowing of skin/eyes, darkening of urine, or numbness/tingling of hands or feet.

Lab tests and eye exams will be required. Keep appointments.

Store at room temperature.

Syrup — store in a tight, light-resistant container.

Isoproterenol

(eye-so-pro-TER-uh-nahl)

Dispos-a-Med Isoproterenol HCl, Isuprel, Isuprel Glossets, Isuprel Mistometer, Medihaler ISO

Used to treat reversible bronchospasm associated with bronchial and nocturnal (nighttime) asthma, chronic bronchitis, emphysema, exercise-induced bronchospasm and other obstructive diseases of the lungs.

Precautions

DO NOT USE if you are allergic to this medicine or have heart rhythm/rate problems.

BEFORE USING THIS MEDICINE, tell your healthcare provider if you are pregnant or breastfeeding; or if you are taking, will be taking or stop taking any prescription or nonprescription medicine; if you have any other medical conditions; or are allergic to sulfites.

Side Effects

Every medicine can cause side effects, but many people have no, or minor, side effects. Tell your healthcare provider if any of the following occurs: nausea; vomiting; appetite changes; heartburn; diarrhea; abdominal pain; dry mouth; pinkish-red saliva; dizziness; lightheadedness; headache; anxiety; tension; twitching or tremor; drowsiness; fatigue; nervousness; confusion; hallucinations; aggressive behaviors; sleeplessness; pounding in the chest; breathing problems; fever; cough; cold sweat; nosebleed; hoarseness (especially in children); flushing; sweating; hives; tingling of the skin; acne; muscle stiffness/rigidity; muscle cramps; unusual or bad taste in mouth; tooth pain, discoloration or discomfort; nightmares; joint and back pain; painful urination; painful menstruation; rapid heartbeat.

Guidelines for Use

USE EXACTLY AS PRESCRIBED.

Read and follow the patient instructions provided with the medicine. If a dose is missed, take it as soon as possible. If several hours have passed or it is nearing time for the next dose, do not double the dose to "catch up," unless advised to do so by your healthcare provider. If more than one dose is missed, contact your healthcare provider.

May cause nervousness, restlessness or sleeplessness. Talk to your healthcare provider if these side effects continue, or if pounding in the chest, chest pain, muscle tremors, dizziness, headache, flushing or difficult urination occurs.

If serious breathing problems occur while using this medicine, stop use and contact your healthcare provider immediately.

If you do not get the usual relief from your normal dose, do not increase your dose or exceed recommended dosage. Excessive use may lead to serious side effects or loss of effectiveness. Do not stop or adjust the dose unless directed by your healthcare provider. If you are using more than 3 treatments in a 24–hour period, keep in close contact with your healthcare provider.

Do not use epinephrine or other inhaled bronchodilators while using this medicine.

Sublingual tablets-Do not crush, chew or swallow. Allow to dissolve under tongue. Do not swallow saliva until absorption has taken place. *Inhalation*-Follow administration and storage instructions exactly. Do not use if solution is cloudy or discolored. Change the solution in the nebulizer daily. *Aerosol*-Shake aerosol canister before each use. Do not spray in eyes or puncture container.

Isosorbide Dinitrate, Oral

(EYE-sos-ORE-bide die-NYE-trate)

Dilatrate-SR, Isordil Tembids, Isordil Titradose, Sorbitrate

This medicine is used to prevent angina attacks.

Precautions

DO NOT USE if you are allergic to this medicine or its relatives.

BEFORE USING THIS MEDICINE, tell your healthcare provider if you are pregnant or breastfeeding; or if you are taking, will be taking or stop taking any prescription or nonprescription medicine; or if you have any other medical conditions.

Side Effects

Every medicine can cause side effects, but many people have no, or minor, side effects. Tell your healthcare provider if any of the following occurs: severe or persistent headache; blurred vision; dry mouth; dizziness; flushing.

Guidelines for Use

USE EXACTLY AS PRESCRIBED.

Take on an empty stomach, with a full glass of water.

Sustained release: Do not crush or chew. Swallow whole.

Too large a dose may produce severe headaches. Lower doses and pain medicines can help control this problem. Headaches tend to become less severe or disappear as therapy continues.

The effectiveness of therapy may decrease over time as tolerance develops. If this occurs, tell your healthcare provider.

Dizziness or weakness can occur when arising from a seated or lying position. Alcohol can worsen this effect. Recovery can be faster by putting the head lower than the heart, or by deep breathing and moving the arms and legs.

Avoid alcohol.

Keep the medicine in its original container.

Isosorbide Dinitrate, Sublingual

EYE-sos-ORE-bide die-NYE-trate)

Isordil, Sorbitrate

Administered under the tongue, this medicine generally is used to prevent angina attacks and may be taken before events or activities that are likely to cause an angina attack.

Precautions

DO NOT USE if you are allergic to this medicine or its relatives.

BEFORE USING THIS MEDICINE, tell your healthcare provider if you are pregnant or breastfeeding; or if you are taking, will be taking or stop taking any prescription or nonprescription medicines; or have any other medical conditions.

Side Effects

Every medicine can cause side effects, but many people have no, or minor, side effects. Tell your healthcare provider if any of the following occurs: severe or persistent headaches; blurred vision; dry mouth; or dizziness and flushing.

Guidelines for Use

USE EXACTLY AS PRESCRIBED.

Too large a dose may produce severe headaches. Lower doses and pain medications can help control this problem. Headaches tend to become less severe or disappear as therapy continues.

The effectiveness of therapy may decrease over time as tolerance develops. If this occurs, tell your healthcare provider.

Dizziness or weakness can occur when arising from a seated or lying position. Alcohol can worsen this effect. Recovery can be hastened by putting the head lower than the heart, or by deep breathing and moving the arms and legs.

Dissolve tablet under tongue. Do not swallow.

A lack of a stinging sensation does not indicate a loss of potency.

Take while sitting at the first sign of an attack (chest pain) before severe pain develops. If pain is not relieved in 5 minutes, dissolve a second tablet under the tongue. If pain is not relieved within another 5 minutes, dissolve a third tablet. If pain continues or gets worse, tell your healthcare provider immediately or go to the nearest hospital emergency room.

Dry mouth decreases absorption and effectiveness.

Keep in the original container. Store at room temperature. Do not use after the expiration date. Protect from moisture. Unused tablets should be discarded 6 months after the original bottle is opened.

Isosorbide Mononitrate

(EYE-sos-ORE-bide MAH-no-NYE-trate)

ISMO Tablets, IMDUR

This medicine is used to prevent angina attacks.

Precautions

DO NOT USE if you are allergic to this medicine or its relatives.

BEFORE USING THIS MEDICINE, tell your healthcare provider if you are pregnant or breastfeeding; or if you are taking, will be taking or stop taking any prescription or nonprescription medicine; or if you have any other medical conditions.

Side Effects

Every medicine can cause side effects, but many people have no, or minor, side effects. Tell your healthcare provider if any of the following occurs: nausea; vomiting; abdominal pain; appetite loss; persistent headache; faintness; apprehension; restlessness; dizziness; muscle twitching; weakness; chest pain; pounding in the chest (palpitations); flushing; excessive sweating; cold sweat; visual disturbances; fever; involuntary passing of urine or feces.

Guidelines for Use

USE EXACTLY AS PRESCRIBED.

Generally, this medication should be taken twice daily, with the two doses 7 hours apart. This can be accomplished by taking the first dose on awakening, and the second dose 7 hours later.

Consult your physician or pharmacist if you have questions about when to take this medication.

Take on an empty stomach with a full glass of water.

May cause daily headaches. Pain medicines such as aspirin or acetaminophen often can help control this problem. Headaches tend to become less severe or disappear as therapy continues. Do not alter your dosing schedule without talking to your healthcare provider.

Transient dizziness or weakness can occur when arising from a seated or lying position. Alcohol can worsen this effect. Recovery can be hastened by putting the head lower than the heart, or by deep breathing and moving the arms and legs.

Avoid alcohol.

Keep the medicine in its original container.

Your healthcare provider also may have you use other forms (under-the-tongue) if an angina attack occurs.

Isotretinoin

(EYE-so-TREH-tih-NO-in)

Accutane

A medicine generally used to treat severe cystic acne unresponsive to conventional therapy.

Precautions

DO NOT USE if you have an allergy to this medicine, parabens (preservatives), vitamin A; if you are or may become pregnant; or if you are breastfeeding.

BEFORE USING THIS MEDICINE, tell your healthcare provider if you are a sexually active woman of childbearing age; if you are taking, will be taking or stop taking any prescription or nonprescription medicine; or have any other medical condition.

Side Effects

Every medicine can cause side effects, but many people have no, or minor, side effects. Tell your healthcare provider if any of the following occurs: visual disturbances; eye irritation; decreased night vision; headache; fatigue; rash; skin sloughing; hair thinning; sensitivity to sunlight; skin pigment changes; hives; dry, fragile skin; itching; brittle nails; bruising; nosebleed; dry nose or mouth; rectal bleeding; severe diarrhea; contact lens intolerance; uncontrolled blood sugar; blood and protein in urine; bone joint or muscle pain; nausea; vomiting; appetite loss.

Guidelines for Use

USE EXACTLY AS PRESCRIBED.

Take with meals.

Do not crush capsules.

Do not take vitamin A supplements while taking this medicine.

Sexually active women of childbearing age should practice contraception 1 month before starting therapy, during therapy and for 1 month after stopping the medicine.

Contact your healthcare provider immediately if pregnancy is suspected during therapy. Major human fetal abnormalities may be caused by this medicine. Discuss continuation of the pregnancy with your healthcare provider.

Worsening of acne may occur during the first part of therapy. This does not suggest failure or a need to stop the medicine.

May cause sensitivity to sunlight. Use sunscreens and wear protective clothing.

Use caution when driving at night as night vision may be decreased.

Do not use with other topical acne preparations.

Avoid alcohol consumption.

Do not donate blood for transfusion during therapy or for 30 days after stopping therapy.

Isoxsuprine Hydrochloride

(eye-SOX-you-preen HIGH-droe-KLOR-ide)

Vasodilan, Voxsuprine

A peripheral vasodilator used to increase blood flow and blood supply to skeletal muscle by relaxing and widening blood vessels in these muscles.

Precautions

DO NOT USE immediately after childbirth or if you have bleeding arteries.

BEFORE USING THIS MEDICINE, tell your healthcare provider if you are pregnant or breastfeeding; or if you are taking, will be taking or stop taking any prescription or nonprescription medicine; or if you have any other medical conditions.

Side Effects

Every medicine can cause side effects, but many people have no, or minor, side effects. Tell your healthcare provider if any of the following occurs: dizziness or lightheadedness when arising from a seated or lying position; fast heartbeat; chest pain; pounding in the chest; severe rash; flushing; weakness; nausea; vomiting; stomach pain.

Guidelines for Use

USE EXACTLY AS PRESCRIBED.

Dizziness or weakness may occur after sudden changes in posture (for example, when rising from a lying position). This can be avoided by getting up slowly or sitting upright for a few minutes before standing.

Isradipine

(iss-RAHD-ih-peen)

DynaCirc

A calcium channel blocker medicine that is used to treat high blood pressure. It may occasionally be prescribed for other reasons.

Precautions

DO NOT USE if you are allergic to this medicine.

BEFORE USING THIS MEDICINE, tell your healthcare provider if you are pregnant or breastfeeding; or if you are taking, will be taking or stop taking any prescription or nonprescription medicine; or if you have any other medical conditions.

Side Effects

Every medicine can cause side effects, but many people have no, or minor, side effects. Tell your healthcare provider if any of the following occurs: irregular heartbeat; increased frequency/severity of angina; shortness of breath; swelling of hands and feet; dizziness; constipation; nausea; low blood pressure or symptoms of a drug allergy (eg, itching, rash, hives, difficult breathing); unusual bleeding or bruising; gum enlargement.

Guidelines for Use

USE EXACTLY AS PRESCRIBED.

If a dose is missed, take it as soon as possible. If several hours have passed or if it is nearing time for the next dose, do not double the dose to catch up, unless advised by your healthcare provider. If more than one dose is missed, contact your healthcare provider.

It is important to brush and floss your teeth and see your dentist regularly.

Do not suddenly stop taking this medicine as this may cause serious chest pains. This can be minimized if the medicine is tapered slowly by your healthcare provider.

Itraconazole

(ih-truh-KAHN-uh-zole)

Sporanox

An antifungal medicine used to treat the fungal infections of blastomycosis and histoplasmosis. It may occasionally be prescribed for other reasons.

Precautions

DO NOT USE if you have an allergy to this medicine or if you are breastfeeding; do not take terfenadine (*Seldane*), astemizole (*Hismanal*), erythromycin or cisapride (*Propulsid*) with this medicine.

BEFORE USING THIS MEDICINE, tell your healthcare provider if you are pregnant; if you are taking, will be taking or stop taking any prescription or nonprescription medicine; or if you have any other medical conditions.

Side Effects

Every medicine can cause side effects, but many people have no, or minor, side effects. Tell your healthcare provider if any of the following occurs: nausea; vomiting; stomach ache; diarrhea; headache; rash; swelling; fever; itching; dizziness; sleepiness; impotence.

Guidelines for Use

USE EXACTLY AS PRESCRIBED.

Take this medicine with food.

If a dose is missed, take it as soon as possible. If several hours have passed or if it is nearing time for the next dose, do not double the dose to catch up unless advised by your healthcare provider. If more than one dose is missed, contact your healthcare provider.

Tell your healthcare provider if you notice unusual fatigue, loss of appetite, nausea, vomiting, yellowing of skin or gums, dark urine or pale stools.

Kanamycin Sulfate Injectable

(kan-uh-MY-sin SULL-fate)

Kantrex

Used to treat infections caused by certain bacteria. It may occasionally be prescribed for other reasons.

Precautions

DO NOT USE if you are allergic to this medicine.

BEFORE USING THIS MEDICINE, tell your healthcare provider if you are pregnant or breastfeeding, or if you are taking, will be taking or stop taking any prescription or nonprescription medicine; or if you have any other medical conditions.

Side Effects

Every medicine can cause side effects, but many people have no, or minor, side effects. Tell your healthcare provider if any of the following occurs: ringing in ears; hearing loss; difficulty breathing; irritation/pain at injection site; diarrhea; dizziness.

Guidelines for Use

USE EXACTLY AS PRESCRIBED.

Complete full course of therapy; take until gone.

If a dose is missed, take it as soon as possible. If several hours have passed or if it is nearing time for the next dose, do not double the dose to "catch up", unless advised by your healthcare provider. If more than one dose is missed, contact your healthcare provider.

Kanamycin Sulfate Oral

(kan-uh-MY-sin SULL-fate)

Kantrex

Used for the suppression of intestinal bacteria and for the treatment of hepatic coma.

Precautions

DO NOT USE if you are allergic to this medicine.

BEFORE USING THIS MEDICINE, tell your healthcare provider if you are pregnant or breastfeeding; or if you are taking, will be taking or stop taking any prescription or nonprescription medicine; or if you have any other medical conditions.

Side Effects

Every medicine can cause side effects, but many people have no, or minor, side effects. Tell your healthcare provider if any of the following occurs: nausea; vomiting; diarrhea; rash; dizziness; difficulty urinating; ringing in ears; hearing loss.

Patient Information

If a dose is missed, take it as soon as possible. If several hours have passed or if it is nearing time for the next dose, do not double the dose to "catch up," unless advised by your healthcare provider. If more than one dose is missed, contact your healthcare provider.

Drink plenty of fluids while taking this medicine.

Continue use until all the prescribed medicine has been taken. Failure to take all of the medicine may prevent complete elimination of bacteria, allowing the infection to return.

Kaolin with Pectin

(KAY-oh-lin/PECK-tin)

Kapectolin

Used to treat diarrhea.

Guidelines for Use

USE EXACTLY AS PRESCRIBED.

Liquids--Shake well before using.

Do not use for diarrhea caused by antibiotics or bacteria.

Do not use for more than 2 days, in the presence of high fever or in infants and children under 3, except under your healthcare provider's supervision.

Ketoconazole Cream

(KEY-toe-KOE-nuh-zole)

Nizoral

Used for the topical treatment of ringworm, jock itch, tinea versicolor (pityriasis), candidiasis (yeast) infections of the skin.

Precautions

DO NOT USE if you are allergic to this medicine.

BEFORE USING THIS MEDICINE, tell your healthcare provider if you are pregnant or breastfeeding; or if you are taking, will be taking or stop taking any prescription or nonprescription medicine; or if you have any other medical conditions.

Side Effects

Every medicine can cause side effects, but many people have no, or minor, side effects. Tell your healthcare provider if any of the following occurs: skin irritation; itching; stinging.

Guidelines for Use

USE EXACTLY AS PRESCRIBED.

Avoid contact with the eyes.

If a dose is missed, apply it as soon as possible. If several hours have passed or if it is nearing time for the next dose, do not double the dose to "catch up," unless advised by your healthcare provider. If more than one dose is missed, contact your healthcare provider.

Apply once daily to cover the affected and immediate surrounding area.

Improvement may be seen soon after treatment is begun.

Jock itch and ringworm should be treated for 2 weeks to reduce the possibility of recurrence.

Patients with tinea versicolor usually exhibit clearing after 2 weeks.

If no improvement is seen after the treatment period, consult your healthcare provider.

Ketoconazole Oral

(KEY-toe-KOE-nuh-zole)

Nizoral

Used to treat internal fungal infections, and to treat severe fungal infections of the skin that do not respond to topical therapy. It may occasionally be prescribed for other reasons.

Precautions

DO NOT USE if you are allergic to this medicine; do not take terfenadine (*Seldane*) or astemizole (*Hismanal*) with this medicine.

BEFORE USING THIS MEDICINE, tell your healthcare provider if you are pregnant or breastfeeding; or if you are taking, will be taking or stop taking any prescription or nonprescription medicine; or if you have any other medical conditions.

Side Effects

Every medicine can cause side effects, but many people have no, or minor, side effects. Tell your healthcare provider if any of the following occurs: nausea; vomiting; stomach ache; diarrhea; headache; fever; dizziness; drowsiness; itching; rash; hives; chills; sensitivity to sunlight; impotence.

Guidelines for Use

USE EXACTLY AS PRESCRIBED.

Do not take with antacids. If necessary, wait 2 hours before taking antacids.

If stomach upset occurs, take with food.

If a dose is missed, take it as soon as possible. If several hours have passed or if it is nearing time for the next dose, do not double the dose to "catch up," unless advised by your healthcare provider. If more than one dose is missed, consult your healthcare provider.

May cause dizziness, drowsiness or headache. Use caution while driving or performing other tasks requiring mental alertness, coordination and dexterity.

Tell your healthcare provider if stomach pain, fever or diarrhea become pronounced or if signs of liver dysfunction (eg, fatigue, loss of appetite, nausea, vomiting, yellowing of skin or eyes, dark urine or pale stools) occurs.

Continue until all the prescribed medicine has been taken. Failure to take all of the medicine may prevent complete elimination of the fungus, allowing the infection to return.

Ketoconazole Shampoo

(KEY-toe-KOE-nuh-zole)

Nizoral

Used to reduce scaling due to dandruff.

Precautions

DO NOT USE if you are allergic to this medicine.

BEFORE USING THIS MEDICINE, tell your healthcare provider if you are pregnant or breastfeeding; or if you are taking, will be taking or stop taking any prescription or nonprescription medicine; or if you have any other medical conditions.

Side Effects

Every medicine can cause side effects, but many people have no, or minor, side effects. Tell your healthcare provider if any of the following occurs: increase in normal hair loss; abnormal hair texture; scalp sores; mild dryness of skin; itching; oiliness/dryness of hair and scalp.

Guidelines for Use

USE EXACTLY AS PRESCRIBED.

If a dose is missed, apply it as soon as possible. If several hours have passed or if it is nearing time for the next dose, do not double the dose to "catch up," unless advised by your healthcare provider. If more than one dose is missed, contact your healthcare provider.

Removal of curl from permanently waved hair may occur.

Continue use until all the prescription has been used. Failure to use all of the medicine may prevent complete elimination of fungus, allowing the infection to return.

Ketoprofen Capsules

(KEY-toe-PRO-fen)

Orudis

A nonsteroidal anti-inflammatory medicine (NSAID) used to relieve mild to moderate pain and inflammation and to treat osteoarthritis (degenerative joint disease), rheumatoid arthritis and dysmenorrhea (cramps). It may occasionally be prescribed for other reasons.

Precautions

DO NOT USE if you are allergic to this medicine, or its relatives, aspirin or iodides.

BEFORE USING THIS MEDICINE, tell your healthcare provider if you are pregnant or breastfeeding; use alcohol chronically; are prone to fluid retention; or if you are taking, will be taking or stop taking any prescription or nonprescription medicine; or have any other medical conditions.

Side Effects

Every medicine can cause side effects, but many people have no, or minor, side effects. Tell your healthcare provider if any of the following occurs: allergic reaction (eg, rash, itching, fever); changes in vision; fluid retention; stomach problems (eg, nausea, vomiting, diarrhea, pain); black stools; constipation; persistent headache; dizziness; nervousness; weakness; drowsiness; ringing in the ears; taste changes; unusual bruising or bleeding.

Guidelines for Use

USE EXACTLY AS PRESCRIBED.

Take with food, milk or antacids.

If stomach pain develops and persists, contact your healthcare provider.

Avoid aspirin and alcoholic beverages while taking this medicine.

If a dose is missed, take it as soon as possible. If several hours have passed or if it is nearing time for the next dose, do not double the dose to "catch up," unless advised by your healthcare provider. If more than one dose is missed, contact your healthcare provider.

May cause drowsiness, dizziness or blurred vision. Use caution while driving or performing other tasks requiring mental alertness, coordination or physical dexterity.

May cause sensitivity to sunlight. Avoid prolonged exposure to the sun. Use sunscreens and wear protective clothing until tolerance is determined.

Store at room temperature (77°F) in a tight container away from moisture.

Ketoprofen Sustained Release

(KEY-toe-PRO-fen)

Oruvail

This medicine is a nonsteroidal anti-inflammatory medicine (NSAID) used to relieve mild to moderate pain and inflammation of rheumatoid arthritis and osteoarthritis. It may occasionally be prescribed for other reasons. This medicine should not be used for acute pain.

Precautions

DO NOT USE if you are allergic to this medicine or its relatives, aspirin or iodides.

BEFORE USING THIS MEDICINE, tell your healthcare provider if you are pregnant or breastfeeding; or if you are taking, will be taking or stop taking any prescription or nonprescription medicine; if you have any other medical conditions; use alcohol chronically; or are prone to fluid retention.

Side Effects

Every medicine can cause side effects, but many people have no, or minor, side effects. Tell your healthcare provider if any of the following occurs: allergic reaction (eg, rash, itching, fever); changes in vision; ringing in the ears; nausea; vomiting; diarrhea; stomach pain; black stools; constipation; persistent headache; dizziness; nervousness; weakness; taste changes; unusual bleeding or bruising; drowsiness; fluid retention (eg, swelling, bloating); gas; hearing changes.

Guidelines for Use

USE EXACTLY AS PRESCRIBED.

Do not crush or chew capsules. Swallow whole.

Take once daily with food or milk.

If stomach upset develops and persists, contact your healthcare provider.

Avoid aspirin and alcoholic beverages while taking this medicine.

If a dose is missed, take it as soon as possible. If several hours have passed or if it is nearing time for the next dose, do not double the dose to "catch up," unless advised by your healthcare provider. If more than one dose is missed, contact your healthcare provider.

May cause drowsiness, dizziness or blurred vision. Use caution while driving or performing other tasks requiring mental alertness, coordination or physical dexterity.

Patients on long-term therapy may require periodic blood tests. Be sure to keep appointments.

May cause sensitivity to sunlight. Avoid prolonged exposure to the sun. Use sunscreens and wear protective clothing until tolerance is determined.

Store at room temperature (77°F) in a tight container away from light.

Ketorolac Tromethamine Ophthalmic

(KEY-TOR-oh-lak tro-METH-uh-meen)

Acular

Used for the relief of ocular itching due to seasonal allergic conjunctivitis.

Precautions

DO NOT USE if you are allergic to this medicine.

BEFORE USING THIS MEDICINE, tell your healthcare provider if you are pregnant or breastfeeding; or if you are taking, will be taking or stop taking any prescription or nonprescription medicine; or if you have any other medical conditions.

Side Effects

Every medicine can cause side effects, but many people have no, or minor, side effects. Tell your healthcare provider if any of the following occurs: temporary burning or stinging; irritation; redness/burning; itching.

Guidelines for Use

USE EXACTLY AS PRESCRIBED.

Consult your healthcare provider if you have experienced bleeding tendencies, are on medicines that prolong bleeding time (eg, blood thinners) or have herpes simplex infection of the eye. Use proper administration technique.

Do not touch the dropper to any surface, including your eye, since it may contaminate the contents or cause damage to the eye.

Mild burning or stinging after instillation is no cause for alarm unless symptoms persist or worsen.

Ketorolac Tromethamine Systemic

(KEY-TOR-oh-lak tro-METH-uh-meen)

Toradol

This medicine is a nonsteroidal anti-inflammatory medicine (NSAID) used to relieve severe pain for no more than 5 days.

Precautions

DO NOT USE if you are allergic to this medicine or any of its relatives, aspirin or iodides; if you are pregnant; have an ulcer, bleeding problems or have not previously had the injection form of this medicine.

BEFORE USING THIS MEDICINE, tell your healthcare provider if you are pregnant or breastfeeding; use alcohol chronically; are prone to fluid retention; or if you are taking, will be taking or stop taking any prescription or nonprescription medicine; or if you have any other medical conditions.

Side Effects

Every medicine can cause side effects, but many people have no, or minor, side effects. Tell your healthcare provider if any of the following occurs: allergic reaction (eg, rash, itching, fever); fluid retention; stomach problems (eg, nausea vomiting, diarrhea, pain); black stools; constipation; headache; dizziness; weakness; unusual bruising or bleeding; difficulty urinating; swelling of the lower legs; gas; inflammation of the mouth; yellow skin or eyes; convulsions; blood in urine.

Injection: pain at the injection site.

Guidelines for Use

USE EXACTLY AS PRESCRIBED.

The injection must be received before the tablets can be taken.

Avoid aspirin and alcoholic beverages while taking this medicine.

If stomach upset occurs, take with food, milk or antacids. If stomach pain continues, contact your healthcare provider.

If a dose is missed, take it as soon as possible. If several hours have passed or if it is nearing time for the next dose, do not double the dose to "catch up," unless advised by your healthcare provider. If more than one dose is missed, contact your healthcare provider.

Tell your healthcare provider if stomach pain, black or bloody stools; rash; itching; swelling of the lower legs; or urination problems occurs.

May cause drowsiness or dizziness. Use caution while driving or performing other tasks requiring mental alertness, coordination and dexterity.

Do not use for more than 5 days. NOT for treatment of acute pain (eg, headaches).

Discard any unused tablets. Do not give the medication to anyone else.

Store at room temperature away from light and moisture.

Labetalol Hydrochloride

(la-BET-uh-lahl HIGH-droe-KLOR-ide)

Normodyne, Trandate

An alpha/beta blocker that lowers blood pressure and prevents increases in blood pressure and pulse rate during exercise. May be used in combination with other medications, including diuretics (water pills).

Precautions

DO NOT USE in you have bronchial asthma; congestive heart failure; heart block or shock; a severely slow heart rate; or if you are breastfeeding.

BEFORE USING THIS MEDICINE, tell your healthcare provider if you are pregnant; or if you are taking, will be taking or stop taking any prescription or nonprescription medicine; or if you have any other medical conditions.

Side Effects

Every medicine can cause side effects, but many people have no, or minor, side effects. Tell your healthcare provider if any of the following occurs: nausea; vomiting; diarrhea; dizziness; headache; drowsiness; difficulty breathing; rash; itching; tingling of scalp/skin; yellowing of skin or eyes; fluid retention; visual disturbances; sexual difficulty; muscle cramps; difficult urination; fever; nasal congestion; hair loss; swelling of lower legs; changes in taste.

Guidelines for Use

USE EXACTLY AS PRESCRIBED.

May be taken with or without food, but should be taken the same way each time.

Usually taken twice a day.

If a dose is missed, take it as soon as possible. If several hours have passed or if it is nearing time for the next dose, do not double the dose to "catch up," unless advised by your healthcare provider. If more than one dose is missed, contact your healthcare provider.

Patients being treated for high blood pressure often feel tired and run down for a few weeks after beginning therapy. It takes time for the body to adjust to lowered blood pressure. Continue taking your medicine even though you may not feel quite normal. Check with your healthcare provider during this time regarding any new symptoms to ensure that these new feelings are a normal consequence of changes in blood pressure. Keep your appointment, even if you feel well.

Do not discontinue medicine except on advice from your healthcare provider.

Transient scalp tingling may occur, especially when treatment is initiated.

Diabetes — This medicine can hide signs of low blood sugar and change blood sugar levels. It may be necessary for your healthcare provider to change your dose of antidiabetic medicine while you are taking this medicine.

May cause dizziness or fainting, especially when rising or standing. If these symptoms should occur, sit or lie down and contact your healthcare provider. Use caution while driving or performing hazardous tasks requiring alertness, coordination or physical dexterity.

Contact your healthcare provider if any of the following occurs: difficulty breathing, chest pain, swelling of the lower legs, itching, dark urine, appetite loss, stomach pain, flu-like symptoms, yellowing of skin or eyes.

Lab tests or exams will be required. Be sure to keep appointments.

Store at room temperature away from moisture.

Lactulose

(LAK-tyoo-lohs)

Cephulac, Cholac, Chronulac, Constilac, Constulose, Duphalac, Enulose, Evalose, Heptalac

A medicine used for the treatment of constipation and to prevent and treat portal-systemic encephalopathy (complication of liver disease), including the stages of hepatic pre-coma and coma.

Precautions

DO NOT USE if you are allergic to this medicine or if you have appendicitis symptoms (nausea, vomiting, stomach pain) or if you require a low galactose diet.

BEFORE USING THIS MEDICINE, tell your healthcare provider if you are pregnant or breastfeeding; or if you are taking, will be taking or stop taking any prescription or nonprescription medicine; or if you have any other medical conditions.

Side Effects

Every medicine can cause side effects, but many people have no, or minor, side effects. Tell your healthcare provider if any of the following occurs: stomach pain; bowel cramping; diarrhea; nausea; vomiting; gas; belching.

Guidelines for Use

USE EXACTLY AS PRESCRIBED.

May be mixed with fruit juice, water or milk to improve taste.

May cause belching, gas or cramps. Notify your healthcare provider if these effects become bothersome or if diarrhea occurs.

Do not take other laxatives while taking this medicine.

If a dose is missed, take it as soon as possible. If several hours have passed or if it is nearing time for the next dose, do not double the dose to "catch up," unless advised by your healthcare provider. If more than one dose is missed, contact your healthcare provider.

Frequent use of laxatives and inadequate fluid intake can cause an imbalance in fluid and electrolyte levels. Symptoms can include muscle cramps, muscle weakness and dizziness.

Rectal bleeding or failure of the laxative to produce a bowel movement can indicate a more serious condition that requires medical attention.

Diabetes — This product contains sugar. Use with caution.

Storage—Store at room temperature. Avoid freezing.

Lamivudine

(lam-MIH-view-deen)

Epivir

An antiviral medicine used in combination with zidovudine (AZT) to treat HIV infection.

Precautions

DO NOT USE if you are allergic to this medicine.

BEFORE USING THIS MEDICATION, tell your healthcare provider if you are pregnant or breastfeeding; if you are taking, will be taking or stop taking any prescription or nonprescription medicine; or if you have any other medical conditions.

Side Effects

Every medicine can cause side effects, but many people have no, or minor, side effects. Tell your healthcare provider if any of the following occurs: nausea; vomiting; diarrhea; appetite loss; stomach pain or cramps; indigestion; sleep disorders; dizziness; headache; fatigue; general body discomfort; fever; chills; nasal congestion; cough; rash; muscle or joint pain; depression; numbness, burning or tingling in the hands or feet.

Guidelines for Use

USE EXACTLY AS PRESCRIBED.

Usually taken twice a day with Retrovir (zidovudine, AZT).

May be taken with or without food.

If a dose is missed, take it as soon as possible. If several hours have passed or if it is nearing time for the next dose, do not double the dose to "catch up," unless advised by your healthcare provider. If more than one dose is missed, contact your healthcare provider.

This medicine is not a cure for HIV infection and patients may continue to acquire illnesses/ infections associated with HIV infection. Patients should remain under the care of their healthcare provider.

This medicine offers no protection from the transmission of HIV (the virus that causes AIDS) to others through sexual contact or blood contamination. HIV-infected mothers should not breastfeed their infants because of the risk of transmitting the HIV infection.

The long-term effects of this medicine are unknown. Children taking this medicine should be monitored for symptoms of pancreatitis (inflammation of the pancreas), such as stomach pain/ tenderness or vomiting. Lab tests/exams will be necessary to monitor treatment. Be sure to keep appointments.

Store at room temperature in a tightly closed container.

Lansoprazole

(lan-SO-pruh-zole)

Prevacid

This medicine is used in adults for the short-term treatment of active duodenal ulcers (up to 4 weeks) and erosive esophagitis (up to 8 weeks), as well as for the long-term treatment of hypersecretory (increased acid secretion) conditions (eg, Zollinger-Ellison syndrome). This medicine should not be used for long-term treatment or prevention of active duodenal ulcers or erosive esophagitis.

Precautions

DO NOT USE if you are allergic to this medicine.

BEFORE USING THIS MEDICINE, tell your healthcare provider if you are pregnant or breastfeeding; if you are taking, will be taking or stop taking any prescription or nonprescription medicine; or if you have any other medical conditions.

Side Effects

Every medicine can cause side effects, but many people have no, or minor, side effects. Tell your healthcare provider if any of the following occurs: diarrhea; stomach pain; nausea; headache.

Guidelines for Use

USE EXACTLY AS PRESCRIBED.

Take this medicine at least 1 hour before eating.

Do not open, chew or crush the capsules. They should be swallowed whole.

If a dose is missed, take it as soon as possible. If several hours have passed or if it is nearing time for the next dose, do not double the dose to "catch up," unless advised by your healthcare provider. If more than one dose is missed, contact your healthcare provider.

Antacids may be used while taking this medicine.

Lab tests will be required. Be sure to keep appointments.

Store at room temperature in a tight container away from moisture.

Leucovorin Calcium

(loo-koe-VORE-in KAL-see-uhm)

Wellcovorin Injection, Wellcovorin Tablets

A fast-acting strong form of folic acid. It is used to treat anemias due to digestive problems, folic acid deficiency, pregnancy and infancy when oral folic acid therapy is not possible.

Precautions

DO NOT USE if you are allergic to this medicine, have pernicious anemia or vitamin B12 deficiencies.

BEFORE USING THIS MEDICINE, tell your healthcare provider if you are pregnant or breastfeeding; or if you are taking, will be taking or stop taking any prescription or nonprescription medicine; or if you have any other medical conditions.

Side Effects

Every medicine can cause side effects, but many people have no, or minor, side effects. Tell your healthcare provider if any of the following occurs: difficulty breathing; itching; skin redness/rash; unexplained ill feeling; irritation at the injection site.

Guidelines for Use

USE EXACTLY AS PRESCRIBED.

Discuss the desired dose and duration of therapy with your healthcare provider.

Leuprolide Acetate

(loo-PRO-lide ASS-uh-TATE)

Lupron, Lupron Depot, Lupron Depot-Ped

Used as an alternative palliative treatment in advanced prostatic cancer when castration or estrogen administration are either not indicated or are unacceptable to the patient. It also is used in the management of endometriosis, including pain relief and reduction of endometriotic lesions.

Used in the treatment of children with central precocious puberty (CPP). It is also used for the treatment of uterine fibroids.

Precautions

DO NOT USE if you are allergic to this medicine or to benzyl alcohol or if you are pregnant or breastfeeding.

BEFORE USING THIS MEDICINE, tell your healthcare provider if you are taking, will be taking or stop taking any prescription or nonprescription medicine; or if you have any other medical conditions.

Side Effects

Every medicine can cause side effects, but many people have no, or minor, side effects. Tell your healthcare provider if any of the following occurs: *Patients with prostatic cancer*—swelling of the extremities; sleeplessness; pain; headache; dizziness/lightheadedness; decreased testicular size; impotence; decreased sex drive; breast tenderness; sweating; hot flashes; loss of appetite; constipation; nausea; vomiting; muscle pain; bone pain; increased urinary frequency; difficulty breathing; sinus congestion; skin reactions; acne; weakness; blood in urine; Patients being treated for endometriosis—swelling; depression; sleeplessness; pain; headache; dizziness; lightheadedness; nervousness; abnormal skin sensations; decreased sex drive; breast tenderness; hot flashes; sweating; stomach pain or upset; nausea; vomiting; joint pain; muscle aches; vaginitis; unusual vaginal bleeding; vaginal discharge; weight change; skin reactions; acne; weakness; *Patients with CPP*—swelling; sleeplessness; pain; headache; nervousness; breast tenderness; nausea; vomiting; vaginitis; vaginal bleeding; vaginal discharge; skin reactions; acne; weight change.

Guidelines for Use

USE EXACTLY AS PRESCRIBED.

Do not discontinue medication except on advice of your healthcare provider.

Prostatic cancer—May cause increased bone pain and increased difficulty in urinating during the first few weeks of treatment.

May cause hot flashes, injection site irritation (eg, burning, itching, swelling) and may cause or aggravate nerve symptoms. Contact your healthcare provider if these become pronounced.

During the first 2 months of therapy a female may experience menses or spotting. If bleeding continues beyond the second month, tell your healthcare provider.

Immediately report any irritation at the injection site to your healthcare provider.

Patient package insert is available with the injection kit.

Report any unusual signs or symptoms to your healthcare provider.

Levamisole Hydrochloride

(lev-AM-ih-sole HIGH-droe-KLOR-ide)

Ergamisol

A medicine used in combination with fluorouracil after surgery in patients with Duke's stage C colon cancer. It may occasionally be prescribed for other reasons.

Precautions

DO NOT USE if you are allergic to this medicine. Use of this medicine may result in decreased red blood cell, white blood cell and platelet counts. Development of flu-like symptoms may be a sign of a serious blood disorder. If such symptoms develop, contact your healthcare provider immediately.

BEFORE USING THIS MEDICINE, tell your healthcare provider if you are pregnant or breastfeeding; or if you are taking, will be taking or stop taking any prescription or nonprescription medicine; or if you have any other medical conditions.

Side Effects

Every medicine can cause side effects, but many people have no, or minor, side effects. Tell your healthcare provider if any of the following occurs: nausea; vomiting; diarrhea; appetite loss; stomach ache; constipation; gas; indigestion; dizziness; drowsiness; lack of coordination; depression; confusion; anxiety; memory loss; weakness; difficulty concentrating; headache; sleep disturbances; nervousness; rash; itching; hair loss; skin discoloration; flu-like symptoms (eg, fatigue, fever, chills); infection; fatigue; fluid retention (edema); changes in taste or smell; vision disturbances; inflammation of the mouth and gums; abnormal tearing; muscle and joint pain.

Guidelines for Use

USE EXACTLY AS PRESCRIBED.

Do not exceed recommended dose or frequency. Side effects may increase.

Notify your healthcare provider immediately if flu-like symptoms occur.

Do not drink alcohol while taking this medication.

If a dose is missed, take it as soon as possible. If several hours have passed or if it is nearing time for the next dose, do not double the dose to "catch up," unless advised by your healthcare provider. If more than one dose is missed, contact your healthcare provider.

Lab tests, including complete blood counts, electrolytes and liver function tests, will be required during therapy. Be sure to keep appointments.

Levobunolol

(LEE-voe-BYOO-no-lahl)

Betagan Liquifilm

A beta blocking agent used to treat glaucoma.

Precautions

DO NOT USE if you have an allergy to this medicine or its relatives.

BEFORE USING THIS MEDICINE, tell your healthcare provider if you are pregnant or breastfeeding; or if you are taking, will be taking or stop taking any prescription or nonprescription medicine; if you have any other medical conditions; or if you are allergic to sulfite preservatives.

Side Effects

Every medicine can cause side effects, but many people have no, or minor, side effects. Tell your healthcare provider if any of the following occurs: temporary stinging or pain when using drops; visual problems or irritation; browache; light sensitivity; depression; slow pulse; palpitations (pounding in the chest); stomach upset; nausea; breathing difficulty; rash.

Guidelines for Use

USE EXACTLY AS PRESCRIBED.

If a dose is missed, take it as soon as possible. If several hours have passed or if it is nearing time for the next dose, do not double the dose to "catch up," unless advised by your healthcare provider. If more than one dose is missed, contact your healthcare provider.

May cause stinging or pain when first instilled in the eye.

Intraocular pressure must be monitored periodically by your healthcare provider to make sure the medicine is working properly.

Tell your healthcare provider if you are using these eye drops and plan to have surgery. You may have to temporarily stop using them.

Levodopa

(LEE-voe-DOE-puh)

Dopar Capsules, Larodopa Tablets

A medicine used to treat parkinsonism. It may occasionally be prescribed for other reasons.

Precautions

DO NOT USE if you are allergic to this medicine or if you are taking monoamine oxidase inhibitors (MAOIs, eg, phenelzine).

BEFORE USING THIS MEDICINE, tell your healthcare provider if you are pregnant or breastfeeding; or if you are taking, will be taking or stop taking any prescription or nonprescription medicine; or if you have any other medical conditions.

Side Effects

Every medicine can cause side effects, but many people have no, or minor, side effects. Tell your healthcare provider if any of the following occurs: uncontrollable movements of the face, eyelids, mouth, tongue, neck, arms, hands or legs; mood or mental changes; irregular heartbeat or palpitations (pounding in the chest); difficult urination; severe or persistent nausea or vomiting; appetite loss; dry mouth; difficulty swallowing; taste distortion; or sudden swings from improved condition to worsened condition.

Guidelines for Use

USE EXACTLY AS PRESCRIBED.

May cause stomach upset. Take with food.

It may take weeks to months to notice benefit. Do not change the dose without first checking with your healthcare provider.

Do not crush or chew sustained-release tablets.

May cause drowsiness. Use caution when driving or performing other tasks requiring mental alertness.

The onset of effect of the first morning dose may be delayed for up to 1 hour. Notify your healthcare provider if this delayed response poses a problem.

Diabetic patients: Medication may interfere with urine tests for sugar or ketones. Report any abnormal results to your doctor before adjusting dosage of antidiabetic medications.

Do not get up quickly after sitting or lying down as this may cause fainting or dizziness. Notify your healthcare provider if this occurs.

May darken urine or sweat. This is not harmful.

Do not take this medication along with vitamins containing vitamin B6.

Levodopa/Carbidopa

(LLE-voe-DOE-puh/CAR-bih-doe-puh)

Sinemet CR

A medicine used to treat parkinsonism.

Precautions

DO NOT USE if you are allergic to these medicines or are taking monoamine oxidase inhibitors (MAOIs, eg, phenelzine, tranylcypromine).

BEFORE USING THIS MEDICINE, tell your healthcare provider if you are pregnant or breastfeeding; or if you are taking, will be taking or stop taking any prescription or nonprescription medicine; or if you have any other medical conditions.

Side Effects

Every medicine can cause side effects, but many people have no, or minor, side effects. Tell your healthcare provider if any of the following occurs: uncontrollable movements of the face, eyelids, mouth, tongue, neck, arms, hands or legs; mood or mental changes; irregular heartbeat or palpitations (pounding in the chest); difficult urination; severe or persistent nausea or vomiting; appetite loss; dry mouth; difficulty swallowing; taste distortion; or sudden swings from improved condition to worsened condition.

Guidelines for Use

USE EXACTLY AS PRESCRIBED.

May cause stomach upset. Take with food.

It may take several weeks to a few months to see benefit from use. The daily dose varies depending on individual needs. Do not adjust the dose without consulting your healthcare provider.

Do not crush or chew sustained-release tablets.

May cause drowsiness. Use caution when driving or performing other tasks requiring mental alertness.

The onset of effect of the first morning dose may be delayed for up to 1 hour. Tell your healthcare provider if this delayed response poses a problem.

Diabetic patients: May interfere with urine tests for sugar or ketones. Report any abnormal results to your healthcare provider before adjusting dosage of antidiabetic medications.

Do not get up quickly after sitting or lying down as this may cause fainting or dizziness. Tell your healthcare provider if this occurs.

May darken urine or sweat. This is not harmful.

Levomethadyl Acetate Hydrochloride

(LEE-voe-METH-uh-dill ASS-uh-TATE HIGH-droe-KLOR-ide)

ORLAAM

A medicine used for opiate addiction. This medicine is intended for use as part of a comprehensive program which includes appropriate medical evaluation, treatment planning and counseling.

Precautions

DO NOT USE if you are allergic to this medicine or if you are pregnant. This medicine may be habit-forming. You will not feel the full effects of the medication for several days.

BEFORE USING THIS MEDICINE, tell your healthcare provider if you are breastfeeding; or if you are taking, will be taking or stop taking any prescription or nonprescription medicine; or if you have any other medical conditions.

Side Effects

Every medicine can cause side effects, but many people have no, or minor, side effects. Tell your healthcare provider if any of the following occurs: weakness; back pain; chills; hot flashes; flu-like symptoms; slow heart rate; abdominal pain; constipation; diarrhea; dry mouth; nausea; vomiting; joint and muscle pain; abnormal dreams; anxiety; decreased sex drive; depression; euphoria; headache; sleeplessness; drowsiness; nervousness; cough; stuffy nose; yawning; rash; sweating; blurred vision; difficult ejaculation; impotence; lightheadedness or fainting upon rising; tearing.

Guidelines for Use

USE EXACTLY AS PRESCRIBED.

This medicine generally is not to be used daily. Such use of the usual doses will lead to serious overdose.

Do not use with alcohol or any mind-altering medications; it could cause a fatal overdose, especially with the first few doses of this medicine either during the start of treatment or after a lapse in treatment. If you are transferring to methadone you should wait 48 hours after the last dose of this medicine before taking the first dose of methadone or other narcotics. All doses must be taken at the clinic.

Use caution while driving or performing other tasks requiring physical dexterity or mental alertness.

Use with caution if you have asthma or any other breathing problem. Tell your healthcare provider if you have problems breathing.

Carry identification (*Medic-Alert*).

Levonorgestrel Implants

(LEE-voe-nor-JESS-truhl)

Norplant System

Used to prevent pregnancy.

Precautions

DO NOT USE if you have blood clots in the leg, certain types of cancer or are pregnant.

BEFORE USING THIS MEDICINE, tell your healthcare provider if you are breastfeeding; if you are taking, will be taking or stop taking any prescription or nonprescription medicine; or if you have any other medical conditions.

Side Effects

Every medicine can cause side effects, but many people have no, or minor, side effects. Tell your healthcare provider if any of the following occurs: bleeding irregularities; absence of menstruation; muscle and bone pain; stomach discomfort; pain or itching near implant site; headache; nervousness; nausea; dizziness; acne; change of appetite; weight gain; excessive hairiness; scalp hair loss; breast discharge.

Patient Information

Capsules can be removed at any time. Capsules must be removed at the end of 5 years.

Contact lens users--If you develop changes in vision or lens intolerance, talk to your ophthalmologist.

Levothyroxine Sodium

(lee-voe-thigh-ROX-een SO-dee-uhm)

Levothroid, Levoxine, Synthroid, Syroxine

A synthetic thyroid hormone substitute used primarily for low thyroid hormone secretion and some other thyroid problems.

Precautions

DO NOT USE if you are allergic to thyroid hormones or the dye tartrazine (for certain products); or as a treatment for obesity.

BEFORE USING THIS MEDICINE, tell your healthcare provider if you are pregnant or breastfeeding; or if you are taking, will be taking or stop taking any prescription or nonprescription medicine; or if you have any other medical conditions.

Side Effects

Every medicine can cause side effects, but many people have no, or minor, side effects. Tell your healthcare provider if any of the following occurs: headache; nervousness; nausea; diarrhea; excessive sweating; heat intolerance; menstrual problems; chest pain; increased pulse rate; pounding in the chest; or any other unusual feeling or symptom. Partial loss of hair may be seen in children in the first few months of therapy, but this is usually temporary.

Guidelines for Use

USE EXACTLY AS PRESCRIBED.

Take as a single daily dose, usually before breakfast.

Be consistent in taking the tablet with or without food.

Do not stop medication except on advice of your healthcare provider.

Dosage is intended to replace the low thyroid secretion. Your response is evaluated by your healthcare provider with laboratory tests. It is important to keep regular appointments with your healthcare provider. Replacement therapy is usually taken for life.

Lidocaine Hydrochloride Mucosal

(LIGH-doe-cane HIGH-droe-KLOR-ide)

Anestacon, Xylocaine

A medicine used to relieve pain or itching of accessible mucous membranes and to treat itching due to hemorrhoids or an inflamed anal or vaginal area. For local anesthesia of mucous membranes including oral, nasal and throat membranes; respiratory tract; digestive tract; and urinary tract. For use during examination of these mucous membranes.

Precautions

DO NOT USE in or around the eyes or if you are allergic to this medicine.

BEFORE USING THIS MEDICINE, tell your healthcare provider if you are pregnant or breastfeeding; or if you are taking, will be taking or stop taking any prescription or nonprescription medicine; or if you have any other medical conditions.

Side Effects

Every medicine can cause side effects, but many people have no, or minor, side effects. Tell your healthcare provider if any of the following occurs: rash; redness; swelling; burning; stinging; irritation.

Guidelines for Use

USE EXACTLY AS PRESCRIBED.

A thin layer of solution, cream, lotion or ointment is all that is necessary. Additional benefit will not be achieved with larger amounts.

Stop therapy if irritation, rash or redness develops. Consult your healthcare provider.

Many topical local anesthetics may be used in the mouth to relieve pain and discomfort. They may interfere with the swallowing reflex. Do not eat for at least 1 hour after use in the mouth or throat. This decreases the risk of choking or aspiration of food into the lungs.

Doses and frequency of use depend on the condition, area being treated, blood supply in the area, individual tolerance and dosage form. Individual products should be reviewed for their use and dosage guidelines. Consult your healthcare provider for product-specific information.

This product temporarily relieves pain but does not treat the cause of it.

Lidocaine Hydrochloride Topical

(LIGH-doe-cane HIGH-droe-KLOR-ide)

Solarcaine, Xylocaine

A medicine used to relieve skin pain, itching and discomfort associated with minor burns, scalds, prickly heat, diaper rash (severe), wounds, abrasions, sunburn, allergy to certain plants (such as poison ivy), insect bites, eczema and other skin conditions.

Precautions

DO NOT USE if you are allergic to this medicine.

BEFORE USING THIS MEDICINE, tell your healthcare provider if you are pregnant or breastfeeding; or if you are taking, will be taking or stop taking any prescription or nonprescription medicine; or if you have any other medical conditions.

Side Effects

Every medicine can cause side effects, but many people have no, or minor, side effects. Tell your healthcare provider if any of the following occurs: allergic contact dermatitis; redness; rash; swelling; burning; stinging; irritation.

Guidelines for Use

USE EXACTLY AS PRESCRIBED.

For external use only.

A thin layer of medicine is all that is necessary. Additional benefit will not be achieved with larger amounts.

This product temporarily relieves pain or itching; it does not treat the cause of it.

Stop therapy if irritation, rash or redness develops. Contact your healthcare provider.

Doses and frequency of use depend on the condition, area being treated, blood supply in the area, individual tolerance and dosage form. Individual products should be reviewed for their use and dosage guidelines. Consult your healthcare provider for product-specific information.

Liothyronine Sodium

(lie-oh-THIGH-row-neen SO-dee-uhm)

Cytomel, Triostat

A synthetic thyroid hormone substitute used primarily for low thyroid hormone secretion and some other thyroid problems.

Precautions

DO NOT USE if you are allergic to thyroid hormones or the dye tartrazine (for certain products) or as a treatment for obesity.

BEFORE USING THIS MEDICINE, tell your healthcare provider if you are pregnant or breastfeeding; or if you are taking, will be taking or stop taking any prescription or nonprescription medicine; or if you have any other medical conditions.

Side Effects

Every medicine can cause side effects, but many people have no, or minor, side effects. Tell your healthcare provider if any of the following occurs: headache; nervousness; nausea; diarrhea; excessive sweating; heat intolerance; menstrual problems; chest pain; increased pulse rate; pounding in the chest or any other unusual feeling or symptom. Partial loss of hair may be seen in children in the first few months of thyroid therapy, but this is usually temporary.

Guidelines for Use

USE EXACTLY AS PRESCRIBED.

Take as a single daily dose, usually before breakfast.

Do not stop medication except on advice of your healthcare provider.

Dosage is intended to replace the low thyroid secretion.

Your response is evaluated by your healthcare provider with laboratory tests. It is important to keep regular appointments with your healthcare provider.

Replacement therapy is usually taken for life.

Lisinopril

(lie-SIN-oh-prill)

Prinivil, Zestril

An angiotensin converting enzyme (ACE) inhibitor medicine generally used to lower high blood pressure or treat heart failure.

Precautions

DO NOT USE if you are allergic to this medicine or if you are pregnant.

BEFORE USING THIS MEDICINE, tell your healthcare provider if you are breastfeeding; or if you are taking, will be taking or stop taking any prescription or nonprescription medicine; or if you have any other medical conditions.

Side Effects

Every medicine can cause side effects, but many people have no, or minor, side effects. Tell your healthcare provider if any of the following occurs: stomach pain; vomiting; diarrhea; constipation, appetite loss; depression; headache; dizziness; nervousness; sleeping difficulties; fatigue; rapid or irregular heartbeat; dizziness/lightheadedness when rising quickly from a sitting or lying position; shortness of breath; cough; nasal congestion; bronchitis; sinus inflammation; rash; sweating; flushing; yellowing of skin or eyes; muscle cramps; weight loss; taste loss; dry mouth; decreased sex drive; back, joint and shoulder pain; urination changes; fever; vision disturbances; numbness/tingling of hands or feet.

Guidelines for Use

USE EXACTLY AS PRESCRIBED.

May be taken without regard to meals.

Patients starting treatment for high blood pressure may feel tired at first. It takes time for the body to adjust. Continue taking medication and check with your healthcare provider.

If a dose is missed, take it as soon as possible. If several hours have passed or if it is nearing time for the next dose, do not double the dose to "catch up," unless advised by your healthcare provider. If more than one dose is missed, contact your healthcare provider. Do not interrupt or stop medication without consulting your healthcare provider.

Do not use salt substitutes without telling your healthcare provider.

A persistent, dry, nonproductive cough may occur. Tell your healthcare provider. Recovery is rapid when the medicine is stopped.

Dizziness, fainting or lightheadedness is most likely after the first dose or in the first days of therapy; avoid sudden changes in posture. If fainting occurs, discontinue medicine until talking to your healthcare provider.

Lithium

(LITH-ee-uhm)

Cibalith-S Syrup, Eskalith Capsules, Eskalith CR Timed Release Tablets, Eskalith Tablets, Lithane Tablets, Lithobid Timed Release Tablets, Lithonate Capsules, Lithotabs Tablets

A medicine used to treat manic episodes of manic-depressive illness. Maintenance therapy prevents or decreases the frequency and intensity of subsequent manic episodes.

Precautions

DO NOT USE if you are allergic to this medicine.

BEFORE USING THIS MEDICINE, tell your healthcare provider if you are pregnant or breastfeeding; or if you are taking, will be taking or stop taking any prescription or nonprescription medicine; or if you have any other medical conditions.

Side Effects

Every medicine can cause side effects, but many people have no, or minor, side effects. Tell your healthcare provider if any of the following occurs: nausea; vomiting; diarrhea; stomach ache; gas; indigestion; headache; fatigue; sleeplessness; slurred speech; confusion; seizures; dizziness; stupor; coma; blackouts; hallucinations; tremors; memory loss; tics; irregular heartbeat; itching; hair loss; acne; vision problems; taste distortion; weight changes; swelling of ankles or wrists; incontinence of urine and stool; changes in sex drive; swollen, painful joints; fever.

Guidelines for Use

USE EXACTLY AS PRESCRIBED.

Take immediately after meals or with milk to avoid stomach upset.

Watch for signs of overdose or toxicity, such as diarrhea, vomiting, unsteady walking, tremor, drowsiness or muscle weakness. Stop the medication and contact your healthcare provider immediately.

If a dose is missed, take it as soon as possible. If several hours have passed or if it is nearing time for the next dose, do not double the dose to "catch up," unless advised by your healthcare provider. If more than one dose is missed, contact your healthcare provider. May cause drowsiness. Use caution while driving or performing other tasks requiring alertness.

Drink 8 to 12 glasses of water or other liquid every day while taking this medicine.

Maintain a regular diet.

Use regular amounts of table salt in food.

If fever or diarrhea occurs, contact your healthcare provider. Regular blood and laboratory tests may be needed. Be sure to keep appointments.

Lomefloxacin Hydrochloride

(low-MUH-FLOX-uh-sin HIGH-droe-KLOR-ide)

Maxaquin

An anti-infection medicine that is used to treat lower respiratory infections and urinary tract infections. It may occasionally be prescribed for other reasons.

Precautions

DO NOT USE if you are allergic to this medicine or its relatives.

BEFORE USING THIS MEDICINE, tell your healthcare provider if you are pregnant or breastfeeding; or if you are taking, will be taking or stop taking any prescription or nonprescription medicine; or if you have any other medical conditions.

Side Effects

Every medicine can cause side effects, but many people have no, or minor, side effects. Tell your healthcare provider if any of the following occurs: nausea; diarrhea; stomach ache; headache; dizziness; sensitivity to light; rash; itching; difficult breathing; tremors; restlessness; confusion.

Guidelines for Use

USE EXACTLY AS PRESCRIBED.

Take with or without meals. Drink plenty of liquids.

Do not take antacids containing magnesium or aluminum, sucralfate (*Carafate*) or iron or zinc-containing products within 2 hours of using this medicine.

Use caution when driving or performing other tasks requiring mental alertness, coordination and dexterity.

Allergy: Discontinue at first appearance of rash or other signs of allergic reactions.

Therapy should not be stopped without consulting your healthcare provider.

If a dose is missed, take it as soon as possible. If several hours have passed or if it is nearing time for the next dose, do not double the dose to "catch up," unless advised by your healthcare provider. If more than one dose is missed, contact your healthcare provider.

Avoid prolonged exposure to the sun. Use sunscreens and wear protective clothing until tolerance is determined.

Lomustine

(LOW-muss-teen)

CeeNu

An anticancer medicine that halts the spread of cancerous cells.

Precautions

DO NOT USE if you are allergic to this medicine, or if you are pregnant or breast-feeding.

BEFORE USING THIS MEDICINE, tell your healthcare provider if you are taking, will be taking or stop taking any prescription or nonprescription medicine; or if you have any other medical conditions.

Side Effects

Every medicine can cause side effects, but many people have no, or minor, side effects. Tell your healthcare provider if any of the following occurs: nausea; vomiting; appetite loss; unusual tiredness; unusual bleeding or bruising; shortness of breath; dry cough; swelling of feet or lower legs; yellowing of eyes and skin; confusion; sores on the mouth or lips; unusual tiredness.

Guidelines for Use

USE EXACTLY AS PRESCRIBED.

Breathing: This medicine may affect the lungs. Report any shortness of breath to your healthcare provider.

Take on an empty stomach to reduce nausea. Nausea and vomiting may occur 3 to 6 hours after an oral dose and usually last less than 24 hours.

This medicine may lower your body's ability to fight infection, therefore notify your health-care provider if fever, sore throat, rashes or chills occur.

Practice effective birth control during therapy.

Loperamide Hydrochloride

(low-PEHR-uh-mide HIGH-droe-KLOR-ide)

Imodium A-D Caplets, Imodium A-D Liquid, Imodium Capsules, Pepto Diarrhea Control Solution

A medicine used to relieve nonspecific diarrhea and chronic diarrhea associated with inflammatory bowel disease. It also is used to decrease the volume of discharge from ileostomies.

Precautions

DO NOT USE if you are allergic to this medicine. Children: Use is not recommended in children under 2 without a doctor's supervision.

BEFORE USING THIS MEDICINE, tell your healthcare provider if you are pregnant or breastfeeding; or if you are taking, will be taking or stop taking any prescription or nonprescription medicine; or if you have any other medical conditions.

Side Effects

Every medicine can cause side effects, but many people have no, or minor, side effects. Tell your healthcare provider if any of the following occurs: constipation; nausea; vomiting; appetite loss; stomach ache; bloating; dry mouth; fever; rash; drowsiness; dizziness.

Guidelines for Use

USE EXACTLY AS PRESCRIBED.

Do not take more than the prescribed dose.

May cause drowsiness or dizziness. Use caution when driving or performing other tasks requiring mental alertness or coordination.

May cause dry mouth. Chew sugarless gum or suck sugarless hard candies if desired.

Tell your healthcare provider if diarrhea does not stop after a few days or if abdominal pain or fever occurs.

Loratadine

(lore-AT-uh-DEEN)

Claritin

A medicine (antihistamine) used for relief of seasonal allergy symptoms.

Precautions

DO NOT USE if you are allergic to this medicine or its relatives, or if you are taking monoamine oxidase inhibitors (MAOIs, eg, *Nardil, Parnate*).

BEFORE USING THIS MEDICINE, tell your healthcare provider if you are pregnant or breastfeeding, or if you are taking, will be taking or stop taking any prescription or nonprescription medicine; or if you have any other medical conditions.

Side Effects

Every medicine can cause side effects, but many people have no, or minor, side effects. Tell your healthcare provider if any of the following occurs: drowsiness; dizziness; dry mouth; stomach upset; constipation; blurred vision; difficult urination; confusion; headache; fainting; irregular heart beats.

Guidelines for Use

USE EXACTLY AS PRESCRIBED.

Take on an empty stomach.

Avoid alcohol and drowsiness-causing medicines (eg, tranquilizers, some pain medicines).

Use caution while driving or performing tasks requiring mental alertness or coordination.

Use alone when sneezing and runny nose exist, but nasal congestion is slight. When nasal congestion occurs with sneezing and runny nose, an oral or topical decongestant also may be used.

Do not take for several days before allergy skin testing.

Lorazepam

(lore-AZE-uh-pam)

Ativan Tablets, Lorazepam Caplets, Lorazepam Intensol Liquid, Lorazepam Tablets

A benzodiazepine medicine generally used to treat anxiety. It may occasionally be prescribed for other reasons.

Precautions

DO NOT USE if you are allergic to this medicine or its relatives, or are breastfeeding.

BEFORE USING THIS MEDICINE, tell your healthcare provider if you are pregnant or breastfeeding, or if you are taking, will be taking or stop taking any prescription or nonprescription medicine; or if you have any other medical conditions.

Side Effects

Every medicine can cause side effects, but many people have no, or minor, side effects. Tell your healthcare provider if any of the following occurs: stomach upset; constipation; diarrhea; change in appetite; vomiting; confusion; depression; nervousness; memory loss; drowsiness; fatigue; dizziness; crying; disorientation; vivid dreams; headache; seizures; changes in heart rate; pounding in the chest; itching; rash; hair growth; yellowing of skin or eyes; visual or hearing disturbances; slurred speech; loss of bladder function; change in sex drive; urine retention; menstrual problems; dry mouth; fever; tremors/uncontrollable muscle movement; difficult breathing; swelling; excessive perspiration; joint pain; weight gain or loss; dehydration; fainting.

Guidelines for Use

USE EXACTLY AS PRESCRIBED.

May be taken with food or water if stomach upset occurs.

If a dose is missed, take it as soon as possible. If several hours have passed or if it is nearing time for the next dose, do not double the dose to "catch up," unless advised by your healthcare provider. If more than one dose is missed, contact your healthcare provider.

This medication can be addictive if used in large doses or for a long time.

Discuss overuse with your healthcare provider.

May cause drowsiness. Use caution while driving or performing other tasks requiring mental alertness, coordination and dexterity.

Avoid alcohol and other medications that cause drowsiness.

Patients on long-term or high-dosage therapy may have withdrawal symptoms if therapy is suddenly stopped. Do not stop therapy abruptly or change dosage without asking your healthcare provider.

Losartan Potassium

(low-SAHR-tan poe-TASS-ee-uhm)

Cozaar

This medicine is an antihypertensive used to lower high blood pressure in patients over 18 years of age. It can be used alone or in combination with other antihypertensive medicines.

Precautions

DO NOT USE if you are allergic to this medicine.

BEFORE USING THIS MEDICINE, tell your healthcare provider if you are pregnant or breastfeeding; if you are taking, will be taking or stop taking any prescription or nonprescription medicine; or if you have any other medical conditions.

Side Effects

Every medicine can cause side effects, but many people have no, or minor, side effects. Tell your healthcare provider if any of the following occurs: diarrhea; indigestion; muscle cramps; stomach, chest, muscle, back or leg pain; dizziness; sleeplessness; stuffy nose; cough; weakness; fatigue; fluid retention (swelling); nausea; headache; sore throat; itching; rash.

Guidelines for Use

USE EXACTLY AS PRESCRIBED.

Notify your healthcare provider if you are pregnant, become pregnant, are planning to become pregnant, or if you are breastfeeding. This medicine can cause injury or death to a developing fetus after the first 3 months of pregnancy.

This medicine may be taken once or twice daily, with or without food.

If a dose is missed, take it as soon as possible. If several hours have passed or if it is nearing time for the next dose, do not double the dose to "catch up," unless advised by your healthcare provider. If more than one dose is missed, contact your healthcare provider.

Maximum effect may take up to 6 weeks.

Dehydration (eg, excess sweating, vomiting, diarrhea) may increase the blood pressure-lowering effect, causing dizziness. Drink plenty of fluids in such situations.

Store at room temperature in a tightly closed container away from light.

Lovastatin

(LOW-vuh-STAT-in)

Mevacor, Mevinolin

A medicine used to lower the level of cholesterol in the blood. It may occasionally be prescribed for other reasons.

Precautions

DO NOT USE if you are pregnant, breastfeeding or allergic to this medicine.

BEFORE USING THIS MEDICINE, tell your healthcare provider if you are taking, will be taking or stop taking any prescription or nonprescription medicine; or if you have any other medical conditions.

Side Effects

Every medicine can cause side effects, but many people have no, or minor, side effects. Tell your healthcare provider if any of the following occurs: nausea; diarrhea; stomach pain; constipation; gas; headache; dizziness; rash; muscle cramps; taste changes.

Guidelines for Use

USE EXACTLY AS PRESCRIBED.

Take with the evening meal.

Report any unexplained muscle pain, tenderness or weakness, especially if accompanied by fever or malaise, to your healthcare provider. Also report any yellowing of the skin or eyes.

Most effective when used with exercise and a diet that reduces the intake of cholesterol and saturated fats.

Magaldrate

(MAG-al-drate)

Isopan, Riopan

Used to treat upset stomach due to too much acid secretion (eg, heartburn, acid indigestion and sour stomach); to treat irritation of the stomach associated with peptic ulcers. It occasionally may be prescribed for other reasons.

Precautions

DO NOT USE if you have kidney disease, stomach emptying disorder or upper digestive tract hemorrhage.

BEFORE USING THIS MEDICINE, tell your healthcare provider if you are pregnant or breastfeeding; or if you are taking, will be taking or stop taking any prescription or nonprescription medicine; or if you have any other medical conditions.

Side Effects

Every medicine can cause side effects, but many people have no, or minor, side effects. Tell your healthcare provider if any of the following occurs: stomach pain; diarrhea; muscle weakness; constipation; lack of energy; headache; confusion; irritability.

Guidelines for Use

USE EXACTLY AS PRESCRIBED.

Antacids reduce acidity for about 30 minutes when taken on an empty stomach. Acidity is reduced for about 3 hours when antacids are taken 1 hour after meals.

Do not take other medications within 1 to 2 hours of taking this medicine.

Tell your healthcare provider if coffee-ground vomiting or black, tar-like stools occur.

Taking too much of these products can cause the stomach to secrete excess stomach acid. Consult your healthcare provider about the appropriate dose.

Long-term use — Do not take for longer than 2 weeks for the relief of indigestion. If discomfort continues, consult your healthcare provider.

Suspension — Shake well before using.

Magnesium Citrate

(mag-NEE-zee-uhm SIH-trate)

Citrate of Magnesia, Citro-Nesia

Used for the short-term treatment of constipation.

Precautions

DO NOT USE if you are allergic to this medicine or have nausea, vomiting or stomach pain.

BEFORE USING THIS MEDICINE, tell your healthcare provider if you are pregnant or breastfeeding; if you are taking, will be taking or stop taking any prescription or nonprescription medicine; or if you have any other medical conditions.

Side Effects

Every medicine can cause side effects, but many people have no, or minor, side effects. Tell your healthcare provider if any of the following occurs: diarrhea; nausea; vomiting; perianal irritation; weakness; dizziness; fainting; pounding in the chest; sweating; bloating; gas; abdominal cramps.

Guidelines for Use

USE EXACTLY AS PRESCRIBED.

Direct attention to proper dietary fiber intake, adequate fluids and regular exercise.

Do not use in the presence of abdominal pain, nausea or vomiting.

Laxative use is only a temporary measure; do not use longer than 1 week. When regularity returns, discontinue use.

Refrigerate to improve taste and retain potency.

Take with a full glass of water or juice.

Notify your healthcare provider if unrelieved constipation, rectal bleeding or symptoms of electrolyte imbalance (eg, muscle cramps or pain, weakness, depression) occurs.

Effects will occur in 30 minutes to 3 hours.

Magnesium Oxide

(mag-NEE-zee-uhm OX-ide)

Mag-Ox 400, Maox 420, Uro-Mag

Used to treat stomach upset due to too much secretion (eg, heartburn, acid indigestion and sour stomach); to treat irritation of the stomach associated with peptic ulcers. It occasionally may be prescribed for other reasons.

Precautions

DO NOT USE if you have kidney disease.

BEFORE USING THIS MEDICINE, tell your healthcare provider if you are pregnant or breastfeeding; or if you are taking, will be taking or stop taking any prescription or nonprescription medicine; or if you have any other medical conditions.

Side Effects

Every medicine can cause side effects, but many people have no, or minor, side effects. Tell your healthcare provider if any of the following occurs: nausea; vomiting; stomach pain; diarrhea; muscular weakness; lack of energy; headache; confusion; irritability.

Guidelines for Use

USE EXACTLY AS PRESCRIBED.

Antacids reduce acidity for about 30 minutes when taken on an empty stomach. Acidity is reduced for about 3 hours when antacids are taken 1 hour after meals.

Do not take other medications within 1 to 2 hours of taking this medicine.

Tell your healthcare provider if coffee-ground vomiting or black, tar-like stools occur.

Taking too much of these products can cause the stomach to secrete excess stomach acid. Talk to your healthcare provider about the appropriate dose.

Long-term use--Do not take for longer than 2 weeks for the relief of indigestion. If discomfort continues, talk to your healthcare provider.

Magnesium Sulfate Injectable

(mag-NEE-zee-uhm SULL-fate)

Magnesium Sulfate

Used as replacement therapy in magnesium deficiency and to correct hypomagnesemia. It also is used for the prevention and control of convulsions due to severe eclampsia, and for control of high blood pressure, brain disease and convulsions associated with kidney problems in children. It occasionally may be prescribed for other reasons.

Precautions

DO NOT USE if you are allergic to this medicine.

BEFORE USING THIS MEDICINE, tell your healthcare provider if you are pregnant or breastfeeding; or if you are taking, will be taking or stop taking any prescription or nonprescription medicine; or if you have any other medical conditions.

Side Effects

Every medicine can cause side effects, but many people have no, or minor, side effects. Tell your healthcare provider if any of the following occurs: flushing; sweating; stupor; difficulty breathing; fainting; irritation at the injection site.

Magnesium Sulfate Oral

(mag-NEE-zee-uhm SULL-fate)

Epsom Salts

For use in short-term constipation or to empty the colon for rectal and bowel examinations. It occasionally may be prescribed for other reasons.

Precautions

DO NOT USE if you are allergic to this medicine; if you have nausea, vomiting or other symptoms of appendicitis; fecal impaction; intestinal obstruction; or undiagnosed abdominal pain.

BEFORE USING THIS MEDICINE, tell your healthcare provider if you are pregnant or breastfeeding; or if you are taking, will be taking or stop taking any prescription or nonprescription medicine; or if you have any other medical conditions.

Side Effects

Every medicine can cause side effects, but many people have no, or minor, side effects. Tell your healthcare provider if any of the following occurs: diarrhea; vomiting; nausea; rectal irritation; weakness; dizziness; fainting; sweating; bloating; gas; abdominal cramps.

Guidelines for Use

USE EXACTLY AS PRESCRIBED.

Take with a full glass of water.

Direct attention to proper dietary fiber intake, adequate fluids and regular exercise.

Do not use in the presence of abdominal pain, nausea or vomiting.

Laxative use is only a temporary measure; do not use longer than 1 week. When regularity returns, discontinue use.

Prolonged, frequent or excessive use may result in dependence or electrolyte imbalance.

Tell your healthcare provider if unrelieved constipation, rectal bleeding or symptoms of electrolyte imbalance (eg, muscle cramps or pain, weakness, dizziness) occurs.

Maprotiline Hydrochloride

(ma-PRO-tih-leen HIGH-droe-KLOR-ide)

Ludiomil

A mood elevating agent usually used for the treatment of depression. It occasionally may be prescribed for other reasons.

Precautions

DO NOT USE if you are allergic to this medicine or to tricyclic antidepressants; or if you are using a monoamine oxidase inhibitor (eg, *Nardil*, *Parnate*).

BEFORE USING THIS MEDICINE, tell your healthcare provider if you are pregnant or breastfeeding; or if you are taking, will be taking or stop taking any prescription or nonprescription medicine; or if you have any other medical conditions.

Side Effects

Every medicine can cause side effects, but many people have no, or minor, side effects. Tell your healthcare provider if any of the following occurs: difficulty breathing; nausea; vomiting; constipation; stomach cramps; diarrhea; confusion; seizures; behavioral changes; nervousness; muscle tremor or stiffness; drowsiness; dizziness; tiredness or weakness; hallucinations; disorientation; delusions; disturbed concentration; panic; sleep disturbances; headache; memory loss; incoordination; rapid pulse; pounding in chest; abnormal heart rhythms; rash; itching; flushing; unusual bleeding or bruising; yellowing of the skin or eyes; hives; sensitivity to light; fever; sweating; hair loss; blurred vision; ringing in the ears; swelling of testicles; painful ejaculation; impotence; changes in sex drive; difficult/frequent urination; irregular menstrual periods; breast enlargement and milk production in females; facial swelling; difficulty swallowing; speech problems; numbness and tingling in arms.

Guidelines for Use

USE EXACTLY AS PRESCRIBED.

If a dose is missed, take it as soon as possible. If several hours have passed or if it is nearing time for the next dose, do not double the dose to "catch up," unless advised by your healthcare provider. If more than one dose is missed, contact your healthcare provider.

May cause drowsiness. Alcohol use may increase this effect. Use caution while driving or performing other tasks requiring alertness until you know how this medication will affect you.

Improvement may not be seen for 2 to 3 weeks.

May cause sensitivity to bright lights. This may be minimized by wearing sunglasses.

Masoprocol

(mass-OH-prah-KOLE)

Actinex

A topical cream used to treat actinic (solar or sun-induced) keratoses (dry, sandpapery places on the skin).

Precautions

DO NOT USE in the eyes; with tight-covering bandages; or if you have an allergy to this medicine.

BEFORE USING THIS MEDICINE tell your healthcare provider if you are pregnant or breastfeeding; or if you are taking, will be taking or stop taking any prescription or nonprescription medicine; or if you have any other medical conditions.

Side Effects

Every medicine can cause side effects, but many people have no, or minor, side effects. Tell your healthcare provider if any of the following occurs: excessive or worsening local skin reactions such as redness, flaking, itching, dryness, swelling, burning or soreness, oozing, blistering, bleeding.

Guidelines for Use

USE EXACTLY AS PRESCRIBED.

For external use only. Do not use in the eyes. If applying near the eyes, nose or mouth, do so carefully.

In case of contact with the eye, promptly wash the eye with water.

Do not use tight-covering bandages over the treated area.

Avoid excessive exposure to the sun.

If cream is applied with fingers, wash hands immediately after use.

This medicine may stain clothing or fabrics.

Generally avoid the use of makeup with this medicine without the advice of your healthcare provider.

To apply, gently wash and dry the areas to be treated, gently rub in cream evenly. Repeat application each morning and evening for 28 days.

A mild burning feeling is common, but should quickly go away. If this feeling worsens or the reactions become more severe, contact your healthcare provider.

Mebendazole

(meh-BEN-duh-zole)

Vermox

A medicine used to treat intestinal parasitic infections such as pinworm, round worm, common hookworm, American hookworm and whipworm.

Precautions

DO NOT USE if you are allergic to this medicine.

BEFORE USING THIS MEDICINE, tell your healthcare provider if you are pregnant or breastfeeding; or if you are taking, will be taking or stop taking any prescription or nonprescription medicine; or if you have any other medical conditions.

Side Effects

Every medicine can cause side effects, but many people have no, or minor, side effects. Tell your healthcare provider if any of the following occurs: stomach ache; diarrhea; fever.

Guidelines for Use

USE EXACTLY AS PRESCRIBED.

Chew or crush and mix with food.

Worm death may be slow. Removal from the digestive tract may take up to 3 days after treatment. Effectiveness depends on factors such as degree of infection, degree of resistance of parasite to treatment, presence of diarrhea and how quickly things pass through the digestive system.

Laxative therapy to remove killed parasites and fasting are not necessary.

If a dose is missed, take it as soon as possible. If several hours have passed or if it is nearing time for the next dose, do not double the dose to "catch up," unless advised by your healthcare provider. If more than one dose is missed, contact your healthcare provider. If not cured in 3 weeks, a second treatment is recommended.

Strict hygiene is essential to prevent reinfection. Disinfect toilet facilities daily. Change and launder undergarments, bed linens, towels and nightclothes daily.

Pinworm infections are easily spread to others. If one family member has a pinworm infection, all family members should be treated.

Meclizine

(MEK-lih-zeen)

Antivert/25 Chewable Tablets, Antivert/25 Tablets, Antivert/50 Tablets, Antrizine Tablets, Bonine Chewable Tablets, Dizmiss Chewable Tablets, En-Vert Tablets, Marezine Tablets, Meni-D Capsules, Ru-Vert-M Tablets

A medicine used for nausea, vomiting, motion sickness and vertigo (feeling of whirling motion).

Precautions

DO NOT USE if you are allergic to this medicine. Do not use in children under 12 years old.

BEFORE USING THIS MEDICINE, tell your healthcare provider if you are pregnant or breastfeeding, or if you are taking, will be taking or stop taking any prescription or nonprescription medicine; or if you have any other medical conditions.

Side Effects

Every medicine can cause side effects, but many people have no, or minor, side effects. Tell your healthcare provider if any of the following occurs: vomiting; constipation; drowsiness (common); nervousness; difficult urination; rash; blurred vision; dry mouth.

Guidelines for Use

USE EXACTLY AS PRESCRIBED.

For motion sickness, the first dose should be taken 30 minutes before exposure to motion.

Avoid alcohol and other depressants (eg, sleeping pills, tranquilizers, narcotic pain relievers, antihistamines).

May cause drowsiness or blurred vision. Use caution while driving or performing other tasks requiring mental alertness.

May cause dry mouth.

Meclofenamate Sodium

(mek-loe-FEN-uh-mate SO-dee-uhm)

Meclomen

A nonsteroidal anti-inflammatory (NSAID) medicine used to relieve mild to moderate pain in conditions such as headache, dental pain, athletic injury, menstrual cramps, acute and chronic rheumatoid arthritis and osteoarthritis. It also is used to treat heavy menstrual blood loss of unknown cause.

Precautions

DO NOT USE if you are allergic to this medicine, or any other nonsteroidal anti-inflammatory medicine or aspirin.

BEFORE USING THIS MEDICINE, tell your healthcare provider if you are pregnant or breastfeeding; use alcohol chronically; or if you are taking, will be taking or stop taking any prescription or nonprescription medicine; or if you have any other medical conditions.

Side Effects

Every medicine can cause side effects, but many people have no, or minor, side effects. Tell your healthcare provider if any of the following occurs: nausea; indigestion; stomach upset or pain; heartburn; diarrhea; cramps; bloating; belching; gas; headache; dizziness; itching; rash; hives; redness (skin); ringing in the ears; rectal bleeding; unexplained bruising or bleeding; yellowing of the skin or eyes; difficulty breathing; fluid retention.

Guidelines for Use

USE EXACTLY AS PRESCRIBED.

If a dose is missed, take it as soon as possible. If several hours have passed, or if it is nearing time for the next dose, do not double the dose to "catch up," unless advised by your healthcare provider. If more than one dose is missed, contact your healthcare provider.

Avoid aspirin and alcoholic beverages while taking this medicine.

If stomach upset occurs, take with food, milk or antacids. If symptoms continue, contact your healthcare provider.

May cause serious effects such as bleeding, ulceration and perforation in patients treated chronically with this medicine. Talk with your healthcare provider about the warning signs of ulceration and perforation.

This medicine may cause dizziness. Use caution while driving or performing other tasks requiring mental alertness, coordination and dexterity.

Tell your healthcare provider if skin rash, itching, visual disturbances, weight gain, swelling of the extremities, stomach pain, black stools or persistent headache, difficulty urinating or urination problems occur.

Medroxyprogesterone Acetate

(meh-DROX-ee-pro-JESS-tuh-rone ASS-uh-TATE)

Amen, Curretab, Cycrin, Provera

A female hormone used to treat amenorrhea (absence of menstrual flow), abnormal bleeding from the uterus and endometriosis. It occasionally may be prescribed for other reasons.

Precautions

DO NOT USE if you are allergic to this medicine; if you are pregnant (during the first four months); if you have a history of blood clots or miscarriage; or if you have breast cancer, liver disease or undiagnosed vaginal bleeding.

BEFORE USING THIS MEDICINE, tell your healthcare provider if you are breastfeeding; or if you are taking, will be taking or stop taking any prescription or nonprescription medicine; or if you have any other medical conditions.

Side Effects

Every medicine can cause side effects, but many people have no, or minor, side effects. Tell your healthcare provider if any of the following occurs: pain in the calves accompanied by swelling; warmth and redness; acute chest pain; sudden shortness of breath; sudden severe headache; vomiting; dizziness; fainting; visual disturbance; numbness in an arm or leg; abnormal vaginal bleeding.

Guidelines for Use

USE EXACTLY AS PRESCRIBED.

If stomach upset occurs, take with food.

If a dose is missed, take as soon as possible. If several hours have passed or if it is nearing time for the next dose, do not double the dose to "catch up," unless advised by your healthcare provider. If more than one dose is missed, contact your healthcare provider.

Discontinue medication pending an eye exam if there is a loss or change in your vision, double vision or migraine.

May cause sensitivity to light. Avoid prolonged exposure to the sun and other ultraviolet light. Use sunscreens and wear protective clothing until tolerance is determined.

Do not change from one brand of medicine to another without consulting your healthcare provider.

Diabetic patients: Glucose tolerance may be decreased. Monitor urine and blood sugar closely and report any abnormal results to your healthcare provider.

Mefenamic Acid

(MEH-fen-AM-ic acid)

Ponstel

A nonsteroidal anti-inflammatory medicine (NSAID) generally used to relieve mild to moderate pain and dysmenorrhea (cramps).

Precautions

DO NOT USE if you are allergic to this medicine or its relatives, aspirin or iodides.

BEFORE USING THIS MEDICINE, tell your healthcare provider if you are pregnant or breastfeeding; use alcohol chronically; are prone to fluid retention; or if you are taking, will be taking or stop taking any prescription or nonprescription medicines; or have any other medical conditions.

Side Effects

Every medicine can cause side effects, but many people have no, or minor, side effects. Tell your healthcare provider if any of the following occurs: allergic reaction (eg, rash, itching, fever); changes in vision; weight gain; fluid retention; stomach problems (eg, nausea, vomiting, diarrhea, pain); black stools; constipation; persistent headache; dizziness; nervousness; weakness; ringing in the ears; taste changes; unusual bruising or bleeding.

Guidelines for Use

USE EXACTLY AS PRESCRIBED.

Avoid aspirin and alcoholic beverages.

If stomach upset occurs, take with food, milk or antacids. If stomach pain continues, tell your healthcare provider.

If a dose is missed, take it as soon as possible. If several hours have passed or if it is nearing time for the next dose, do not double the dose to "catch up," unless advised by your healthcare provider. If more than one dose is missed, contact your healthcare provider.

May cause drowsiness or dizziness. Observe caution while driving or performing other tasks requiring mental alertness, coordination and dexterity.

May cause sensitivity to sunlight. Avoid prolonged exposure to the sun. Use sunscreens and wear protective clothing until tolerance is determined.

Megestrol Acetate

(meh-JESS-trole ASS-uh-TATE)

Megace

A medicine used for the treatment of advanced cancer of the breast or endometrium (recurrent, inoperable metastatic disease). It also has been used as an appetite stimulant in AIDS-related malnutrition.

Precautions

DO NOT USE if you are allergic to this medicine; as a diagnostic test for pregnancy; if you are pregnant; or as a preventative method to avoid weight loss.

BEFORE USING THIS MEDICINE, tell your healthcare provider if you are pregnant or breastfeeding; or if you are taking, will be taking or stop taking any prescription or nonprescription medicine; or if you have any other medical conditions.

Side Effects

Every medicine can cause side effects, but many people have no, or minor, side effects. Tell your healthcare provider if any of the following occurs: weight gain (due to increased appetite); nausea; vomiting; fluid retention; indigestion; hair loss; carpal tunnel syndrome; rash; difficulty breathing; vaginal bleeding at abnormal times; headache; sleeplessness; dry mouth; increased salivation; mouth sores; gas; sexual function changes; cough; sore throat; vision problems; unusual bleeding or bruising; chest, back or stomach pain; breast tenderness; diarrhea; constipation.

Guidelines for Use

USE EXACTLY AS PRESCRIBED.

Take on an empty stomach 1 hour before or 2 hours after eating with a full glass of water. However, if stomach upset occurs, take with food.

Use of this medicine during the first four months of pregnancy is not recommended because of possible birth defects.

Birth control measures are recommended during treatment.

May cause back or stomach pain, headache, nausea, vomiting or breast tenderness. Tell your healthcare provider if these become severe.

If a dose is missed, take it as soon as possible. If several hours have passed or if it is nearing time for the next dose, do not double the dose to "catch up," unless advised by your healthcare provider. If more than one dose is missed, contact your healthcare provider.

Do not stop taking this medicine without consulting your healthcare provider.

Storage — Tablets and solution: Store in a well-closed container at room temperature.

Oral: Shake well before using. Store below 77 degrees in a tight container. Protect from light. Do not freeze.

Contact your healthcare provider if vaginal bleeding occurs.

Melphalan

(MELL-fuh-lan)

Alkeran

A medicine used to treat multiple myeloma and cancer of the ovaries.

Precautions

DO NOT USE if you are allergic or have prior resistance to this medicine.

BEFORE USING THIS MEDICINE, tell your healthcare provider if you are pregnant or breastfeeding; or if you are taking, will be taking or stop taking any prescription or nonprescription medicine; or if you have any other medical conditions.

Side Effects

Every medicine can cause side effects, but many people have no, or minor, side effects. Tell your healthcare provider if any of the following occurs: nausea; vomiting; diarrhea; mouth sores; skin reactions; hair loss; skin ulceration at the injection site; breakdown of the skin; allergy symptoms (hives, itching, difficulty breathing, rapid heart rate, fluid retention); difficulty breathing; painful veins; weakness.

Guidelines for Use

USE EXACTLY AS PRESCRIBED.

Take under close medical supervision. Tell your healthcare provider of unusual bleeding or bruising, black tarry stools, nausea, vomiting, weight loss, fever, chills, sore throat, rash, cough, shortness of breath, lack of menstrual flow, unusual lumps or masses, sores in the mouth or on the lips.

Birth control measures are strongly recommended for both men and women.

If a dose is missed, take it as soon as possible. If several hours have passed or if it is nearing time for the next dose, do not double the dose to "catch up," unless advised by your healthcare provider. If more than one dose is missed, contact your healthcare provider.

Response may be gradual over many months; repeated courses or continuous therapy is important. The maximum benefit may be missed if treatment is ended too soon.

Protect tablets from light. Dispense in glass container.

Laboratory blood counts will need to be taken periodically. Keep your appointments with your healthcare provider.

Meperidine Hydrochloride

(meh-PEHR-ih-deen HIGH-droe-KLOR-ide)

Demerol Hydrochloride Syrup, Demerol Hydrochloride Tablet

A narcotic pain reliever used for moderate to severe pain.

Precautions

DO NOT USE if you are allergic to this medicine or its relatives. Do not use within 14 days of monoamine oxidase inhibitor (phenelzine, tranylcypromine) treatment.

BEFORE USING THIS MEDICINE, tell your healthcare provider if you are pregnant or breastfeeding; or if you are taking, will be taking or stop taking any prescription or nonprescription medicine; or if you have any other medical conditions. Long term, regular use of narcotic pain relievers may lead to dependence and physical tolerance. Withdrawal symptoms may occur when therapy is stopped.

Side Effects

Every medicine can cause side effects, but many people have no, or minor, side effects. Tell your healthcare provider if any of the following occurs: lightheadedness; dizziness; drowsiness; nausea; vomiting; sweating; abdominal pain; cramps; constipation; diarrhea; urine retention; appetite loss; indigestion; gas; excitability; vision problems; difficult breathing.

Guidelines for Use

USE EXACTLY AS PRESCRIBED.

Take with food if stomach upset occurs.

May cause drowsiness, dizziness or blurred vision. Use caution while driving or performing other tasks requiring mental alertness, judgment and coordination.

Avoid alcohol and other medicines that cause drowsiness (eg, sleeping pills, antihistamines).

May cause nausea, vomiting or constipation. Constipation may be avoided by using a stool softener or fiber laxative.

This medicine works best if taken regularly. It is more effective in preventing pain than in treating pain after it occurs.

Give the medicine ample time to work before taking more (approximately 30 minutes to 1 hour).

If a dose is missed, take it as soon as possible. If several hours have passed or if it is nearing time for the next dose, do not double the dose to "catch up," unless advised by your healthcare provider. If more than one dose is missed, contact your healthcare provider.

Orthostatic hypotension (dizziness or lightheadedness when rising quickly from a seated or lying position) may occur. Avoid sudden changes in posture.

Meprobamate

(meh-pro-BAM-ate)

Equanil, Meprospan, Miltown

A medicine used to manage anxiety disorders and to provide short-term relief of symptoms of anxiety. Anxiety and tension associated with everyday stress usually does not require treatment with an antianxiety agent.

Precautions

DO NOT USE if you are allergic to this medicine, carisoprodol or its relatives.

BEFORE USING THIS MEDICINE, tell your healthcare provider if you are pregnant or breastfeeding; or if you are taking, will be taking or stop taking any prescription or nonprescription medicine; or if you have any other medical conditions.

Side Effects

Every medicine can cause side effects, but many people have no, or minor, side effects. Tell your healthcare provider if any of the following occurs: stomach upset; nausea; vomiting; diarrhea; drowsiness; dizziness; feeling of whirling motion; incoordination; headache; weakness; overstimulation; exaggerated sense of well–being; pounding in the chest; rash; chills; hives; unusual bleeding or bruising; slurred speech; fever; blurred vision; shortness of breath; tingling and numbness.

Guidelines for Use

USE EXACTLY AS PRESCRIBED.

If a dose is missed, take it as soon as possible. If several hours have passed, or if it is nearing time for the next dose, do not double the dose to "catch up," unless advised by your healthcare provider. If more than one dose is missed, contact your healthcare provider.

If you become pregnant during therapy or intend to become pregnant, consult your healthcare provider about use of this medicine.

This medicine may cause drowsiness, dizziness or blurred vision. Use caution while driving or performing other tasks requiring mental alertness, coordination and dexterity.

Discontinue at first appearance of rash or other sign of allergy. In some instances, rash may be accompanied by more severe allergy reactions (see side effects). If this occurs, tell your healthcare provider immediately.

Avoid alcohol and medicines that cause drowsiness during therapy.

Do not suddenly stop taking this medicine after long-term use. Talk with your healthcare provider.

Physical and psychological dependence and abuse may occur.

Mercaptopurine

(mer-cap-toe-PURE-een)

Purinethol

An anticancer medicine. It is generally used to treat acute lymphatic leukemia.

Precautions

DO NOT USE if you have shown prior resistance to this medicine or thioguanine, or if you are pregnant or breastfeeding.

BEFORE USING THIS MEDICINE, tell your healthcare provider if you are taking, will be taking or stop taking any prescription or nonprescription medicine; or if you have any other medical conditions.

Side Effects

Every medicine can cause side effects, but many people have no, or minor, side effects. Tell your healthcare provider if any of the following occurs: stomach discomfort; appetite loss; diarrhea; fever; sore throat; chills; nausea; vomiting; unusual bleeding or bruising; black, tarry stools; cough or shortness of breath; darkened or bloody urine; yellowing of skin or eyes; mouth sores or swelling; flank or joint pain; swelling of feet or legs.

Guidelines for Use

USE EXACTLY AS PRESCRIBED.

If a dose is missed, take it as soon as possible. If several hours have passed or if it is nearing time for the next dose, do not double the dose to "catch up," unless advised by your healthcare provider. If more than one dose is missed, contact your healthcare provider.

Practice effective birth control during therapy.

Mesalamine

(me-SAL-uh-MEEN)

Asacol Delayed-Release Tablets, Pentasa Delayed-Release Capsules, Rowasa Suppositories, Rowasa Rectal Suspension

A medicine used for the treatment of various forms of mild to moderate ulcerative colitis.

Precautions

DO NOT USE if you are allergic to this medicine or its relatives or salicylates (eg, aspirin).

BEFORE USING THIS MEDICINE, tell your healthcare provider if you are pregnant or breastfeeding; or if you are taking, will be taking or stop taking any prescription or nonprescription medicine; or if you have any other medical conditions.

Side Effects

Every medicine can cause side effects, but many people have no, or minor, side effects. Tell your healthcare provider if any of the following occurs: diarrhea; constipation; nausea; vomiting; abdominal pain; loss of appetite; headache; rash; fever; worsening of ulcerative colitis; acne; dizziness; back/muscle pain.

Guidelines for Use

USE EXACTLY AS PRESCRIBED.

Sustained released: Swallow whole. Do not crush or chew tablets. If intact or partially intact tablets appear in the stool, notify your healthcare provider.

Suppositories: If you do not know the correct way to insert a suppository, ask your health-car provider.

Suspension: Patient instructions are included. Shake well. Remove protective sheath from applicator tip; gently insert applicator tip into the rectum.

If a dose is missed, take as soon as possible. If several hours have passed or if it is nearing time for the next dose, do not double the dose to "catch up," unless advised by your healthcare provider. If more than one dose is missed, contact your healthcare provider.

Metaproterenol Sulfate

(MEH-tuh-pro-TEHR-uh-nahl SULL-fate)

Alupent, Arm-a-Med, Metaprel, Prometa

A medicine that makes breathing easier by widening breathing passages of the lungs and by removing (expectorating) mucus and other debris that cause congestion in the lungs. It may be used to treat asthma, bronchitis or emphysema.

Precautions

DO NOT USE if you are allergic to this medicine or have heart rhythm disturbances associated with a rapid heart rate.

BEFORE USING THIS MEDICINE, tell your healthcare provider if you are pregnant or breastfeeding; or if you are taking, will be taking or stop taking any prescription or nonprescription medicine; or have any other medical conditions.

Side Effects

Every medicine can cause side effects, but many people have no, or minor, side effects. Tell your healthcare provider if any of the following occurs: nausea; vomiting; loss of appetite; heartburn; nervousness; restlessness; dizziness; lightheadedness; headache; anxiety; tension; tremor; drowsiness; weakness; sleeplessness; chest pain; pounding in chest (palpitations); breathing problems; coughing; flushing; sweating; hives; muscle cramps; unusual or bad taste in mouth; drying or irritation of mouth or throat.

Guidelines for Use

USE EXACTLY AS PRESCRIBED.

Patient instructions are available with products.

If a dose is missed, take it as soon as possible. If several hours have passed or if it is nearing time for the next dose, do not double the dose to "catch up," unless advised to do so by your healthcare provider.

Do not exceed recommended dosage. Excessive use may lead to side effects or loss of effectiveness.

Do not stop or adjust the dose except on the recommendation of your healthcare provider.

Tell your healthcare provider if pounding in the chest, chest pain, muscle tremors, dizziness, headache, flushing or difficult urination occurs, or if breathing difficulty or nervousness persists.

Oral: If stomach upset occurs, take with food.

Inhalation: Administer pressurized inhalation during the second half of breath intake. If more than one inhalation per dose is necessary, wait at least one full minute between doses. (Give second inhalation at 10 minutes). If you do not get the usual relief from your normal dose, do not increase your dose, but call your healthcare provider immediately.

Do not use epinephrine or other inhaled bronchodilators within 4 hours of using this medicine.

Storage: Store at room temperature. Avoid excessive heat. Protect from light. Do not use if solution is cloudy or discolored. Change solution in nebulizer daily.

Aerosol storage: Refrigerate unit dose nebulizer vials at 35–46 degrees F. Avoid excessive heat. Protect from light.

Metformin

(met-FORE-min)

Glucophage

An oral antidiabetic used to treat non-insulin-dependent diabetes mellitus in adults who cannot manage blood sugar levels by diet and exercise alone. It may also be prescribed with other hypoglycemic drugs.

Precautions

DO NOT USE if you are allergic to this medicine, have kidney or liver problems, or a metabolism imbalance. This medicine could slightly increase the risk of heart problems compared to treatment with diet alone or diet plus insulin. Lactic acidosis may occur while taking this medicine. Stop taking this medicine and contact your healthcare provider immediately if the following occur: general body discomfort; muscle pain; difficulty breathing; drowsiness; stomach pain; chills; dizziness; lightheadedness; slow heartbeat.

BEFORE USING THIS MEDICINE, tell your healthcare provider if you are pregnant or breastfeeding; if you are taking, will be taking or stop taking any prescription or nonprescription medicine; or if you have any other medical conditions.

Side Effects

Every medicine can cause side effects, but many people have no, or minor, side effects. Tell your healthcare provider if any of the following occurs: diarrhea; nausea; vomiting; gas; stomach bloating; appetite loss; unpleasant/metallic taste; rash; weakness; and any of the symptoms of lactic acidosis listed above.

Guidelines for Use

USE EXACTLY AS PRESCRIBED.

This medicine is usually taken twice daily with the morning and evening meals.

Follow dosage instructions, diet and exercise program prescribed by your healthcare provider.

If a dose is missed, take it as soon as possible. If several hours have passed or if it is nearing time for the next dose, do not double the dose to "catch up," unless advised by your healthcare provider. If more than one dose is missed, contact your healthcare provider.

Contact your healthcare provider if unexplained breathing problems, muscle aches, body discomfort, drowsiness or fever occur. Nausea, vomiting, diarrhea, gas and appetite loss generally stop with continued use. If they continue, contact your healthcare provider.

Avoid drinking alcohol.

The effectiveness of this medicine may decrease over time. If you feel that it is losing its effectiveness, contact your healthcare provider.

Lab tests will be required to monitor therapy. Keep appointments.

Store at room temperature.

Methadone Hydrochloride

(METH-uh-dohn HIGH-droe-KLOR-ide)

Dolophine Hydrochloride Tablets, Methadone Hydrochloride Intensol Liquid, Methadone Hydrochloride Solution, Methadone Hydrochloride Tablets

A narcotic pain reliever used for moderate to severe pain, detoxification and temporary maintenance treatment of narcotic addicts.

Precautions

DO NOT USE if you are allergic to this medicine or its relatives.

BEFORE USING THIS MEDICINE, tell your healthcare provider if you are pregnant or breastfeeding; or if you are taking, will be taking or stop taking any prescription or nonprescription medicine; or if you have any other medical conditions. Long-term, regular use of narcotic pain relievers may lead to dependence and physical tolerance. Withdrawal symptoms may occur when therapy is stopped. Some products may contain sulfite preservatives that can cause allergic reactions in some people. Ask your healthcare provider.

Side Effects

Every medicine can cause side effects, but many people have no, or minor, side effects. Tell your healthcare provider if any of the following occurs: lightheadedness; dizziness; drowsiness; nausea; vomiting; sweating; abdominal pain; cramps; constipation; diarrhea; urine retention; appetite loss; indigestion; gas; excitability; vision problems; difficult breathing.

Guidelines for Use

USE EXACTLY AS PRESCRIBED.

Take with food if stomach upset occurs.

May cause drowsiness, dizziness or blurred vision. Use caution while driving or performing other tasks requiring mental alertness, judgment and coordination.

Avoid alcohol and other medicines that cause drowsiness (eg, sleeping pills, antihistamines).

May cause nausea, vomiting or constipation. Constipation may be avoided by using a stool softener or fiber laxative.

This medicine works best if taken regularly. It is more effective in preventing pain than in treating pain after it occurs.

Give the medicine ample time to work before taking more (approximately 30 minutes to 1 hour).

If a dose is missed, take it as soon as possible. If several hours have passed or if it is nearing time for the next dose, do not double the dose to "catch up," unless advised by your healthcare provider. If more than one dose is missed, contact your healthcare provider.

Methamphetamine Hydrochloride

(meth-am-FET-uh-meen HIGH-droe-KLOR-ide)

Desoxyn, Desoxyn Gradumets

A medicine used to treat narcolepsy, a rare sleep disorder that causes people to uncontrollably fall asleep, attention deficit disorder in children, and for short-term use as part of an overall diet plan to reduce weight.

Precautions

DO NOT USE if you are allergic to this medicine, with monoamine oxidase inhibitors (MAOIs) or within 14 days following MAOI use.

BEFORE USING THIS MEDICINE, tell your healthcare provider if you are pregnant or breastfeeding; or if you are taking, will be taking or stop taking any prescription or nonprescription medicine; or if you have any other medical conditions.

Side Effects

Every medicine can cause side effects, but many people have no, or minor, side effects. Tell your healthcare provider if any of the following occurs: diarrhea; constipation; stomach cramps; appetite loss; psychological problems; headache; nervousness; dizziness; depression (between doses or after stopping); inability to sleep; excessive restlessness; irritability; pounding in the chest; rash; hives; itching; muscle tremor or twitching; dry mouth/bad taste; sexual problems; fatigue between doses or after stopping; weight loss (children); stunted growth (children).

Guidelines for Use

USE EXACTLY AS PRESCRIBED.

Take early in the day to avoid nighttime sleep loss. Do not chew or crush long-acting tablets.

Do not increase dosage, except on your healthcare provider's advice.

May impair ability to drive or perform other tasks requiring alertness. May mask extreme fatigue.

May cause nervousness, restlessness, sleeplessness, dizziness, appetite loss, dry mouth and digestive tract disturbances. Tell your healthcare provider if these effects become pronounced.

If a dose is missed, take it as soon as possible. If several hours have passed or if it is nearing time for the next dose, do not double the dose to "catch up," unless advised by your healthcare provider. If more than one dose is missed, contact your healthcare provider.

Attention deficit disorder in children—Your healthcare provider may occasionally interrupt therapy to determine if there is a recurrence of symptoms.

Methenamine and Methenamine Salts

(meh-THEN-uh-meen and meh-THEN-uh-meen salts)

Hiprex, Urex

A medicine used to eliminate or suppress the bacteria in the urine that causes urinary tract infections.

Precautions

DO NOT USE if you are allergic to this medicine or if you are taking sulfonamide antibiotics.

BEFORE USING THIS MEDICINE, tell your healthcare provider if you are pregnant or breastfeeding; or if you are taking, will be taking or stop taking any prescription or nonprescription medicine; or if you have any other medical conditions.

Side Effects

Every medicine can cause side effects, but many people have no, or minor, side effects. Tell your healthcare provider if any of the following occurs: painful urination; frequent urination; nausea; vomiting; stomach cramps; appetite loss; rash; hives; itching; headache; difficult breathing; fluid retention; mouth sores; blood in urine.

Guidelines for Use

USE EXACTLY AS PRESCRIBED.

May cause stomach upset. Take with food.

Drink plenty of fluids to ensure good flow of urine.

Take the full course of therapy to ensure best results. Do not stop the medicine without consulting your healthcare provider.

It may be necessary to attempt to acidify the urine in order to get the best clinical response. Ascorbic acid (vitamin C) at doses of 2 g/day or administration of 8 to 12 g of ammonium chloride per day may acidify the urine. Intake of cranberries, plums, prunes or cranberry juice may help slightly in producing an acid urine. Check with your healthcare provider.

Avoid heavy intake of citrus fruit or juice and milk products or medications such as bicarbonate and acetazolamide. They may change the urine from acid to alkaline.

If a dose is missed, take it as soon as possible. If several hours have passed or if it is nearing time for the next dose, do not double the dose to "catch up," unless advised by your healthcare provider. If more than one dose is missed, contact your healthcare provider.

Large doses (up to 8 g/day for 3 to 4 weeks) may cause bladder irritation, painful and frequent urination, and protein or blood in the urine. Tell your healthcare provider if rash, painful urination or severe stomach upset occurs.

Methenamine hippurate—has been associated with liver toxicity. With long-term therapy, periodic liver function tests need to be performed.

Methenamine mandelate—Administer with caution in the elderly or others with poor reflexes who might inhale the liquid into the lungs and develop pneumonia.

Oral suspension-Shake well before using.

Gout or high serum uric acid levels—This medicine may cause uric acid crystals to form in urine.

Store at room temperature.

Methicillin Sodium

(meth-ih-SILL-in SO-dee-uhm)

Staphcillin

Used for the treatment of infections.

Precautions

DO NOT USE if you are allergic to this medicine or any penicillins.

Side Effects

Every medicine can cause side effects, but many people have no, or minor, side effects. Tell your healthcare provider if any of the following occurs: pain/irritation at the injection site; hallucinations; convulsions; seizures; nausea; vomiting; diarrhea; rash; difficulty breathing; difficulty urinating; drowsiness.

Guidelines for Use

USE EXACTLY AS PRESCRIBED.

If symptoms of an allergic reaction develop (eg, difficulty breathing, facial swelling, rash, itching), stop taking this medicine and contact your healthcare provider.

If a dose is missed, take it as soon as possible. If several hours have passed, or if it is nearing time for the next dose, do not double to the dose to "catch up," unless advised by your healthcare provider. If more than one dose is missed, contact your healthcare provider.

Continue to take until all of the prescribed medicine is gone. Failure to take all of the medicine may prevent complete elimination of bacteria, causing the infection to return.

Methimazole

(meth-IMM-uh-zole)

Tapazole

A medicine used to treat hyperthyroidism (overactive thyroid gland) and to treat or prepare the overactive thyroid for surgery.

Precautions

DO NOT USE if you are allergic to this medicine or if you are breastfeeding.

BEFORE USING THIS MEDICINE, tell your healthcare provider if you are pregnant; or if you are taking, will be taking or stop taking any prescription or nonprescription medicine; or if you have any other medical conditions.

Side Effects

Every medicine can cause side effects, but many people have no, or minor, side effects. Tell your healthcare provider if any of the following occurs: blood disorders; nausea; vomiting; tingling in arms/legs; headache; dizziness; drowsiness; rash; itching; bruising/bleeding; yellowing of skin/eyes; hair loss; joint/muscle pain; swelling.

Guidelines for Use

USE EXACTLY AS PRESCRIBED.

Take at regular intervals around the clock (usually every 8 hours), unless directed otherwise by your healthcare provider.

Methocarbamol

(meth-oh-CAR-buh-mahl)

Delaxin, Robaxin

A medicine used to relieve muscle discomfort due to strain and sprain.

Precautions

DO NOT USE if you are allergic to this medicine or its relatives.

BEFORE USING THIS MEDICINE, tell your healthcare provider if you are pregnant or breastfeeding; or if you are taking, will be taking or stop taking any prescription or nonprescription medicine; or if you have any other medical conditions.

Side Effects

Every medicine can cause side effects, but many people have no, or minor, side effects. Tell your healthcare provider if any of the following occurs: stomach upset; constipation; diarrhea; appetite change; vomiting; lightheadedness; confusion; nervousness; drowsiness; fatigue; dizziness; headache; changes in heart rate; itching; rash; visual disturbances; slurred speech; change in bladder function; dry mouth; fever; tremors; difficulty breathing; swelling; fainting.

Guidelines for Use

USE EXACTLY AS PRESCRIBED.

May be taken with food or water if stomach upset occurs.

If a dose is missed, take it as soon as possible. If several hours have passed or if it is nearing time for the next dose, do not double the dose to "catch up," unless advised by your healthcare provider. If more than one dose is missed, contact your healthcare provider.

This medication can be addictive if used in large doses or for a long time. Discuss overuse with your healthcare provider.

May cause drowsiness, dizziness, or blurred vision. Use caution while driving or performing other tasks requiring mental alertness, coordination and dexterity.

Avoid alcohol and medications that cause drowsiness while taking this medicine (eg, sleeping pills, tranquilizers, antihistamines).

Patients on long-term or high dosage therapy may have withdrawal symptoms if therapy is suddenly stopped. Do not stop therapy abruptly or change dosage without asking your healthcare provider.

May color urine brown, black or green.

Methotrexate

(meth-oh-TREK-sate)

Abitrexate, Rheumatrex Dose Pack

An anticancer medicine used to treat cancer as well as to control severe psoriasis and severe rheumatoid arthritis. It occasionally may be prescribed for other reasons.

Precautions

DO NOT USE if you are allergic to this medicine; or if you are pregnant or breastfeeding.

BEFORE USING THIS MEDICINE, tell your healthcare provider if you are pregnant or breastfeeding; or if you are taking, will be taking or stop taking any prescription or nonprescription medicine; or if you have any other medical conditions.

Side Effects

Every medicine can cause side effects, but many people have no, or minor, side effects. Tell your healthcare provider if any of the following occurs: nausea; vomiting; stomach discomfort; appetite loss; dizziness; headache; hair loss; rash; boils; acne; fever; sore throat; chills; unusual bleeding or bruising; black, tarry stools; diarrhea; cough or shortness of breath; darkened or bloody urine; yellow discoloration of the skin or eyes; mouth sores; flank or joint pain; swelling of the feet or legs.

Guidelines for Use

USE EXACTLY AS PRESCRIBED.

Drink plenty of liquids.

If a dose is missed, take it as soon as possible. If several hours have passed or if it is nearing time for the next dose, do not double the dose to "catch up," unless advised by your healthcare provider. If more than one dose is missed, contact your healthcare provider.

This medicine may cause sensitivity to light. Avoid prolonged exposure to sunlight or sunlamps. Use sunscreens and wear protective clothing.

Methyldopa and Methyldopate Hydrochloride

(meth-ill-DOE-puh and meth-ill-DOE-pate HIGH-droe-KLOR-ide)

Aldomet, Amodopa, Methyldopate Hydrochloride Injection

A medicine used to lower high blood pressure by relaxing and widening blood vessels.

Precautions

DO NOT USE if you are allergic to this medicine or if you are breastfeeding.

BEFORE USING THIS MEDICINE, tell your healthcare provider if you are pregnant; or if you are taking, will be taking or stop taking any prescription or nonprescription medicine; or if you have any other medical conditions.

Side Effects

Every medicine can cause side effects, but many people have no, or minor, side effects. Tell your healthcare provider if any of the following occurs: nausea; vomiting; diarrhea; constipation; gas; colitis; dizziness; nightmares; depression; drowsiness; headache; tingling of fingers and toes; unusual body movements; slow heart rate, chest pain; difficulty breathing; rash; yellowing of skin or eyes; easy bruising or bleeding; joint pain; fluid retention; sore or black tongue; absence of menstrual period; impotence/decreased sex drive; breast swelling/milk production; muscle aches; anemia; fever.

Guidelines for Use

USE EXACTLY AS PRESCRIBED.

May cause drowsiness or dizziness when beginning treatment or increasing the dose. Use caution when driving or performing other tasks requiring mental alertness.

If a dose is missed, take it as soon as possible. If several hours have passed or if it is nearing time for the next dose, do not double the dose to "catch up," unless advised by your healthcare provider. If more than one dose is missed, contact your healthcare provider.

Avoid alcohol while taking this medicine; it may cause excessive drowsiness.

Regular blood and laboratory tests may be necessary to make sure your medicine is working as it should.

Patients being treated for high blood pressure often feel tired for a few weeks after beginning therapy. Continue taking your medicine even though you may not feel quite normal. Have your blood pressure checked regularly, and keep your appointments with your healthcare provider even if you feel well.

When urine is exposed to air after voiding, it may darken. This is not a problem.

Methylphenidate Hydrochloride

(meth-ill-FEN-ih-date HIGH-droe-KLOR-ide)

Ritalin, Ritalin-SR

A central nervous system stimulant used to treat narcolepsy and to aid in the treatment of children with attention deficit disorder.

Precautions

DO NOT USE if you are allergic to this medicine.

BEFORE USING THIS MEDICINE, tell your healthcare provider if you are pregnant or breastfeeding; or if you are taking, will be taking or stop taking any prescription or nonprescription medicines; or if you have any other medical conditions.

Side Effects

Every medicine can cause side effects, but many people have no, or minor, side effects. Tell your healthcare provider if any of the following occurs: nervousness; difficulty sleeping; chest pain; palpitations (pounding in the chest); rapid heart rate; vomiting; fever; skin rash; headache; appetite loss; increase in blood pressure; perspiration; confusion.

Guidelines for Use

USE EXACTLY AS PRESCRIBED.

It is important to keep regular appointments with your healthcare provider so laboratory tests and blood pressure can be checked to make sure the medicine is working properly.

Take the last dose early in the day, before 6:00 p.m., to avoid insomnia (sleeplessness).

May disguise tiredness, impair physical coordination or cause dizziness or drowsiness.

Use caution when driving or performing other tasks requiring mental alertness, coordination and dexterity.

Prolonged use may cause tolerance to the medication.

Dose may need to be adjusted. Your healthcare provider may recommend medicine-free days to evaluate the need for continued use and to return potency of the medication.

Consult your healthcare provider before withdrawing the medication.

Sustained release: Do not crush or chew this medicine.

Methylprednisolone

(METH-ill-pred-NIH-suh-lone)

Medrol

A hormone used as replacement therapy when the adrenal cortex gland is not functioning properly. It also is used for its anti-inflammatory action. It occasionally may be prescribed for other reasons.

Precautions

DO NOT USE if you are allergic to this medicine or its relatives, or if you are breastfeeding.

BEFORE USING THIS MEDICINE, tell your healthcare provider if you are pregnant; or breastfeeding; or if you are taking, will be taking or stop taking any prescription or nonprescription medicine; if you have any other medical conditions; or if you are allergic to tartrazine or sulfite preservatives.

Side Effects

Every medicine can cause side effects, but many people have no, or minor, side effects. Tell your healthcare provider if any of the following occurs: appearance of round, swollen moonface; fat deposits (eg, shoulders, midsection); nausea; vomiting; increased appetite; weight gain; stomach pain; rectal bleeding with black, tarry stools; seizures; dizziness; headache; behavior changes; sleeplessness; hiccups; fluid retention; low or high blood pressure; irregular heart rhythm; impaired wound healing; thinning of skin; excessive darkening of skin; acne; excessive body hair growth; rash; hives; loss of muscle mass; bone fractures; menstrual irregularities; growth suppression in children; higher blood sugar levels.

Guidelines for Use

USE EXACTLY AS PRESCRIBED.

May cause stomach upset. Take with meals or snacks.

Take single daily or alternate day doses in the morning prior to 9 a.m. Take multiple doses at evenly spaced intervals throughout the day.

Patients on long-term therapy with this medicine should carry identification.

High dose or long-term therapy: DO NOT change or stop therapy unless directed by your healthcare provider.

If a dose is missed, take it as soon as possible. If several hours have passed or if it is nearing time for the next dose, do not double the dose to "catch up," unless advised by your healthcare provider. If more than one dose is missed, contact your healthcare provider.

Diabetes — May require increased doses of insulin or oral diabetes medications.

Methysergide Maleate

(METH-ih-SIR-jide MAL-ee-ate)

Sansert

This medicine is used to prevent or reduce the strength and frequency of migraine headaches in those patients who suffer regular attacks.

Precautions

DO NOT USE if you are allergic to this medicine or tartrazine; are pregnant or breastfeeding.

Side Effects

Every medicine can cause side effects, but many people have no, or minor, side effects. Tell your healthcare provider if any of the following occurs: nausea; vomiting; diarrhea; abdominal pain; fatigue; weight loss; sleeplessness; drowsiness; euphoria; weakness; dizziness; hallucinations.

Guidelines for Use

USE EXACTLY AS PRESCRIBED.

May cause stomach upset. Take with food or milk.

May cause drowsiness. Use caution while driving or performing other tasks requiring mental alertness.

Do not stop taking this medicine suddenly.

This medicine may cause weight gain. Watch your diet.

Continuous treatment should not exceed 6 months. Maintain a medicine-free interval of 3 to 4 weeks after each 6 month treatment course. Reduce dosage gradually during last 2 to 3 weeks of treatment period to avoid headache rebound. Allow 1 to 2 days for protective effects to develop. The protective effects will subside 1 to 2 days after stopping the medicine.

Notify your healthcare provider of cold, numb or painful extremities, leg cramps when walking, girdle, flank or chest pain, painful urination or shortness of breath.

Metoclopramide Hydrochloride

(MET-oh-kloe-PRA-MIDE HIGH-droe-KLOR-ide)

Maxolon Tablets, Metoclopramide Hydrochloride Tablets, Octamide PFS, Reglan Syrup, Reglan Tablets

A medicine used to treat symptoms of delayed stomach emptying, diabetic digestive problems (eg, nausea, vomiting, heartburn, persistent fullness after meals and appetite loss), the nausea and vomiting associated with cancer chemotherapy and bubbling of stomach contents into the esophagus.

Precautions

DO NOT USE if you are allergic to this medicine.

BEFORE USING THIS MEDICINE, tell your healthcare provider if you are pregnant or breastfeeding; or if you are taking, will be taking or stop taking any prescription or nonprescription medicine; or if you have any other medical conditions.

Side Effects

Every medicine can cause side effects, but many people have no, or minor, side effects. Tell your healthcare provider if any of the following occurs: involuntary movement of the eyes, face or limbs; restlessness; drowsiness; fatigue; weakness; dizziness; headache; depression.

Guidelines for Use

USE EXACTLY AS PRESCRIBED.

Take 30 minutes before each meal.

May cause drowsiness. Use caution when driving or performing other tasks requiring mental alertness.

Do not take regularly or for more than 12 weeks without discussing this with your healthcare provider.

This medicine should not be used routinely for uncomplicated nausea or vomiting.

Do not consume alcohol while taking this medicine without discussing it with your healthcare provider.

Metolazone

(meh-TOLE-uh-ZONE)

Mykrox, Zaroxolyn

Used to treat edema and high blood pressure. It occasionally may be prescribed for other reasons.

Precautions

DO NOT USE if you are allergic to this medicine.

BEFORE USING THIS MEDICINE, tell your healthcare provider if you are pregnant or breastfeeding; or if you are taking, will be taking or stop taking any prescription or nonprescription medicine; or if you have any other medical conditions.

Side Effects

Every medicine can cause side effects, but many people have no, or minor, side effects. Tell your healthcare provider if any of the following occurs: chest pain; cold hands/feet; bitter taste; dry skin; joint pain; back pain; cough; sinus congestion; sore throat; chills; eye itching; ringing in the ears; headache; pounding in the chest; dizziness; lightheadedness; weakness; anxiety depression; nervousness; nausea; vomiting; abdominal pain/cramping; bloating; dry mouth; excessive urination; impotence; reduced sex drive; rash; itching; muscle cramps/spasm; change in taste; numbness; trouble sleeping; yellow eyes or skin; diarrhea; constipation; loss of appetite; vision change.

Guidelines for Use

USE EXACTLY AS PRESCRIBED.

May cause stomach upset; take with food or milk.

May be taken with other antihypertensive medications.

If a dose is missed, take it as soon as possible. If several hours have passed or if it is nearing time for the next dose, do not double the dose to "catch up," unless advised by your healthcare provider. If more than one dose is missed, contact your healthcare provider.

Dehydration (eg, excess sweating, vomiting, diarrhea) may increase the blood pressure-lowering effect, causing dizziness. Drink plenty of fluids in such situations.

This medicine will initially increase urination, which will subside after a few weeks.

Take early in the day or as directed.

Tell your healthcare provider if muscle pain, weakness or cramps, nausea, vomiting, restlessness, excessive thirst, tiredness, drowsiness, or diarrhea occurs.

May cause dizziness, fainting or lightheadedness, especially after the first dose or during the first day of therapy; avoid sudden changes in posture.

May cause sensitivity to sunlight. Avoid prolonged exposure to the sun. Use sunscreens and protective clothing until tolerance is determined.

Diabetes — May increase blood sugar levels.

Avoid alcohol and medicines that cause drowsiness, including medicines for appetite control, asthma, colds, cough, hay fever or sinus problems.

Do not stop, interrupt or alter the dose of this medicine even if you are feeling well.

May cause gout attacks. Tell your healthcare provider if sudden joint pain occurs.

Store at room temperature in a tight container away from light.

Metoprolol

(meh-TOE-pro-lahl)

Betapace Tablets, Lopressor Tablets, Toprol XL Tablets

A medicine used to treat irregular heartbeats.

Precautions

DO NOT USE if you are allergic to this medicine; if you have bronchial asthma, bronchospasm, certain heart disorders or if you are breastfeeding.

BEFORE USING THIS MEDICINE, tell your healthcare provider if you are pregnant or breastfeeding; or if you are taking, will be taking or stop taking any prescription or nonprescription medicine; or if you have any other medical conditions.

Side Effects

Every medicine can cause side effects, but many people have no, or minor, side effects. Tell your healthcare provider if any of the following occurs: difficulty breathing, especially on exertion or when lying down; night cough; swelling of the extremities; slow pulse rate; dizziness; confusion or depression; rash; fever; sore throat; unusual bleeding or bruising.

Guidelines for Use

USE EXACTLY AS PRESCRIBED.

Take consistently with or without food at the same time each day.

Use caution while driving or performing other tasks requiring mental alertness.

Do not discontinue use of this medicine without consulting your healthcare provider.

Diabetes: These products can mask signs of hypoglycemia (low blood sugar) and alter blood sugar levels. It may be necessary for your healthcare provider to alter your dose of diabetic medications while taking this medicine.

Sustained release: Do not crush or chew.

Metronidazole Gel

(meh-troe-NID-uh-zole)

MetroGel

A medicine used to treat inflammatory papules, pustules and erythema of acne rosacea. It occasionally may be prescribed for other reasons.

Precautions

DO NOT USE if you are allergic to this medicine or if you are in the first trimester (13 weeks) of pregnancy. Safety and effectiveness in children have not been established.

Breastfeeding — A nursing mother should express and discard any breast milk produced while using this medicine and resume breastfeeding 24 to 48 hours after the medicine is stopped.

BEFORE USING THIS MEDICINE, tell your healthcare provider if you are pregnant or breastfeeding; or if you are taking, will be taking or stop taking any prescription or nonprescription medicine; or if you have any other medical conditions.

Side Effects

Every medicine can cause side effects, but many people have no, or minor, side effects. Tell your healthcare provider if any of the following occurs: tearing of the eyes (if medicine is applied too close to the eye); redness; mild dryness, burning or irritation of the skin.

Guidelines for Use

USE EXACTLY AS PRESCRIBED.

For external use only. Avoid contact with the eyes.

Wash area before application. Rub on a thin film twice daily. Results should be seen within three weeks.

Avoid alcoholic beverages while using this medicine.

Metronidazole Systemic

(meh-troe-NID-uh-zole)

Flagyl, Metro I.V., Protostat

A medicine used to treat serious infections caused by susceptible bacteria. These infections may include: abdominal infections (peritonitis, abscess, liver abscess); skin and skin structure infections; gynecologic infections; meningitis and brain abscess. It also is used to treat amebiasis and trichomoniasis (protozoal infections). It occasionally may be prescribed for other reasons.

Precautions

DO NOT USE if you are allergic to this medicine or if you are in the first trimester (13 weeks) of pregnancy.

Breastfeeding — A nursing mother should express and discard any breast milk produced while on this medicine and resume breastfeeding 24 to 48 hours after the medicine is stopped.

BEFORE USING THIS MEDICINE, tell your healthcare provider if you are pregnant or breastfeeding; or if you are taking, will be taking or stop taking any prescription or nonprescription medicine; or if you have any other medical conditions.

Side Effects

Every medicine can cause side effects, but many people have no, or minor, side effects. Tell your healthcare provider if any of the following occurs: nausea; vomiting; appetite loss; diarrhea; stomach ache; constipation; seizures; vertigo (feeling or whirling motion); depression; lack of coordination; confusion; irritability; weakness; inability to sleep; headache; rash; hives; flushing; dry mouth; joint pain; metallic taste; nasal congestion; painful and frequent urination; darkened urine; tingling in hands and feet.

Guidelines for Use

USE EXACTLY AS PRESCRIBED.

May cause stomach upset. Take with food.

Avoid alcoholic beverages. Do not consume alcohol for at least one full day after therapy is stopped.

Some patients report a metallic taste while taking this medicine. This is not cause for alarm and disappears when therapy is stopped.

During treatment for trichomoniasis, refrain from sexual intercourse or use a condom to avoid reinfection. Sexual partners of patients with trichomoniasis should be treated simultaneously, whether they have symptoms or not.

Metronidazole Vaginal

(meh-troe-NID-uh-zole)

MetroGel Vaginal Gel

A medicine used to treat bacterial vaginosis.

Precautions

DO NOT USE if you are allergic to this medicine or if you are in the first trimester (13 weeks) of pregnancy or if you are taking disulfiram.

Breastfeeding — A nursing mother should express and discard any breast milk produced while on this medicine and resume breastfeeding 24 to 48 hours after the medicine is stopped.

BEFORE USING THIS MEDICINE, tell your healthcare provider if you are pregnant or breastfeeding; or if you are taking, will be taking or stop taking any prescription or nonprescription medicine; or if you have any other medical conditions.

Side Effects

Every medicine can cause side effects, but many people have no, or minor, side effects. Tell your healthcare provider if any of the following occurs: tearing of the eyes (if medicine is applied too close to the eye); redness; mild dryness, burning or irritation of the skin; cramps; abdominal pain; change in white blood cell count.

Guidelines for Use

USE EXACTLY AS PRESCRIBED.

Avoid contact with the eyes.

Patient instructions are included with product.

Insert high into the vagina (with applicator provided). Use of an applicator may not be recommended during pregnancy.

Use only on the advice of your healthcare provider. Complete full course of therapy.

Do not engage in vaginal sexual intercourse during treatment.

Mexiletine Hydrochloride

(MEX-ih-leh-teen HIGH-droe-KLOR-ide)

Mexitil

A heart medicine that is used to correct or prevent various types of irregular heartbeats.

Precautions

DO NOT USE if you are allergic to this medicine.

BEFORE USING THIS MEDICINE, tell your healthcare provider if you are pregnant or breastfeeding; or if you are taking, will be taking or stop taking any prescription or nonprescription medicine; or if you have any other medical conditions.

Side Effects

Every medicine can cause side effects, but many people have no, or minor, side effects. Tell your healthcare provider if any of the following occurs: nausea; vomiting; heartburn; stomach pain; constipation or diarrhea; dizziness; tremor; lightheadedness; nervousness; confusion; coordination difficulties; headache; tingling or numbness; changes in sleep habits; weakness; fatigue; depression; pounding in the chest; chest pain; joint pain or stiffness; dry mouth; fever; vision problems; ringing in the ears; speech difficulties; rash; uncomfortable or painful breathing.

Guidelines for Use

USE EXACTLY AS PRESCRIBED.

Do not discontinue therapy unless instructed by your healthcare provider.

Take this medication at evenly spaced intervals around the clock.

Take medication with food or an antacid.

Notify your healthcare provider if unexplained general tiredness, yellowing of the skin or eyes, fever or sore throat occurs.

Avoid changes in diet that could drastically acidify or alkalinize the urine.

Mezlocillin Sodium

(MEZZ-low-SILL-in SO-dee-uhm)

Mezlin

An antibiotic used to treat severe infections.

Precautions

DO NOT USE if you are allergic to any penicillins.

BEFORE USING THIS MEDICINE, tell your healthcare provider if you are pregnant or breastfeeding; if you are taking, will be taking or stop taking any prescription or nonprescription medicine; or if you have any other medical conditions.

Side Effects

Every medicine can cause side effects, but many people have no, or minor, side effects. Tell your healthcare provider if any of the following occurs: pain/irritation at the injection site; fatigue; prolonged muscle relaxation; convulsions and seizures; nausea; vomiting; diarrhea; rash; itching; fever; difficulty breathing; change in taste.

Guidelines for Use

USE EXACTLY AS PRESCRIBED.

If symptoms of an allergic reaction develop (eg, difficulty breathing, facial swelling, rash, itching), stop taking this medicine and contact your healthcare provider.

If a dose is missed, inject it as soon as possible. If several hours have passed or if it is nearing time for the next dose, do not double the dose to "catch up," unless advised by your healthcare provider. If more than one dose is missed, contact your healthcare provider.

Continue to take until all of the prescribed medicine is gone. Failure to take all of the medicine may prevent complete elimination of bacteria, causing the infection to return.

Miconazole

(my-KAHN-uh-zole)

Micatin, Micatin Liquid, Monistat i.v., Monistat-Derm,

Vaginal: used to treat vaginal yeast infections. Topical: used to treat athlete's foot; tinea cruris (jock itch) and tinea corporis (ringworm); cutaneous candidiasis (moniliasis); tinea versicolor. Injectable: used to treat severe fungal infections.

Precautions

DO NOT USE if you have an allergy to this medicine.

BEFORE USING THIS MEDICINE, tell your healthcare provider if you are pregnant or breastfeeding; or if you are taking, will be taking or stop taking any prescription or nonprescription medicine; or if you have any other medical conditions.

Side Effects

Every medicine can cause side effects, but many people have no, or minor, side effects. Tell your healthcare provider if any of the following occurs: nausea; vomiting; diarrhea; loss of appetite; fever and chills; drowsiness; headache; body aches; local irritation and burning; irritation at the injection site; burning; itching; sensitivity to light; foul smelling vaginal discharge; rash; hives.

Guidelines for Use

USE EXACTLY AS PRESCRIBED.

Vaginal: Patient instructions for proper use are enclosed in each package.

Complete a full course of therapy.

Keep using, even during your menstrual period.

If a dose is missed contact your healthcare provider for instructions.

If the medicine causes burning or irritation, or if symptoms worsen, contact your healthcare provider.

Refrain from sexual intercourse during treatment. The base in this formulation may interact with (weaken) certain latex products such as condoms or diaphragms. This interaction could last up to 72 hours. Do not rely on condoms or diaphragms to prevent pregnancy or sexually transmitted diseases.

A sanitary napkin or mini-pad may be used to prevent staining of clothing due to seepage or leakage. Do not use tampons.

If infection recurs, see your healthcare provider, as other factors may be involved. Factors that increase the risk of infection include AIDS, diabetes, chronic antibiotic therapy, pregnancy, steroid use and oral contraceptive use.

Topical: For external use only.

If condition worsens, or if irritation (burning, itching, stinging, redness) occurs, discontinue use and notify your healthcare provider.

Use for full treatment time, even if symptoms improve.

Tell your healthcare provider if there is no improvement after 2 weeks (candida infections, tinea cruris and corporis) or 4 weeks (tinea pedis).

For best results: Follow instructions exactly; wear cotton underwear and loose clothing; dry vaginal area thoroughly after bathing; wipe away from the vagina after bowel movements or urination; do not douche; do not scratch area.

If your partner experiences penile itching, redness, or discomfort, he should contact his healthcare provider and mention that you are using this medication.

Milk of Magnesia (Magnesia, Magnesium Hydroxide)

(milk of mag-NEE-zhuh)

Phillip's Milk of Magnesia

Used to treat upset stomach due to too much acid secretion (eg, heartburn, acid indigestion and sour stomach); to treat irritation of the stomach associated with peptic ulcers. It may occasionally be prescribed for other reasons.

Precautions

DO NOT USE if you have kidney disease.

BEFORE USING THIS MEDICINE, tell your healthcare provider if you are pregnant or breastfeeding; or if you are taking, will be taking or stop taking any prescription or nonprescription medicine; or if you have any other medical conditions.

Side Effects

Every medicine can cause side effects, but many people have no, or minor, side effects. Tell your healthcare provider if any of the following occurs: nausea; vomiting; stomach pain; diarrhea; muscular weakness; lack of energy; headache; confusion; irritability.

Guidelines for Use

USE EXACTLY AS PRESCRIBED.

Antacids reduce acidity for about 30 minutes when taken on an empty stomach. Acidity is reduced for about 3 hours when antacids are taken 1 hour after meals.

Do not take other medications within 1 to 2 hours of taking this medicine.

Tell your healthcare provider if coffee-ground vomiting or black, tar-like stools occur.

Taking too much of these products can cause the stomach to secrete excess stomach acid. Talk to your healthcare provider about the appropriate dose.

Long-term use—Do not take for longer than 2 weeks for the relief of indigestion. If discomfort continues, talk to your healthcare provider.

Chewable tablets—Chew thoroughly before swallowing. Follow with a glass of water.

Liquids—Shake well before using. Refrigeration of liquid antacids may improve the flavor (avoid freezing).

If the taste of one antacid product is not satisfactory, talk to your healthcare provider about switching to another product.

Minocycline

(min-oh-SIGH-kleen)

Dynacin, Minocin, Minocin IV

An anti-infection medicine used to treat infections caused by certain bacteria.

Precautions

DO NOT USE if you are allergic to this medicine or its relatives; if you are pregnant; in children under 8 years of age; or if the medicine is out of date.

BEFORE USING THIS MEDICINE, tell your healthcare provider if you are pregnant or breastfeeding; or if you are taking, will be taking or stop taking any prescription or nonprescription medicine; or if you have any other medical conditions.

Side Effects

Every medicine can cause side effects, but many people have no, or minor, side effects. Tell your healthcare provider if any of the following occurs: headache; lightheadedness; dizziness; nausea; diarrhea; vaginal infections; vomiting; visual disturbances.

Guidelines for Use

USE EXACTLY AS PRESCRIBED.

Take with a full glass of water or other fluid, with or without meals.

Avoid use with antacids, laxatives, dairy products or iron-containing products.

If an antacid must be taken, take 2 to 3 hours before or after this medicine.

If a dose is missed, take it as soon as possible. If several hours have passed or if it is nearing time for the next dose, do not double the dose to "catch up," unless advised by your healthcare provider. If more than one dose is missed, contact your healthcare provider .

Continue to take until all the prescribed medicine is gone. Failure to take all of the medicine may prevent complete elimination of bacteria, causing the infection to return.

May cause sensitivity to sunlight. Avoid prolonged exposure to the sun and other ultraviolet light. Use sunscreens and wear protective clothing until tolerance is determined.

Do not use outdated medicine since it may be highly toxic.

May cause lightheadedness or dizziness. Use caution while driving or performing other tasks requiring mental alertness, coordination and dexterity.

Minoxidil Oral

(min-OX-ih-dill)

Loniten

A medicine used to treat high blood pressure.

Precautions

DO NOT USE if you are allergic to this medicine.

BEFORE USING THIS MEDICINE, tell your healthcare provider if you are pregnant or breastfeeding; or if you are taking, will be taking or stop taking any prescription or nonprescription medicine; or if you have any other medical conditions.

Side Effects

Every medicine can cause side effects, but many people have no, or minor, side effects. Tell your healthcare provider if any of the following occurs: rash; nausea; vomiting; dizziness, lightheadedness or fainting when rising from a lying or sitting position; fatigue; unusual hair growth.

Guidelines for Use

USE EXACTLY AS PRESCRIBED.

Do not take more often than prescribed or increase the dosage unless directed by your healthcare provider. Do not stop taking this medicine unless directed by your healthcare provider.

If a dose is missed, take it as soon as possible. If several hours have passed or if it is nearing time for the next dose, do not double the dose to "catch up," unless advised by your healthcare provider. If more than one dose is missed, contact your healthcare provider.

Notify your healthcare provider if any of the following occurs: rapid heart rate; rapid weight gain of greater than 5 pounds; unusual swelling of the legs, face or abdomen; or difficulty breathing (especially when lying down).

Dizziness or lightheadedness when rising quickly from a seated or lying position may occur. Avoid sudden changes in posture.

Hypertension (high blood pressure) is a long-term or life-long disease. This medicine is not a cure for high blood pressure, but helps to control it. Do not stop taking or change your dose, even if you feel well, without your doctor's consent. It is important not to miss any doses, and to follow your healthcare provider's instructions to monitor your condition at home. You may be asked to monitor your diet, weight or sodium intake.

Minoxidil, Topical

(min-OX-ih-dill)

Loniten, Rogaine

A scalp medicine generally used to treat male pattern baldness and female hair loss or thinning.

Precautions

DO NOT USE if you are allergic to this medicine.

BEFORE USING THIS MEDICINE, tell your healthcare provider if you are pregnant or breastfeeding; or if you are taking, will be taking or stop taking any prescription or nonprescription medicine or if you have any other medical conditions.

Side Effects

Every medicine can cause side effects, but many people have no, or minor, side effects. Tell your healthcare provider if any of the following occurs: bronchitis; upper respiratory infection; sinusitis; skin irritation; vomiting; diarrhea; headache; dizziness; swelling; vision changes; weight gain.

Guidelines for Use

USE EXACTLY AS PRESCRIBED.

For external use only. Avoid contact with the eyes.

Specific instructions for use should come with this medicine.

Apply 1 ml to the area of desired hair growth 2 times daily. If applied with fingertips, wash hands afterwards.

First hair growth may be soft, downy, colorless and barely visible. After further treatment, the new hair should be the color and thickness of other scalp hair.

Apply to a healthy scalp only. Damaged scalp skin (eg, scrapes, sunburn) may increase absorption of the medicine and increase the risk of side effects.

Contains alcohol—may cause burning or irritation of sensitive skin, eyes and mucous membranes; if contact occurs, bathe the area with large amounts of cool tap water.

Do not use with other topical scalp medications.

At least 4 months of continuous use generally is required before hair growth is seen and continues through 1 year of treatment.

The new hair growth is not permanent; stopping treatment will lead to hair loss within a few months. If one or two daily applications are missed, restart twice-daily applications and return to the usual schedule. Do not make up for missed applications.

Avoid inhalation of the spray mist. Accidental oral ingestion could produce significant side effects.

Misoprostol

(MY-so-PRAHST-ole)

Cytotec

An anti-ulcer medicine used to prevent the formation of stomach ulcers in patients who are taking nonsteroidal anti-inflammatory drugs, including aspirin.

Precautions

DO NOT USE if you are allergic to this medicine or its relatives; or if you are pregnant.

Children: Safety and effectiveness in patients under 18 have not been established.

Elderly: The dose should be reduced if it is not well tolerated.

Women: This medicine may cause miscarriage and bleeding of the uterus.

BEFORE USING THIS MEDICINE, tell your healthcare provider if you are pregnant or breastfeeding; or if you are taking, will be taking or stop taking any prescription or nonprescription medicine; or if you have any other medical conditions.

Side Effects

Every medicine can cause side effects, but many people have no, or minor, side effects. Tell your healthcare provider if any of the following occurs: diarrhea; nausea; vomiting; constipation; abdominal pain; gas; indigestion; menstrual irregularities; painful menstruation; vaginal bleeding or spotting; headache.

Guidelines for Use

USE EXACTLY AS PRESCRIBED.

Contraceptive measures (birth control) are recommended during therapy.

If a dose is missed, take it as soon as possible. If several hours have passed or if it is nearing time for the next dose, do not double the dose to "catch up," unless advised by your healthcare provider. If more than one dose is missed, contact your healthcare provider.

Diarrhea may occur early in the course of therapy. It may be minimized by taking after meals and at bedtime.

Discontinue the medicine and tell your healthcare provider immediately if pregnancy is suspected. This medicine produces contractions of the uterus that may cause a miscarriage.

Avoid magnesium-containing antacids.

Mitomycin

(MY-toe-MY-sin)

Mutamycin

Used for the treatment for cancer of the stomach or pancreas. It may occasionally be prescribed for other reasons.

Precautions

DO NOT USE if you are pregnant.

Side Effects

Every medicine can cause side effects, but many people have no, or minor, side effects. Tell your healthcare provider if any of the following occurs: irritation at the injection site; hair loss; fever; loss of appetite; nausea; vomiting; headache; blurred vision; confusion; drowsiness; fainting; diarrhea; pain; difficulty breathing; infection; inflammation of the mouth; weakness; swelling of the lower legs.

Guidelines for Use

USE EXACTLY AS PRESCRIBED.

Inform your healthcare provider if you are pregnant, become pregnant, are planning to become pregnant; or if you are breastfeeding.

This medicine may lower your body's ability to fight infection. Notify your healthcare provider of any signs of infection including fever, sore throat, rash or chills.

Lab testing is required during therapy. Be sure to keep appointments.

Mitotane

(MY-toe-TANE)

Lysodren

A medicine used to treat inoperable cancer of the adrenal gland.

Precautions

DO NOT USE if you are allergic to this medicine.

Long-term use: Continuous use may lead to brain and nervous system damage. Talk with your healthcare provider.

BEFORE USING THIS MEDICINE, tell your healthcare provider if you are pregnant or breastfeeding; or if you are taking, will be taking or stop taking any prescription or nonprescription medicine; or if you have any other medical conditions.

Side Effects

Every medicine can cause side effects, but many people have no, or minor, side effects. Tell your healthcare provider if any of the following occurs: joint and muscle aches/pain; muscle twitching; darkening of the skin; headache; appetite loss; diarrhea; nausea; vomiting; dizziness; drowsiness; disorders of consciousness; general body discomfort; sleep problems; fatigue; depression; feeling of whirling motion; skin disorders; hot flashes; abnormal vision; blood in urine; fever.

Guidelines for Use

USE EXACTLY AS PRESCRIBED.

Birth control measures are recommended during therapy with this medicine. Tell your healthcare provider immediately if you suspect pregnancy.

May cause drowsiness or dizziness. Use caution while driving or performing other tasks requiring mental alertness, coordination or dexterity.

If a dose is missed, take it as soon as possible. If several hours have passed or if it is nearing time for the next dose, do not double the dose to "catch up," unless advised by your healthcare provider. If more than one dose is missed, contact your healthcare provider.

Notify your healthcare provider if nausea, vomiting, appetite loss, diarrhea, mental depression or skin rash or darkening of skin occurs.

Medication may cause muscle aches, fever, flushing or muscle twitching; contact your healthcare provider if these become pronounced.

Storage--Store in tight, light-resistant container at room temperature.

Mitoxantrone Hydrochloride

(MY-toe-ZAN-trone HIGH-droe-KLOR-ide)

Novantrone

Used in combination with other medicines for the treatment of certain types of leukemia. It may occasionally be prescribed for other reasons.

Side Effects

Every medicine can cause side effects, but many people have no, or minor, side effects. Tell your healthcare provider if any of the following occurs: nausea; vomiting; diarrhea; stomach pain; yellowing of the skin or eyes; cough; difficulty breathing; seizures; headache; eye irritation; fever; hair loss; black/bloody stools; inflammation of the mouth; difficult/painful urination; pain at injection site.

Guidelines for Use

USE EXACTLY AS PRESCRIBED.

This medicine may turn the urine blue-green in color for 24 hours after administration. A bluish discoloration to eyeball might develop.

This medicine may lower your body's ability to fight infection. Notify your healthcare provider of any signs of infection including fever, sore throat, rash or chills.

Moexipril Hydrochloride

(moe-EX-ah-pril HIGH-droe-KLOR-ide)

Univasc

An angiotensin converting enzyme (ACE) inhibitor medicine used to treat high blood pressure in adults.

Precautions

DO NOT USE if you have a history of angioedema (throat or tongue swelling with difficult breathing), are allergic to this medicine or other ACE inhibitors, or are pregnant.

BEFORE USING THIS MEDICINE, tell your healthcare provider if you are pregnant or breastfeeding; or if you are taking, will be taking or stop taking any prescription or nonprescription medicine; or if you have any other medical conditions.

Side Effects

Every medicine can cause side effects, but many people have no, or minor, side effects. Tell your healthcare provider if any of the following occurs: increased cough; dizziness; diarrhea; flu syndrome; fatigue; sore throat; flushing; rash; muscle or chest pain; headache; pain; nasal congestion; runny nose; indigestion; nausea; swelling of the arms or legs; sinus infection; changes in urinary frequency.

Guidelines for Use

USE EXACTLY AS PRESCRIBED.

Take one tablet 1 hour before meal, once daily. Dosage may need to be adjusted by your healthcare provider depending upon your response.

If a dose is missed, take it as soon as possible. If several hours have passed or if it is nearing time for the next dose, do not double the dose to "catch up," unless advised by your healthcare provider. If more than one dose is missed, contact your healthcare provider.

This medicine can cause damage to a developing fetus, especially in the second and third trimester. Contact your healthcare provider immediately if you are pregnant or plan to become pregnant.

The effects of this medicine may decrease toward the end of the dosing interval.

Take your blood pressure just prior to taking this medicine. If your blood pressure is not satisfactory, contact your healthcare provider, a dosage adjustment may be required.

Inform your healthcare provider if you are taking any type of diuretic. Taking this medicine along with a diuretic can cause low blood pressure. A dosage adjustment may be required.

Contact your healthcare provider immediately and stop taking this medicine if any of the following occurs: swelling of the face, arms, legs, eyes, lips or tongue, difficulty breathing, signs of infection (eg, sore throat, fever).

This medicine can cause lightheadedness, fainting or dizziness especially during the first few days of treatment. Avoid sudden changes in posture. If you faint, stop taking the medicine and contact your healthcare provider. Excessive sweating, dehydration, vomiting and diarrhea also can cause low blood pressure. Contact your healthcare provider if any of these occur.

Do not take potassium supplements or salt substitutes containing potassium without checking with your healthcare provider first.

A persistent, dry, nonproductive cough may occur. Tell your healthcare provider if this occurs. Recovery is rapid when the medicine is stopped.

Store at room temperature in a tightly-closed container away from moisture.

Mometasone Furoate

(moe-MET-uh-SONE- FYU-roh-ate)

Elocon Cream, Elocon Lotion, Elocon Ointment

A topical anti-inflammatory agent used to treat rash or skin irritation.

Precautions

DO NOT USE near eyes or eyelids or if you have an allergy to this medicine.

BEFORE USING THIS MEDICINE, tell your healthcare provider if you are pregnant or breastfeeding; or if you are taking, will be taking or stop taking any prescription or nonprescription medicine; or if you have any other medical conditions.

Side Effects

Every medicine can cause side effects, but many people have no, or minor, side effects. Tell your healthcare provider if any of the following occurs: burning; itching; irritation; redness; dryness; acne; streaks in skin; stinging and cracking; elevated blood sugar; cataracts and glaucoma (prolonged use near eyes); numbness of fingers.

Guidelines for Use

USE EXACTLY AS PRESCRIBED.

Apply sparingly as a thin film. Rub in lightly.

Wash or soak the affected area before application as this may increase medicine penetration.

Avoid contact with the eyes.

Avoid prolonged use, especially near the eyes, on the face, on genital and rectal areas, and in skin folds.

Do not use tight-fitting diapers or plastic pants on children being treated in the diaper area.

Do not wrap the treated area with bandages or tight-fitting clothing unless specifically directed by your physician. Skin infections may worsen.

It may be necessary to stop the corticosteroid and treat the infection.

Skin wasting may occur in 3 to 4 weeks.

Do not mix these products with other products. Allergic reactions may occur.

If the condition being treated gets worse or irritation, burning, redness, swelling or stinging persists, do not reapply the medicine. Contact your healthcare provider.

Alcohol-containing preparations may cause drying, burning or irritation of open lesions.

Morphine

(MORE-feen)

Astromorph, Duramorph, MS Contin Timed Release Tablets, MSIR Solution, Oramorph SR Timed Release Tablets, RMS Suppositories, Roxanol SR Timed Release Tablets, Roxanol UD Solution, Roxanol 100

A narcotic pain reliever used for moderate to severe pain.

Precautions

DO NOT USE if you are allergic to this medicine or its relatives.

BEFORE USING THIS MEDICINE, tell your healthcare provider if you are pregnant or breastfeeding; or if you are taking, will be taking or stop taking any prescription or nonprescription medicine; if you have any other medical conditions; or if you are allergic to sulfites. Long-term, regular use of narcotic pain relievers may lead to dependence and physical tolerance. Withdrawal symptoms may occur when therapy is stopped.

Side Effects

Every medicine can cause side effects, but many people have no, or minor, side effects. Tell your healthcare provider if any of the following occurs: lightheadedness; dizziness; drowsiness; nausea; vomiting; sweating; abdominal pain; cramps; constipation; diarrhea; urine retention; appetite loss; indigestion; gas; excitability; vision problems; difficulty breathing.

Guidelines for Use

USE EXACTLY AS PRESCRIBED.

Take with food if stomach upset occurs.

May cause drowsiness, dizziness or blurred vision. Use caution while driving or performing other tasks requiring mental alertness, judgment and coordination.

Avoid alcohol and other medicines that cause drowsiness (eg, sleeping pills, antihistamines).

May cause nausea, vomiting or constipation. Constipation may be avoided by using a stool softener or fiber laxative.

This medicine works best if taken regularly. It is more effective in preventing pain than in treating pain after it occurs. Give the medicine ample time to work before taking more.

If a dose is missed, take it as soon as possible. If several hours have passed or if it is nearing time for the next dose, do not double the dose to "catch up," unless advised by your healthcare provider. If more than one dose is missed, contact your healthcare provider.

Controlled release: Do not crush or chew this medicine.

Suppositories: If you do not know the correct way to insert a suppository, ask your healthcare provider.

Mupirocin

(myoo-PIHR-oh-sin)

Bactroban

An ointment used to treat impetigo.

Precautions

DO NOT USE if you are allergic to this medicine.

BEFORE USING THIS MEDICINE, tell your healthcare provider if you are pregnant or breastfeeding; or if you are taking, will be taking or stop taking any prescription or nonprescription medicine; or if you have any other medical conditions.

Side Effects

Every medicine can cause side effects, but many people have no, or minor, side effects. Tell your healthcare provider if any of the following occurs: burning; stinging; pain; itching; rash; dry skin; tenderness; swelling; redness; nausea.

Guidelines for Use

USE EXACTLY AS PRESCRIBED.

For external use only.

Generally apply a small amount of the ointment to the affected area 3 times daily. A loose-fitting dressing may be used to cover the area. If improvement is not seen in 3 to 5 days, contact your healthcare provider.

Do not use in or near the eyes.

Muromonab-CD3

(MYOO-row-MOE-nab—CD3)

Orthoclone OKT3

Use to prevent the rejection of new organs in kidney, heart and liver transplant patients.

Side Effects

Every medicine can cause side effects, but many people have no, or minor, side effects. Tell your healthcare provider if any of the following occurs: difficulty breathing; nausea; vomiting; chest pain; diarrhea; tremor; wheezing; headache; fever; chills; flu-like symptoms; fatigue; general body discomfort; weakness; loss of appetite; muscle aches; joint pain; arthritis; stiffness; vision problems; hearing loss; ringing in the ears; feeling of a whirling motion; nasal and ear stuffiness; rash; pain at injection site.

Patient Information

Tell your healthcare provider if skin rash, hives, difficulty in swallowing and breathing or any swelling occurs.

This medicine may lower your body's ability to fight infection. Notify your healthcare provider if any signs of infection including fever, sore throat, rash or chills.

Lab tests may be required to monitor therapy. Be sure to keep appointments.

Mycophenolate Mofetil

(my-koe-FEN-oh-late MOE-feh-till)

CellCept

An immunosuppressant used to prevent kidney transplant rejection in adults. This medicine is taken along with cyclosporine and corticosteroids.

Precautions

DO NOT USE if you are allergic to this medicine, its ingredients or mycophenolic acid.

BEFORE USING THIS MEDICINE, tell your healthcare provider if you are pregnant or breastfeeding; if you are taking, will be taking or stop taking any presription or nonprescription medicine; or if you have any other medical conditions.

Side Effects

Every medicine can cause side effects, but many people have no, or minor, side effects. Tell your healthcare provider if any of the following occurs: diarrhea; nausea; vomiting; constipation; indigestion; cramps; decreased appetite; gas; swollen gums; black or bloody stools; headache; nervousness; depression; tremors; sleep changes; dizziness; weakness; blood in urine; painful urination; changes in urinary frequency; sexual difficulties; chills; fever; flushing; stomach, chest, joint, muscle or back pain; eye, mouth, sinus or skin infections; difficulty breathing; cough; sore throat; rash; hives; acne; sweating; hair changes; swelling in face, legs or arms; unusual bruising; vision changes.

Guidelines for Use

USE EXACTLY AS PRESCRIBED.

Do not open or crush capsules. Do not inhale or have skin contact with the powder in the capsules. If skin or eye contact occurs, wash thoroughly with soap and water, rinse eyes with plain water.

Take this medicine twice a day on an empty stomach (1 hour before or 2 hours after meals).

Do not take antacids at the same time as this medicine.

If a dose is missed, take it as soon as possible. If several hours have passed or if it is nearing time for the next dose, do not double the dose to "catch up," unless advised by your healthcare provider. If more than one dose is missed, contact your healthcare provider.

Female patients must use effective contraception before beginning this medicine, during therapy and for 6 weeks after therapy has stopped. Contact your doctor if you become pregnant.

This medicine increases the chances of infections, lymphomas and other malignancies, particularly of the skin. Tell your healthcare provider if any of the following occur: fever, chills, tiredness, bruising or bleeding, sore throat, mouth sores.

Lab tests will be required. Be sure to keep appointments.

Store at room temperature.

Nabumetone

(nab-YOU-meh-TONE)

Relafen

A nonsteroidal anti-inflammatory medicine (NSAID) generally used to treat osteoarthritis (degenerative joint disease) and rheumatoid arthritis. It may occasionally be prescribed for other reasons.

Precautions

DO NOT USE if you are allergic to this medicine or its relatives, aspirin or iodides.

BEFORE USING THIS MEDICINE, tell your healthcare provider if you are pregnant or breastfeeding; use alcohol chronically; are prone to fluid retention; or if you are taking, will be taking or stop taking any prescription or nonprescription medicines; or if you have any other medical conditions.

Side Effects

Every medicine can cause side effects, but many people have no, or minor, side effects. Tell your healthcare provider if any of the following occurs: allergic reaction (eg, rash, itching, fever); changes in vision; weight gain; fluid retention; stomach problems (eg, nausea, vomiting, diarrhea, pain); black stools; constipation; persistent headache; dizziness; nervousness; weakness; ringing in the ears; taste changes; unusual bruising or bleeding.

Guidelines for Use

USE EXACTLY AS PRESCRIBED.

Avoid aspirin and alcoholic beverages.

If stomach upset occurs, take with food, milk or antacids. If stomach pain continues, tell your healthcare provider.

If a dose is missed, take it as soon as possible. If several hours have passed or if it is nearing time for the next dose, do not double the dose to "catch up," unless advised by your healthcare provider. If more than one dose is missed, contact your healthcare provider.

May cause drowsiness or dizziness. Observe caution while driving or performing other tasks requiring mental alertness, coordination and dexterity.

May cause sensitivity to sunlight. Avoid prolonged exposure to the sun. Use sunscreens and wear protective clothing until tolerance is determined.

Nadolol

(nay-DOE-lahl)

Corgard

A beta blocker medicine used to lower high blood pressure and to treat angina and heart attack.

Precautions

DO NOT USE if you are allergic to this medicine or its relatives, or if you are breastfeeding.

BEFORE USING THIS MEDICINE, tell your healthcare provider if you are pregnant; or if you are taking, will be taking or stop taking any prescription or nonprescription medicine; or if you have any other medical conditions.

Side Effects

Every medicine can cause side effects, but many people have no, or minor, side effects. Tell your healthcare provider if any of the following occurs: nausea; vomiting; stomach ache; diarrhea; constipation; appetite changes; indigestion; depression; anxiety; hallucinations; short-term memory loss; behavior changes; disorientation; fainting; dizziness; lightheadedness; tiredness; sleep disturbances; decreased concentration; headache; nightmares; emotional instability; changes in heart rate; chest pain; chills; cold or numb extremities; pounding in the chest; difficulty breathing; cough; nasal congestion; rash; hives; fluid retention; flushing or paleness; increased pigmentation; itching; hair loss; sweating; dry skin; psoriasis; painful and aching joints and muscles; painful, frequent or difficult urination; blurred vision; dry, burning or irritated eyes; ringing in the ears; taste changes; sore throat; dry mouth; slurred speech; fever; weight gain; changes in blood sugar levels.

Guidelines for Use

USE EXACTLY AS PRESCRIBED.

Ask your healthcare provider before using other medicines including nasal decongestants, diet aids or nonprescription cold preparations.

Do not stop this medicine suddenly, it could cause a worsening of disease including worse angina (chest pain), irregular heartbeats and increased risk of heart attack and death.

Withdraw these medications slowly over 1 to 2 weeks by gradually decreasing the dose.

Diabetes — These products can mask signs of low blood sugar and change blood sugar levels. It may be necessary for your healthcare provider to change your dose of diabetic medications.

Use caution while driving or performing other tasks requiring mental alertness, coordination and dexterity.

Nafarelin Acetate

(NAFF-uh-RELL-in ASS-uh-TATE)

Synarel

A hormone that is used for the management of endometriosis in women 18 years and older for a period not to exceed 6 consecutive months of therapy.

Precautions

DO NOT USE if you are allergic to this medicine or its relatives, are pregnant or may become pregnant during therapy or if you are breastfeeding.

BEFORE USING THIS MEDICINE, tell your healthcare provider if you are taking, will be taking or stop taking any prescription or nonprescription medicine; or if you have any other medical conditions.

Side Effects

Every medicine can cause side effects, but many people have no, or minor, side effects. Tell your healthcare provider if any of the following occurs: depression; headache; insomnia; emotional instability; acne; excessive body hair growth; excessively oily skin; weight gain or loss; fluid retention; hot flashes; vaginal dryness; decreased breast size; changes in sex drive; muscle pain; lack of menstruation.

Guidelines for Use

USE EXACTLY AS PRESCRIBED.

Treatment should begin between the second and fourth day of the menstrual period.

When used regularly at the recommended dose, this medicine usually interferes with ovulation and stops menstruation. However, use of the medicine should not be considered a reliable form of birth control. Other birth control measures (eg, condom, diaphragm) should be used during therapy.

Do not use if pregnancy is suspected.

May cause breakthrough bleeding if doses are missed. However, if regular menstruation persists, notify your healthcare provider.

If the use of a topical nasal decongestant is necessary during treatment, do not use the decongestant until at least 30 minutes after taking this medicine.

The usual course of therapy is 6 months. Retreatment is not currently recommended.

Nalbuphine Hydrochloride

(NAL-byoo-FEEN HIGH-droe-KLOR-ide)

Nubain

This medicine is used for the relief of moderate to severe pain. May be used during surgery or labor.

Side Effects

Every medicine can cause side effects, but many people have no, or minor, side effects. Tell your healthcare provider if any of the following occurs: sedation; sweaty/clammy feeling; nausea; vomiting; dizziness; feeling of a whirling motion; dry mouth; headache; pain at injection site.

Patient Information

May cause drowsiness or dizziness. Use caution while driving or performing other tasks requiring mental alertness, coordination and dexterity.

Nalidixic Acid

(nal-ih-DIK-sik acid)

NegGram

A medicine used to treat urinary tract infections caused by susceptible bacteria.

Precautions

DO NOT USE if you are allergic to this medicine or have a history of convulsive disorders.

BEFORE USING THIS MEDICINE, tell your healthcare provider if you are pregnant or breastfeeding; or if you are taking, will be taking or stop taking any prescription or nonprescription medicine; or if you have any other medical conditions.

Side Effects

Every medicine can cause side effects, but many people have no, or minor, side effects. Tell your healthcare provider if any of the following occurs: drowsiness; weakness; headache; dizziness; feeling of a whirling motion; brief convulsions; abdominal pain; nausea; vomiting; diarrhea; rash; itching; hives; visual disturbances; joint pain; abnormal skin sensations; yellowing of the skin or eyes; unusual bleeding and bruising.

Guidelines for Use

USE EXACTLY AS PRESCRIBED.

Suspension — Shake well before using.

May cause stomach upset; take with food.

This medicine may cause drowsiness, dizziness or blurred vision. Use caution while driving or performing other tasks requiring mental alertness, coordination and dexterity.

If a dose is missed, take it as soon as possible. If several hours have passed or if it is nearing time for the next dose, do not double the dose to "catch up," unless advised by your healthcare provider. If more than one dose is missed, contact your healthcare provider.

May cause sensitivity to sunlight. Avoid prolonged exposure to the sun. Use sunscreen and wear protective clothing until tolerance is determined.

If seizures, psychotic behavior (eg, hallucinations, incoherent speech, confusion) or severe headaches occur, tell your healthcare provider immediately.

Storage—Keep in tightly closed container at room temperature.

Suspension—Do not freeze.

Naproxen

(nay-PROX-ehn)

Aleve, Anaprox, EC-Naprosyn, Naprosyn

A nonsteroidal anti-inflammatory medicine (NSAID) used to relieve mild to moderate pain and inflammation and to treat osteoarthritis (degenerative joint disease), rheumatoid arthritis, spinal problems, tendinitis, bursitis, gout, symptoms of premenstrual syndrome (PMS), dysmenorrhea (cramps) and to treat juvenile rheumatoid arthritis in children over 2 years of age. It may occasionally be prescribed for other reasons.

Precautions

DO NOT USE if you are allergic to this medicine or its relatives, aspirin or iodides.

BEFORE USING THIS MEDICINE, tell your healthcare provider if you are pregnant or breastfeeding; use alcohol chronically; are prone to fluid retention; or if you are taking, will be taking or stop taking any prescription or nonprescription medicines; or have any other medical conditions.

Side Effects

Every medicine can cause side effects, but many people have no, or minor, side effects. Tell your healthcare provider if any of the following occurs: allergic reaction (eg, rash, itching, fever); changes in vision; weight gain; fluid retention; stomach problems (eg, nausea, vomiting, diarrhea, pain); black stools; constipation; persistent headache; dizziness; nervousness; weakness; ringing in the ears; taste changes; unusual bruising or bleeding; heartburn; indigestion; inflammation of the mouth; drowsiness; lightheadedness; feeling of a whirling motion; sweating; thirst; difficulty breathing; pounding in the chest.

Guidelines for Use

USE EXACTLY AS PRESCRIBED.

Avoid aspirin and alcoholic beverages.

Take with food, milk or antacids. If stomach pain occurs, tell your healthcare provider.

If a dose is missed, take it as soon as possible. If several hours have passed or if it is nearing time for the next dose, do not double the dose to "catch up," unless advised by your healthcare provider. If more than one dose is missed, contact your healthcare provider.

Do not take more than one medicine containing naproxen at one time.

May cause drowsiness or dizziness. Observe caution while driving or performing other tasks requiring mental alertness, coordination and dexterity.

May cause sensitivity to sunlight. Avoid prolonged exposure to the sun. Use sunscreens and wear protective clothing until tolerance is determined.

Delayed release: Do not crush or chew.

Oral Suspension: Shake well before using.

Store at room temperature in a tightly closed container.

Natamycin

(NAT-uh-MY-sin)

Natacyn

An ophthalmic medicine used for the treatment of fungal eye infections caused by susceptible fungi.

Precautions

DO NOT USE if you are allergic to this medicine or benzalkonium chloride.

BEFORE USING THIS MEDICINE, tell your healthcare provider if you are pregnant or breastfeeding; or if you are taking, will be taking or stop taking any prescription or nonprescription medicine; or if you have any other medical conditions.

Side Effects

Every medicine can cause side effects, but many people have no, or minor, side effects. Tell your healthcare provider if any of the following occurs: redness or swelling.

Guidelines for Use

USE EXACTLY AS PRESCRIBED.

Continue therapy for 14 to 21 days or until the fungal infection disappears. If no improvement occurs after 7 to 10 days of therapy, the infection may be caused by an organism that is not susceptible to this medicine. Consult your healthcare provider.

Tell your healthcare provider if eye pain, itching, changes in vision or a sense of foreign body in the eye occurs.

If a dose is missed, take it as soon as possible. If it is nearing time for the next dose, do not double the dose to "catch up," unless advised by your healthcare provider. If more than one dose is missed, contact your healthcare provider.

Instillation--Wash hands thoroughly before administration. Tilt head backward or lie down and gaze upward. Gently grasp lower eyelid before eyelashes and pull the eyelid away from the eye to form a pouch. Place a dropper directly over eye. Avoid contact of the dropper with the eye, finger or any surface, since this may contaminate the suspension. Look upward just before applying a drop. After instilling the drop, look downward for several seconds. Release the lid slowly. With eyes closed, apply gentle pressure with fingers to the inside corner of eye for 3 to 5 minutes. Do not rub the eye, and minimize blinking.

Do not rinse the dropper.

Do not use eye drops that have changed color.

If more than one type of ophthalmic drop is used, wait at least 5 more minutes before administering the second medicine.

Shake well before using.

Storage—Avoid exposure to sunlight and excessive heat. Store at room temperature (not more than 75 degrees) or refrigerate. Do not freeze.

Nedocromil Sodium

((NEH-doe-KROE-mill SO-dee-uhm)

Tilade

A medicine used to prevent asthma attacks.

Precautions

DO NOT USE if you are allergic to this medicine. This medicine will not relieve acute asthma attacks (bronchospasms).

BEFORE USING THIS MEDICINE, tell your healthcare provider if you are pregnant or breastfeeding; or if you are taking, will be taking or stop taking any prescription or nonprescription medicine; or if you have any other medical conditions.

Side Effects

Every medicine can cause side effects, but many people have no, or minor, side effects. Tell your healthcare provider if any of the following occurs: unpleasant taste; coughing; difficult breathing; nose or throat irritation; nausea; headache; chest pain.

Guidelines for Use

USE EXACTLY AS PRESCRIBED.

Proper inhalation technique is very important. Follow the directions that are in the patient information leaflet, which is included with the medicine.

To achieve the most benefit from this medicine, it must be taken at regular intervals on a daily basis, even during symptom-free periods. This medicine should be added to your existing treatment.

Once a positive response is made to the inhaler and the asthma is under good control, your healthcare provider may gradually reduce your other medicines.

Do not expect this medicine to work quickly. Sometimes two or more weeks of regular treatment are required before improvement in your asthma control will be noticed.

If an inhaled bronchodilator medicine also is prescribed, use it first.

Nefazodone Hydrochloride

(neff-AZE-oh-dohn HIGH-droe-KLOR-ide)

Serzone

An antidepressant medicine used to relieve mental depression in patients over 18 years of age.

Precautions

DO NOT USE if you are allergic to this medicine or other similar antidepressants (eg, *Desyrel*); or if you are using or have recently used astemizole (*Hismanal*), terfenadine (*Seldane*) or a monoamine oxidase inhibitor (MAOIs, eg, *Nardil, Parnate*).

BEFORE USING THIS MEDICINE, tell your healthcare provider if you are pregnant or breastfeeding; or if you are taking, will be taking or stop taking any prescription or nonprescription medicine; or if you have any other medical conditions.

Side Effects

Every medicine can cause side effects, but many people have no, or minor, side effects. Tell your healthcare provider if any of the following occurs: nausea; constipation; indigestion; diarrhea; appetite changes; vomiting; dizziness; sleep disorders; weakness; lightheadedness; confusion; headache; cough; runny nose; difficulty breathing; sinus infection; bronchitis; itching; rash; chills; fever; stiff neck; stomach pain; gas; tremors; anxiety; depression; chest pain; pounding in the chest; flushing; sweating; prolonged or inappropriate erections; decreased sexual drive; changes in urinary frequency; breast pain; painful menstruation; impotence; painful urination; vision problems; swelling; sore throat; ringing in the ears; eye pain; taste changes; body pain; weight gain; cramping.

Guidelines for Use

USE EXACTLY AS PRESCRIBED.

Take in two divided doses on an empty stomach, or as directed.

Do not stop or change the dose unless directed by your healthcare provider.

Notify your healthcare provider immediately if you develop a rash, hives or other type of allergic reaction.

If a dose is missed, take it as soon as possible. If several hours have passed or if it is nearing time for the next dose, do not double the dose in order to "catch up," unless advised by your healthcare provider. If more than one dose is missed, contact your healthcare provider.

Do not use in combination with MAOIs (monoamine oxidase inhibitors) or within 14 days of discontinuing treatment with an MAOI. After stopping this medicine, wait at least 1 week before starting an MAOI.

Improvement may take several weeks.

Exams may be necessary; keep appointments.

May impair judgement, thinking or motor skills. Use caution while driving or performing other tasks requiring alertness, coordination or physical dexterity until effects are known.

Avoid alcohol while using this medicine.

Store in a dry place at room temperature.

Neostigmine

(nee-oh-STIGG-meen)

Prostigmin

A medicine used to diagnose and treat myasthenia gravis and as an antidote for certain muscle relaxant medicines. It also is used for the prevention of postoperative distention and urinary retention.

Precautions

DO NOT USE if you are allergic to this medicine or any other anticholinesterase medicine.

BEFORE USING THIS MEDICINE, tell your healthcare provider if you are pregnant or breastfeeding; or if you are taking, will be taking or stop taking any prescription or nonprescription medicine; or if you have any other medical conditions.

Side Effects

Every medicine can cause side effects, but many people have no, or minor, side effects. Tell your healthcare provider if any of the following occurs: muscle cramps and spasms; muscle twitching; joint pain; tearing; blurred vision; double vision; visual changes; nausea; vomiting; diarrhea; stomach pain or cramping; gas; convulsions; loss of consciousness; dizziness; drowsiness; weakness; headache; rash; itching; hair loss; sweating; flushing; vocal problems or difficulty speaking; difficulty swallowing; uncontrolled urination; increased urination; increased saliva; difficult or painful breathing; allergic reaction.

Guidelines for Use

USE EXACTLY AS PRESCRIBED.

Close supervision by a healthcare provider is required during treatment to avoid overdosage.

Do not change the dosing schedule without consulting your healthcare provider.

Frequently, therapy is required day and night. Keep a daily record of doses and note times of greatest fatigue.

Contact your healthcare provider immediately if you experience periods of extreme muscle weakness, diarrhea or difficulty speaking or swallowing.

Niacin (Vitamin B_3)

(NYE-uh-sin)

A vitamin supplement used to correct niacin deficiency and to prevent or treat pellagra. Also used to treat high cholesterol.

Precautions

DO NOT USE if you are allergic to this medicine, have liver disease, low blood pressure, an active peptic ulcer or a bleeding disorder.

BEFORE USING THIS MEDICINE, tell your healthcare provider if you are pregnant or breastfeeding; or if you are taking, will be taking or stop taking any prescription or nonprescription medicine; or if you have any other medical conditions.

Side Effects

Every medicine can cause side effects, but many people have no, or minor, side effects. Tell your healthcare provider if any of the following occurs: nausea; vomiting; stomach ache; diarrhea; headache; restlessness; hives; itching; flushing of face, neck or chest; tingling of skin; yellowing of skin; sensation of warmth; low blood pressure; dimming of vision.

Guidelines for Use

USE EXACTLY AS PRESCRIBED.

May cause stomach upset. Take with meals.

If dizziness occurs, avoid sudden changes in posture.

Skin flushing and a sensation of warmth, especially in the area of the face, neck and ears, may occur within the first 2 hours. Itching or tingling and headache also may occur. These effects are temporary and will gradually diminish with continued therapy. If flushing is distressing or persistent, 300 mg aspirin given 30 minutes before each dose of vitamin B_3 or slow upward adjustment of dose may help relieve this reaction.

Most people on balanced diets do not need vitamin supplements. Common sources of this vitamin are chicken, steak, milk products, beans and eggs.

Nicardipine Hydrochloride Injectable

(NYE-CAR-dih-peen HIGH-droe-KLOR-ide)

Cardene IV Injection

A calcium channel blocker medicine that is used to treat high blood pressure. It may occasionally be prescribed for other reasons.

Precautions

DO NOT USE if you are allergic to this medicine.

BEFORE USING THIS MEDICINE, tell your healthcare provider if you are pregnant or breastfeeding; or if you are taking, will be taking or stop taking any prescription or nonprescription medicine; or if you have any other medical conditions.

Side Effects

Every medicine can cause side effects, but many people have no, or minor, side effects. Tell your healthcare provider if any of the following occurs: irregular heartbeat; increased frequency/severity of angina; shortness of breath; swelling of hands and feet; dizziness; constipation; nausea or low blood pressure; itching; rash; hives; difficult breathing; unusual bruising or bleeding; gum enlargement; irritation at the injection site.

Guidelines for Use

USE EXACTLY AS PRESCRIBED.

Nicardipine Hydrochloride Oral

(NYE-CAR-dih-peen HIGH-droe-KLOR-ide)

Cardene Capsules, Cardene SR Timed Release Capsules

A calcium channel blocker medicine that is used to treat high blood pressure. It may occasionally be prescribed for other reasons.

Precautions

DO NOT USE if you are allergic to this medicine.

BEFORE USING THIS MEDICINE, tell your healthcare provider if you are pregnant or breastfeeding; or if you are taking, will be taking or stop taking any prescription or nonprescription medicine; or if you have any other medical conditions.

Side Effects

Every medicine can cause side effects, but many people have no, or minor, side effects. Tell your healthcare provider if any of the following occurs: irregular heartbeat, increased frequency/severity of angina; shortness of breath; swelling of hands and feet; dizziness; constipation; nausea or low blood pressure; itching; rash; hives; difficulty breathing; unusual bruising or bleeding; gum enlargement.

Guidelines for Use

USE EXACTLY AS PRESCRIBED.

If a dose is missed, take it as soon as possible. If several hours have passed or if it is nearing time for the next dose, do not double the dose to "catch up," unless advised by your healthcare provider. If more than one dose is missed, contact your healthcare provider.

Abrupt withdrawal of calcium channel blockers may cause a withdrawal syndrome characterized by chest pains. Rebound angina (chest pain) can be minimized if the drug is slowly tapered under medical supervision.

It is important to brush and floss your teeth and see your dentist regularly.

Nicotine Gum

(NIK-oh-TEEN)

Nicorette, Nicorette DS

This medicine helps prevent physical signs of nicotine withdrawal after stopping smoking. It is a smoking deterrent to be used as part of a comprehensive behavioral smoking-cessation program.

Precautions

DO NOT USE if you are pregnant, or if you have an allergy to this medicine. This medicine can poison children. Keep this medicine out of the reach of children. It is possible to become dependent on and abuse this medicine.

BEFORE USING THIS MEDICINE, tell your healthcare provider if you are pregnant or breastfeeding; or if you are taking, will be taking or stop taking any prescription or nonprescription medicine; or if you have any other medical problems.

Side Effects

Every medicine can cause side effects, but many people have no, or minor, side effects. Tell your healthcare provider if any of the following occurs: constipation; indigestion; diarrhea; nausea; belching; excess saliva; hiccups; dizziness; nervousness; headache; insomnia; dreams; weakness (overdose); cough; sore throat; changes in taste perception; joint or muscle pain; back pain; painful menstruation; sore mouth or throat; jaw muscle ache; injury to teeth or lining of the mouth; burning; itching; redness; rash.

Guidelines for Use

USE EXACTLY AS PRESCRIBED.

Read patient information sheet carefully.

Most patients require approximately 10 to 12 pieces of gum per day during the first month of treatment.

Do not exceed 30 pieces of gum per day.

Do not start using nicotine gum until you have stopped smoking completely. It may take a few days to adjust to the unpleasant taste.

Slowly chew one piece of gum whenever there is an urge to smoke. Chew each piece slowly and intermittently for about 30 minutes. Chewing quickly can release the nicotine too rapidly, causing effects similar to oversmoking (eg, nausea, hiccups or throat irritation).

Stop using the gum or gradually withdraw after 3 months of usage and complete by 6 months.

The use of nicotine gum beyond 6 months is not recommended.

Nicotine Transdermal

(NIK-oh-TEEN)

Habitrol Transdermal System, Nicoderm Transdermal System, Nicotrol Transdermal System, ProStep Transdermal System

This medicine helps prevent physical signs of nicotine withdrawal after stopping smoking. It is a smoking deterrent to be used as part of a comprehensive behavioral smoking-cessation program.

Precautions

DO NOT USE if you are pregnant, or if you have an allergy to this medicine. This medicine can poison children. Keep this medicine out of the reach of children.

BEFORE USING THIS MEDICINE, tell your healthcare provider if you are pregnant or breastfeeding; or if you are taking, will be taking or stop taking any prescription or nonprescription medicine; or have any other medical problems.

Side Effects

Every medicine can cause side effects, but many people have no, or minor, side effects. Tell your healthcare provider if any of the following occurs: constipation; indigestion; diarrhea; nausea; belching; excess saliva; hiccups; dizziness; nervousness; headache; insomnia; dreams; weakness (overdose); burning; itching; redness; rash; cough; sore throat; changes in taste perception; joint or muscle pain; back pain; painful menstruation.

Guidelines for Use

USE EXACTLY AS PRESCRIBED.

Stop smoking completely. Do not smoke when using this medicine.

Apply promptly upon removal from the protective pouch. Use only if pouch is intact.

Apply once a day to a non-hairy, clean, dry skin site on the upper body or upper outer arm.

After removing the used system, apply a new system to an alternate skin site.

Following application or removal, wash hands with water only.

Avoid contact with eyes. Skin sites should not be reused for at least a week. Do not use the same system for more than 24 hours.

Dosage may vary. Once the appropriate dosage has been selected, continue therapy at that dosage for 4 to 8 weeks.

If you are unable to stop smoking within 4 weeks, therapy should be discontinued. Do not use for longer than 3 months after you have stopped smoking because of the harmful and addictive effects of nicotine.

Discontinue use and consult your healthcare provider if you experience severe or persistent skin reactions.

Nifedipine Capsules

(nye-FED-ih-peen)

Adalat, Procardia

A calcium channel blocker medicine that is used to treat various types of angina. It may occasionally be prescribed for other reasons.

Precautions

DO NOT USE if you are allergic to this medicine.

BEFORE USING THIS MEDICINE, tell your healthcare provider if you are pregnant or breastfeeding; or if you are taking, will be taking or stop taking any prescription or nonprescription medicine; or if you have any other medical conditions.

Side Effects

Every medicine can cause side effects, but many people have no, or minor, side effects. Tell your healthcare provider if any of the following occurs: irregular heartbeat; increased frequency/severity of angina; shortness of breath; swelling of hands and feet; dizziness; constipation; nausea; low blood pressure or symptoms of a drug allergy (eg, itching, rash, hives, difficult breathing); unusual bruising or bleeding; gum enlargement.

Guidelines for Use

USE EXACTLY AS PRESCRIBED.

Swallow whole; do not crush, divide or chew.

If a dose is missed, take it as soon as possible. If several hours have passed or if it is nearing time for the next dose, do not double the dose to "catch up," unless advised by your healthcare provider. If more than one dose is missed, contact your healthcare provider.

Do not suddenly stop taking this medicine as this may cause serious chest pains. This can be minimized if the medicine is tapered slowly by your healthcare provider.

It is important to brush and floss your teeth and see your dentist regularly.

Nifedipine Extended Release

(nye-FED-ih-peen)

Adalat CC, Nifedipine (GITS), Procardia XL

A calcium channel blocker medicine that is used to treat various types of angina and high blood pressure. It may occasionally be prescribed for other reasons.

Precautions

DO NOT USE if you are allergic to this medicine.

BEFORE USING THIS MEDICINE, tell your healthcare provider if you are pregnant or breastfeeding; or if you are taking, will be taking or stop taking any prescription or nonprescription medicines; or if you have any other medical conditions.

Side Effects

Every medicine can cause side effects, but many people have no, or minor, side effects. Tell your healthcare provider if any of the following occurs: irregular heartbeat; increased frequency/severity of angina; shortness of breath; swelling of hands and feet; dizziness; constipation; nausea; low blood pressure; symptoms of a medicine allergy (eg, itching, rash, hives, difficulty breathing); unusual bruising or bleeding; gum enlargement.

Guidelines for Use

USE EXACTLY AS PRESCRIBED.

May be taken without regard to meals.

Swallow whole; do not chew, divide or crush.

An empty tablet may appear in the stool; this is no cause for concern.

If a dose is missed, take it as soon as possible. If several hours have passed or if it is nearing time for the next dose, do not double the dose to "catch up," unless advised by your healthcare provider. If more than one dose is missed, contact your healthcare provider.

Do not suddenly stop taking this medicine as this may cause serious chest pains. This can be minimized if the medicine is tapered slowly by your healthcare provider.

It is important to brush and floss your teeth and see your dentist regularly.

Nimodipine

(NYE-MOE-dih-peen)

Nimotop

A medicine that is used to improve neurologic deficits following bleeding in the brain. It may occasionally be prescribed for other reasons.

Precautions

DO NOT USE if you are allergic to this medicine.

BEFORE USING THIS MEDICINE, tell your healthcare provider if you are pregnant or breastfeeding; or if you are taking, will be taking or stop taking any prescription or nonprescription medicine; or if you have any other medical conditions.

Side Effects

Every medicine can cause side effects, but many people have no, or minor, side effects. Tell your healthcare provider if any of the following occurs: irregular heartbeat, increased frequency/severity of angina, shortness of breath, swelling of hands and feet, dizziness, headache, flushing, diarrhea, nausea, low blood pressure or symptoms of a drug allergy (eg, itching, rash, hives, difficult breathing); unusual bleeding or bruising.

Guidelines for Use

USE EXACTLY AS PRESCRIBED.

If a dose is missed, take it as soon as possible. If several hours have passed or if it is nearing time for the next dose, do not double the dose to catch up, unless advised by your healthcare provider. If more than one dose is missed, contact your healthcare provider.

This medicine alone, and with aspirin, may cause unusual episodes of bruising or bleeding. Report these to your healthcare provider.

Nitrofurantoin

(nye-troe-FYOOR-an-toyn)

Furadantin Suspension, Furadantin Tablets, Furalan Tablets, Furan Tablets, Furanite Tablets, Macrobid Capsules, Macrodantin Capsules, Macrodantin MACPAC Capsules, Nitrofan Capsules

An anti-infective medicine used to treat urinary tract infections caused by susceptible bacteria.

Precautions

DO NOT USE if you are allergic to this medicine, or if you are a pregnant woman at term.

BEFORE USING THIS MEDICINE, tell your healthcare provider if you are pregnant or breastfeeding; or if you are taking, will be taking or stop taking any prescription or nonprescription medicine; or if you have any other medical conditions.

Side Effects

Every medicine can cause side effects, but many people have no, or minor, side effects. Tell your healthcare provider if any of the following occurs: vomiting; appetite loss; stomach ache; diarrhea; headache; dizziness; drowsiness; seizures; cough; difficulty breathing; rash; itching; chills; chest pain; fever; joint pain; muscle aches or weakness; tingling or numbness in hands or feet; fluid retention; yellowing of skin or eyes.

Guidelines for Use

USE EXACTLY AS PRESCRIBED.

Take with food or milk.

Contact your healthcare provider immediately if numbness or tingling in feet or hands, muscle weakness, seizures or paralysis occurs.

A harmless brownish discoloration of the urine may occur.

Take the full course of therapy. Do not stop therapy unless told to do so by your healthcare provider.

Report chest pain, difficulty breathing, chills, fever and cough to your healthcare provider. These side effects tend to disappear soon after the medicine is stopped. If these side effects occur once, they will probably occur again if therapy is resumed. Tell your healthcare provider if you have experienced this reaction to this medicine in the past.

Contact your healthcare provider if rash, yellowing of skin or eyes, or severe stomach upset occurs.

Oral suspension: Shake well before using.

Nitroglycerin Oral

(nye-troe-GLIH-suh-rin)

Nitro-Bid SR Capsules, Nitrocine SR Capsules, Nitrogard Buccal Controlled Release Tablets, Nitroglyn SR Capsules, Nitrolingual Spray, Nitrong SR Tablets, Nitrostat Sublingual Tablets

A medicine generally used to prevent angina attacks and may be taken before events or activities that are likely to cause an angina attack.

Precautions

DO NOT USE if you are allergic to this medicine or its relatives.

BEFORE USING THIS MEDICINE, tell your healthcare provider if you are pregnant or breastfeeding; or if you are taking, will be taking or stop taking any prescription or nonprescription medicines; or have any other medical conditions.

Side Effects

Every medicine can cause side effects, but many people have no, or minor, side effects. Tell your healthcare provider if any of the following occurs: severe or persistent headaches; blurred vision; dry mouth; dizziness; flushing.

Guidelines for Use

USE EXACTLY AS PRESCRIBED.

Do not crush or chew this medicine. Follow your healthcare provider's instructions on the proper use of your medicine.

Excessive dosages may produce severe headaches. Lower doses and pain medications can help control this problem. Headaches tend to become less severe or disappear as therapy continues.

The effectiveness of nitrate therapy may decrease over time as tolerance develops. If this occurs, tell your healthcare provider.

Transient dizziness or weakness can occur when arising from a seated or lying position. Avoid sudden changes in posture.

Alcohol can worsen this effect. Recovery can be hastened by putting the head lower than the heart, or by deep breathing and moving the arms and legs.

Keep in the original container. Store at room temperature. Do not use after the expiration date. Protect from moisture.

Unused tablets should be discarded 6 months after the original bottle is opened.

Nitroglycerin Topical

(nye-troe-GLIH-suh-rin)

Deponit, Minitran, Nitro-Bid, Nitrodisc, Nitro-Dur, Nitrol, Transderm-Nitro

A medicine generally used to prevent angina attacks and may be taken before events or activities that are likely to cause an angina attack.

Precautions

DO NOT USE if you are allergic to this medicine or its relatives.

BEFORE USING THIS MEDICINE, tell your healthcare provider if you are pregnant or breastfeeding; or if you are taking, will be taking or stop taking any prescription or nonprescription medicines; or have any other medical conditions.

Side Effects

Every medicine can cause side effects, but many people have no, or minor, side effects. Tell your healthcare provider if any of the following occurs: severe or persistent headaches; blurred vision; dry mouth; dizziness; flushing.

Guidelines for Use

USE EXACTLY AS PRESCRIBED.

Patient instructions are provided with this product.

Excessive dosages may produce severe headaches. Lower doses and pain medications can help control this problem. Headaches tend to become less severe or disappear as therapy continues.

The effectiveness of nitrate therapy may decrease over time as tolerance develops. If this occurs, tell your healthcare provider.

Transient dizziness or weakness can occur when arising from a seated or lying position. Avoid sudden posture changes.

Alcohol can worsen this effect. Recovery can be hastened by putting the head lower than the heart, or by deep breathing and moving the arms and legs.

Nizatidine

(nye-ZAT-ih-deen)

Axid

An anti-ulcer medicine used to treat stomach and duodenal (upper small intestine) ulcers, and gastroesophageal reflux disease (GERD, or the bubbling of stomach contents into the food pipe, which causes heartburn). It may occasionally be prescribed for other reasons.

Precautions

DO NOT USE if you are allergic to this medicine, cimetidine, ranitidine or famotidine.

BEFORE USING THIS MEDICINE, tell your healthcare provider if you are pregnant or breastfeeding; or if you are taking, will be taking or stop taking any prescription or nonprescription medicine; or if you have any other medical conditions.

Side Effects

Every medicine can cause side effects, but many people have no, or minor, side effects. Tell your healthcare provider if any of the following occurs: headache; nausea; diarrhea; dizziness; joint pain; behavioral changes; rash; itching; unusual bleeding or bruising; sore throat; difficulty breathing; shortness of breath; fever; sleep disturbances.

Guidelines for Use

USE EXACTLY AS PRESCRIBED.

Take without regard to meals.

May be taken with antacids, if needed.

If a dose is missed, take it as soon as possible. If several hours have passed or if it is nearing time for the next dose, do not double the dose to "catch up," unless advised by your healthcare provider. If more than one dose is missed, contact your healthcare provider.

It may be necessary to make significant lifestyle changes to assist in the treatment and prevention of ulcers and other digestive problems that can include stress-reduction programs, exercise and dietary changes.

Notify your healthcare provider if there are any symptoms that suggest a bleeding ulcer, such as black, tarry stools or coffee-ground vomit.

Never self-diagnose or self-treat ulcers with this or any other medicine.

Lab tests or exams may be required. Be sure to keep appointments.

Store at room temperature.

Norfloxacin

(nor-FLOX-uh-SIN)

Chibroxin, Noroxin

A quinolone antibiotic medicine used to treat certain urinary tract infections or gonorrhea.

Precautions

DO NOT USE if you are allergic to this medicine or any of its relatives.

BEFORE USING THIS MEDICINE, tell your healthcare provider if you are pregnant or breastfeeding; or if you are taking, will be taking or stop taking any prescription or nonprescription medicine; or if you have any other medical conditions.

Side Effects

Every medicine can cause side effects, but many people have no, or minor, side effects. Tell your healthcare provider if any of the following occurs: nausea; rash; hives; itching; diarrhea; difficulty breathing; wheezing; dizziness; headache; or other signs of allergic reaction.

Guidelines for Use

USE EXACTLY AS PRESCRIBED.

Tell your healthcare provider if you suspect pregnancy.

Take on an empty stomach at least 1 hour before or 2 hours after a meal with a glass of fluid. Drink plenty of liquids.

Do not take antacids containing sucralfate (*Carafate*), or iron or zinc-containing products within 4 hours before or 2 hours after using these agents.

If a dose is missed, take it as soon as possible. If several hours have passed or if it is nearing time for the next dose, do not double the dose to "catch up," unless advised by your healthcare provider. If more than one dose is missed, contact your healthcare provider.

May cause dizziness or lightheadedness. Use caution when driving or performing other tasks requiring mental alertness, coordination or physical dexterity.

Continue use until all the prescribed medicine has been taken. Failure to take a full course of therapy may cause a relapse of the infection.

May cause sensitivity to sunlight. Avoid prolonged exposure to the sun. Use sunscreens and wear protective clothing until tolerance is determined.

Nortriptyline Hydrochloride

(nor-TRIP-tih-leen HIGH-droe-KLOR-ide)

Aventyl Hydrochloride Capsules, Aventyl Hydrochloride Liquid, Pamelor Capsules, Pamelor Solution

A tricyclic antidepressant generally used to relieve mental depression. It may occasionally be prescribed for other reasons.

Precautions

DO NOT USE if you are allergic to this medicine or its relatives, or if you are using monoamine oxidase inhibitors (MAOIs, eg, phenelzine, tranylcypromine).

BEFORE USING THIS MEDICINE, tell your healthcare provider if you are pregnant or breastfeeding; or if you are taking, will be taking or stop taking any prescription or nonprescription medicine; or if you have any other medical conditions.

Side Effects

Every medicine can cause side effects, but many people have no, or minor, side effects. Tell your healthcare provider if any of the following occurs: nausea; vomiting; dry mouth; blurred vision; dizziness; increased heart rate; impaired coordination; difficult urination; constipation; skin rash; excessive sedation; seizures; mental confusion.

Guidelines for Use

USE EXACTLY AS PRESCRIBED.

If a dose is missed, take it as soon as possible. If several hours have passed or if it is nearing time for the next dose, do not double the dose to "catch up," unless advised by your healthcare provider. If more than one dose is missed, contact your healthcare provider.

These medications may not reach full effectiveness for 2 to 3 weeks.

Using these medications with alcohol or other central nervous system depressants (eg, pain relievers, sedatives, antihistamines) may cause added drowsiness.

May cause drowsiness or blurred vision. Use caution while driving or performing other tasks requiring mental alertness, coordination and dexterity.

Symptoms of nausea, headache or fatigue may develop after abruptly stopping the medicine after long-term use.

May cause sensitivity to sunlight. Avoid prolonged exposure to the sun. Use sunscreens and wear protective clothing until tolerance is determined.

Taking these medicines at bedtime may help reduce side effects (eg, daytime drowsiness).

Nystatin Mouth and Throat

(nye-STAT-in)

Mycostatin Troche, Nilstat, Nystat

A medicine used to treat oral fungal infections (thrush) due to Candida species (yeast).

Precautions

DO NOT USE if you are allergic to this medicine.

BEFORE USING THIS MEDICINE, tell your healthcare provider if you are pregnant or breastfeeding; if you are taking, will be taking or stop taking any prescription or nonprescription medicine; or if you have any other medical conditions.

Side Effects

Every medicine can cause side effects, but many people have no, or minor, side effects. Tell your healthcare provider if any of the following occurs: nausea; vomiting; stomach ache; diarrhea.

Guidelines for Use

USE EXACTLY AS PRESCRIBED.

Retain in mouth as long as possible.

Troche: Dissolve slowly Do not chew or swallow whole.

Continue therapy for at least two days after symptoms have disappeared.

If a dose is missed, take it as soon as possible. If several hours have passed or if it is nearing time for the next dose, do not double the dose to "catch up," unless advised by your healthcare provider. If more than one dose is missed, contact your healthcare provider.

If symptoms worsen, contact your healthcare provider.

Nystatin Oral

(nye-STAT-in)

Mycostain, Nilstat

A medicine used to treat intestinal fungal infection due to Candida species (yeast).

Precautions

DO NOT USE if you are allergic to this medicine.

BEFORE USING THIS MEDICINE, tell your healthcare provider if you are pregnant or breastfeeding; or if you are taking, will be taking or stop taking any prescription or nonprescription medicine; or if you have any other medical conditions.

Side Effects

Every medicine can cause side effects, but many people have no, or minor, side effects. Tell your healthcare provider if any of the following occurs: nausea; vomiting; stomach ache; diarrhea.

Guidelines for Use

USE EXACTLY AS PRESCRIBED.

Continue therapy for at least two days after symptoms have disappeared. If symptoms worsen, contact your healthcare provider.

Nystatin Topical

(nye-STAT-in)

Mycostatin, Nilstat, Nystex

A medicine used to treat skin and mucous membrane fungal infections due to Candida species (yeast).

Precautions

DO NOT USE if you are allergic to this medicine.

BEFORE USING THIS MEDICINE, tell your healthcare provider if you are pregnant or breastfeeding; or if you are taking, will be taking or stop taking any prescription or nonprescription medicine; or if you have any other medical conditions.

Side Effects

Every medicine can cause side effects, but many people have no, or minor, side effects. Tell your healthcare provider if any of the following occurs: irritation; itching.

Guidelines for Use

USE EXACTLY AS PRESCRIBED.

Avoid contact with the eyes. Wash and dry the affected area before applying the medicine.

If your condition worsens, contact your healthcare provider.

Continue therapy for at least two days after symptoms have disappeared.

Nystatin Vaginal

(nye-STAT-in)

Mycostatin

A medicine used to treat vaginal yeast infections.

Precautions

DO NOT USE if you have an allergy to this medicine.

BEFORE USING THIS MEDICINE, tell your healthcare provider if you are pregnant or breastfeeding; or if you are taking, will be taking or stop taking any prescription or nonprescription medicine; or if you have any other medical conditions.

Side Effects

Every medicine can cause side effects, but many people have no, or minor, side effects. Tell your healthcare provider if any of the following occurs: headache; body aches; local irritation; burning; itching; sensitivity to light.

Guidelines for Use

USE EXACTLY AS PRESCRIBED.

Patient instructions for proper use are enclosed in each package.

Insert high into the vagina, except during pregnancy.

Complete a full course of therapy.

Keep using, even during the menstrual period.

If the medicine causes burning or irritation, or if symptoms worsen, contact your healthcare provider.

Refrain from sexual intercourse during treatment or the male sexual partner should use a condom to avoid the risk of reinfection.

A sanitary napkin or mini-pad may be used to prevent staining of clothing due to seepage or leakage of the medicine. If infection recurs, other factors may be involved.

Factors that increase the risk of infection include AIDS, diabetes, chronic antibiotic therapy, pregnancy, corticosteroid use and oral contraceptive use.

Octreotide Acetate

(ock-TREE-oh-tide ASS-uh-TATE)

Sandostatin

Used to reduce blood levels of growth hormone and IGF-I in acromegaly patients; used for the treatment of patients with metastatic carcinoid tumors in certain situations; used for the treatment of profuse watery diarrhea associated with VIP-secreting tumors. It may occasionally be prescribed for other reasons.

Precautions

DO NOT USE if you are allergic to this medicine.

BEFORE USING THIS MEDICINE, tell your healthcare provider if you are pregnant or breastfeeding; or if you are taking, will be taking or stop taking any prescription or nonprescription medicine; or if you have any other medical conditions.

Side Effects

Every medicine can cause side effects, but many people have no, or minor, side effects. Tell your healthcare provider if any of the following occurs: diarrhea; nausea; stomach pain; headache; dizziness; fatigue; weakness; cold symptoms; pain at the injection site; flushing; swelling in the legs; itching; hair loss; joint pain; vomiting; constipation; difficulty breathing; difficulty urinating; blurred vision; backache.

Ofloxacin Ophthalmic

(oh-FLOX-uh-SIN)

Ocuflox Ophthalmic

A medicine used for the treatment of certain eye infections caused by susceptible bacteria.

Precautions

DO NOT USE if you are allergic to this medicine or any of its relatives.

BEFORE USING THIS MEDICINE, tell your healthcare provider if you are pregnant or breastfeeding; or if you are taking, will be taking or stop taking any prescription or nonprescription medicine; or if you have any other medical conditions.

Side Effects

Every medicine can cause side effects, but many people have no, or minor, side effects. Tell your healthcare provider if any of the following occurs: burning; eye discomfort; stinging; redness; itching; tearing; dryness; sensitivity to sunlight; dizziness.

Guidelines for Use

USE EXACTLY AS PRESCRIBED.

Keep the applicator tip clean; avoid touching the eye or fingers. Ask your healthcare provider about proper instillation technique.

This medicine has caused severe allergic reactions in some patients, even following a single dose. Immediately discontinue use at the first sign of a rash or allergic reaction and contact your healthcare provider.

Ofloxacin Oral

(oh-FLOX-uh-SIN)

Floxin

A quinolone antibiotic medicine used to treat certain urinary tract infections or gonorrhea.

Precautions

DO NOT USE if you are allergic to this medicine or any of its relatives.

BEFORE USING THIS MEDICINE, tell your healthcare provider if you are pregnant or breastfeeding; or if you are taking, will be taking or stop taking any prescription or nonprescription medicine; or if you have any other medical conditions.

Side Effects

Every medicine can cause side effects, but many people have no, or minor, side effects. Tell your healthcare provider if any of the following occurs: nausea; rash; hives; itching; diarrhea; difficulty breathing; wheezing; dizziness; headache; or other signs of allergic reaction.

Guidelines for Use

USE EXACTLY AS PRESCRIBED.

Tell your healthcare provider if you suspect pregnancy.

Take on an empty stomach at least 1 hour before or 2 hours after a meal with a glass of fluid.

Drink plenty of liquids.

Do not take antacids containing sucralfate (*Carafate*), or iron or zinc-containing products within 4 hours before or 2 hours after using these agents.

If a dose is missed, take it as soon as possible. If several hours have passed or if it is nearing time for the next dose, do not double the dose to "catch up," unless advised by your healthcare provider. If more than one dose is missed, contact your healthcare provider.

May cause dizziness or lightheadedness. Use caution when driving or performing other tasks requiring mental alertness, coordination or physical dexterity.

Continue use until all the prescribed medicine has been taken. Failure to take a full course of therapy may cause a relapse of the infection.

May cause sensitivity to sunlight. Avoid prolonged exposure to the sun. Use sunscreens and wear protective clothing until tolerance is determined.

Olsalazine Sodium

(OLE-SAL-uh-zeen SO-dee-uhm)

Dipentum

A medicine used to reduce the chances that ulcerative colitis will reoccur in patients who cannot take sulfasalazine.

Precautions

DO NOT USE if you are allergic to this medicine or its relatives or salicylates (eg, aspirin).

BEFORE USING THIS MEDICINE, tell your healthcare provider if you are pregnant or breastfeeding; or if you are taking, will be taking or stop taking any prescription or nonprescription medicine; or if you have any other medical conditions.

Side Effects

Every medicine can cause side effects, but many people have no, or minor, side effects. Tell your healthcare provider if any of the following occurs: diarrhea; cramps, nausea; indigestion; bloating; appetite loss; headache; tiredness; drowsiness; depression; dizziness; sleeplessness; joint pain; upper respiratory infection; itching.

Guidelines for Use

USE EXACTLY AS PRESCRIBED.

Take with food.

Take in evenly divided doses.

May cause diarrhea in some patients. Contact your healthcare provider if diarrhea occurs.

If a dose is missed, take as soon as possible. If several hours have passed or if it is nearing time for the next dose, do not double the dose to "catch up," unless advised by your healthcare provider. If more than one dose is missed, contact your healthcare provider.

Omeprazole

(oh-MEH-pray-ZAHL)

Prilosec

This medicine suppresses gastric acid secretion and is used for short-term treatment (4 to 8 weeks) of severe gastroesophageal reflux disease (bubbling of stomach contents into the esophagus), active duodenal ulcer, severe erosive esophagitis and long-term treatment of hypersecretory (increased acid secretion) conditions (eg, Zollinger-Ellison Syndrome). It may occasionally be prescribed for other reasons.

Precautions

DO NOT USE if you are allergic to this medicine or its relatives.

BEFORE USING THIS MEDICINE, tell your healthcare provider if you are pregnant or breastfeeding; are taking, will be taking or stop taking any prescription or nonprescription medicine; or have any other medical conditions.

Side Effects

Every medicine can cause side effects, but many people have no, or minor, side effects. Tell your healthcare provider if any of the following occurs: headache; nausea; vomiting; diarrhea; stomach pain; dizziness; rash; itching; difficulty breathing; shortness of breath; joint or muscle pain; fever; sleep disturbances; constipation; cough; gas; back pain.

Guidelines for Use

USE EXACTLY AS PRESCRIBED.

Take one hour before eating.

Antacids may be used with this medicine.

Swallow capsule whole. Do not open, chew or crush.

Normal daily dose is 20 mg (1 capsule); larger doses may occasionally be prescribed.

If a dose is missed, take it as soon as possible. If several hours have passed or if it is nearing time for the next dose, do not double the dose to "catch up," unless advised by your healthcare provider. If more than one dose is missed, contact your healthcare provider.

Do not take this medicine any longer than recommended by your healthcare provider.

Exams may be necessary. Be sure to keep appointments.

Store at room temperature in a tight container away from moisture and light.

Ondansetron Hydrochloride

(ahn-DAN-SEH-trahn HIGH-droe-KLOR-ide)

Zofran

A medicine used to treat nausea and vomiting associated with cancer chemotherapy in patients over 4 years of age, as well as for post-operative conditions in adult patients. It may occasionally be prescribed for other reasons.

Precautions

DO NOT USE if you are allergic to this medicine.

BEFORE USING THIS MEDICINE, tell your healthcare provider if you are pregnant or breastfeeding; or if you are taking, will be taking or stop taking any prescription or nonprescription medicine; or if you have any other medical conditions.

Side Effects

Every medicine can cause side effects, but many people have no, or minor, side effects. Tell your healthcare provider if any of the following occurs: constipation; diarrhea; headache; weakness; pain at the injection site (injection only); general discomfort; dizziness; stomach pain; dry mouth; rash; fatigue; drowsiness.

Guidelines for Use

USE EXACTLY AS PRESCRIBED.

May use without regard to food.

May cause dizziness. Use caution while driving or performing other tasks requiring alertness, coordination or physical dexterity.

Injection: This medicine will be injected by a healthcare professional just prior to certain cancer medicine therapies, then 1 or 2 doses following therapy.

Oral: *Chemotherapy Dose* (take for 1–2 days starting 30 minutes before chemotherapy): Over 12–years-old, one 8 mg tablet is given twice a day; 4– to 11–years-old, one 4 mg tablet is given three times a day. *Radiotherapy Dose* (adults only): One 8 mg tablet three times a day starting 1–2 hours before radiation. *Postoperative Dose* (adults only): Two 8 mg tablets 1 hour before anesthesia.

Do not exceed 8 mg per day in patients with liver disease.

If a dose is missed, take is as soon as possible. If several hours have passed or if it is nearing time for the next dose, do not double the dose to "catch up," unless advised by your healthcare provider. If more than one dose is missed, contact your healthcare provider.

Store at room temperature, away from light.

Oral Contraceptives, Combination Products

Brevicon 21-Day, Brevicon 28-Day, Demulen 1/35-21, Demulen 1/35-28, Demulen 1/50-21, Demulen 1/50-28, Desogen, Ethinyl Estradiol/Norethindrone, GenCept, Genora 0.5/35, Genora 1/35, Genora 1/50, Jenest-28, Levlen 21, Levlen 28, Lo/Ovral-21, Lo/Ovral-28, Loestrin 21 1.5/30, Loestrin 21 1/20, Loestrin Fe 1.5/30, Loestrin Fe 1/20, Modicon 21, Modicon 28, N.E.E., Nelova 0.5/35 21 day, Nelova 0.5/35 28 day, Nelova 1/35E 21 day, Nelova 1/35E 28 day, Nelova 1/50M, Nelova 10/11, Nelulen 1/35 E, Nelulen 1/50 E, Norcept-E 1/35, Nordette-21, Nordette-28, Norethin 1/35 E 21 day, Norethin 1/35 E 28 day, Norethin 1/50M, Norgestimate and Ethinyl Estradiol, Norinyl 1 + 35 21 day, Norinyl 1 + 35 28 day, Norinyl 1 + 50, Norlestrin 21, Norlestrin 28, Norlestrin FE, Ortho Tri-Cyclen, Ortho-Cept, Ortho-Cyclen, Ortho-Novum 1/35 21, Ortho-Novum 1/35 28, Ortho-Novum 1/50 21, Ortho-Novum 1/50 28, Ortho-Novum 10/11-21, Ortho-Novum 10/11-28, Ortho-Novum 7/7/7, Ovcon-35, Ovcon-50, Ovral-21, Ovral-28, Tri-Levlen-21, Tri-Levlen-28, Tri-Norinyl 28 day, Tri-Norinyl 21 day, Triphasil-21, Triphasil-28

A birth control pill used to prevent pregnancy by hormonal alteration.

Precautions

DO NOT USE if you are allergic to this medicine.

BEFORE USING THIS MEDICINE, tell your healthcare provider if you have a family history of heart disease or cancer; high blood pressure; age over 35 years; overweight; more than 10 years oral contraceptive use; smoke more than 15 cigarettes/day; if you are pregnant or breastfeeding; or if you are taking, will be taking or stop taking any prescription or nonprescription medicine; or if you have any other medical conditions.

Side Effects

Every medicine can cause side effects, but many people have no, or minor, side effects. Tell your healthcare provider if any of the following occurs: blood clots; stroke; high blood pressure; heart attack; gall bladder disease; vision changes; menstrual changes; mid-cycle vaginal bleeding; breast fullness; contact lens intolerance; depression.

Guidelines for Use

USE EXACTLY AS PRESCRIBED.

Take every 24 hours with a meal or at bedtime. Use additional birth control for at least the first week after starting this medicine.

Take once daily for 21 or 28 days depending on the brand.

Sunday-start Packaging: Take the first tablet on the first Sunday after the menstrual period begins. If the menstrual period begins on Sunday, take the first tablet on that day.

Missed Dose: Ovulation is not likely to occur if one tablet is missed but spotting or mid-cycle bleeding is increased. The possibility of ovulation occurring increases each day that tablets are missed. Any time one or more tablets are missed, use additional birth control for at least 7 to 14 days or until the start of the next menstrual period. One tablet missed, take as soon as remembered or take 2 tablets the next day, and continue; two tablets missed, take 2 tablets as soon as remembered with the next pill at the usual time, or take 2 tablets daily for the next 2 days, then resume regular schedule.

Oral Contraceptives, Progestin only

Micronor, Nor-Q.D., Norethindrone (mini-pill), Norgestrel, Ovrette

A hormone used to prevent pregnancy. It may occasionally be prescribed for other reasons.

Precautions

DO NOT USE if you are allergic to this medicine; are pregnant; have a personal or family history of cancer of the uterus or breast, heart attack or stroke, liver disease, tumors or blood clots.

BEFORE USING THIS MEDICINE, tell your healthcare provider if you are pregnant or breastfeeding; if you smoke; or if you are taking, will be taking or stop taking any prescription or nonprescription medicine; or if you have any other medical conditions.

Side Effects

Every medicine can cause side effects, but many people have no, or minor, side effects. Tell your healthcare provider if any of the following occurs: chest pain; calf pain; difficulty breathing; blood clots; Raynaud's syndrome; high blood pressure; gallbladder disease; fetal defects; liver problems; changes in vision; change in menstrual flow; abnormal vaginal bleeding; temporary infertility after discontinuing medicine; unusual vaginal secretions; vaginal infection; growth of uterine cysts; nausea; vomiting; stomach cramps; bloating; migraine; depression; yellowing of skin or eyes; patchy discoloration of skin; rash; breast tenderness/enlargement/secretions; contact lens intolerance; fluid retention (edema); weight gain or loss.

Guidelines for Use

USE EXACTLY AS PRESCRIBED.

Take exactly as directed at intervals not greater than 24 hours.

Take regularly with a meal or at bedtime.

Take every day for as long as you wish to avoid pregnancy.

May cause spotting or breakthrough bleeding during the first months of therapy. If it continues past the second month, tell your healthcare provider.

Use an additional form of birth control for at least the first week after you begin taking oral contraceptives.

Missed dose: Take as soon as you remember, then take the next pill at the regularly scheduled time. If two pills in a row are missed, take one, discard the other and resume the usual dosage pattern. If more than two pills are missed, stop taking completely until a menstrual period occurs or results of a pregnancy test are known. Anytime a dose of the mini-pill is missed, use another method of birth control until the next menstrual period.

This information is advisory only; it does not contain all information about this medicine. If you have any questions about your medicine, ask your healthcare provider.

Orphenadrine Citrate

(ore-FEN-uh-dreen SIH-trate)

Banflex, Flexoject, Flexon, Myolin, Norflex

A medicine used to relieve muscle discomfort due to strain and sprain.

Precautions

DO NOT USE if you are allergic to this medicine or its relatives.

BEFORE USING THIS MEDICINE, tell your healthcare provider if you are pregnant or breastfeeding; or if you are taking, will be taking or stop taking any prescription or nonprescription medicine; or if you have any other medical conditions.

Side Effects

Every medicine can cause side effects, but many people have no, or minor, side effects. Tell your healthcare provider if any of the following occurs: stomach upset; constipation; vomiting; lightheadedness; confusion; nervousness; drowsiness; fatigue; dizziness; headache; changes in heart rate; itching; rash; visual disturbances; slurred speech; change in bladder function; dry mouth; fever; tremors; difficulty breathing; swelling; fainting.

Guidelines for Use

USE EXACTLY AS PRESCRIBED.

May be taken with food or water if stomach upset occurs.

If a dose is missed, take it as soon as possible. If several hours have passed or if it is nearing time for the next dose, do not double the dose to "catch up," unless advised by your healthcare provider. If more than one dose is missed, contact your healthcare provider.

May cause drowsiness, dizziness or blurred vision. Use caution while driving or performing other tasks requiring mental alertness, coordination and dexterity.

Avoid alcohol and other medication that cause drowsiness while taking this medication (eg, sleeping pills, tranquilizers, antihistamines). Patients on long-term or high dosage therapy may have withdrawal symptoms if therapy is suddenly stopped.

Do not stop therapy abruptly or change dosage without asking your pharmacist or healthcare provider.

Solution: Shake well before using.

Oxacillin Sodium

(OX-uh-SILL-in SO-dee-uhm)

Bactocill, Prostaphlin

A penicillin antibiotic used to treat infections caused by certain bacteria.

Precautions

DO NOT USE if you are allergic to any cephalosporin or penicillin.

BEFORE USING THIS MEDICINE, tell your healthcare provider if you are pregnant or breastfeeding; or if you are taking, will be taking or stop taking any prescription or nonprescription medicine; or if you have any other medical conditions.

Side Effects

Every medicine can cause side effects, but many people have no, or minor, side effects. Tell your healthcare provider if any of the following occurs: rash; itching; hives; severe diarrhea; shortness of breath; wheezing; dizziness; black tongue; sore throat; nausea; vomiting; fever; swollen joints; or any unusual bleeding or bruising.

Guidelines for Use

USE EXACTLY AS PRESCRIBED.

Oral: Take on an empty stomach approximately 30 minutes to one hour before meals or two hours after a meal.

Take at even intervals, preferably around the clock.

If a dose is missed, take it as soon as possible. If several hours have passed or if it is nearing time for the next dose, do not double the dose to "catch up," unless advised by your healthcare provider. If more than one dose is missed, contact your healthcare provider.

Continue until all the prescribed medicine has been taken. Failure to take a full course of therapy may cause a relapse of the infection.

Solution: Shake well before using.

Oxaprozin

(ox-uh-PRO-zin)

Daypro

A nonsteroidal anti-inflammatory medicine (NSAID) used to relieve mild to moderate pain and inflammation due to osteoarthritis (degenerative joint disease) and rheumatoid arthritis. It may occasionally be prescribed for other reasons.

Precautions

DO NOT USE if you are allergic to this medicine or its relatives, aspirin or iodides.

BEFORE USING THIS MEDICINE, tell your healthcare provider if you are pregnant or breastfeeding; use alcohol chronically; are prone to fluid retention; if you are taking, will be taking or stop taking any prescription or nonprescription medicines; or have any other medical conditions.

Side Effects

Every medicine can cause side effects, but many people have no, or minor, side effects. Tell your healthcare provider if any of the following occurs: allergic reaction (eg, rash, itching, fever, difficulty breathing); changes in vision; weight gain; fluid retention; stomach problems (eg, nausea, vomiting, diarrhea, pain); black stools; constipation; persistent headache; dizziness; nervousness; drowsiness; difficult urination; weakness; ringing in the ears; taste or appetite changes; unusual bruising or bleeding.

Guidelines for Use

USE EXACTLY AS PRESCRIBED.

Avoid aspirin and alcoholic beverages.

If stomach upset occurs, take with food, milk or antacids. If stomach pain continues, tell your healthcare provider.

If a dose is missed, take it as soon as possible. If several hours have passed or if it is nearing time for the next dose, do not double the dose to "catch up," unless advised by your healthcare provider. If more than one dose is missed, contact your healthcare provider.

May cause drowsiness or dizziness. Observe caution while driving or performing other tasks requiring mental alertness, coordination and dexterity.

May cause sensitivity to sunlight. Avoid prolonged exposure to the sun. Use sunscreens and wear protective clothing until tolerance is determined.

Oxazepam

(ox-AZE-uh-pam)

Serax

A benzodiazepine medicine that is a sleeping pill to treat insomnia for a short period of time (1 to 2 weeks). Long-term use generally is not recommended.

Precautions

DO NOT USE if you are allergic to this medicine or its relatives; or if you are pregnant.

BEFORE USING THIS MEDICINE, tell your healthcare provider if you are pregnant or breastfeeding; or if you are taking, will be taking or stop taking any prescription or nonprescription medicine; or if you have any other medical conditions.

Side Effects

Every medicine can cause side effects, but many people have no, or minor, side effects. Tell your healthcare provider if any of the following occurs: vision changes; irregular heartbeat; headache; chest pain; yellowing of skin or eyes; rash; unusual bleeding or bruising; vomiting; heartburn; diarrhea; constipation; appetite loss; nervousness; irritability; memory loss; sleeplessness; ringing in the ears; sore throat; joint pain.

Guidelines for Use

USE EXACTLY AS PRESCRIBED.

Do not exceed prescribed dosage.

Take with a full glass of water.

Use caution while driving or performing other tasks requiring mental alertness, coordination and dexterity.

May cause morning drowsiness, unusual tiredness in the morning or daytime sleepiness after using these medications for sleep. The elderly are particularly sensitive to these effects.

Avoid alcohol and medications that cause drowsiness (eg, pain relievers, sedatives, antihistamines).

Nighttime sleep may be disturbed for 1 or 2 nights following stopping of the medication.

May be habit-forming. Do not discontinue medicine abruptly, especially if you have a history of seizures, regardless of other antiseizure medications you may be taking.

Long-term use may result in dependence. Withdrawal symptoms may occur when the medication is stopped.

Oxybutynin Chloride

(OX-ee-BYOO-tih-nin KLOR-ide)

Ditropan

A medicine used for the relief of certain bladder conditions, such as frequent or painful urination, incontinence or urinary leakage.

Precautions

DO NOT USE if you are allergic to this medicine.

Diarrhea may be a sign of partial intestinal obstruction. If you develop this symptom discontinue use and tell your healthcare provider.

BEFORE USING THIS MEDICINE, tell your healthcare provider if you are pregnant or breastfeeding; or if you are taking, will be taking or stop taking any prescription or nonprescription medicine; or if you have any other medical conditions.

Side Effects

Every medicine can cause side effects, but many people have no, or minor, side effects. Tell your healthcare provider if any of the following occurs: nausea; vomiting; constipation; dizziness; sleeplessness; weakness; restlessness; drowsiness; hallucinations; palpitations (pounding in the chest); rapid heart rate; difficulty or inability to urinate; impotence; decreased tearing of eyes; vision problems; suppression of breast milk production; decreased sweating; dry mouth; rash.

Guidelines for Use

USE EXACTLY AS PRESCRIBED.

May cause drowsiness or blurred vision. Alcohol or sedatives may enhance these effects.

Use caution when driving or performing other tasks requiring alertness, coordination or physical dexterity.

Use caution in hot weather. This medicine can cause fever and heatstroke due to decreased sweating.

Oxycodone Hydrochloride

(OX-ee-KOE-dohn HIGH-droe-KLOR-ide)

Roxicodone Intensol Solution, Roxicodone Solution, Roxicodone Tablets

A narcotic pain reliever used for moderate to severe pain.

Precautions

DO NOT USE if you are allergic to this medicine or its relatives.

BEFORE USING THIS MEDICINE, tell your healthcare provider if you are pregnant or breastfeeding; or if you are taking, will be taking or stop taking any prescription or nonprescription medicine; or if you have any other medical conditions. Long-term, regular use of narcotic pain relievers may lead to dependence and physical tolerance. Withdrawal symptoms may occur when therapy is stopped.

Side Effects

Every medicine can cause side effects, but many people have no, or minor, side effects. Tell your healthcare provider if any of the following occurs: lightheadedness; dizziness; drowsiness; nausea; vomiting; sweating; abdominal pain; cramps; constipation; diarrhea; urine retention; appetite loss; indigestion; gas; excitability; vision problems; difficult breathing.

Guidelines for Use

USE EXACTLY AS PRESCRIBED.

Take with food if stomach upset occurs.

May cause drowsiness, dizziness or blurred vision. Use caution while driving or performing other tasks requiring mental alertness, judgment and coordination.

Avoid alcohol and other medicines that cause drowsiness (eg, sleeping pills, antihistamines).

May cause nausea, vomiting or constipation. Constipation may be avoided by using a stool softener or fiber laxative.

This medicine works best if taken regularly. It is more effective in preventing pain than in treating pain after it occurs. Give the medicine ample time to work before taking more (approximately 30 minutes to 1 hour).

If a dose is missed, take it as soon as possible. If several hours have passed or if it is nearing time for the next dose, do not double the dose to "catch up," unless advised by your healthcare provider. If more than one dose is missed, contact your healthcare provider.

Oxycodone/Acetaminophen

(OX-ee-KOE-dohn/ass-cet-ah-MEE-noe-fen)

Acetaminophen w/Oxycodone Tablets, Apap with Oxycodone Tablets, Percocet Tablets, Roxicet Solution, Roxilox Capsules, Tylox Capsules

A nonaspirin pain reliever plus a narcotic pain reliever for the relief of mild to moderate pain.

Precautions

DO NOT USE if you are allergic to either of these medications or if you have acute bronchial asthma. Long-term use may be habit-forming or lead to physical tolerance.

BEFORE USING THIS MEDICATION, tell your healthcare provider if you are pregnant or breastfeeding; or if you are taking, will be taking or stop taking any prescription or nonprescription medicine; or if you have any other medical conditions.

Side Effects

Every medicine can cause side effects, but many people have no, or minor, side effects. Tell your healthcare provider if any of the following occurs: drowsiness; dizziness; blurred vision; urinary retention; nausea; vomiting; constipation; shortness of breath; difficulty breathing; yellowing of the skin, eyes or gums.

Guidelines for Use

USE EXACTLY AS PRESCRIBED.

Take with food.

Avoid drinking alcohol and use caution with other drowsiness-causing medicines (eg, sleeping pills, antihistamines).

This medicine may cause drowsiness; use caution while driving or performing any tasks requiring mental alertness, coordination and dexterity.

If pain is severe, persistent or recurrent, contact your healthcare provider.

Wait 30 to 60 minutes for the medicine to take effect before deciding if more is needed.

If a dose is missed, you do not need to make it up.

If constipation becomes a problem, a stool softener or bulk laxative may help.

Overdosage with this medicine can be very dangerous. If this occurs, contact your healthcare provider, pharmacist or poison control center immediately.

Oxytocin Nasal

(ox-ih-TOE-sin)

Syntocinon

Used for initial milk letdown when nursing. It may occasionally be prescribed for other reasons.

Precautions

DO NOT USE if you are allergic to this medicine or if you are pregnant.

BEFORE USING THIS MEDICINE, tell your healthcare provider if you are pregnant or breastfeeding; or if you are taking, will be taking or stop taking any prescription or nonprescription medicine; or if you have any other medical conditions.

Side Effects

Every medicine can cause side effects, but many people have no, or minor, side effects. Tell your healthcare provider if any of the following occurs: nausea; vomiting.

Guidelines for Use

USE EXACTLY AS PRESCRIBED.

Initial milk letdown — One spray into one or both nostrils 2 to 3 minutes before nursing or pumping of the breasts.

Hold the squeeze bottle upright when administering the medicine to the nose; the patient should be sitting rather than lying down.

If preferred, the solution can be instilled in drop form by inverting the squeeze bottle and exerting gentle pressure.

Paclitaxel Injection

(pak-lih-TAX-uhl)

Taxol

A medicine used to treat cancer of the ovary.

Precautions

DO NOT USE if you are allergic to this medicine or polyoxyethylated castor oil; if you are pregnant, breastfeeding or have severe anemia. Lab tests will be required during treatment.

BEFORE USING THIS MEDICINE, tell your healthcare provider if you are pregnant or breastfeeding; or if you are taking, will be taking or stop taking any prescription or nonprescription medicines; or have any other medical conditions.

Side Effects

Every medicine can cause side effects, but many people have no, or minor, side effects. Tell your healthcare provider if any of the following occurs: *Common:* fever; chills; drowsiness; tiredness; sore throat; joint and muscle aches/pain; headache. *Other:* appetite loss; diarrhea; constipation; stomach pain; nausea; vomiting; gas; heartburn; dizziness; confusion; forgetfulness; incoordination; mood disorders; nervousness; sleep problems; weakness; depression; abnormal thinking; tingling of extremities; chest pain; pounding in chest; bleeding; difficulty breathing; pneumonia; coughing; bronchitis; sinusitis; hair loss; redness; rash; dry skin; skin disorders; sweating; muscle twitching; allergic reaction; swelling of extremities; back pain; weight loss; taste changes; dehydration; thirst; dry/swollen mouth; pain; hot flashes; cold sores; nosebleeds; numbness and tingling; runny nose; abnormal vision.

Guidelines for Use

USE EXACTLY AS PRESCRIBED.

Contraceptive measures (birth control) are recommended during therapy with this medicine.

Notify your healthcare provider immediately if you suspect pregnancy.

May cause drowsiness or dizziness. Use caution while driving or performing other tasks requiring alertness.

Infections — This medicine may lower your body's ability to fight infection. Notify your healthcare provider immediately of any signs of infection (fever, sore throat, rash or chills).

Before treatment with this medicine, you must be pretreated with medication to prevent serious allergic reactions.

Lab tests will be required during treatment; be sure to keep appointments.

Pamidronate Disodium

(pam-IH-DROE-nate die-SO-dee-uhm)

Aredia

Used to treat bone lesions of multiple myeloma in patients with moderate to severe Paget's disease. It also is used in conjunction with adequate hydration for the treatment of moderate to severe high calcium levels associated with malignancy.

Side Effects

Every medicine can cause side effects, but many people have no, or minor, side effects. Tell your healthcare provider if any of the following occurs: fever; irritation at the injection site; fatigue; swelling; nausea; loss of appetite; constipation; diarrhea; upset stomach; vomiting; sleeplessness; inflammation of the mouth; difficulty breathing; muscle pain; drowsiness; difficult urination; pain at the injection site.

Patient Information

May cause loss of potassium. If signs of potassium loss occurs (weakness, cramps, nausea; dizziness, etc), contact your healthcare provider.

Pancrelipase

(pan-KREE-lih-pace)

Cotazym, Cotazym-S, Creon, Dizymes, Donnazyme, Entozyme, Hi-Vegi-Lip, Ilozyme, Ku-Zyme HP, Pancrease, Pancrease MT 4, Pancrease MT 10, Pancrease MT 16, 4X Pancreatin 600 mg, 8X Pancreatin 900 mg, Protilase, Ultrase MT12, Ultrase MT24, Viokase, Zymase

A medicine used to replace the pancreatic enzymes in patients who do not normally produce enough enzymes (eg, cystic fibrosis, chronic pancreatitis, removal of the pancreas, obstruction of the pancreatic duct and pancreatic insufficiency). It also is used to treat excess fat in the bowel movement due to malabsorption syndrome and to test pancreatic function.

Precautions

DO NOT USE if you are allergic to pork.

BEFORE USING THIS MEDICINE, tell your healthcare provider if you are pregnant or breastfeeding; or if you are taking, will be taking or stop taking any prescription or nonprescription medicine; or if you have any other medical conditions.

Side Effects

Every medicine can cause side effects, but many people have no, or minor, side effects. Tell your healthcare provider if any of the following occurs: rash; sneezing, tearing, difficulty breathing (exposure to powder only); nausea; abdominal cramps; diarrhea; gout.

Guidelines for Use

USE EXACTLY AS PRESCRIBED.

Take before or with meals.

Do not inhale or spill powder on skin. The powder may irritate skin, nose or lungs if spilled or inhaled.

Inhaling may cause an asthma attack.

Do not crush or chew coated tablets or capsules.

Avoid using antacids while taking digestive enzymes. Antacids may negate the beneficial effect of the enzymes.

If a dose is missed, take it as soon as possible. If several hours have passed or if it is nearing time for the next dose, do not double the dose to catch up, unless advised by your healthcare provider. If more than one dose is missed, contact your healthcare provider.

Report any rash or persistent gastric upset to your healthcare provider.

Do not change brands without consulting your healthcare provider.

Storage: Store in a dry place in a tightly closed container at room temperature.

Papaverine Hydrochloride

(pap-PAV-uhr-een HIGH-droe-KLOR-ide)

Cerespan Timed Release, Pavabid HP Tablets, Pavased, Pavasule, Pavatine, Pavatym, Paverolan

A peripheral vasodilator used to relax and widen blood vessels to increase blood flow. Increased blood flow allows more oxygen to reach the brain, heart and muscles. It may occasionally be prescribed for other reasons.

Precautions

DO NOT USE if you are allergic to this medicine or if you have heart block.

BEFORE USING THIS MEDICINE, tell your healthcare provider if you are pregnant or breastfeeding; or if you are taking, will be taking or stop taking any prescription or nonprescription medicine; or if you have any other medical conditions.

Side Effects

Every medicine can cause side effects, but many people have no, or minor, side effects. Tell your healthcare provider if any of the following occurs: nausea; stomach ache; appetite loss; constipation; diarrhea; headache; dizziness; drowsiness; increased pulse/heart rate; increased blood pressure; yellowing of skin or eyes; sweating; flushing of face; rash; fatigue and general body aches; increase in depth of respirations.

Guidelines for Use

USE EXACTLY AS PRESCRIBED.

May cause drowsiness or dizziness. Use caution when driving or performing tasks requiring alertness.

Alcohol may intensify these effects.

Oral: Take at evenly spaced intervals throughout the day.

Sustained release: Swallow whole; do not crush or chew.

Paromomycin

(par-oh-moe-MY-sin)

Humatin

A medicine used to treat intestinal parasites (amebiasis) and to treat hepatic coma.

Precautions

DO NOT USE if you are allergic to this medicine.

BEFORE USING THIS MEDICINE, tell your healthcare provider if you are pregnant or breastfeeding; or if you are taking, will be taking or stop taking any prescription or nonprescription medicine; or if you have any other medical conditions.

Side Effects

Every medicine can cause side effects, but many people have no, or minor, side effects. Tell your healthcare provider if any of the following occurs: increased urination; ringing in the ears; hearing impairment; dizziness; rash; itching; nausea; vomiting; diarrhea; cramping; fatty stools.

Guidelines for Use

USE EXACTLY AS PRESCRIBED.

Complete full course of therapy. Take until all medication is used.

May cause nausea, vomiting or diarrhea.

Tell your healthcare provider if ringing in the ears, hearing impairment, rash, problems urinating, or dizziness occurs.

Drink plenty of fluids.

If a dose is missed, take it as soon as possible. If several hours have passed or if it is nearing time for the next dose, do not double the dose to "catch up," unless advised by your healthcare provider. If more than one dose is missed, contact your healthcare provider.

This medicine may be associated with significant hearing and kidney damage.

Toxicity may develop particularly in people with kidney disease and pre-existing hearing loss. Evidence of toxicity requires discontinuation of the medicine.

Use of this medicine may result in bacterial or fungal overgrowth of organisms. Such overgrowth may lead to a second infection. The medicine may need to be stopped and another antibiotic may need to be prescribed for the second infection.

Paroxetine Hydrochloride

(puh-ROKS-uh-teen HIGH-droe-KLOR-ide)

Paxil

A mood elevating medicine (antidepressant).

Precautions

DO NOT USE if you are allergic to this medicine.

BEFORE USING THIS MEDICINE, tell your healthcare provider if you are pregnant or breastfeeding; or if you are taking, will be taking or stop taking any prescription or nonprescription medicine; or if you have any other medical conditions.

Side Effects

Every medicine can cause side effects, but many people have no, or minor, side effects. Tell your healthcare provider if any of the following occurs: nausea; vomiting; diarrhea; constipation; headache; dizziness; fatigue; nervousness; insomnia; chest pain or pounding; dry mouth; vision disturbance; ringing in the ears; sexual problems; difficult urination; hot flashes; rash; manic symptoms; tingling; fever; fainting; belching; drowsiness; tremors; confusion; sweating; cough; runny nose; muscle aches; weight loss.

Guidelines for Use

USE EXACTLY AS PRESCRIBED.

Do not use in combination with monoamine oxidase inhibitors (MAOIs, eg, phenelzine, tranylcypromine) or within 14 days of discontinuing treatment with an MAOI.

If a dose is missed, take it as soon as possible. If several hours have passed or if it is nearing time for the next dose, do not double the dose to "catch up," unless advised by your healthcare provider. If more than one dose is missed, contact your healthcare provider.

May cause drowsiness or dizziness. Use caution while driving or performing other tasks requiring alertness or coordination.

Avoid alcohol or other drowsiness-causing agents (eg, narcotic pain relievers, tranquilizers, antihistamines).

Improvement may not occur for several weeks. Do not stop taking your medicine without telling your healthcare provider.

Pemoline

(PEM-oh-leen)

Cylert

A medicine used to treat attention-deficit hyperactivity disorder in adults and children over 6 years old. It may occasionally be prescribed for other reasons.

Precautions

DO NOT USE if you are allergic to this medicine or have liver problems.

BEFORE USING THIS MEDICINE, tell your healthcare provider if you are pregnant or breastfeeding; or if you are taking, will be taking or stop taking any prescription or nonprescription medicine; or if you have any other medical conditions.

Side Effects

Every medicine can cause side effects, but many people have no, or minor, side effects. Tell your healthcare provider if any of the following occurs: yellowing of the skin or eyes; dark urine; convulsive seizures; hallucinations; uncoordinated or involuntary movements of tongue, lips, face, arms and legs; jerky eye movement; rolling back of eyes into a fixed position; dizziness; increased irritability; headache; drowsiness; appetite loss; weight loss; nausea; stomach ache; growth suppression in children.

Guidelines for Use

USE EXACTLY AS PRESCRIBED.

Take once daily in the morning. The dosage may be gradually increased by your healthcare provider to the most effective dosage.

If a dose is missed, take it as soon as possible. If several hours have passed, or if it is nearing time for the next dose, do not double the dose to "catch up," unless advised by your healthcare provider. If more than one dose is missed, contact your healthcare provider.

Do not stop or change the dose unless advised to do so by your healthcare provider.

Improvement with this medicine is gradual. It may by 3–4 weeks before significant benefit is observed.

This medicine may need to be interrupted occasionally to determine the need for continued use and to allow "catch up," growth.

If dizziness occurs, use caution while driving or performing other tasks requiring mental alertness.

This medicine may cause growth suppression in children on long-term therapy.

This medicine may aggravate behavior problems in children.

This medicine should be given with caution to emotionally unstable patients who may increase the dosage without contacting their healthcare provider.

Contact your healthcare provider if sleeplessness occurs and continues.

Lab tests may be required. Be sure to keep appointments.

Store at room temperature.

Penbutolol Sulfate

(pen-BYOO-toe-lole SULL-fate)

Levatol

A "beta blocker" medicine used to lower high blood pressure and to treat angina and heart attack.

Precautions

DO NOT USE if you are allergic to this medicine or its relatives, or if you are breastfeeding.

BEFORE USING THIS MEDICINE, tell your healthcare provider if you are pregnant; or if you are taking, will be taking or stop taking any prescription or nonprescription medicine; or if you have any other medical conditions.

Side Effects

Every medicine can cause side effects, but many people have no, or minor, side effects. Tell your healthcare provider if any of the following occurs: nausea; vomiting; stomach ache; diarrhea; constipation; appetite changes; indigestion; depression; anxiety; hallucinations; short-term memory loss; behavior changes; disorientation; fainting; dizziness; lightheadedness; tiredness; sleep disturbances; decreased concentration; headache; nightmares; emotional lability; changes in heart rate; chest pain; chills; cold or numb extremities; pounding in the chest; difficulty breathing; cough; nasal congestion; rash; hives; fluid retention; flushing or paleness; increased pigmentation; itching; hair loss; sweating; dry skin; psoriasis; painful and aching joints and muscles; painful, frequent or difficult urination; blurred vision; dry, burning or irritated eyes; ringing in the ears; taste changes; sore throat; dry mouth; slurred speech; fever; weight gain; changes in blood sugar levels.

Guidelines for Use

USE EXACTLY AS PRESCRIBED.

Ask your healthcare provider before using other medicines including nasal decongestants, diet aids or nonprescription cold preparations.

Do not stop this medicine suddenly, it could cause a worsening of disease including worse angina (chest pain), irregular heartbeats and increased risk of heart attack and death.

Withdraw these medications slowly over 1 to 2 weeks by gradually decreasing the dose.

These products can mask signs of low blood sugar and change blood sugar levels. It may be necessary for your healthcare provider to change your dose of diabetic medications.

Use caution while driving or performing other tasks requiring mental alertness, coordination and dexterity.

Penicillin G

(pen-ih-SILL-in G)

Bicillin L-A, Crysticillin, Pentids, Permapen, Pfizerpen, Pfizerpen-AS, Wycillin

A penicillin antibiotic used to treat infections caused by certain bacteria.

Precautions

DO NOT USE if you are allergic to any cephalosporin or penicillin.

BEFORE USING THIS MEDICINE, tell your healthcare provider if you are pregnant or breastfeeding; or if you are taking, will be taking or stop taking any prescription or nonprescription medicine; or if you have any other medical conditions.

Side Effects

Every medicine can cause side effects, but many people have no, or minor, side effects. Tell your healthcare provider if any of the following occurs: rash; itching; hives; severe diarrhea; shortness of breath; wheezing; dizziness; black tongue; sore throat; nausea; vomiting; fever; swollen joints; or any unusual bleeding or bruising.

Guidelines for Use

USE EXACTLY AS PRESCRIBED.

Oral: Take on an empty stomach approximately 30 minutes to one hour before meals or two hours after a meal.

Take at even intervals, preferably around the clock.

If a dose is missed, take it as soon as possible. If several hours have passed or if it is nearing time for the next dose, do not double the dose to "catch up," unless advised by your healthcare provider. If more than one dose is missed, contact your healthcare provider.

Continue until all the prescribed medicine has been taken. Failure to take a full course of therapy may cause a relapse of the infection.

Solution: Store in the refrigerator. Do not freeze. Shake well before using.

Penicillin V

(pen-ih-SILL-in V)

Beepen-VK, Betapen-VK, Ledercillin VK, Pen VK, Pen-Vee K, Robicillin VK, V-Cillin K, Veetids

A penicillin antibiotic used to treat infections caused by certain bacteria.

Precautions

DO NOT USE if you are allergic to any penicillin (eg, ampicillin, amoxicillin) or cephalosporin.

BEFORE USING THIS MEDICINE, tell your healthcare provider if you are pregnant or breastfeeding; if you are taking, will be taking or stop taking any prescription or nonprescription medicine; or if you have any other medical conditions.

Side Effects

Every medicine can cause side effects, but many people have no, or minor, side effects. Tell your healthcare provider if any of the following occurs: rash; itching; hives; severe diarrhea; shortness of breath; wheezing; dizziness; black tongue; sore throat; nausea; vomiting; fever; swollen joints; any unusual bleeding or bruising.

Guidelines for Use

USE EXACTLY AS PRESCRIBED.

To help absorption of the medicine, take on an empty stomach approximately 30 minutes to one hour before meals or two hours after a meal.

Take at even intervals, preferably around the clock.

If a dose is missed, take it as soon as possible. If several hours have passed or if it is nearing time for the next dose, do not double the dose to "catch up," unless advised by your healthcare provider. If more than one dose is missed, contact your healthcare provider.

Continue use until all the prescribed medicine has been taken. Failure to take a full course of therapy may cause a relapse of the infection.

Solution: Shake well before using. Store in the refrigerator. Do not freeze.

Pentamidine Isethionate Injectable

(pen-TAM-ih-deen ice-uh-THIGH-uh-nate)

Pentacarinat, Pentam 300

A medicine used for the treatment of *Pneumocystis carinii* pneumonia (PCP).

Precautions

DO NOT USE if you are allergic to this medicine.

BEFORE USING THIS MEDICINE, tell your healthcare provider if you are pregnant or breastfeeding; or if you are taking, will be taking or stop taking any prescription or nonprescription medicine; or if you have any other medical conditions.

Side Effects

Every medicine can cause side effects, but many people have no, or minor, side effects. Tell your healthcare provider if any of the following occurs: pain at injection site; nausea; loss of appetite; fever; rash; bad taste in mouth; confusion; hallucinations.

Guidelines for Use

USE EXACTLY AS PRESCRIBED.

Laboratory tests will need to be performed before, during and after therapy.

Pentamidine Isethionate Inhalation

(pen-TAM-ih-deen ice-uh-THIGH-uh-nate)

NebuPent, Pentacarinat

A medicine used to prevent pneumocystis pneumonia (PCP) infection in high-risk AIDS patients or HIV infected patients who either have had a previous episode of PCP infection or whose T4 cell count is equal to or less than 200 cu mm. Doctors occasionally may prescribe it for other reasons.

Precautions

DO NOT USE if you are allergic to this medicine.

BEFORE USING THIS MEDICINE, tell your healthcare provider if you are pregnant or breastfeeding; or if you are taking, will be taking or stop taking any prescription or nonprescription medicine; or if you have any other medical conditions.

Side Effects

Every medicine can cause side effects, but many people have no, or minor, side effects. Tell your healthcare provider if any of the following occurs: nausea; vomiting; appetite loss; diarrhea; stomach ache; dizziness; fatigue; headache; shortness of breath; chest pain; congestion; cough; rash; night sweats; chills; bad taste; muscle ache; fluid retention; throat irritation.

Guidelines for Use

USE EXACTLY AS PRESCRIBED.

Store at room temperature and protect from light. The solution is stable for 48 hours. Discard unused portion after this time.

Administer the medicine only by the Respigard 2 nebulizer with a high-pressure compressor at a flow rate of 5 to 7 L/min. Treatment usually takes 30 to 45 minutes and is given once a month.

Use of a bronchodilator medicine prior to treatment may reduce breathing side effects.

Laboratory tests will need to be performed before, during and after therapy.

Pentazocine Oral

(pen-TAZ-oh-seen)

Talwin NX

A medicine used for the treatment of moderate to severe pain.

Precautions

DO NOT USE if you are allergic to this medicine.

BEFORE USING THIS MEDICINE, tell your healthcare provider if you are pregnant or breastfeeding; or if you are taking, will be taking or stop taking any prescription or nonprescription medicine; or if you have any other medical conditions.

Side Effects

Every medicine can cause side effects, but many people have no, or minor, side effects. Tell your healthcare provider if any of the following occurs: nausea; dizziness; lightheadedness; vomiting; euphoria (exaggerated sense of well-being); constipation; cramps; abdominal distress; loss of appetite; diarrhea; dry mouth; taste change; sedation; headache; weakness; faintness; depression; disturbing dreams; sleeplessness; fainting; hallucinations; tremor; irritability; excitement; ringing in the ears; disorientation; confusion; blurred vision; difficulty focusing; rapid eye movement; double vision; facial swelling; sweating; rash; hives; flushed skin; skin inflammation; itching; difficulty breathing; urinary retention; abnormal skin sensations; chills; tremors.

Guidelines for Use

USE EXACTLY AS PRESCRIBED.

This medicine may cause drowsiness or dizziness. Use caution while driving or performing other tasks requiring mental alertness, coordination and dexterity.

Avoid alcohol and medicines that may cause drowsiness.

Contact your healthcare provider if skin rash, confusion or disorientation occurs.

If a dose is missed, take it as soon as possible. If several hours have passed or if it is nearing time for the next dose, do not double the dose to catch up, unless advised by your healthcare provider. If more than one dose is missed, contact your healthcare provider.

This medicine may be addictive if used in large doses or for a long time. Do not exceed prescribed dose.

Discuss overuse with your healthcare provider.

Store at room temperature and protect from sunlight.

Pentobarbital Sodium

(pen-toe-BAR-bih-tal SO-dee-uhm)

Nembutal

A barbiturate central nervous system depressant that can produce mild sedation, sleep and up to deep coma. Usually used to treat insomnia, to calm agitated people and to treat certain seizure disorders.

Precautions

DO NOT USE if you are allergic to this medicine or its relatives. This medicine may be habit-forming. Tolerance and dependence may occur, especially following prolonged use of high doses. Withdrawal symptoms can be severe.

BEFORE USING THIS MEDICINE, tell your healthcare provider if you are pregnant or breastfeeding; or if you are taking, will be taking or stop taking any prescription or nonprescription medicine; or if you have any other medical conditions.

Side Effects

Every medicine can cause side effects, but many people have no, or minor, side effects. Tell your healthcare provider if any of the following occurs: sleepiness; tired feeling; nausea; vomiting; morning hangover.

Guidelines for Use

USE EXACTLY AS PRESCRIBED.

Take only the amount of medicine prescribed by your healthcare provider.

This medicine contains alcohol. It may decrease alertness or physical ability. Use caution when driving or performing tasks requiring mental alertness.

Avoid alcohol and other mental depressants (eg, narcotics, tranquilizers, antihistamines) while you are taking this medicine.

Use as an aid to sleep is limited; generally not for use longer than 2 weeks.

Seizure control: Do not stop therapy suddenly.

Pentostatin

(PEN-toe-STAT-in)

Nipent

Used to treat adult patients with certain types of leukemia.

Precautions

DO NOT USE if you are allergic to this medicine.

Side Effects

Every medicine can cause side effects, but many people have no, or minor, side effects. Tell your healthcare provider if any of the following occurs: nausea; vomiting; loss of appetite; diarrhea; constipation; gas; rash; skin disorder; dry skin; itching; fever; fatigue; pain; chills; chest pain; stomach pain; back pain; flu-like syndrome; weakness; general body discomfort; weight loss; swelling; cough; difficulty breathing; headache; anxiety; confusion; depression; dizziness; sleeplessness; nervousness; abnormal skin sensations; drowsiness; muscle aches; joint pain; abnormal vision; ear pain; eye pain; inflammation of the mouth; skin discoloration; sweating; swelling of the lower legs; blood in the urine.

Pentoxifylline

(pen-TOX-IH-fill-in)

Trental

This medicine improves blood flow and generally is used to treat circulation problems (eg, intermittent claudication) that cause leg discomfort. It may occasionally be prescribed for other reasons.

Precautions

DO NOT USE if you have an allergy to this medicine, caffeine (coffee, tea), theophylline or theobromine (chocolate).

BEFORE USING THIS MEDICINE, tell your healthcare provider if you are pregnant or breastfeeding; or if you are taking, will be taking or stop taking any prescription or nonprescription medicine; or if you have any other medical conditions.

Side Effects

Every medicine can cause side effects, but many people have no, or minor, side effects. Tell your healthcare provider if any of the following occurs: indigestion; nausea; vomiting; gas; loss of appetite; dizziness; headache; tremor; anxiety; nose and throat irritation/problems. Skin rash or itching may mean you are allergic to the medicine.

Guidelines for Use

USE EXACTLY AS PRESCRIBED.

Take with meals.

Improvement may take 2 to 4 weeks to notice and up to 8 weeks for maximum relief.

Pergolide Mesylate

(PURR-go-lide MEH-sih-LATE)

Permax

An antiparkinson agent used to manage the signs and symptoms of Parkinson's disease.

Precautions

DO NOT USE if you are allergic to this medicine.

BEFORE USING THIS MEDICINE, tell your healthcare provider if you are pregnant or breastfeeding; or if you are taking, will be taking or stop taking any prescription or nonprescription medicine; or if you have any other medical conditions.

Side Effects

Every medicine can cause side effects, but many people have no, or minor, side effects. Tell your healthcare provider if any of the following occurs: nausea; vomiting; constipation; diarrhea; indigestion; abdominal pain; appetite loss; hallucinations; difficult or abnormal movement; restlessness; twitching; confusion; dizziness; drowsiness; fainting; sleeplessness; anxiety; tremor; depression; abnormal dreams; personality changes; headache; weakness; incoordination; palpitations (pounding in the chest); irregular heartbeat; inflammation of the nose; difficulty breathing; rash; sweating; abnormal sensations; dry mouth; taste changes; general body pain; joint, muscle or nerve pain; abnormal vision; double vision; frequent urination; urinary tract infections; blood in urine; edema (fluid retention); back, neck and chest pain; flu-like symptoms; nosebleed; hiccups; weight gain; chills; difficulty speaking.

Guidelines for Use

USE EXACTLY AS PRESCRIBED.

Dizziness or lightheadedness may occur when getting up or standing too quickly from a seated or lying position. Avoid sudden changes in posture while taking this medicine.

May cause drowsiness. Use caution while driving or performing other tasks requiring alertness.

Perphenazine

(per-FEN-uh-zeen)

Trilafon

A medicine used to control nausea and vomiting. It also is used to improve concentration and self-control in patients with psychotic behavior. It may occasionally be prescribed for other reasons.

Precautions

DO NOT USE if you are allergic to this medicine or its relatives. Laboratory tests may be needed including eye exams, blood counts and kidney and liver tests.

BEFORE USING THIS MEDICINE, tell your healthcare provider if you are pregnant or breastfeeding; or if you are taking, will be taking or stop taking any prescription or nonprescription medicine; if you have any other medical conditions; or if you are allergic to tartrazine.

Side Effects

Every medicine can cause side effects, but many people have no, or minor, side effects. Tell your healthcare provider if any of the following occurs: tremors; drooling; shuffling gait; restlessness; muscle spasms; aching or numbness; sore throat; fever; unusual bleeding or bruising; skin rash; weakness; impaired vision; dark-colored urine; pale stools; yellow skin or eyes.

Guidelines for Use

USE EXACTLY AS PRESCRIBED.

Oral: Take routinely as directed; it controls illness symptoms and is not habit-forming.

Improvement may not be seen for several weeks.

If a dose is missed, take it as soon as possible. If several hours have passed or if it is nearing time for the next dose, do not double the dose to "catch up," unless advised by your healthcare provider. If more than one dose is missed, contact your healthcare provider.

May cause drowsiness; use caution while driving. Avoid alcohol and medicines that cause drowsiness (eg, sleeping pills).

May cause sunlight sensitivity. Use sunscreens and protective clothing until tolerance is known.

May discolor the urine pink or reddish brown. This is not harmful.

If dizziness or fainting occurs (more common during first week of therapy), avoid sudden changes in posture.

Caution in hot weather: may increase risk of heat-stroke.

Perphenazine/Amitriptyline

(per-FEN-uh-zeen/am-ee-TRIP-tih-leen)

Etrafon, Triavil

A medicine used to treat moderate to severe anxiety or agitation and depression.

Precautions

DO NOT USE if you are allergic to this medicine or its relatives (eg, antidepressants) or concurrent use of a monoamine oxidase inhibitor (MAOI) or if you have bone marrow suppression.

BEFORE USING THIS MEDICINE, tell your healthcare provider if you are pregnant or breastfeeding; or if you are taking, will be taking or stop taking any prescription or nonprescription medicine; or if you have any other medical conditions.

Side Effects

Every medicine can cause side effects, but many people have no, or minor, side effects. Tell your healthcare provider if any of the following occurs: seizures; trouble breathing; fever; sweating; muscle stiffness or weakness; unusual tiredness; lightheadedness; yellowing of the skin or eyes; nausea; vomiting; constipation; blurred vision; dry mouth; restlessness; drowsiness; incoordination; sleeplessness; dizziness; frequent urination; urinary retention; stuffy nose; wheezing; appetite loss; hives; itching; flushing; changes in menstrual cycle; spontaneous flow of breast milk; false-positive pregnancy test; breast enlargement in females and males; changes in sex drive.

Guidelines for Use

USE EXACTLY AS PRESCRIBED.

The initial dose is given 3 to 4 times daily and may be decreased by your healthcare provider over time.

May be taken without regard to food.

If a dose is missed, take it as soon as possible. If several hours have passed or if it is nearing time for the next dose, do not double the dose to "catch up," unless advised by your healthcare provider. If more than one dose is missed, contact your healthcare provider.

Contact your healthcare provider if sore throat or other signs of infection appear.

This medicine should be discontinued several days before surgery; consult your healthcare provider.

May cause drowsiness or dizziness, and response to alcohol and sedative medicines may be enhanced.

Use caution while driving or performing other tasks requiring mental alertness, coordination and dexterity.

This medication may cause sensitivity to sunlight. Avoid prolonged exposure to the sun. Use sunscreen and wear protective clothing until tolerance is determined.

Phenazopyridine Hydrochloride

(fen-AZZ-oh-PIE-rih-deen HIGH-droe-KLOR-ide)

AZO-Standard, Baridium, Eridium, Geridium, Phenazodine, Pyridiate, Pyridiate #2, Pyridium, Urodine, Urogesic

A medicine used for the relief of short-term (up to two days) pain, burning, frequent urination and other discomforts due to infection or inflammation of the lower urinary tract.

Precautions

DO NOT USE if you are allergic to this medicine or if you have kidney disease.

BEFORE USING THIS MEDICINE, tell your healthcare provider if you are pregnant or breastfeeding; or if you are taking, will be taking or stop taking any prescription or nonprescription medicine; or if you have any other medical conditions.

Side Effects

Every medicine can cause side effects, but many people have no, or minor, side effects. Tell your healthcare provider if any of the following occurs: headache; rash; itching; stomach upset; dizziness; breathing difficulty; lack of energy.

Guidelines for Use

USE EXACTLY AS PRESCRIBED.

May cause stomach upset. Take with food or after meals.

May cause urine to turn reddish-orange. May stain bedding or undergarments.

Treatment for urinary tract infection with this medicine should not exceed two days.

Use of an antibiotic can continue alone after two days.

Provides symptomatic pain relief only.

This medication should not be administered to children under 12 years old unless recommended by their healthcare provider.

Phenelzine Sulfate

(FEN-uhl-zeen SULL-fate)

Nardil Tablets

A monoamine oxidase inhibitor (MAOI) that generally is used to treat mental depression.

Precautions

DO NOT USE if you are allergic to this medicine, taking sympathomimetics, tricyclic antidepressants, selective serotonin reuptake inhibitors (SSRIs, eg, fluoxetine) or carbamazepines.

BEFORE USING THIS MEDICINE, tell your healthcare provider if you are pregnant or breastfeeding; or if you are taking, will be taking or stop taking any prescription or nonprescription medicines; or if you have any other medical conditions.

Side Effects

Every medicine can cause side effects, but many people have no, or minor, side effects. Tell your healthcare provider if any of the following occurs: severe headache; skin rash; darkening of the urine; pale stools; yellowing of skin or eyes; dizziness; constipation; diarrhea; nausea; weight gain.

Guidelines for Use

USE EXACTLY AS PRESCRIBED.

It may take a few weeks for the medicine to work. Do not discontinue this medication or take any other medication, except on the advice of your healthcare provider.

If a dose is missed, take it as soon as possible. If several hours have passed or if it is nearing time for the next dose, do not double the dose to "catch up," unless advised by your healthcare provider. If more than one dose is missed, contact your healthcare provider.

May cause drowsiness or blurred vision. Use caution while driving or performing other tasks requiring mental alertness.

Initially, dizziness, weakness or fainting may occur when arising from a horizontal or sitting position. If this occurs, get up slowly.

Tyramine-containing foods should be avoided including: any high protein food that is aged or undergoes breakdown by putrefaction process to improve flavor: many dairy products, some fish, alcohol products (especially beers, ales and red wines), some fruits/vegetables (eg, avocado, yeast extracts, bananas, figs, fava beans) and any caffeine-containing products or tyramine. Do not drink alcoholic beverages or self-medicate with cold, hay fever or weight-reducing preparations while undergoing therapy. Report promptly the occurrence of headache or other unusual symptoms.

Wear or carry identification saying that you take an MAOI.

Phenobarbital

(fee-no-BAR-bih-tahl)

Luminal, Solfoton

A barbiturate central nervous system depressant that can produce mild sedation, sleep and up to deep coma. Usually used to treat insomnia, to calm agitated people and to treat certain seizure disorders.

Precautions

DO NOT USE if you are allergic to this medicine or its relatives. This medicine may be habit-forming. Tolerance and dependence may occur, especially following prolonged use of high doses. Withdrawal symptoms can be severe.

BEFORE USING THIS MEDICINE, tell your healthcare provider if you are pregnant or breastfeeding; or if you are taking, will be taking or stop taking any prescription or nonprescription medicine; or if you have any other medical conditions.

Side Effects

Every medicine can cause side effects, but many people have no, or minor, side effects. Tell your healthcare provider if any of the following occurs: sleepiness; tired feeling; nausea; vomiting; morning hangover.

Guidelines for Use

USE EXACTLY AS PRESCRIBED.

Oral: Take only the amount of medicine prescribed by your healthcare provider.

This medicine contains alcohol. May decrease alertness or physical ability. Use caution when driving or performing tasks requiring mental alertness.

Avoid alcohol and other mental depressants (eg, narcotics, tranquilizers, antihistamines) while you are taking this medicine.

Use as an aid to sleep is limited; generally not for use longer than 2 weeks. Seizure control: Do not stop therapy suddenly.

Phenolphthalein

(fee-nahl-THAY-leen)

Alophen, Espotabs, Evac-U-Gen, Evac-U-Lax, Ex-Lax, Feen-A-Mint, Lax Pills, Laxative Pills, Medilax, Modane, Phenolax, Prulet

A medicine used for short-term treatment of constipation and to clean out the bowel before bowel examinations or bowel surgery.

Precautions

DO NOT USE if you are allergic to this medicine.

BEFORE USING THIS MEDICINE, tell your healthcare provider if you are pregnant or breastfeeding; or if you are taking, will be taking or stop taking any prescription or nonprescription medicine; or if you have any other medical conditions.

Side Effects

Every medicine can cause side effects, but many people have no, or minor, side effects. Tell your healthcare provider if any of the following occurs: nausea; vomiting; stomach ache; bowel cramping; diarrhea; weakness; dizziness; fainting; facial swelling, redness and discomfort; rectal bleeding; muscle cramps or pain; irritation of the rectal area; sweating; pounding in the chest.

Guidelines for Use

USE EXACTLY AS PRESCRIBED.

Take with a full glass of water or juice.

Laxative use is only a temporary measure. When normal bowel habits return, stop use of this medicine.

Frequent use of laxatives and inadequate fluid intake can cause an imbalance in fluid and electrolyte levels. Symptoms can include muscle cramps, muscle weakness and dizziness.

Effects will occur in 6 to 10 hours.

Pink-red, red-violet or red-brown discoloration of the urine may occur.

Phenoxybenzamine Hydrochloride

(fen-ox-ee-BEN-zuh-meen HIGH-droe-KLOR-ide)

Dibenzyline

Used to control episodes of high blood pressure and sweating. It may occasionally be prescribed for other reasons.

Precautions

DO NOT USE if you are allergic to this medicine.

BEFORE USING THIS MEDICINE, tell your healthcare provider if you are pregnant or breastfeeding; or if you are taking, will be taking or stop taking any prescription or nonprescription medicine; or if you have any other medical conditions.

Side Effects

Every medicine can cause side effects, but many people have no, or minor, side effects. Tell your healthcare provider if any of the following occurs: nasal congestion; stomach discomfort; drowsiness; fatigue; sexual difficulty; fainting; pin point pupils.

Patient Information

Avoid alcohol.

If dizziness occurs, avoid sudden changes in posture.

Avoid cough, cold or allergy medications that may cause dizziness, unless advised not to by your healthcare provider.

Phenylephrine Hydrochloride Ophthalmic

(fen-ill-EFF-rin HIGH-droe-KLOR-ide)

AK-Dilate, AK-Nefrin, Isopto Frin, Mydfrin, Neo-Synephrine Plain Ophthalmic, Neo-Synephrine Viscous Ophthalmic, Phenoptic Ophthalmic, Prefrin Liquifilm Ophthalmic, Relief Ophthalmic

A vasoconstrictor that causes the pupil to dilate (widen) and reduces redness. It is used as an ophthalmic decongestant to relieve minor eye irritations.

Precautions

DO NOT USE if you are allergic to this medicine.

BEFORE USING THIS MEDICINE, tell your healthcare provider if you are pregnant or breastfeeding; or if you are taking, will be taking or stop taking any prescription or nonprescription medicine; if you have any other medical conditions; or if you are allergic to sulfite preservatives.

Side Effects

Every medicine can cause side effects, but many people have no, or minor, side effects. Tell your healthcare provider if any of the following occurs: temporary stinging; blurred vision; redness; eye pain; tremor; faintness; pounding in the chest; collapse; headache; pale skin; sweating.

Guidelines for Use

USE EXACTLY AS PRESCRIBED.

May cause temporary blurred vision. Use caution when driving or performing other tasks requiring mental alertness.

Phenylephrine Hydrochloride Systemic

(fen-ill-EFF-rin HIGH-droe-KLOR-ide)

Alconefrin Nasal Solution, Rhinall

A decongestant used to treat nasal congestion due to the common cold, sinusitis, hay fever and other allergies. It also is used to relieve air block and pressure pain during air travel. It may occasionally be prescribed for other reasons.

Precautions

DO NOT USE if you have an allergy to this medicine.

BEFORE USING THIS MEDICINE, tell your healthcare provider if you are pregnant or breastfeeding; or if you are taking, will be taking or stop taking any prescription or nonprescription medicine; if you have any other medical conditions; or if you are allergic to sulfites.

Side Effects

Every medicine can cause side effects, but many people have no, or minor, side effects. Tell your healthcare provider if any of the following occurs: nausea; vomiting; appetite loss; anxiety; restlessness; tremors; headache; dizziness; drowsiness; sleeplessness; hallucinations; convulsions; depression; palpitations (pounding in the chest); sweating; pallor; difficulty breathing; chest pain; tearing; eye irritation; sensitivity of eyes to light; urinary retention; painful urination; nasal burning, stinging or dryness; sneezing; local irritation; rebound congestion.

Guidelines for Use

USE EXACTLY AS PRESCRIBED.

Do not take more than recommended dosage and do not use longer than 3 to 5 days.

Stinging, burning or drying of the nose may occur.

Excessive use may cause certain side effects (nervousness, dizziness or sleeplessness) that are more likely in the elderly and children.

Long-term, high-dose therapy may be habit-forming. Rebound congestion may occur after the dose wears off.

Stop using the medicine gradually; stop using the medicine in one nostril, then both nostrils. An oral decongestant may be substituted.

Phenylpropanolamine Hydrochloride

(fen-ill-pro-pan-OLE-uh-meen HIGH-droe-KLOR-ide)

Propagest

A decongestant used to treat nasal and sinus congestion due to the common cold, hay fever, sinusitis and other allergies.

Precautions

DO NOT USE if you are allergic to this medicine; have high blood pressure; or are breastfeeding.

BEFORE USING THIS MEDICINE, tell your healthcare provider if you are pregnant or breastfeeding; or if you are taking, will be taking or stop taking any prescription or nonprescription medicine; if you have any other medical conditions; or if you are allergic to sulfites.

Side Effects

Every medicine can cause side effects, but many people have no, or minor, side effects. Tell your healthcare provider if any of the following occurs: nausea; vomiting; appetite loss; anxiety; restlessness; tremors; headache; dizziness; drowsiness; sleeplessness; hallucinations; convulsions; irregular heartbeat; changes in blood pressure; palpitations (pounding in the chest); tearing; eye irritation; sensitivity of eyes to light; urinary retention; painful urination.

Guidelines for Use

USE EXACTLY AS PRESCRIBED.

If symptoms do not improve within 7 days or are accompanied by a high fever, consult your healthcare provider before continuing use.

Do not exceed recommended dosage. Higher doses may cause nervousness, dizziness or sleeplessness.

If a dose is missed, take it as soon as possible. If several hours have passed or if it is nearing time for the next dose, do not double the dose to "catch up," unless advised by your healthcare provider. If more than one dose is missed, contact your healthcare provider.

Phenylpropanolamine/Guaifenesin

(fen-ill-pro-pan-OLE-uh-meen/GWHY-fen-ah-sin)

Dura-Gest Capsules, Enomine Capsules, Entex LA, Vanex LA

A combination medicine of a nasal and sinus decongestant and expectorant that thins mucus in the lungs and makes the mucus easier to cough up, reducing chest congestion and making coughs more productive. This medicine is used to relieve symptoms of colds and allergies where congestion of the head and chest are prominent.

Precautions

DO NOT USE if you are breastfeeding; allergic to this medicine; or if you are taking monoamine oxidase (MAO) inhibitors.

BEFORE USING THIS MEDICINE, tell your healthcare provider if you are pregnant or breastfeeding; or if you are taking, will be taking or stop taking any prescription or nonprescription medicine; or if you have any other medical conditions.

Side Effects

Every medicine can cause side effects, but many people have no, or minor, side effects. Tell your healthcare provider if any of the following occurs: anxiety; restlessness; dizziness; insomnia; increased pulse or blood pressure; nausea; vomiting; loss of appetite; difficulty urinating.

Guidelines for Use

USE EXACTLY AS PRESCRIBED.

Do not exceed recommended dosage.

Drink a glass of water or other fluid with each dose of expectorant. A well-hydrated body (due to fluid intake) thins respiratory tract mucus and may be as valuable or more so than the medicine itself.

Do not take this product for persistent or chronic cough such as occurs with smoking, asthma, chronic bronchitis or emphysema, or when cough is accompanied by excessive phlegm, unless directed by your healthcare provider. A persistent cough may be a sign of a serious condition.

If symptoms persist for more than one week, tend to recur or are accompanied by fever, rash or persistent headache, consult your healthcare provider.

Sustained release: Swallow whole; do not crush or chew.

Phenytoin

(FEN-ih-toe-in)

Dilantin-125, Dilantin-30 Pediatric, Diphenylan

A medicine that helps control epilepsy and seizures. It may occasionally be prescribed for other reasons.

Precautions

DO NOT USE if you are allergic to this medicine or its relatives.

BEFORE USING THIS MEDICINE, tell your healthcare provider if you are pregnant or breastfeeding. Inform your healthcare provider if you become pregnant; or if you are taking, will be taking or stop taking any prescription or nonprescription medicines; or have any other medical conditions.

Side Effects

Every medicine can cause side effects, but many people have no, or minor, side effects. Tell your healthcare provider if any of the following occurs: skin rash; severe nausea or vomiting; swollen glands; bleeding, swollen or tender gums; yellowing of skin or eyes; joint pain; unexplained fever; sore throat; unusual bleeding or bruising; persistent headache; general body discomfort; infection or bleeding tendency; drowsiness; slurred speech; incoordination.

Guidelines for Use

USE EXACTLY AS PRESCRIBED.

May cause stomach upset; take with food.

Do not change the dose or stop taking this medication without consulting your healthcare provider.

Keep scheduled appointments with your healthcare provider and carry identification listing your medical condition and medication.

May cause drowsiness, dizziness, blurred vision. Use caution while driving or performing other tasks requiring mental alertness.

Maintain good oral hygiene (regular brushing and flossing).

Diabetes—Monitor urine sugar regularly and report any abnormal results to your healthcare provider.

Solution: Shake well before using.

Phytonadione (Vitamin K_1) Injection

(fye-toe-nuh-DIE-ohn)

AquaMEPHYTON, Konakion

A medicine used to correct coagulation (clotting) disorders caused by: anticoagulants, salicylates, antibiotics, or obstructive jaundice and biliary fistulas and other intestinalionditons limiting absorption of vitamin K; for prevention and therapy of hemorrhagic disease of the newborn.

Precautions

DO NOT USE if you are allergic to this medicine.

BEFORE USING THIS MEDICINE, tell your healthcare provider if you are pregnant or breastfeeding; or if you are taking, will be taking or stop taking any prescription or nonprescription medicine; or if you have any other medical conditions.

Side Effects

Every medicine can cause side effects, but many people have no, or minor, side effects. Tell your healthcare provider if any of the following occurs: pain, swelling and tenderness at the injection site; flushing sensations; taste perversion; anaphylactoid reactions (hives, redness of skin, difficulty breathing).

Phytonadione (Vitamin K_1) Oral

(fye-toe-nuh-DIE-ohn)

Mephyton

A medicine used to correct coagulation (clotting) disorders caused by: anticoagulants; salicylates, antibiotics or obstructive jaundice and biliary fistulas.

Precautions

DO NOT USE if you are allergic to this medicine.

BEFORE USING THIS MEDICINE, tell your healthcare provider if you are pregnant or breastfeeding; or if you are taking, will be taking or stop taking any prescription or nonprescription medicine; or if you have any other medical conditions.

Side Effects

Every medicine can cause side effects, but many people have no, or minor, side effects. Tell your healthcare provider if any of the following occurs: anaphylactoid reactions (hives, redness of skin, difficulty breathing).

Guidelines for Use

USE EXACTLY AS PRESCRIBED.

Protect from light at all times.

This information is advisory only; it does not contain all information about this medicine. If you have any questions about your medicine, ask your healthcare provider.

Pilocarpine Ophthalmic

(pie-low-CAR-peen)

Carbachol Solution, Miochol Solution, Miostat Solution, Pilopine HS Gel, Piloptic-1 Solution, Piloptic-2 Solution, Pilostat Solution

A direct-acting miotic that decreases high eye pressure in glaucoma; it helps reduce the blurred vision caused by medicines used in eye examinations or eye surgery.

Precautions

DO NOT USE if you are allergic to this medicine.

BEFORE USING THIS MEDICINE, tell your healthcare provider if you are pregnant or breastfeeding; or if you are taking, will be taking or stop taking any prescription or nonprescription medicine; or if you have any other medical conditions.

Side Effects

Every medicine can cause side effects, but many people have no, or minor, side effects. Tell your healthcare provider if any of the following occurs: burning; itching; tearing; blurring; inflammation of lids and conjunctiva; reduced vision in poor light; nausea; vomiting; diarrhea; excess watering of the mouth; sweating; headache; browache; abnormal heart rhythm.

Guidelines for Use

USE EXACTLY AS PRESCRIBED.

May sting when administered, especially the first few times.

Use caution while driving at night or performing tasks in poor lighting as vision may be reduced.

Report any changes in vision to your healthcare provider immediately.

Storage: Refrigerate; Do not freeze.

Pilocarpine Hydrochloride Systemic

(pie-low-CAR-peen HIGH-droe-KLOR-ide)

Salagen

A medicine used to treat dry mouth associated with radiation therapy for cancer of the head and neck.

Precautions

DO NOT USE if you are allergic to this medicine; have uncontrolled asthma; or any condition where contraction of the pupil is undesirable, such as narrow-angle glaucoma.

BEFORE USING THIS MEDICINE, tell your healthcare provider if you are pregnant or breastfeeding; if you are taking, will be taking or stop taking any prescription or nonprescription medicine; or if you have any other medical conditions.

Side Effects

Every medicine can cause side effects, but many people have no, or minor, side effects. Tell your healthcare provider if any of the following occurs: sweating; nausea; nasal congestion; chills; flushing; frequent urination; dizziness; weakness; headache; indigestion; tearing; diarrhea; edema (fluid retention).

Guidelines for Use

USE EXACTLY AS PRESCRIBED.

This medicine may be taken with or without food.

If a dose is missed, take it as soon as possible. If several hours have passed or if it is nearing time for the next dose, do not double the dose to "catch up," unless advised by your healthcare provider. If more than one dose is missed, contact your healthcare provider.

This medicine may cause vision problems, especially at night, that could affect your ability to drive safely.

If you sweat a lot while taking this medicine and cannot drink enough liquid, consult your healthcare provider.

Pindolol

(PIN-doe-lahl)

Visken

A beta blocker medicine used to lower high blood pressure and to treat angina and heart attack.

Precautions

DO NOT USE if you are allergic to this medicine or its relatives, or if you are breastfeeding.

BEFORE USING THIS MEDICINE, tell your healthcare provider if you are pregnant or breastfeeding; or if you are taking, will be taking or stop taking any prescription or nonprescription medicine; or if you have any other medical conditions.

Side Effects

Every medicine can cause side effects, but many people have no, or minor, side effects. Tell your healthcare provider if any of the following occurs: nausea; vomiting; stomach ache; diarrhea; constipation; appetite changes; indigestion; depression; anxiety; hallucinations; short-term memory loss; behavior changes; disorientation; fainting; dizziness; lightheadedness; tiredness; sleep disturbances; decreased concentration; headache; nightmares; emotional instability; chest pain; chills; cold or numb extremities; pounding in the chest; difficulty breathing; cough; nasal congestion; rash; hives; fluid retention; flushing or paleness; increased pigmentation; itching; hair loss; sweating; dry skin; painful and aching joints and muscles; painful, frequent or difficult urination; blurred vision; dry, burning or irritated eyes; ringing in the ears; taste changes; sore throat; dry mouth; slurred speech; fever; weight gain; changes in blood sugar levels.

Guidelines for Use

USE EXACTLY AS PRESCRIBED.

Ask your healthcare provider before using other medicines including nasal decongestants, diet aids or nonprescription cold preparations.

Do not stop this medicine suddenly; it could cause a worsening of disease including worse angina (chest pain), irregular heartbeats and increase risk of heart attack and death. Withdraw these medications slowly over one to two weeks by gradually decreasing the dose.

Diabetes — These products can mask signs of low blood sugar and change blood sugar levels. It may be necessary for your healthcare provider to change your dose of diabetic medications.

Use caution while driving or performing other tasks requiring mental alertness, coordination and dexterity.

Piperacillin

(PIH-per-uh-SILL-in)

Pipracil

Used to treat serious infections.

Precautions

DO NOT USE if you are allergic to penicillin or cephalosporins.

BEFORE USING THIS MEDICINE, tell your healthcare provider if you are pregnant or breastfeeding; or if you are taking, will be taking or stop taking any prescription or nonprescription medicine; or if you have any other medical conditions.

Side Effects

Every medicine can cause side effects, but many people have no, or minor, side effects. Tell your healthcare provider if any of the following occurs: pain/irritation at the injection site; itchy eyes; dizziness; fatigue; diarrhea; difficult breathing; rash; headache; unusual bleeding or bruising.

Guidelines for Use

USE EXACTLY AS PRESCRIBED.

If symptoms of an allergic reaction develop (eg, difficult breathing, facial swelling, rash, itching), stop taking the medicine and contact your healthcare provider.

If a dose is missed, take it as soon as possible. If several hours have passed or if it is nearing time for the next dose, do not double the dose to "catch up," unless advised by your healthcare provider. If more than one dose is missed, contact your healthcare provider.

Continue until all the prescribed medicine has been taken. Failure to take a full course of therapy may cause a relapse of the infection.

Pirbuterol Acetate

(pihr-BYOO-tuh-role ASS-uh-TATE)

Maxair

A medicine that makes breathing easier by widening breathing passages of the lung and by removing (expectorating) mucus and other debris causing congestion in the lungs. This medicine may be used along with theophylline or corticosteroids. It may be used to treat or prevent asthma attacks.

Precautions

DO NOT USE if you are allergic to this medicine or have heart rhythm disturbances associated with a rapid heart rate.

BEFORE USING THIS MEDICINE, tell your healthcare provider if you are pregnant or breastfeeding; or if you are taking, will be taking or stop taking any prescription or nonprescription medicine; or if you have any other medical conditions.

Side Effects

Every medicine can cause side effects, but many people have no, or minor, side effects. Tell your healthcare provider if any of the following occurs: nausea; vomiting; loss of appetite; heartburn; nervousness; restlessness; dizziness; lightheadedness; headache; anxiety; tension; tremor; drowsiness; weakness; sleeplessness; chest pain; pounding in chest (palpitations); breathing problems; coughing; flushing; sweating; hives; muscle cramps; unusual or bad taste in mouth; drying or irritation of mouth; diarrhea.

Guidelines for Use

USE EXACTLY AS PRESCRIBED.

Solution: Shake well before using.

Tell your healthcare provider if pounding in chest, chest pain, muscle tremors, dizziness, headache, flushing or difficult urination occurs, or if breathing difficulty or nervousness persists.

Patient instructions are available with products.

Do not exceed recommended dosage. Excessive use may lead to side effects or loss of effectiveness. Do not stop or adjust the dose except on the recommendation of your healthcare provider. If you do not get the usual relief from your normal dose, do not increase your dose, but call your healthcare provider immediately.

Aerosol — Usual dose: 2 inhalations (puffs) every 4–6 hours. One inhalation may be enough for some patients. Do not exceed a total daily dose of 12 inhalations. Administer pressurized inhalation during the second half of breath intake.

If more than one inhalation per dose is necessary, wait at least one full minute between doses. (Administer second inhalation at 3 to 5 minutes.)

This medicine is effective for 5 hours or longer. If a dose is missed, inhale it as soon as possible. If several hours have passed or if it is nearing time for the next dose, do not double the dose to "catch up," unless advised by your healthcare provider. If more than one dose is missed, contact your healthcare provider.

If serious breathing problems occur while taking this medicine, stop using and contact your healthcare provider immediately.

Do not use epinephrine or other bronchodilators while using this medicine.

Do not spray in eyes.

Store at room temperature and out the reach of children. Do not puncture container, use or store near heat or open flame.

Piroxicam

(pihr-OX-ih-kam)

Feldene

A nonsteroidal anti-inflammatory medicine (NSAID) used to relieve mild to moderate pain and inflammation of rheumatoid arthritis and osteoarthritis (degenerative joint disease). Doctors occasionally may prescribe it for other reasons.

Precautions

DO NOT USE if you are allergic to this medicine or its relatives, aspirin or iodides.

BEFORE USING THIS MEDICINE, tell your healthcare provider if you are pregnant or breastfeeding; or if you are taking, will be taking or stop taking any prescription or nonprescription medicines; if you have any other medical conditions; if you are prone to fluid retention; or if you use alcohol chronically.

Side Effects

Every medicine can cause side effects, but many people have no, or minor, side effects. Tell your healthcare provider if any of the following occurs: allergic reaction (eg, rash, itching, fever); changes in vision; weight gain; fluid retention; stomach problems (eg, nausea, vomiting, diarrhea, pain); black stools; constipation; persistent headache; dizziness; nervousness; weakness; ringing in the ears; taste changes; unusual bruising or bleeding.

Guidelines for Use

USE EXACTLY AS PRESCRIBED.

Avoid aspirin and alcoholic beverages.

If stomach upset occurs, take with food, milk or antacids. If stomach pain continues, tell your healthcare provider.

If a dose is missed, take it as soon as possible. If several hours have passed or if it is nearing time for the next dose, do not double the dose to catch up, unless advised by your healthcare provider. If more than one dose is missed, contact your healthcare provider.

May cause drowsiness or dizziness. Use caution while driving or performing other tasks requiring mental alertness, coordination and dexterity.

May cause sensitivity to sunlight. Avoid prolonged exposure to the sun. Use sunscreens and wear protective clothing until tolerance is determined.

Plicamycin

(PLY-kae-MY-sin)

Mithracin

Used to treat malignant testicular tumors when surgery or radiation is not possible. It also is used to treat high blood levels of calcium and calcium in the urine associated with advanced tumors.

Side Effects

Every medicine can cause side effects, but many people have no, or minor, side effects. Tell your healthcare provider if any of the following occurs: nausea; vomiting; loss of appetite; diarrhea; fever; drowsiness; weakness; overall body discomfort; headache; depression; facial flushing; skin rash; inflammation of the mouth; unusual bleeding or bruising; pain at the injection site.

Patient Information

Tell your healthcare provider if the following occurs: fever, sore throat, rashes, chills, unusual bleeding or bruising, bloody nose, black tarry stools, dark urine, yellowing of skin or eyes.

To avoid nausea, vomiting or upset stomach: Avoid sweet, fried or fatty foods. Eat smaller light meals several times a day. Dry foods (eg, crackers, toast) and liquids (eg, soup, unsweetened apple juice) may be more easily digested. Do not lie down after eating. If this does not help, antinausea medicine may be prescribed.

Contraceptive (birth control) measures are recommended during therapy.

Calcium supplements may be needed; discuss this with your healthcare provider.

Polyethylene Glycol Solution (PEG)

(poli-eth-uh-leen gli-cawl)

Colovage, CoLyte, GoLYTELY, OCL

An agent used for bowel cleansing prior to examination of the digestive tract.

Precautions

DO NOT USE if you are allergic to this medicine.

BEFORE USING THIS MEDICINE, tell your healthcare provider if you are pregnant or breastfeeding; or if you are taking, will be taking or stop taking any prescription or nonprescription medicine.

Side Effects

Every medicine can cause side effects, but many people have no, or minor, side effects. Tell your healthcare provider if any of the following occurs: nausea; abdominal fullness; bloating; cramps; vomiting; anal irritation.

Guidelines for Use

USE EXACTLY AS PRESCRIBED.

Do not add flavoring or additional ingredients to the solution before use, but solution will taste better if chilled before drinking.

Fasting 3 to 4 hours before drinking the solution is the best approach. However, under no circumstances should solid foods be eaten less than 2 hours before solution is administered.

No foods except clear liquids are permitted after administration of solution until the examination has been completed.

Adult dosage is 4 liters (approximately 132 oz) of solution prior to exam.

Drink 8 oz every 10 minutes until 4 liters are consumed or until a watery stool is clear.

Rapid drinking of each portion is preferred to drinking small amounts continuously.

The first bowel movement should occur in about one hour.

For midmorning examination — Allow 3 hours for drinking and 1 hour to complete bowel evacuation. Or drink the solution the evening before the examination, particularly if you are to have a barium enema.

Storage — Refrigerate the solution

Potassium Chloride

(poe-TASS-ee-uhm KLOR-ide)

Effer-K, K + 10, Kaon-Cl, Kaon Cl-10, K-Dur 10, K-Dur 20, Klor-Con, Klor-Con/EF, K-Lease, Klotrix, K-Lyte, K-Lyte DS, K-Norm, K-Tab, Micro-K, Micro-K 18, Slow-K, Ten-K

Used for the treatment of low potassium levels in various situations. It also is used for the prevention of potassium depletion when dietary intake is inadequate. Injectable — Used for the prevention and treatment of moderate or severe potassium deficiency when oral replacement therapy is not feasible. It may occasionally be prescribed for other reasons.

Precautions

DO NOT USE if you are allergic to this medicine.

BEFORE USING THIS MEDICINE, tell your healthcare provider if you are pregnant or breastfeeding; or if you are taking, will be taking or stop taking any prescription or nonprescription medicine; or if you have any other medical conditions.

Side Effects

Every medicine can cause side effects, but many people have no, or minor, side effects. Tell your healthcare provider if any of the following occurs: nausea; vomiting; diarrhea; gas; stomach discomfort; rash; irritation at the injection site; difficulty breathing; weakness; black or bloody stools; lack of energy; mental confusion; weakness and heaviness in the legs.

Guidelines for Use

USE EXACTLY AS PRESCRIBED.

May cause stomach upset; take after meals, or with food and a full glass of water.

Do not use salt substitutes concurrently, except on the advice of your healthcare provider.

Tell your healthcare provider if the following occurs: tingling of the hands and feet; unusual tiredness or weakness; a feeling of heaviness in the legs; severe nausea; vomiting; abdominal pain or black stools.

Tablets — Do not crush or chew; swallow whole.

Oral liquids, soluble powders and effervescent tablets; Mix or dissolve completely in 3 to 8 ounces of cold water, juice or other suitable beverage and drink slowly.

Following release of potassium chloride, the wax covering is excreted in the stool. This is normal and is not a cause for concern.

Pravastatin Sodium

(PRUH-vuh-stuh-tin SO-dee-uhm)

Pravachol

A medicine used to lower the level of cholesterol in the blood. It may occasionally be prescribed for other reasons.

Precautions

DO NOT USE if you are pregnant; breastfeeding; or allergic to this medicine.

BEFORE USING THIS MEDICINE, tell your healthcare provider if you are pregnant or breastfeeding; or if you are taking, will be taking or stop taking any prescription or nonprescription medicine; or if you have any other medical conditions.

Side Effects

Every medicine can cause side effects, but many people have no, or minor, side effects. Tell your healthcare provider if any of the following occurs: nausea; diarrhea; stomach pain; constipation; gas; headache; dizziness; rash; muscle cramps; taste changes.

Guidelines for Use

USE EXACTLY AS PRESCRIBED.

Take in the evening. May be taken without regard to meals.

Report any unexplained muscle pain, tenderness or weakness, especially if accompanied by fever or malaise, to your healthcare provider.

Notify your healthcare provider of any yellowing of the skin or eyes.

Most effective when used with exercise and a diet that reduces the intake of cholesterol and saturated fats.

Praziquantel

(pray-zih-KWAHN-tuhl)

Biltricide

A medicine used to treat worm infections (anthelmintic).

Precautions

DO NOT USE if you are allergic to this medicine or if the infection is in the eye.

BEFORE USING THIS MEDICINE, tell your healthcare provider if you are pregnant or breastfeeding; or if you are taking, will be taking or stop taking any prescription or nonprescription medicine; or if you have any other medical conditions.

Side Effects

Every medicine can cause side effects, but many people have no, or minor, side effects. Tell your healthcare provider if any of the following occurs: headache; dizziness; nausea; fever; general body discomfort; stomach pain.

Guidelines for Use

USE EXACTLY AS PRESCRIBED.

Take with meals.

Do not crush or chew tablets. This medicine is taken as 3 separate doses in one day.

The interval between doses should be no less than 4 hours or greater than 6 hours.

Continue use until all the prescribed medicine has been taken. Failure to take all of the medicine may prevent complete elimination of the worms, causing the infection to return.

May cause drowsiness or dizziness. Do not drive a car or operate machinery on the day you receive this medicine and on the following day.

Store at room temperature.

Prazosin

(PRAY-zoe-sin)

Minipress

A medicine for adults used to lower high blood pressure. It may occasionally be prescribed for other reasons.

Precautions

DO NOT USE if you are allergic to this medicine or its relatives or are breastfeeding.

BEFORE USING THIS MEDICINE, tell your healthcare provider if you are pregnant; or if you are taking, will be taking or stop taking any prescription or nonprescription medicine; or if you have any other medical conditions.

Side Effects

Every medicine can cause side effects, but many people have no, or minor, side effects. Tell your healthcare provider if any of the following occurs: dizziness; lightheadedness; pounding in the chest; nausea; shortness of breath; nasal congestion; sinus inflammation; muscle pain; blurred vision; drowsiness; fatigue; nervousness; numbness of fingers/toes; impotence; headache; swelling; urinary changes; weakness.

Guidelines for Use

USE EXACTLY AS PRESCRIBED.

Take the first dose at bedtime to reduce the risk of dizziness.

If a dose is missed, contact your healthcare provider immediately.

Do not increase the dose without consulting your healthcare provider. Patients being treated for high blood pressure often feel tired and run down for a few weeks after beginning therapy. Continue taking your medication even though you may not feel quite normal.

May cause drowsiness, dizziness, lightheadedness or blurred vision. Use caution when driving or performing other tasks requiring mental alertness.

Avoid engaging in any hazardous tasks for at least 24 hours after taking the first dose, missing several doses, increasing the dose or taking other high blood pressure medications.

Use caution when rising from a sitting or lying position.

If dizziness, lightheadedness or pounding in the chest become a problem, contact your healthcare provider.

Do not take nonprescription decongestants; weight loss products; or cold, sinus or allergy medications without first consulting your healthcare provider.

Prednisolone Ophthalmic

(pred-NISS-oh-lone)

AK Pred, Econopred, Inflamase Forte, Inflamase Mild, Pred Forte, Pred Mild

An anti-inflammatory agent for the eye. It works by inhibiting the inflammatory response of tissues to mechanical, chemical, or allergy-causing agents.

Precautions

DO NOT USE if you are allergic to this medicine.

BEFORE USING THIS MEDICINE, tell your healthcare provider if you are pregnant or breastfeeding; or if you are taking, will be taking or stop taking any prescription or nonprescription medicine; or if you have any other medical conditions.

Side Effects

Every medicine can cause side effects, but many people have no, or minor, side effects. Tell your healthcare provider if any of the following occurs: visual defects; temporary stinging or burning; muscle weakness.

Guidelines for Use

USE EXACTLY AS PRESCRIBED.

Do not stop using this medicine without consulting your healthcare provider.

May cause sensitivity to light. This may be reduced by wearing sunglasses.

Notify your healthcare provider if improvement is not seen after 7 or 8 days, if condition worsens, or if pain, itching or swelling occurs.

Some of these products may contain sulfite preservatives that can cause allergic reactions in certain individuals.

Check package label when available or consult your healthcare provider.

Prednisolone Systemic

(pred-NISS-oh-lone)

Delta-Cortef Tablets, Hydeltrasol, Hydeltrasol Injection, Hydeltra-T.B.A., Key-Pred, Pediapred Liquid, Predcor, Predicort, Predlone T.B.A., Prelone Syrup

A hormone used as replacement therapy when the adrenal cortex is not functioning properly. It is also used for its anti-inflammatory action. It may be prescribed for a variety of other uses.

Precautions

DO NOT USE if you have an allergy to this medicine or its relatives.

BEFORE USING THIS MEDICINE, tell your healthcare provider if you are pregnant or breastfeeding; or if you are taking, will be taking or stop taking any prescription or nonprescription medicine; or if you have any other medical conditions.

Side Effects

Every medicine can cause side effects, but many people have no, or minor, side effects. Tell your healthcare provider if any of the following occurs: unusual weight gain; swelling of the lower extremities; muscle weakness; black tarry stools; vomiting of blood; burning, puffing of the face; menstrual irregularities; prolonged sore throat; fever; cold.

Guidelines for Use

USE EXACTLY AS PRESCRIBED.

May cause stomach upset. Take with meals or snacks.

Take single daily or alternate day doses in the morning prior to 9 a.m. Take multiple doses at evenly spaced intervals throughout the day.

Patients on long-term therapy should carry *Medic-Alert* identification indicating that you are taking this medication.

High-dose or long-term therapy: DO NOT change or stop therapy unless directed by your healthcare provider. Sudden withdrawal of therapy may cause symptoms of fatigue, loss of appetite, nausea, vomiting, diarrhea, weight loss, weakness, dizziness and low blood sugar. It is important to keep regular appointments with your healthcare provider.

Alternate day therapy: Used to retain beneficial drug effects while lowering the risk of side effects. Twice the usual daily dose is given every other day in the morning before 9 a.m.

Diabetics may require increased doses of insulin or oral diabetes medications while taking this medication.

Prednisone

(PRED-nih-sone)

Deltasone Tablets, Intensol Solution, Liquid Pred Syrup, Meticorten Tablets, Orasone Tablets, Panasol-S Tablets, Prednicen-M Film Coated Tablets, Sterapred DS Tablets, Sterapred Tablets

A hormone used as replacement therapy when the adrenal cortex is not functioning properly. It also is used for its anti-inflammatory action. It may be prescribed for other reasons.

Precautions

DO NOT USE if you are allergic to this medicine; have a systemic fungal infection; or if you are receiving a live virus vaccine (eg, smallpox).

BEFORE USING THIS MEDICINE, tell your healthcare provider if you are pregnant or breastfeeding; or if you are taking, will be taking or stop taking any prescription or nonprescription medicine; or if you have any other medical conditions.

Side Effects

Every medicine can cause side effects, but many people have no, or minor, side effects. Tell your healthcare provider if any of the following occurs: unusual weight gain; swelling of the lower extremities; muscle weakness; black tarry stools; vomiting of blood; burning, puffing of the face; menstrual irregularities; prolonged sore throat; fever; cold.

Guidelines for Use

USE EXACTLY AS PRESCRIBED.

May cause stomach upset. Take with meals or snacks.

Take single daily or alternate day doses in the morning prior to 9 a.m. Take multiple doses at evenly spaced intervals throughout the day.

Patients on long-term therapy should carry *Medic-Alert* identification indicating that you are taking this medication.

High-dose or long-term therapy: DO NOT change or stop therapy unless directed by your healthcare provider. Sudden withdrawal of therapy may cause symptoms of fatigue, loss of appetite, nausea, vomiting, diarrhea, weight loss, weakness, dizziness and low blood sugar.

It is important to keep regular appointments with your healthcare provider.

Alternate day therapy: Used to retain beneficial drug effects while lowering the risk of side effects. Twice the usual daily dose is given every other day in the morning before 9 a.m.

Diabetics may require increased doses of insulin or oral diabetes medications while taking this medication.

Primaquine

(PRIM-uh-kween)

A medicine used to treat a malaria attack or prevent it from coming back. It may occasionally be prescribed for other reasons.

Precautions

DO NOT USE if you are allergic to this medicine or if you are taking quinacrine.

BEFORE USING THIS MEDICINE, tell your healthcare provider if you are pregnant or breastfeeding; or if you are taking, will be taking or stop taking any prescription or nonprescription medicine; or if you have any other medical conditions.

Side Effects

Every medicine can cause side effects, but many people have no, or minor, side effects. Tell your healthcare provider if any of the following occurs: nausea; vomiting; stomach pain/cramps; unusual tiredness; darkening of urine; vision or hearing changes; diarrhea; rash.

Guidelines for Use

USE EXACTLY AS PRESCRIBED.

If stomach upset occurs, take with food.

If a dose is missed, take it as soon as possible. If several hours have passed or if it is nearing time for the next dose, do not double the dose to "catch up," unless advised by your healthcare provider. If more than one dose is missed, contact your healthcare provider.

Continue use until all the prescribed medicine has been taken. Failure to take all of the medicine may prevent complete elimination of the active malaria, causing it to return.

If stomach upset (nausea, vomiting or stomach pain) continues, contact your healthcare provider.

Contact your healthcare provider if a darkening of the urine occurs.

Lab test may be required; keep regular appointments.

Store in tightly closed container and protect from light.

Primidone

(PRIM-ih-dohn)

Mysoline

Used to control grand mal, psychomotor or focal epileptic seizures, alone or with other medications. It may occasionally be prescribed for other reasons.

Precautions

DO NOT USE if you are allergic to this medicine.

BEFORE USING THIS MEDICINE, tell your healthcare provider if you are pregnant or breastfeeding; or if you are taking, will be taking or stop taking any prescription or nonprescription medicine; or if you have any other medical conditions.

Side Effects

Every medicine can cause side effects, but many people have no, or minor, side effects. Tell your healthcare provider if any of the following occurs: feeling of a whirling motion; fatigue; irritability; emotional disturbances; double vision; rapid eye movement; drowsiness; mood and personality changes; nausea; vomiting; loss of appetite; impotence; weakness; rash.

Guidelines for Use

USE EXACTLY AS PRESCRIBED.

May cause drowsiness, dizziness or change in vision. Use caution while driving or performing other tasks requiring mental alertness, coordination and dexterity.

If stomach upset occurs, take with food.

Do not discontinue medication abruptly or change dosage, except on advice of your doctor.

Tell your healthcare provider if skin rash or fever occurs.

Tell your healthcare provider immediately if you become pregnant.

Patients should carry identification (*Medic-Alert*) indicating medication usage and epilepsy.

Oral suspension: Shake well before using.

Probenecid

(pro-BEN-uh-sid)

Benemid, Probalan

Used to prevent gout attacks. May also be used with some antibiotics to make them more effective in treating infections.

Precautions

DO NOT USE with aspirin or other salicylates because these could make your condition worse. Do not start therapy until an acute gouty attack has subsided.

BEFORE USING THIS MEDICINE, tell your healthcare provider if you are pregnant or breastfeeding; or if you are taking, will be taking or stop taking any prescription or nonprescription medicine; or if you have any other medical conditions.

Side Effects

Every medicine can cause side effects, but many people have no, or minor, side effects. Tell your healthcare provider if any of the following occurs: nausea; vomiting; headache; rash; trouble breathing; fever; sore gums; dizziness; unusual tiredness; painful or frequent urination; blood in urine; loss of appetite; redness of face.

Guidelines for Use

USE EXACTLY AS PRESCRIBED.

The initial dose, for gout, is given twice daily and may be decreased by your healthcare provider over time.

If stomach upset occurs, take with food.

If nausea, vomiting or loss of appetite persists, notify your healthcare provider.

Drink plenty of water, at least 6 to 8 full glasses daily, to prevent kidney stones.

If a dose is missed, take it as soon as possible. If several hours have passed or if it is nearing time for the next dose, do not double the dose to "catch up," unless advised by your healthcare provider. If more than one dose is missed, contact your healthcare provider.

Store at room temperature (below 86 degrees F).

Probucol

(PRO-byoo-kahl)

Lorelco

A medicine used to lower cholesterol after weight loss and change in diet have not worked.

Precautions

DO NOT USE if you are allergic to this medicine.

BEFORE USING THIS MEDICINE, tell your healthcare provider if you are pregnant or breastfeeding; or if you are taking, will be taking or stop taking any prescription or nonprescription medicine; or if you have any other medical conditions.

Side Effects

Every medicine can cause side effects, but many people have no, or minor, side effects. Tell your healthcare provider if any of the following occurs: diarrhea; nausea; vomiting; gas; chest pain; headache; ringing in the ears; rash; vision changes; dark stools; stomach pain; fainting; dizziness; tingling or numbness in hands or feet.

Guidelines for Use

USE EXACTLY AS PRESCRIBED.

This medicine is usually taken 1 to 2 times daily with meals.

If a dose is missed, take it as soon as possible. If several hours have passed or it is nearing the time for the next dose, do not double the dose to "catch up," unless advised by your helathcare provider. If more than one dose is missed, contact your healthcare provider.

Female patients should avoid becoming pregnant for at least 6 months after stopping this medicine.

May cause diarrhea, gas, stomach pain, nausea or vomiting. Tell your healthcare provider if they persist.

Continue to control your diet while taking this medication.

Store at room temperature (below 86 degrees F).

Protect from light and moisture.

Lab tests will be required; be sure to keep appointments.

Procainamide Hydrochloride

(pro-CANE-uh-mide HIGH-droe-KLOR-ide)

Procan, Pronestyl

A heart medicine used to correct or prevent various types of irregular heartbeats and to treat heart rhythm disturbances.

Precautions

DO NOT USE if you are allergic to this medicine or its relatives.

BEFORE USING THIS MEDICINE, tell your healthcare provider if you are pregnant or breastfeeding; or if you are taking, will be taking or stop taking any prescription or nonprescription medicine; if you have any other medical conditions; or if you are allergic to tartrazine.

Side Effects

Every medicine can cause side effects, but many people have no, or minor, side effects. Tell your healthcare provider if any of the following occurs: joint pain or stiffness; skin lesions; muscle aches; chest pain with breathing; unexplained fever and chills; weakness and fatigue; headache; nausea; abdominal pain; appetite loss; vomiting; diarrhea; depression; dizziness; weakness; giddiness; hallucinations; rash; itching; hives; flushing; fluid retention; bitter taste in mouth.

Guidelines for Use

USE EXACTLY AS PRESCRIBED.

Do not discontinue medication unless instructed by your healthcare provider.

Administer this medication at evenly spaced intervals around the clock.

Notify your healthcare provider if soreness of the mouth, throat or gums, or symptoms of upper respiratory tract infection occurs.

Procarbazine Hydrochloride

(pro-CAR-buh-ZEEN HIGH-droe-KLOR-ide)

Matulane

A medicine used alone or with other antineoplastics for the treatment of Hodgkin's disease. It may occasionally be prescribed for other reasons.

Precautions

DO NOT USE if you are allergic to this medicine.

BEFORE USING THIS MEDICINE, tell your healthcare provider if you are pregnant or breastfeeding; or if you are taking, will be taking or stop taking any prescription or nonprescription medicine; or if you have any other medical conditions.

Side Effects

Every medicine can cause side effects, but many people have no, or minor, side effects. Tell your healthcare provider if any of the following occurs: nausea; vomiting; unusual tiredness; mouth sores; diarrhea; blood in urine; rash; yellow skin or eyes; dizziness; headache; nervousness; hallucinations; confusion; sleeplessness; nightmares; chills; hair loss; fainting; hearing changes; slurred speech; cough; sore throat; fever; unusual bleeding or bruising; trouble breathing; loss of appetite; muscle or joint pain; frequent urination.

Guidelines for Use

USE EXACTLY AS PRESCRIBED.

Contraceptive measures (birth control) for both men and women are recommended during treatment.

May be taken with or without food.

Blood and urine tests will be required; be sure to keep appointments.

This medicine may lower your body's ability to fight infection. Tell your doctor about any signs of infection including fever, sore throat, rashes or chills.

May cause sensitivity to sunlight. Avoid prolonged exposure to the sun. Use sunscreens and wear protective clothing until tolerance is determined.

May cause drowsiness or dizziness. Use caution when driving or performing other tasks requiring mental alertness, coordination or dexterity.

May cause muscle or joint pain, nausea, vomiting, sweating, tiredness, weakness, constipation, headache, difficulty swallowing, loss of appetite, loss of hair and depression. Notify your healthcare provider if these become pronounced.

Even though the medication might cause nausea and vomiting, it is important that you continue to take it.

Avoid alcohol.

Avoid foods with high amounts of tyramine (eg, red wine, yogurt, aged cheese, bananas).

Wash your hands immediately after touching the medication.

Store at room temperature (below 86 degrees F).

Prochlorperazine

(pro-klor-PURR-uh-zeen)

Compazine, Compazine Spansules Timed Release

A medicine used to control nausea and vomiting. It is also used to improve concentration and self-control in patients with psychotic behavior. It may occasionally be prescribed for other purposes.

Precautions

DO NOT USE if you are allergic to this medicine, its relatives or tartrazine. Laboratory tests may be needed.

BEFORE USING THIS MEDICINE, tell your healthcare provider if you are pregnant or breastfeeding; or if you are taking, will be taking or stop taking any prescription or nonprescription medicine; or if you have any other medical conditions.

Side Effects

Every medicine can cause side effects, but many people have no, or minor, side effects. Tell your healthcare provider if any of the following occurs: tremors; drooling; shuffling gait; restlessness; muscle spasms; aching or numbness; sore throat; fever; unusual bleeding or bruising; skin rash; weakness; impaired vision; dark-colored urine; pale stools; yellow skin or eyes; drowsiness.

Guidelines for Use

USE EXACTLY AS PRESCRIBED.

Take this medicine routinely as directed; it controls illness symptoms and is not habit-forming.

If a dose is missed, take it as soon as possible. If several hours have passed or if it is nearing time for the next dose, do not double the dose to "catch up," unless advised by your healthcare provider. If more than one dose is missed, contact your healthcare provider.

Improvement may not be seen for several weeks.

May cause drowsiness. Use caution while driving or performing other tasks requiring mental alertness. Avoid alcohol and medicines that cause drowsiness.

May cause sunlight sensitivity. Avoid long exposure to the sun. Use sunscreens and protective clothing until tolerance is known.

If dizziness or fainting occurs, avoid sudden changes in posture and use caution when climbing stairs, etc (more common during first week of therapy).

This medicine may increase risk of heat-stroke.

Sustained release: Do not crush or chew.

Procyclidine

(pro-SIGH-klih-deen)

Kemadrin

A medicine used to treat the symptoms of parkinsonism, and parkinsonism disorders. This agent is not a cure for parkinsonism, it only helps control the symptoms.

Precautions

DO NOT USE if you are allergic to this medicine or its relatives (eg, anticholinergics).

BEFORE USING THIS MEDICINE, tell your healthcare provider if you are pregnant or breastfeeding; or if you are taking, will be taking or stop taking any prescription or nonprescription medicine; or if you have any other medical conditions.

Side Effects

Every medicine can cause side effects, but many people have no, or minor, side effects. Tell your healthcare provider if any of the following occurs: rash; confusion; nervousness; lightheadedness; dizziness; drowsiness; dry mouth; nausea; vomiting; vision changes; painful or difficult urination; racing heart.

Guidelines for Use

USE EXACTLY AS PRESCRIBED.

Take after meals or a snack.

Usually taken 3 times a day; occasionally a bedtime dose is used.

May cause drowsiness, dizziness or blurred vision. Use caution when driving or performing other tasks requiring mental alertness, coordination or dexterity.

Use caution when rising from a seated or lying position.

If a dose is missed, take it as soon as possible. If several hours have passed or it is nearing time for the next dose, do not double the dose to "catch up," unless advised by your healthcare provider. If more than one dose is missed, consult your healthcare provider.

Avoid alcohol and medicines (eg, tranquilizers, antihistamines, some pain medicines) that cause drowsiness.

Sucking on hard candy, drinking fluids, or maintaining good dental hygiene can relieve dry mouth.

If constipation occurs, use stool softeners if necessary. If constipation or difficult urination persists notify your healthcare provider.

Notify your healthcare provider if rapid or pounding heartbeat, confusion, eye pain occurs.

Progesterone Injectable

(pro-JESS-ter-ohn)

Gesterol, Progestaject

Used to treat abnormal uterine bleeding, amenorrhea (absence of menstrual bleeding) and endometriosis.

Precautions

DO NOT USE if you are allergic to this medicine or if you are pregnant.

BEFORE USING THIS MEDICINE, tell your healthcare provider if you are pregnant or breastfeeding; or if you are taking, will be taking or stop taking any prescription or nonprescription medicine; or if you have any other medical conditions.

Side Effects

Every medicine can cause side effects, but many people have no, or minor, side effects. Tell your healthcare provider if any of the following occurs: breakthrough bleeding; spotting; change in menstrual flow; absence of menstrual flow; breast changes; swelling; changes in weight; rash (with or without itching); acne; mental depression; hair loss; hives; abnormal hairiness; irritation at the injection site.

Patient Information

Tell your healthcare provider if you suspect you are pregnant or if any of the following occurs: pain in the calves accompanied by swelling, warmth and redness; sudden severe headache; visual disturbance; numbness in an arm or leg.

Diabetes — Glucose tolerance may be decreased; monitor urine sugar closely and report any abnormalities to your healthcare provider.

Progesterone Intrauterine System

(pro-JESS-ter-ohn)

Progestasert

An intrauterine contraceptive device (IUD) for use in women who have had at least one child, are in a stable, mutually monogamous relationship, and have no history of pelvic inflammatory disease (PID). The device should be replaced every 12 months. It may occasionally be used for other conditions.

Precautions

DO NOT USE if you are pregnant or suspect pregnancy; have the presence or history of PID; if you or your partner have multiple sex partners; have a sexually transmitted disease; have postpartum endometriosis or infected abortion; have uterine or cervical cancer; have had an unresolved pap smear; have genital bleeding of unknown cause; have a vaginal or cervical infection, unless infection has been completely controlled and is nongonococcal and nonchlamydial; have a previously inserted IUD still in place; have a condition or are undergoing a treatment associated with increased risk of infection (eg, leukemia, diabetes); or if you are an IV drug user.

Side Effects

Every medicine can cause side effects, but many people have no, or minor, side effects. Tell your healthcare provider if any of the following occurs: abnormal or excessive bleeding; severe cramping; abnormal or odorous vaginal discharge; fever or flu-like symptoms; pain; genital lesions or sores; missed period.

Guidelines for Use

USE EXACTLY AS PRESCRIBED.

Pregnancy must be ruled out prior to insertion. Conduct pregnancy tests whenever pregnancy is suspected. If pregnancy occurs, the device must be removed.

Bleeding and cramps may occur during the first few weeks after insertion; if symptoms continue or are severe, contact your healthcare provider.

Patient package insert and patient instructions available with product. Patient must read and initial each section of the Patient Information Leaflet, and the Informed Choice Statement must be signed by the patient and by the physician.

Promethazine Hydrochloride

(pro-METH-uh-zeen HIGH-droe-KLOR-ide)

Anergan 25, K-Phen-50, Pentazine, Phenameth, Phenazine, Phencen-50, Phenergan, Phenergan Fortis, Phenoject-50, Pro-50, Prometh 50, Prorex-25, Prorex-50, Prothazine, V-Gan 25, V-Gan 50

Used to control nausea and vomiting and to treat motion sickness.

Precautions

DO NOT USE if you are allergic to this medicine.

BEFORE USING THIS MEDICINE, tell your healthcare provider if you are pregnant or breastfeeding; or if you are taking, will be taking or stop taking any prescription or nonprescription medicines; or if you have any other medical conditions.

Side Effects

Every medicine can cause side effects, but many people have no, or minor, side effects. Tell your healthcare provider if any of the following occurs: sore throat; fever; unusual bleeding; bruising; skin rash; weakness; tremors; impaired vision; headache; behavior changes; breast changes; difficult breathing; stomach upset; dark-colored urine; pale stools; yellowing of skin or eyes; involuntary muscle twitching or movement.

Guidelines for Use

USE EXACTLY AS PRESCRIBED.

Do not change from one brand of this medicine to another without consulting your healthcare provider.

May cause drowsiness, use caution while driving or performing other tasks requiring mental alertness, coordination or physical dexterity.

Avoid alcohol or medicines that cause drowsiness, in particular medicines with anticholinergic actions.

Taking this medicine with lithium may cause severe confusion and disorientation.

May discolor the urine pink or reddish-brown. This is not harmful.

If dizziness or fainting occurs, avoid sudden changes in posture and use caution when climbing stairs, etc.

Use with caution in hot weather. May increase susceptibility to heat stroke. Avoid prolonged exposure to the sun. Use sunscreens and wear protective clothing until tolerance is determined.

Suppository: If unsure about proper insertion procedure, consult your healthcare provider. Store suppositories in the refrigerator.

Propantheline Bromide

(pro-PAN-thuh-leen BROE-mide)

Pro-Banthine

Used for the treatment of peptic ulcers. Usually used in combination with other medications. It may occasionally be prescribed for other reasons.

Precautions

DO NOT USE if you are allergic to this medicine or its relatives (eg, anticholinergics).

BEFORE USING THIS MEDICINE, tell your healthcare provider if you are pregnant or breastfeeding; or if you are taking, will be taking or stop taking any prescription or nonprescription medicine; or if you have any other medical conditions.

Side Effects

Every medicine can cause side effects, but many people have no, or minor, side effects. Tell your healthcare provider if any of the following occurs: vision changes; eye pain; nausea; constipation; vomiting; dry mouth; headache; nervousness; confusion; drowsiness; weakness; dizziness; rash; painful or difficult urination; racing heart; pounding in the chest.

Guidelines for Use

USE EXACTLY AS PRESCRIBED.

Take 30 minutes before each meal and at bedtime.

May cause drowsiness, dizziness or blurred vision. Use caution when driving or performing other tasks requiring mental alertness.

If a dose is missed, take it as soon as possible. If several hours have passed or it is nearing time for the next dose, do not double the dose to "catch up," unless advised by your healthcare provider. If more than one dose is missed, consult your healthcare provider.

Avoid alcohol and medicines (eg, tranquilizers, antihistamines, some pain medicines) that cause drowsiness.

Sucking on hard candy, drinking fluids, or maintaining good dental hygiene can relieve dry mouth.

Notify your healthcare provider if skin rash, flushing, rapid heartbeat or eye pain occurs.

If constipation occurs, use stool softeners if necessary. If constipation or difficult urination persists, notify your healthcare provider.

This medicine can reduce the ability to sweat, an important function by which overheating is prevented. Avoid excess sun and exercise.

Propoxyphene

(pro-POX-ee-feen)

Darvon Capsules, Darvon-N Suspension, Darvon-N Tablets, Dolene Capsules

A narcotic pain reliever used for mild to moderate pain.

Precautions

DO NOT USE if you are allergic to this medicine or its relatives.

BEFORE USING THIS MEDICINE, tell your healthcare provider if you are pregnant or breastfeeding; or if you are taking, will be taking or stop taking any prescription or nonprescription medicine; or if you have any other medical conditions. Long-term, regular use of narcotic pain relievers may lead to dependence and physical tolerance. Withdrawal symptoms may occur when therapy is stopped.

Side Effects

Every medicine can cause side effects, but many people have no, or minor, side effects. Tell your healthcare provider if any of the following occurs: lightheadedness; dizziness; drowsiness; nausea; vomiting; sweating; abdominal pain; cramps; constipation; diarrhea; urine retention; appetite loss; indigestion; gas; excitability; vision problems; difficult breathing.

Guidelines for Use

USE EXACTLY AS PRESCRIBED.

Take with food if stomach upset occurs.

May cause drowsiness, dizziness or blurred vision. Use caution while driving or performing other tasks requiring mental alertness, judgment and coordination.

Avoid alcohol and other medicines that cause drowsiness (eg, sleeping pills, antihistamines).

May cause nausea, vomiting or constipation. Constipation may be avoided by using a stool softener or fiber laxative.

This medicine works best if taken regularly. It is more effective in preventing pain than in treating pain after it occurs. Give the medicine ample time to work before taking more (approximately 30 minutes to 1 hour).

If a dose is missed, take it as soon as possible. If several hours have passed or if it is nearing time for the next dose, do not double the dose to "catch up," unless advised by your healthcare provider. If more than one dose is missed, contact your healthcare provider.

Propoxyphene/Acetaminophen

(pro-POX-ee-feen/ass-cet-ah-MEE-noe-fen)

Darvocet-N Tablets, Propacet 100 Tablets, Propoxyphene Napsylate w/Acetaminophen Caplet, Propoxyphene Napsylate w/Acetaminophen Tablet

A medicine used to relieve moderate to severe pain.

Precautions

DO NOT USE if you are allergic to this medicine.

BEFORE USING THIS MEDICINE, tell your healthcare provider if you are pregnant or breastfeeding; or if you are taking, will be taking or stop taking any prescription or nonprescription medicine; or if you have any other medical conditions.

Side Effects

Every medicine can cause side effects, but many people have no, or minor, side effects. Tell your healthcare provider if any of the following occurs: drowsiness; dizziness; blurred vision; nausea; vomiting; constipation; difficulty breathing; rash; yellowing of the skin.

Guidelines for Use

USE EXACTLY AS PRESCRIBED.

May cause nausea. Take with food.

May cause drowsiness, dizziness or blurred vision. Use caution while driving or performing other tasks requiring mental alertness. Avoid alcohol and other sedatives or drowsiness-causing substances.

Long-term use may lead to addiction. An early sign of this is medicine ineffectiveness. Dependence is not an issue in terminal illness pain where patient comfort is more important.

May cause constipation with long-term use. Use stool softener or fiber laxative.

Narcotics are more effective in preventing pain than in treating pain after it occurs. Significant overdosage requires emergency treatment.

Propranolol Hydrochloride

(pro-PRAN-oh-lahl HIGH-droe-KLOR-ide)

Inderal, Inderal LA CapsuleTimed Release

An antihypertensive medicine used to lower high blood pressure; treat angina; treat narrowing of the aortic valve in the heart; treat irregular heartbeats; treat heart attack; prevent migraines. It may occasionally be prescribed for other reasons.

Precautions

DO NOT USE if you are allergic to this medicine or its relatives or if you are breastfeeding.

BEFORE USING THIS MEDICINE, tell your healthcare provider if you are pregnant; or if you are taking, will be taking or stop taking any prescription or nonprescription medicines; or have any other medical conditions.

Side Effects

Every medicine can cause side effects, but many people have no, or minor, side effects. Tell your healthcare provider if any of the following occurs: difficult breathing, especially on exertion or when lying down; night cough; swelling of the extremities; slow pulse rate; dizziness; confusion or depression; rash; fever; sore throat; unusual bleeding or bruising.

Guidelines for Use

USE EXACTLY AS PRESCRIBED.

Take consistently with or without food at the same time each day.

Consult your healthcare provider before using other products including nasal decongestants, diet aids or nonprescription cold preparations.

Use caution while driving or performing other tasks requiring mental alertness.

Discontinuing therapy—If discontinued suddenly, this medicine may mask the signs of hyperthyroidism (overactive thyroid). If thyroid patients stop taking this medicine too suddenly symptoms of hyperthyroidism (eg, a rapid pulse) may occur. Sudden discontinuation also has caused worsening of angina (chest pain), heart attacks, irregular heartbeats and death.

Other serious withdrawal symptoms include: sweating; pounding in the chest; headache.

Withdraw this medicine slowly over one to two weeks.

Diabetes—This medicine can mask signs of hypoglycemia (low blood sugar) and alter blood sugar levels. It may be necessary for your healthcare provider to alter your medicine.

Sustained release: Swallow whole; do not crush or chew.

Propylthiouracil

(pro-puhl-thigh-oh-YOU-rah-sill)

Propyl-Thyracil

A medicine used to treat hyperthyroidism (overactive thyroid gland) and to treat or prepare the overactive thyroid for surgery.

Precautions

DO NOT USE if you are allergic to this medicine or if you are breastfeeding.

BEFORE USING THIS MEDICINE, tell your healthcare provider if you are pregnant or breastfeeding; or if you are taking, will be taking or stop taking any prescription or nonprescription medicine; or if you have any other medical conditions.

Side Effects

Every medicine can cause side effects, but many people have no, or minor, side effects. Tell your healthcare provider if any of the following occurs: blood disorders; nausea; vomiting; tingling in arms/legs; headache; dizziness; drowsiness; rash; itching; bruising/bleeding; yellowing of skin; hair loss; joint/muscle pain; swelling.

Guidelines for Use

USE EXACTLY AS PRESCRIBED.

Take at regular intervals around the clock (usually every 8 hours), unless directed otherwise by your healthcare provider.

Protriptyline Hydrochloride

(pro-TRIP-tih-leen HIGH-droe-KLOR-ide)

Vivactil

A mood elevating medicine usually used for the relief of depression. It may occasionally be prescribed for other reasons.

Precautions

DO NOT USE if you are allergic to this medicine or its relatives, or if you are using monoamine oxidase inhibitors (eg, *Nardil, Parnate*).

BEFORE USING THIS MEDICINE, tell your healthcare provider if you are pregnant or breastfeeding; or if you are taking, will be taking or stop taking any prescription or nonprescription medicine; or if you have any other medical conditions.

Side Effects

Every medicine can cause side effects, but many people have no, or minor, side effects. Tell your healthcare provider if any of the following occurs: dry mouth; blurred vision; impaired coordination; difficult urination; excessive sedation; seizures.

Guidelines for Use

USE EXACTLY AS PRESCRIBED.

Take as directed with a full glass of water, with or without food.

If a dose is missed, take it as soon as possible. If several hours have passed or if it is nearing time for the next dose, do not double the dose to "catch up," unless advised by your healthcare provider. If more than one dose is missed, contact your healthcare provider.

This medicine may not be effective for 2 to 3 weeks.

Using this medicine with alcohol or other central nervous system depressants (eg, pain relievers, sedatives, antihistamines) may cause added drowsiness.

May cause drowsiness or blurred vision. Use caution while driving or performing other tasks requiring mental alertness.

May cause sensitivity to sunlight. Avoid prolonged exposure to the sun. Use sunscreens and wear protective clothing until tolerance is determined.

Taking this medicine at bedtime may help reduce side effects (eg, daytime drowsiness). Discuss this possibility with your healthcare provider.

Symptoms of nausea, headache or fatigue may develop; talk to your healthcare provider if these become severe.

Pseudoephedrine Hydrochloride

(SUE-doe-eh-FED-rin HIGH-droe-KLOR-ide)

Congestion Relief, Halofed, Novafed Capsule Timed Release, PediaCare Decongestant, Pseudo-Gest, Sudafed, Sudafed 12–Hour

A decongestant used to treat nasal and sinus congestion due to the common cold, hay fever, sinusitis and other allergies.

Precautions

DO NOT USE use if you are allergic to this medicine; have high blood pressure; or are breastfeeding.

BEFORE USING THIS MEDICINE, tell your healthcare provider if you are pregnant or breastfeeding; or if you are taking, will be taking or stop taking any prescription or nonprescription medicine; if you have any other medical conditions; or if you are allergic to sulfites.

Side Effects

Every medicine can cause side effects, but many people have no, or minor, side effects. Tell your healthcare provider if any of the following occurs: nausea; vomiting; appetite loss; anxiety; restlessness; tremors; headache; dizziness; drowsiness; sleeplessness; hallucinations; convulsions; irregular heartbeat; changes in blood pressure; pounding in the chest; tearing; eye irritation; sensitivity of eyes to light; urinary retention; painful urination.

Guidelines for Use

USE EXACTLY AS PRESCRIBED.

If symptoms do not improve within 7 days or are accompanied by a high fever, consult your healthcare provider before continuing use.

Do not exceed recommended dosage. Higher doses may cause nervousness, dizziness or sleeplessness.

If a dose is missed, take it as soon as possible. If several hours have passed or if it is nearing time for the next dose, do not double the dose to "catch up," unless advised by your healthcare provider. If more than one dose is missed, contact your healthcare provider.

Pseudoephedrine Sulfate

(SUE-doe-eh-FED-rin SULL-fate)

Afrin, Chlor-Trimeton, Drixoral Non-Drowsy Formula

Used for the temporary relief of nasal congestion due to the common cold, hay fever or other upper respiratory allergies and nasal congestion associated with sinusitis; to promote nasal or sinus drainage; relief of eustachian tube congestion.

Precautions

DO NOT USE if you are allergic to this medicine.

BEFORE USING THIS MEDICINE, tell your healthcare provider if you are pregnant or breastfeeding; or if you are taking, will be taking or stop taking any prescription or nonprescription medicine; or if you have any other medical conditions.

Side Effects

Every medicine can cause side effects, but many people have no, or minor, side effects. Tell your healthcare provider if any of the following occurs: fear; anxiety; restlessness; headache; lightheadedness; dizziness; drowsiness; tremor; insomnia; hallucinations; weakness; pounding in the chest; nausea; vomiting; difficulty breathing; sweating.

Guidelines for Use

USE EXACTLY AS PRESCRIBED.

Patients with hypertension or other cardiovascular diseases, hyperthyroidism, diabetes mellitus or prostatic hypertrophy should use this medicine only on the advice of your healthcare provider.

Do not exceed recommended dosage; higher doses may cause nervousness; dizziness or sleeplessness.

If symptoms do not improve within 7 days or are accompanied by a high fever, consult your healthcare provider before continuing use.

Pyrazinamide

(peer-uh-ZIN-uh-mide)

Tebrazid

Used to treat active tuberculosis. Usually used in combination with other medications. It may occasionally be prescribed for other reasons.

Precautions

DO NOT USE if you are allergic to this medicine.

BEFORE USING THIS MEDICINE, tell your healthcare provider if you are pregnant or breastfeeding; or if you are taking, will be taking or stop taking any prescription or nonprescription medicine; or if you have any other medical conditions.

Side Effects

Every medicine can cause side effects, but many people have no, or minor, side effects. Tell your healthcare provider if any of the following occurs: fever; joint pain; nausea; vomiting; loss of appetite; rash; acne; darkened urine; yellowing of the skin or eyes; stomach pain.

Guidelines for Use

USE EXACTLY AS PRESCRIBED.

May be taken with or without food.

Take at even intervals around the clock as prescribed, avoid missing a dose.

If a dose is missed, take it as soon as possible. If several hours have passed or if it is nearing time for the next dose, do not double the dose to "catch up," unless advised by your healthcare provider.

Continue use until all the prescribed medicine has been taken.

Notify your healthcare provider promptly of: fever, loss of appetite, general body discomfort, nausea and vomiting, darkened urine, yellowish discoloration of skin or eyes, pain or swelling of the joints.

May cause sensitivity to sunlight. Avoid prolonged exposure to the sun. Use sunscreens and wear protective clothing until tolerance is determined.

Failure to take all of the medicine may prevent complete elimination of the active tuberculosis, allowing the infection to return.

Store at room temperature (below 86 degrees F).

Pyridoxine (Vitamin B_6)

(peer-ih-DOX-een)

Beesix, Nestrex

A medicine used to treat pyridoxine (vitamin B_6) deficiency. It may occasionally be prescribed for other reasons.

Precautions

DO NOT USE if you are allergic to this medicine.

BEFORE USING THIS MEDICINE, tell your healthcare provider if you are pregnant or breastfeeding; or if you are taking, will be taking or stop taking any prescription or nonprescription medicine; or if you have any other medical conditions.

Side Effects

Every medicine can cause side effects, but many people have no, or minor, side effects. Tell your healthcare provider if any of the following occurs: numbness or tingling of skin or in fingers and toes; numbness around mouth; unstable walk; awkwardness of hands; decreased touch, temperature and vibration perception; drowsiness.

Guidelines for Use

USE EXACTLY AS PRESCRIBED.

Most people on balanced diets do not need vitamin supplements. People who are malnourished, those on certain prescription medicines (eg, isoniazid, estrogen-containing contraceptives) and those with specific metabolic problems are at risk for pyridoxine deficiency.

Recommended Dietary Allowances (RDA)--Adult males: 2 mg; Adult females: 1.6 mg; Pregnancy and lactation: 2.1 to 2.2 mg.

Common sources of pyridoxine--Fish, chicken, liver, kidney, pork, eggs, beans, unmilled rice, oats, whole-wheat products and nuts.

Quazepam

(KWAY-zuh-pam)

Doral

A benzodiazepine medicine that is a sleeping pill used to treat insomnia for a short period of time (1 to 2 weeks). Long-term use generally is not recommended.

Precautions

DO NOT USE if you are allergic to this medicine or its relatives or if you are pregnant.

BEFORE USING THIS MEDICINE, tell your healthcare provider if you are breastfeeding; or if you are taking, will be taking or stop taking any prescription or nonprescription medicine; or if you have any other medical conditions.

Side Effects

Every medicine can cause side effects, but many people have no, or minor, side effects. Tell your healthcare provider if any of the following occurs: vision changes; irregular heartbeat; headache; chest pain; yellowing of skin or eyes; rash; unusual bleeding or bruising; vomiting; heartburn; diarrhea; constipation; appetite loss; nervousness; irritability; memory loss; sleeplessness; ringing in the ears; sore throat; joint pain.

Guidelines for Use

USE EXACTLY AS PRESCRIBED.

Do not exceed prescribed dosage.

Take with a full glass of water.

Use caution while driving or performing other tasks requiring mental alertness, coordination and dexterity.

May cause morning drowsiness, unusual tiredness in the morning or daytime sleepiness after using these medications for sleep. The elderly are particularly sensitive to these effects.

Avoid alcohol and other medications that cause drowsiness (eg, pain relievers, sedatives, antihistamines).

Nighttime sleep may be disturbed for 1 or 2 nights following stopping of the medication.

May be habit forming. Do not discontinue medicine abruptly, especially if you have a history of seizures, regardless of other antiseizure medications you may be taking.

Long-term use may result in dependence. Withdrawal symptoms may occur when the medication is stopped.

Quinacrine Hydrochloride

(KWIN-uh-kreen HIGH-droe-KLOR-ide)

Atabrine Hydrochloride

Used to either treat a malaria attack or prevent it from coming back. It does not cure malaria. It is also used for the treatment of worms. It may occasionally be prescribed for other reasons.

Precautions

DO NOT USE if you are allergic to this medicine or if you are taking primaquine.

BEFORE USING THIS MEDICINE, tell your healthcare provider if you are pregnant or breastfeeding; or if you are taking, will be taking or stop taking any prescription or nonprescription medicine; or if you have any other medical conditions.

Side Effects

Every medicine can cause side effects, but many people have no, or minor, side effects. Tell your healthcare provider if any of the following occurs: vision changes; nausea; vomiting; diarrhea; stomach pain/cramps; convulsions; headache; dizziness; rash; nervousness;

Guidelines for Use

USE EXACTLY AS PRESCRIBED.

Take after meals with a full glass of water.

The tablet may be crushed and put into honey or jam.

This medication may cause a yellow color to skin or urine.

If a dose is missed, take it as soon as possible. If several hours have passed or if it is nearing time for the next dose, do not double the dose to "catch up," unless advised by your healthcare provider. If more than one dose is missed, contact your healthcare provider.

Continue use until all the prescribed medicine has been taken.

Failure to take all of the medicine may prevent complete elimination of the active malaria or the worms, allowing the infection to return.

Promptly report any visual disturbances to your healthcare provider.

If you are receiving long-term treatment, periodic eye examinations will be required; be sure to keep appointments.

Quinapril Hydrochloride

(KWIN-uh-PRILL HIGH-droe-KLOR-ide)

Accupril

An angiotensin converting enzyme (ACE) inhibitor medicine generally used to lower high blood pressure.

Precautions

DO NOT USE if you are allergic to this medicine or if you are pregnant.

BEFORE USING THIS MEDICINE, tell your healthcare provider if you are breastfeeding; or if you are taking, will be taking or stop taking any prescription or nonprescription medicine; or if you have any other medical conditions.

Side Effects

Every medicine can cause side effects, but many people have no, or minor, side effects. Tell your healthcare provider if any of the following occurs: stomach pain; vomiting; diarrhea; constipation; appetite loss; depression; headache; dizziness; nervousness; sleeping difficulties; fatigue; rapid or irregular heartbeat; dizziness/lightheadedness when rising quickly from a sitting or lying position; shortness of breath; cough; nasal congestion; bronchitis; sinus inflammation; rash; sweating; flushing; yellowing of skin or eyes; muscle cramps; weight loss; taste loss; dry mouth; decreased sex drive; back, joint and shoulder pain; urination changes; fever; vision disturbances; numbness/tingling of hands or feet.

Guidelines for Use

USE EXACTLY AS PRESCRIBED.

Avoid taking with meals that have a high fat content.

Patients starting treatment for high blood pressure may at first feel tired. It takes time for the body to adjust. Continue taking medication and check with your healthcare provider.

If a dose is missed, take it as soon as possible. If several hours have passed or if it is nearing time for the next dose, do not double the dose to "catch up," unless advised by your healthcare provider. If more than one dose is missed, contact your healthcare provider.

Do not interrupt or stop medication without consulting your healthcare provider.

Do not use salt substitutes without telling your healthcare provider.

A persistent, dry, nonproductive cough may occur. Tell your healthcare provider. Recovery is rapid when the medicine is stopped.

Dizziness, fainting or lightheadedness is most likely after the first dose or in the first days of therapy; avoid sudden changes in posture. If fainting occurs, discontinue medicine until talking to your healthcare provider.

Quinidine

(KWIN-ih-deen)

Cardioquin Tablets, Quinora Tablets

A heart medicine that is used to treat abnormal heart rhythms. It may occasionally be prescribed for other reasons.

Precautions

DO NOT USE if you are allergic to this medicine, or have discoloration or bruising associated with this medicine.

BEFORE USING THIS MEDICINE, tell your healthcare provider if you are pregnant or breastfeeding; or if you are taking, will be taking or stop taking any prescription or nonprescription medicine; or if you have any other medical conditions.

Side Effects

Every medicine can cause side effects, but many people have no, or minor, side effects. Tell your healthcare provider if any of the following occurs: nausea; vomiting; stomach pain; diarrhea; appetite loss; dizziness; delirium; headache; depression; lack of coordination; confusion; apprehension; fainting; low blood pressure; changes in heart rate or rhythm; difficult breathing; asthma (allergic reaction); rash; itching; sensitivity to sunlight; flushing; vision disturbances; hearing disturbances; joint or muscle pain.

Guidelines for Use

USE EXACTLY AS PRESCRIBED.

Do not discontinue medication unless instructed by your healthcare provider.

May cause stomach upset. Take with food.

Notify your healthcare provider if ringing in the ears, visual disturbances, dizziness or headache occurs.

Quinine Sulfate

(KWIE-nine SULL-fate)

Formula-Q Capsules, Legatrin Tablets, M-KYA Capsules, Q-vel Caplets, Quin-Amino Tablets, Quinamm Tablets, Quinine Sulfate Capsules, Quinine Sulfate Tablets, Quiphile Tablets

A medicine used to treat malaria. It also is used to prevent and treat nighttime leg cramps.

Precautions

DO NOT USE if you are allergic to this medicine or if you are pregnant.

BEFORE USING THIS MEDICINE, tell your healthcare provider if you are breastfeeding; or if you are taking, will be taking or stop taking any prescription or nonprescription medicine; or if you have any other medical conditions.

Side Effects

Every medicine can cause side effects, but many people have no, or minor, side effects. Tell your healthcare provider if any of the following occurs: ringing in the ears; headache; nausea; disturbed vision; disturbed color vision; sensitivity to light; blurred vision; night blindness; double vision; dilated pupil; optic nerve damage; nausea; vomiting; stomach ache; headache; vertigo (feeling of whirling motion); restlessness; confusion; excitement; apprehension; delirium; seizures; chest pain; rash; itching; flushing; sweating; hearing loss; facial swelling; fever; hepatitis (inflammation of the liver); anemia; other blood disorders; lowered body temperature; fainting.

Guidelines for Use

USE EXACTLY AS PRESCRIBED.

May cause stomach upset. Take with food or after meals.

May cause nausea, vomiting, diarrhea, stomach cramps or pain.

Use caution when driving or performing other tasks requiring alertness.

Stop this medicine if there is any evidence of allergy such as flushing, itching, rash, fever, stomach pain, difficult breathing, ringing in the ears or vision problems.

This medicine has been replaced as the primary medicine employed to treat malaria because safer and more effective medicines are currently available.

Ramipril

(ruh-MIH-pril)

Altace

An angiotensin converting enzyme (ACE) inhibitor medicine generally used to lower high blood pressure.

Precautions

DO NOT USE if you are allergic to this medicine or if you are pregnant.

BEFORE USING THIS MEDICINE, tell your healthcare provider if you are breastfeeding; or if you are taking, will be taking or stop taking any prescription or nonprescription medicine; or if you have any other medical conditions.

Side Effects

Every medicine can cause side effects, but many people have no, or minor, side effects. Tell your healthcare provider if any of the following occurs: stomach pain; vomiting; diarrhea; constipation; appetite loss; depression; headache; dizziness; nervousness; sleeping difficulties; fatigue; rapid or irregular heartbeat; dizziness/lightheadedness when rising quickly from a sitting or lying position; shortness of breath; cough; nasal congestion; bronchitis; sinus inflammation; rash; sweating; flushing; yellowing of skin or eyes; muscle cramps; weight loss; taste loss; dry mouth; decreased sex drive; back, joint and shoulder pain; urination changes; fever; vision disturbances; numbness/tingling of hands or feet.

Guidelines for Use

USE EXACTLY AS PRESCRIBED.

May be taken without regard to meals.

Patients starting treatment for high blood pressure may at first feel tired. It takes time for the body to adjust. Continue taking your medication and check with your healthcare provider.

If a dose is missed, take it as soon as possible. If several hours have passed or if it is nearing time for the next dose, do not double the dose to "catch up," unless advised by your healthcare provider. If more than one dose is missed, contact your healthcare provider.

Do not interrupt or stop medication without consulting your healthcare provider.

Do not use salt substitutes without telling your healthcare provider.

A persistent, dry, nonproductive cough may occur. Tell your healthcare provider. Recovery is rapid when the medicine is stopped.

Dizziness, fainting or lightheadedness is most likely after the first dose or in the first days of therapy; avoid sudden changes in posture. If fainting occurs, discontinue medicine until talking to your healthcare provider.

Ranitidine

(ran-EYE-tih-DEEN)

Zantac

An anti-ulcer medicine that blocks acid production by the stomach. It is used to treat stomach and duodenal ulcers, hypersecretory (increased acid secretion) conditions (eg, Zollinger-Ellison syndrome), erosive esophagitis and gastroesophageal reflux (bubbling of stomach contents into the esophagus, which causes heartburn).

Precautions

DO NOT USE if you are allergic to this medicine.

BEFORE USING THIS MEDICINE, tell your healthcare provider if you are pregnant or breastfeeding; or if you are taking, will be taking or stop taking any prescription or nonprescription medicine; or if you have any other medical conditions.

Side Effects

Every medicine can cause side effects, but many people have no, or minor, side effects. Tell your healthcare provider if any of the following occurs: headache; nausea; diarrhea; dizziness; joint pain; behavioral changes; rash; itching; unusual bleeding or bruising; sore throat; difficult breathing; shortness of breath; fever; sleep disturbances; constipation.

Guidelines for Use

USE EXACTLY AS PRESCRIBED.

Take without regard to meals.

Efferdose: Dissolve in 6–8 oz of water before drinking.

Do not take directly with antacids; separate doses by at least an hour.

Store between 39 degrees and 77 degrees F. Keep in its original container.

If a dose is missed, take it as soon as possible. If several hours have passed or if it is nearing time for the next dose, do not double the dose to "catch up," unless advised by your healthcare provider. If more than one dose is missed, contact your healthcare provider.

Never self-diagnose or self-treat ulcers with this or any other medicine.

It may be necessary to make significant lifestyle changes to assist in the treatment and prevention of ulcers and other digestive problems that can include stress-reduction programs, exercise and dietary changes.

Notify your healthcare provider if there are any symptoms that suggest a bleeding ulcer, such as black, tarry stools or coffee-ground vomit.

Lab tests or exams may be required. Be sure to keep appointments.

Store at room temperature.

Riboflavin, Vitamin B_2

(RYE-boh-FLAY-vin)

Used to treat and prevent riboflavin deficiency.

Patient Information

May cause yellow/orange discoloration of the urine.

Recommended Daily Allowances: Adult males--1.4 mg to 1.8 mg; adult females--1.2 mg to 1.3 mg.

Common sources of riboflavin—meats, poultry, fish, milk products, fortified cereals, yeast and green vegetables (eg, broccoli).

Most people on balanced diets do not need vitamin supplements.

Rifabutin

(RIFF-uh-BYOO-tin)

Ansamycin, Mycobutin

A medicine used to prevent tuberculosis infections in patients with advanced HIV infection.

Precautions

DO NOT USE if you are allergic to this medicine or any other rifamycin.

BEFORE USING THIS MEDICINE, tell your healthcare provider if you are pregnant; or if you are taking, will be taking or stop taking any prescription or nonprescription medicines; or have any other medical conditions.

Side Effects

Every medicine can cause side effects, but many people have no, or minor, side effects. Tell your healthcare provider if any of the following occurs: nausea; vomiting; appetite loss; diarrhea; stomach pain; dizziness; unusual tiredness; weakness; drowsiness; confusion; rash; itching; hives; muscle pain or arthritis; headache; vision problems; fever; abnormal lab tests (eg, liver function, blood count); numbness, pain or tingling in hands or feet; general body discomfort; chest pain; indigestion; belching; gas; sleeplessness; taste perversion; discolored urine.

Guidelines for Use

USE EXACTLY AS PRESCRIBED.

Take on an empty stomach. If nausea or vomiting occurs, take with food.

Do not stop taking the medicine before consulting your healthcare provider.

Avoid missing doses; however, if a dose is missed, take it as soon as possible. If several hours have passed, or if it is nearing time for the next dose, do not double the dose to "catch up," unless advised to do so by your healthcare provider. If more than one dose is missed, contact your healthcare provider.

May cause a brownish-orange discoloration of urine, stools, saliva, tears, sweat, sputum and skin. This is not harmful.

May also discolor soft contact lenses.

Oral contraceptives may not be as effective. Consider a nonhormonal method of birth control.

Rifampin

(RIFF-am-pin)

Rifadin, Rimactane

Used to treat tuberculosis and asymptomatic carriers of *Neisseria meningitidis*. It may occasionally be prescribed for other reasons.

Precautions

DO NOT USE if you are allergic to this medicine.

BEFORE USING THIS MEDICINE, tell your healthcare provider if you are pregnant or breastfeeding; or if you are taking, will be taking or stop taking any prescription or nonprescription medicine; or if you have any other medical conditions.

Side Effects

Every medicine can cause side effects, but many people have no, or minor, side effects. Tell your healthcare provider if any of the following occurs: flu-like symptoms; heartburn; loss of appetite; nausea; vomiting; gas; cramps; diarrhea; sore mouth and tongue; rash; hives; itching; flushing; headache; drowsiness; fatigue; dizziness; inability to concentrate; mental confusion; generalized numbness; behavioral changes; incoordination; pain in extremities; visual disturbances; menstrual changes; fever; swelling of the face and extremities; shortness of breath; wheezing; stomach pain; blood in the urine.

Guidelines for Use

USE EXACTLY AS PRESCRIBED.

Take on an empty stomach, at least 1 hour before or 2 hours after meals.

Take medication on a regular basis; avoid missing doses.

Do not discontinue therapy except on advice of your healthcare provider.

May cause a reddish-orange discoloration of urine, stools, saliva, tears, sweat and sputum. This is to be expected and is not harmful.

May also permanently discolor soft contact lenses.

Tell your healthcare provider if you experience flu-like symptoms (fever, chills, muscle and bone pain, headache), excessive tiredness or weakness, loss of appetite, nausea and vomiting, sore throat, unusual bleeding or bruising, yellowish discoloration of the skin or eyes, skin rash or itching.

Oral contraceptives may not be effective. Consider a nonhormonal method of birth control.

Riluzole

(RILL-you-zole)

Rilutek

A drug to prolong survival in patients with amyotrophic lateral sclerosis (ALS, Lou Gehrig's disease) in adults.

Precautions

DO NOT USE if you are allergic to this medicine or its ingredients.

BEFORE USING THIS MEDICINE, tell your healthcare provider if you are pregnant or breastfeeding; if you are taking, will be taking or stop taking any prescription or nonprescription medicine; or if you have any other medical conditions, especially liver or kidney disease.

Side Effects

Every medicine can cause side effects, but many people have no, or minor, side effects. Tell your healthcare provider if any of the following occurs: nausea; vomiting; constipation; weight loss; diarrhea; appetite loss; stomach pain; gas; dry, inflamed or sore mouth; numbness/tingling around mouth; yellowing of skin or eyes; general body discomfort; dizziness; feeling of whirling motion; headache; weakness; depression; drowsiness; sleeplessness; abnormal skin sensations; itching; rash; joint or back pain; inflexibility; difficulty breathing; cough; nasal congestion; high blood pressure; fast heartbeat; difficult or painful urination.

Guidelines for Use

USE EXACTLY AS PRESCRIBED.

Usual dose is 1 tablet every 12 hours. Take at the same time of day (eg, in the morning and evening). Women and Japanese patients may require a lower dose.

Take on an empty stomach, at least 1 hour before or 2 hours after a meal.

Taking with a high fat meal may decrease absorption of this medicine.

If a dose is missed, take the next tablet as originally planned.

This medicine may cause drowsiness or dizziness. Use caution while driving or performing other tasks requiring mental alertness, coordination or dexterity.

Inform your healthcare provider if you smoke (smoking may reduce effectiveness of this medicine).

Avoid drinking exessive alcohol while taking this medicine to reduce the risk of liver damage.

Contact your healthcare provider immediately if any illness with fever or yellowing of skin or eyes occurs.

Lab tests will be required to monitor therapy. Be sure to keep appointments.

Store at room temperature, away from bright light.

Rimantadine Hydrochloride

(rih-MAN-tuh-deen HIGH-droe-KLOR-ide)

Flumadine

This medicine is used for the prevention and treatment of illness caused by various strains of influenza A virus in adults and for prevention of illness caused by various strains of influenza A in children.

Precautions

DO NOT USE if you are allergic to this medicine or any of its relatives or if you are breastfeeding.

BEFORE USING THIS MEDICINE, tell your healthcare provider if you are pregnant; or if you are taking, will be taking or stop taking any prescription or nonprescription medicine; or if you have any other medical conditions.

Side Effects

Every medicine can cause side effects, but many people have no, or minor, side effects. Tell your healthcare provider if any of the following occurs: insomnia; dizziness; headache; seizures; nervousness; fatigue; nausea; vomiting; anorexia; dry mouth; abdominal pain; general body discomfort; depression; inability to concentrate.

Guidelines for Use

USE EXACTLY AS PRESCRIBED.

Therapy should be started as soon as possible, preferably within 48 hours after onset of signs and symptoms of influenza A infection.

Therapy should be continued for approximately 7 days from the start of symptoms.

If a dose is missed, take it as soon as possible. If several hours have passed or if it is nearing time for the next dose, do not double the dose to "catch up," unless advised by your healthcare provider. If more than one dose is missed, contact your healthcare provider.

An increased incidence of seizures has been reported in patients with a history of epilepsy who received the related medicine amantadine. If seizures develop, stop taking the medicine and contact your healthcare provider immediately.

Risperidone

(RISS-PURR-ih-dohn)

Risperdal

A medicine used for the management of the symptoms of certain mental (psychotic) disorders.

Precautions

DO NOT USE if you are allergic to this medicine or if you are breastfeeding.

BEFORE USING THIS MEDICINE, tell your healthcare provider if you are pregnant; or if you are taking, will be taking or stop taking any prescription or nonprescription medicine; or if you have any other medical conditions.

Side Effects

Every medicine can cause side effects, but many people have no, or minor, side effects. Tell your healthcare provider if any of the following occurs: sleeplessness; sleepiness; agitation; anxiety; dizziness (especially when rising quickly from a sitting or lying position); fatigue; constipation; nausea; upset stomach; vomiting; changes in saliva; coughing; chest pain; fever; rash; dry skin; upper respiratory infection; abnormal vision; joint and muscle aches; increased dream activity; sexual problems; increased pigmentation; sensitivity to light; frequent or difficult urination; heavy menstrual bleeding; vaginal dryness; uncontrollable movements; rigid muscles; inflammation in the nose or throat; rapid heartbeat.

Guidelines for Use

USE EXACTLY AS PRESCRIBED.

May be taken with or without food.

Avoid alcohol while using this medicine.

May cause drowsiness or dizziness. Use caution when driving or performing other tasks requiring mental alertness or physical coordination.

If a dose is missed, take it as soon as possible. If several hours have passed or if it is nearing time for the next dose, do not double the dose to "catch up," unless advised by your healthcare provider. If more than one dose is missed, contact your healthcare provider.

Dizziness or lightheadedness may occur if you stand up too fast from a lying or sitting position. If this occurs, get up slowly and avoid sudden changes in posture.

Ritodrine Hydrochloride

(RIH-toe-dreen HIGH-droe-KLOR-ide)

Yutopar

A medicine used in the management of preterm labor.

Precautions

DO NOT USE if you are allergic to this medicine or before the 20th week of pregnancy.

BEFORE USING THIS MEDICINE, tell your healthcare provider if you are taking, will be taking or stop taking any prescription or nonprescription medicine; or if you have any other medical conditions.

Side Effects

Every medicine can cause side effects, but many people have no, or minor, side effects. Tell your healthcare provider if any of the following occurs: injection--pounding in the chest; tremor; nausea; vomiting; headache; nervousness; jitteriness; restlessness; emotional upset; anxiety; chest pain or tightness in the chest; bloating; constipation; diarrhea; difficulty breathing; sweating; chills; drowsiness; weakness; Oral--pounding in the chest; tremor; nausea; jitteriness; rash.

Guidelines for Use

USE EXACTLY AS PRESCRIBED.

Ritonavir

(rih-TON-a-veer)

Norvir

An antiviral used to slow the progression of HIV in adults and children over 12 years of age. This medicine may be used in combination with other HIV medicines.

Precautions

DO NOT USE if you are allergic to this medicine or its ingredients; or if you are taking alprazolam (*Xanax*), amiodarone (*Cordarone*), astemizole (*Hismanal*), bepridil (*Vascor*), bupropion (*Wellbutrin*), cisapride (*Propulsid*), clorazepate (eg, *Tranxene*), clozapine (*Clozaril*), diazepam (eg, *Valium*), encainide (*Enkaid*), estazolam (*ProSom*), flecainide (*Tambocor*), flurazepam (eg, *Dalmane*), meperidine (eg, *Demerol*), midazolam (*Versed*), piroxicam (eg, *Feldene*), propafenone (*Rythmol*), propoxyphene (eg, *Darvon*), quinidine, rifabutin (*Mycobutin*), terfenadine (*Seldane*), triazolam (*Halcion*) or zolpidem (*Ambien*).

BEFORE USING THIS MEDICINE, tell your healthcare provider if you are pregnant or breastfeeding; if you are taking, will be taking or stop taking any prescription or nonprescription medicine; or if you have any other medical conditions.

Side Effects

Every medicine can cause side effects, but many people have no, or minor, side effects. Tell your healthcare provider if any of the following occurs: weakness; headache; general body discomfort; nausea; diarrhea; vomiting; constipation; appetite loss; stomach or muscle pain; sore throat; taste changes; rash; sweating; tingling sensations; dizziness; drowsiness; seeplessness.

Guidelines for Use

USE EXACTLY AS PRESCRIBED.

The usual dose is 600 mg twice daily.

Take with food, if possible.

If nausea persists, talk with your healthcare provider about starting at a lower dose and gradually increasing dose as tolerated. Do not change the dose or stop taking unless advised by your healthcare provider.

If a dose is missed, take it as soon as possible. If several hours have passed or if it is nearing time for the next dose, do not double the dose to "catch up," unless advised by your healthcare provider. If more than one dose is missed, contact your healthcare provider.

This medicine is not a cure for HIV infection and patients may still acquire illnesses/infections associated with HIV infection.

This medicine offers no protection from the transmission of HIV to others through sexual contact or blood contamination. HIV-infected mothers should not breastfeed their infants because of the risk of transmitting the HIV infection.

Lab tests will be required to monitor therapy. Be sure to keep appointments.

Store refrigerated, away from light.

Salicylate Combinations

(suh-LIS-uh-late combinations)

Trisilate

Used for the treatment of pain, fever or inflammation (eg, arthritis). It may occasionally be prescribed for other reasons.

Precautions

DO NOT USE if you are allergic to aspirin or its relatives (eg, nonsteroidal anti-inflammatory medicine) or to tartrazine.

BEFORE USING THIS MEDICINE, tell your healthcare provider if you are pregnant or breastfeeding; or if you are taking, will be taking or stop taking any prescription or nonprescription medicine; or if you have any other medical conditions.

Side Effects

Every medicine can cause side effects, but many people have no, or minor, side effects. Tell your healthcare provider if any of the following occurs: nausea; heartburn; unusual tiredness; rash; rapid or trouble breathing; fever; vision changes; ringing in the ears; diminished hearing; headache; confusion; thirst; black or bloody stools.

Guidelines for Use

USE EXACTLY AS PRESCRIBED.

Take with a full glass of water.

May cause GI upset; take with or after meals or snack.

Tell your healthcare provider immediately if ringing in the ears or persistent stomach or intestinal pain occurs while taking this medication.

Do not take aspirin if it has a strong vinegar-like odor.

If on a dosing schedule and a dose is missed, take it as soon as possible. If several hours have passed, or if it is nearing time for the next dose, do not double the dose to "catch up," unless advised by your healthcare provider. If more than one dose is missed, contact your healthcare provider.

Do not crush, chew or open sustained release products.

Store at room temperature (below 86 degrees F). Protect from moisture.

Salmeterol Xinafoate

(sal-MEET-ah-rahl zin-AF-oh-ate)

Serevent

Used for long-term treatment of asthma (including night-time asthma); to prevent exercise-induced bronchospasm; and to prevent other breathing problems in patients over 12 years of age.

Precautions

DO NOT USE to treat acute asthma symptoms; if you are allergic to this medicine; have significantly worsening or rapidly deteriorating asthma; or as a substitute for short-acting bronchodilators.

BEFORE USING THIS MEDICINE, tell your healthcare provider if you are pregnant or breastfeeding; if you are taking, will be taking or stop taking any prescription or nonprescription medicine; or if you have any other medical conditions (eg, heart problems).

Side Effects

Every medicine can cause side effects, but many people have no, or minor, side effects. Tell your healthcare provider if any of the following occurs: pounding in chest; runny nose; nausea; vomiting; diarrhea; stomach pain; rash; tooth, muscle, joint or back pain; muscle cramps; nervousness; fatigue; painful menstruation; tremors; cough; headache; chest discomfort; rapid heartbeat; unusual or bad taste in mouth; drying or irritation of mouth or throat.

Guidelines for Use

USE EXACTLY AS PRESCRIBED.

Follow the instructions on the package insert exactly.

Always have a short-acting bronchodilator on hand to treat sudden, acute breathing problems. If increased breathing problems occur, stop use immediately and contact your healthcare provider.

Shake well before use.

For long-term treatment of asthma and other breathing problems: Use 2 inhalations (puffs) twice daily about 12 hours apart (morning and evening). Do not exceed recommended dose and do not stop or adjust dose without your healthcare provider's advice.

If a dose is missed, inhale it as soon as possible. If several hours have passed or if it is nearing time for the next dose, do not double the dose to "catch up," unless advised by your healthcare provider. If more than one dose is missed, contact your healthcare provider.

To prevent exercise-induced breathing problems—Use 2 inhalations (puffs) at least 30-60 minutes before exercise. Do not use additional doses for 12 hours.

If using this medicine twice daily, do not use additional doses.

Contact your healthcare provider if any of the following occurs when using a short-acting bronchodilator along with this medicine: Use of 4 or more inhalations per day for more than 2 days; use of more than 1 canister in an 8-week period; increased inhalations; loss of effectiveness.

Do not spray in eyes.

Store canister with the nozzle pointed down and at room temperature, away from direct sunlight and the reach of children. Do not freeze, store near open flame or puncture. This medicine is not as effective if cold.

Saquinavir Mesylate

(sack-KWIN-uh-vihr MEH-sih-LATE)

Invirase

An antiviral medicine used in combination with zidovudine (AZT) to treat HIV infection in adults over 16 years of age.

Precautions

DO NOT USE if you are allergic to this medicine.

BEFORE USING THIS MEDICATION, tell your healthcare provider if you are pregnant or breastfeeding; if you are taking, will be taking or stop taking any prescription or non-prescription medicine; or if you have any other medical conditions.

Side Effects

Every medicine can cause side effects, but many people have no, or minor, side effects. Tell your healthcare provider if any of the following occurs: nausea; diarrhea; stomach discomfort or pain; indigestion; mouth sores; headache; abnormal skin sensations; numbness or tingling of hands and feet; weakness; rash; muscle pain.

Guidelines for Use

USE EXACTLY AS PRESCRIBED.

Do not take with food. Take no sooner than 2 hours after a full meal.

If a dose is missed, take it as soon as possible. If several hours have passed or if it is nearing time for the next dose, do not double the dose to "catch up," unless advised by your healthcare provider. If more than one dose is missed, contact your healthcare provider.

This medicine is not a cure for HIV infection and patients may continue to acquire illnesses/infections associated with HIV infection. Patients should remain under the care of their healthcare provider while using this medicine.

This medicine offers no protection from the transmission of HIV (the virus that causes AIDS) to others through sexual contact or blood contamination. HIV-infected mothers should not breastfeed their infants because of the risk of transmitting the HIV infection.

The long-term effects of this medicine are unknown.

May cause sensitivity to sunlight. Avoid prolonged exposure to the sun. Use sunscreen and wear protective clothing until tolerance is determined.

Lab tests will be required to monitor treatment. Be sure to keep appointments.

Store at room temperature in a tightly sealed container.

Sargramostim

(sar-GRUH-moe-STIM)

Leukine

Used during bone marrow transplants to speed up the recovery or when the bone marrow transplants have failed. It may occasionally be prescribed for other reasons.

Side Effects

Every medicine can cause side effects, but many people have no, or minor, side effects. Tell your healthcare provider if any of the following occurs: fever; weakness; general body discomfort; swelling; nausea; diarrhea; vomiting; loss of appetite; stomach or abdominal pain or discomfort; hair loss; rash; difficulty breathing; headache; joint pain; muscle pain.

Guidelines for Use

USE EXACTLY AS PRESCRIBED.

Scopolamine Injectable

(skoe-PAHL-uh-meen)

Used before surgery, to calm delirium and to treat motion sickness.

Side Effects

Every medicine can cause side effects, but many people have no, or minor, side effects. Tell your healthcare provider if any of the following occurs: altered taste; nausea; vomiting; difficulty in swallowing; heartburn; constipation; bloated feeling; urinary difficulties; impotence; vision problems; pounding in the chest; headache; flushing; nervousness; drowsiness; weakness; dizziness; confusion; sleeplessness; fever; mental confusion; excitement; hallucinations.

Patient Information

May cause drowsiness, dizziness or blurred vision. Use caution while driving or performing activities requiring coordination and dexterity.

Tell your healthcare provider if skin rash, flushing or eye pain occurs.

May cause dry mouth, difficulty in urination, constipation or increased sensitivity to light; tell your healthcare provider if these become severe.

Scopolamine Ophthalmic

(skoe-PAHL-uh-meen)

Isopto Hyoscine

A pupil dilator used when there is eye inflammation or when an eye exam is performed. It works by relaxing the muscles of the eye to cause the pupil to dilate (widen) and prevent the eye from focusing.

Precautions

DO NOT USE if you are allergic to this medicine or its relatives.

BEFORE USING THIS MEDICINE, tell your healthcare provider if you are pregnant or breastfeeding; or if you are taking, will be taking or stop taking any prescription or nonprescription medicine; or if you have any other medical conditions.

Side Effects

Every medicine can cause side effects, but many people have no, or minor, side effects. Tell your healthcare provider if any of the following occurs: increased intraocular (fluid) pressure; stinging; redness; swelling; sensitivity to light; blurred vision; headache; drowsiness; slurred speech; loss of coordination; incoherent speech; restlessness; hallucinations; hyperactivity; seizures; disorientation; rapid irregular pulse; flushing; dryness; rash; lack of sweating; dryness of mouth and nose; bladder distention; fever.

Guidelines for Use

USE EXACTLY AS PRESCRIBED.

May produce drowsiness, loss of coordination, blurred vision or sensitivity to light (due to dilated pupils).

Use caution while driving or performing other tasks requiring mental alertness.

If eye pain occurs, stop using the drops and contact your healthcare provider.

Scopolamine Transdermal

(skoe-PAHL-uh-meen)

Transderm-Scop

Used for the prevention of nausea and vomiting associated with motion sickness in adults.

Precautions

DO NOT USE if you are allergic to this medicine or if you have glaucoma.

BEFORE USING THIS MEDICINE, tell your healthcare provider if you are pregnant or breastfeeding; or if you are taking, will be taking or stop taking any prescription medicine; or if you have any other medical conditions.

Side Effects

Every medicine can cause side effects, but many people have no, or minor, side effects. Tell your healthcare provider if any of the following occurs: dry mouth; drowsiness; vision changes; disorientation; memory disturbances; dizziness; restlessness; hallucinations; confusion; difficulty urinating; rash; flushing; dry, itchy eyes.

Guidelines for Use

USE EXACTLY AS PRESCRIBED.

Patient package insert is available with this medicine.

May cause drowsiness or dizziness. Use caution while driving or performing other activities requiring coordination and dexterity.

Wash hands thoroughly after handling the transdermal disc.

Avoid contact with the eyes. Temporary dilation of the pupils and blurred vision may occur if the disc comes in contact with the eyes.

Secobarbital Sodium

(see-koe-BAR-bih-tahl SO-dee-uhm)

Seconal Injection, Seconal Sodium Capsules

A barbiturate central nervous system depressant that can produce mild sedation, sleep and up to deep coma. Usually used to treat insomnia, to calm agitated people and to treat certain seizure disorders.

Precautions

DO NOT USE if you are allergic to this medicine or its relatives. This medicine may be habit-forming. Tolerance and dependence may occur, especially following prolonged use of high doses. Withdrawal symptoms can be severe.

BEFORE USING THIS MEDICINE, tell your healthcare provider if you are pregnant or breastfeeding; or if you are taking, will be taking or stop taking any prescription or nonprescription medicine; or if you have any other medical conditions.

Side Effects

Every medicine can cause side effects, but many people have no, or minor, side effects. Tell your healthcare provider if any of the following occurs: sleepiness; tired feeling; nausea; vomiting; morning hangover.

Guidelines for Use

USE EXACTLY AS PRESCRIBED.

Take only the amount of medicine prescribed by your healthcare provider.

May decrease alertness or physical ability. Use caution when driving or performing tasks requiring mental alertness.

Avoid alcohol and other mental depressants (eg, narcotics, tranquilizers, antihistamines) while you are taking this medicine.

Use as an aid to sleep is limited; generally not for use longer than 2 weeks.

Seizure control - Do not stop therapy suddenly.

Selegiline Hydrochloride

(seh-LEH-jih-leen HIGH-droe-KLOR-ide)

Eldepryl

A medicine used to treat Parkinson's disease in conjunction with levodopa/carbidopa in patients whose response to levodopa/carbidopa is deteriorating. There is no evidence that it has any benefit without the concurrent use of levodopa.

Precautions

DO NOT USE if you are allergic to this medicine; or with meperidine; or with tyramine-containing foods. Children: Safety and effectiveness have not been established.

BEFORE USING THIS MEDICINE, tell your healthcare provider if you are pregnant or breastfeeding; or if you are taking, will be taking or stop taking any prescription or non-prescription medicine; or if you have any other medical conditions.

Side Effects

Every medicine can cause side effects, but many people have no, or minor, side effects. Tell your healthcare provider if any of the following occurs: increased or decreased urination (especially at night); difficult urination; nausea; vomiting; diarrhea; rectal bleeding; constipation; loss of appetite; heartburn; difficulty swallowing; dry mouth; weakness; confusion; anxiety; dreams and nightmares; headache; affected speech; tremor; restlessness; involuntary movements; loss of balance; spasms of eyelid; hallucinations; dizziness when arising quickly from a seated or lying position; changes in blood pressure; pounding in the chest; irregular pulse; angina (chest pain); irregular heartbeats; shortness of breath; asthma; increased sweating; hair loss; sensitivity to sunlight; facial hair growth; rash; bruising.

Guidelines for Use

USE EXACTLY AS PRESCRIBED.

Do not exceed the recommended daily dose.

Immediately report any severe headache or unusual symptoms to your healthcare provider.

Avoid food with high amounts of tyramine (eg, red wine, yogurt, aged cheese, bananas).

Senna

(SEN-ah)

Black-Draught, Dr. Caldwell Senna Laxative, Fletcher's Castoria, Gentlax, Senexon, Senna-Gen, Senokot, Senokotxtra, Senolax, X-prep

A medicine used for short-term treatment of constipation and to clean out the bowel before bowel examinations or bowel surgery.

Precautions

DO NOT USE if you are allergic to this medicine.

BEFORE USING THIS MEDICINE, tell your healthcare provider if you are pregnant or breastfeeding; or if you are taking, will be taking or stop taking any prescription or nonprescription medicine; or if you have any other medical conditions.

Side Effects

Every medicine can cause side effects, but many people have no, or minor, side effects. Tell your healthcare provider if any of the following occurs: nausea; vomiting; stomach ache; bowel cramping; diarrhea; weakness; dizziness; fainting; facial swelling, redness and discomfort; rectal bleeding; muscle cramps or pain; irritation of the rectal area; sweating; pounding in the chest.

Guidelines for Use

USE EXACTLY AS PRESCRIBED.

Take with a full glass of water or juice.

Laxative use is only a temporary measure. When normal bowel habits return, stop use of this medicine.

Frequent use of laxatives and inadequate fluid intake can cause an imbalance in fluid and electrolyte levels. Symptoms can include muscle cramps, muscle weakness and dizziness.

Effects will occur in 6 to 10 hours.

Pink-red, red-violet or red-brown discoloration of the urine may occur.

Sertraline Hydrochloride

(SIR-truh-leen HIGH-droe-KLOR-ide)

Zoloft

Used for the treatment of depression. It may occasionally be prescribed for other reasons.

Precautions

DO NOT USE if you are allergic to this medicine, if you are taking a monoamine oxidase inhibitor (MAOI) or if you have taken an MAOI within the last 14 days.

BEFORE USING THIS MEDICINE, tell your healthcare provider if you are pregnant or breastfeeding; or if you are taking, will be taking or stop taking any prescription or nonprescription medicine; or if you have any other medical conditions.

Side Effects

Every medicine can cause side effects, but many people have no, or minor, side effects. Tell your healthcare provider if any of the following occurs: headache; stomach pain; fever; chills; hot flushes; pounding in the chest; sleeplessness; sleepiness; nervousness; anxiety; dizziness; tremor; decreased sexual function; twitching; agitation; abnormal skin sensations; fatigue; overall body discomfort; decreased concentration; decreased sensitivity to touch; nausea; vomiting; diarrhea; upset stomach; dry mouth; loss of appetite; constipation; increased appetite; gas; thirst; muscle aches; yawning; increased sweating; rash; vision changes; taste changes; ringing in the ears; frequent urination; back pain; menstrual changes; runny nose; difficulty urinating.

Guidelines for Use

USE EXACTLY AS PRESCRIBED.

If a dose is missed, take it as soon as possible. If several hours have passed or if it is nearing time for the next dose, do not double the dose to "catch up," unless advised by your healthcare provider. If more than one dose is missed, contact your healthcare provider.

May cause drowsiness or dizziness. Use caution while driving or performing other tasks requiring mental alertness, coordination or dexterity.

Avoid alcohol or other drowsiness-causing agents (eg, narcotic pain relievers, tranquilizers, antihistamines).

Tell your healthcare provider if rash or hives develop.

Continue taking your medication even if you notice improvement.

Store at room temperature (59–86° F).

This information is advisory only; it does not contain all information about this medicine. If you have any questions about your medicine, ask your healthcare provider.

Simethicone

(sih-METH-ih-kone)

Flatulex, Gas Relief, Gas-X, Gas-X (Extra Strength), Major-Con, Maximum Strength Phazyme 125, Mylanta Gas, Mylanta Gas (Maximum Strength), Mylicon, Phazyme, Phazyme 95

Used for the relief of the painful symptoms and pressure of excess gas in the stomach. It may occasionally be prescribed for other reasons.

Guidelines for Use

USE EXACTLY AS PRESCRIBED.

Drops--Shake well before using.

Chewable tablets--Chew thoroughly before swallowing.

Simvastatin

(SIM-vuh-STAT-in)

Zocor

A medicine used to lower the level of cholesterol in the blood. It may occasionally be prescribed for other reasons.

Precautions

DO NOT USE if you are pregnant; breastfeeding; or allergic to this medicine.

BEFORE USING THIS MEDICINE, tell your healthcare provider if you are taking, will be taking or stop taking any prescription or nonprescription medicine; or if you have any other medical conditions

Side Effects

Every medicine can cause side effects, but many people have no, or minor, side effects. Tell your healthcare provider if any of the following occurs: nausea; diarrhea; stomach pain; constipation; gas; headache; dizziness; rash; muscle cramps; taste changes.

Guidelines for Use

USE EXACTLY AS PRESCRIBED.

Take in the evening.

May be taken without regard to meals.

Report any unexplained muscle pain, tenderness or weakness, especially if accompanied by fever or malaise, to your healthcare provider. Also report any yellowing of the skin or eyes.

Most effective when used with exercise and a diet that reduces the intake of cholesterol and saturated fats.

Sodium Bicarbonate

(SO-dee-uhm by-CAR-boe-nate)

BellJans, Citrocarbonate, Neut

Used to treat upset stomach due to too much acid secretion (eg, heartburn, acid indigestion and sour stomach); to treat irritation of the stomach associated with peptic ulcers. It may occasionally be prescribed for other reasons.

Precautions

DO NOT USE if you are allergic to this medicine.

BEFORE USING THIS MEDICINE, tell your healthcare provider if you are pregnant or breastfeeding; or if you are taking, will be taking or stop taking any prescription or nonprescription medicine; or if you have any other medical conditions.

Side Effects

Every medicine can cause side effects, but many people have no, or minor, side effects. Tell your healthcare provider if any of the following occurs: nausea; vomiting; stomach pain; muscular weakness; lack of energy; headache; confusion; irritability.

Guidelines for Use

USE EXACTLY AS PRESCRIBED.

Antacids reduce acidity for about 30 minutes when taken on an empty stomach. Acidity is reduced for about 3 hours when antacids are taken 1 hour after meals.

Do not take other medications within 1 to 2 hours of taking this medicine.

Tell your healthcare provider if coffee-ground vomiting or black, tar-like stools occur.

Taking too much of these products can cause the stomach to secrete excess stomach acid. Talk to your healthcare provider about the appropriate dose.

Long-term use—Do not take for longer than 2 weeks for the relief of indigestion. If discomfort continues, talk to your healthcare provider.

Sodium Phosphate/Sodium Biphosphate

(SO-dee-uhm FOSS-fate/SO-dee-uhm by-FOSS-fate)

Fleet (enema), Fleet Phospho-soda, Sodium Phosphates

Used for short-term treatment of constipation; to clean out the bowel before bowel examinations or bowel surgery; to eliminate foods or medicines from the digestive tract in suspected poisonings.

Precautions

DO NOT USE if you are allergic to this medicine; after abdominal surgery; if you have appendicitis symptoms (nausea, vomiting, abdominal pain), a bowel obstruction or stool impaction.

BEFORE USING THIS MEDICINE, tell your healthcare provider if you are pregnant or breastfeeding; or if you are taking, will be taking or stop taking any prescription or nonprescription medicine; or if you have any other medical conditions.

Side Effects

Every medicine can cause side effects, but many people have no, or minor, side effects. Tell your healthcare provider if any of the following occurs: nausea; vomiting; stomach pain/cramps; diarrhea; weakness; dizziness; fainting; rectal bleeding; irritation of the rectal area; sweating; pounding in the chest; gas; bloating.

Guidelines for Use

USE EXACTLY AS PRESCRIBED.

Take with a full glass of water or juice.

Do not take in the presence of abdominal pain, nausea or vomiting.

Laxative use is only a temporary measure. When normal bowel habits return, stop use of these products.

Prolonged use may result in dependence or electrolyte imbalance.

Tell your healthcare provider if unrelieved constipation, rectal bleeding or symptoms of electrolyte imbalance (muscle cramps or pain, weakness, dizziness) occurs.

Effects will occur in 2 to 15 minutes.

Sodium Polystyrene Sulfonate

(SO-dee-uhm pah-lee-STYE-reen SULL-fuh-nate)

Kayexalate, SPS

A medicine used for the treatment of hyperkalemia.

Precautions

DO NOT USE if you are allergic to this medicine or if you have low blood potassium.

BEFORE USING THIS MEDICINE, tell your healthcare provider if you are pregnant or breastfeeding; or if you are taking, will be taking or stop taking any prescription or nonprescription medicine; or if you have any other medical conditions.

Side Effects

Every medicine can cause side effects, but many people have no, or minor, side effects. Tell your healthcare provider if any of the following occurs: stomach pain; loss of appetite; nausea; vomiting; constipation; diarrhea.

Guidelines for Use

USE EXACTLY AS PRESCRIBED.

Be sure to shake bottle thoroughly before using.

Talk to your healthcare provider before taking any laxatives or antacids.

Report any sign of constipation or water retention to your healthcare provider.

Somatrem

(so-muh-TREM)

Protropin

Used for long-term treatment in children who have growth failure due to a lack of growth hormone secretion.

Precautions

DO NOT USE if you are allergic to this medicine or to benzyl alcohol.

BEFORE USING THIS MEDICINE, tell your healthcare provider if you are pregnant or breastfeeding; or if you are taking, will be taking or stop taking any prescription or nonprescription medicine; or if you have any other medical conditions.

Side Effects

Every medicine can cause side effects, but many people have no, or minor, side effects. Tell your healthcare provider if any of the following occurs: pain at the injection site.

Guidelines for Use

USE EXACTLY AS PRESCRIBED.

Do not shake vials.

If home use is prescribed, your healthcare provider will provide you with a puncture-resistant container for the disposal of used syringes and needles. Follow your healthcare provider's instructions on the safe disposal of used syringes and needles. Do not reuse syringes or needles.

If a dose is missed, take it as soon as possible. If several hours have passed, or if it is nearing time for the next dose, do not double the dose to "catch up," unless advised by your healthcare provider. If more than one dose is missed, contact your healthcare provider.

Discard after 14 days.

Store in the refrigerator.

Somatropin

(SO-muh-TROE-pin)

Humatrope, Nutropin

Used for long-term treatment in children who have growth failure due to a lack of adequate hormone secretion. It also is prescribed for children who have growth failure associated with chronic kidney problems up to the time of kidney transplantation.

Precautions

DO NOT USE if you are allergic to this medicine or to benzyl alcohol.

BEFORE USING THIS MEDICINE, tell your healthcare provider if you are pregnant or breastfeeding; or if you are taking, will be taking or stop taking any prescription or nonprescription medicine; or if you have any other medical conditions.

Side Effects

Every medicine can cause side effects, but many people have no, or minor, side effects. Tell your healthcare provider if any of the following occurs: pain at the injection site.

Guidelines for Use

USE EXACTLY AS PRESCRIBED.

If home use is prescribed, your healthcare provider will provide you with a puncture-resistant container for the disposal of used syringes and needles. Follow your healthcare provider's instructions on the safe disposal of used syringes and needles. Do not reuse syringes or needles.

Do not shake vials.

If a dose is missed, take it as soon as possible. If several hours have passed, or if it is nearing time for the next dose, do not double the dose to "catch up," unless advised by your healthcare provider. If more than one dose is missed, contact your healthcare provider.

Store in the refrigerator.

Discard after 14 days.

Sotalol Hydrochloride

(SOTT-uh-lahl HIGH-droe-KLOR-ide)

Betapace

A medicine used to treat irregular heartbeats.

Precautions

DO NOT USE if you are allergic to this medicine; if you have bronchial asthma; bronchospasm; certain heart disorders; or if you are breastfeeding.

BEFORE USING THIS MEDICINE, tell your healthcare provider if you are pregnant or breastfeeding; or if you are taking, will be taking or stop taking any prescription or nonprescription medicine; or if you have any other medical conditions.

Side Effects

Every medicine can cause side effects, but many people have no, or minor, side effects. Tell your healthcare provider if any of the following occurs: difficult breathing, especially on exertion or when lying down; night cough; swelling of the extremities; slow pulse rate; dizziness; confusion or depression; rash; fever; sore throat; unusual bleeding or bruising.

Guidelines for Use

USE EXACTLY AS PRESCRIBED.

Take consistently with or without food at the same time each day.

Use caution while driving or performing other tasks requiring mental alertness.

Do not discontinue use of this medicine without consulting your healthcare provider.

Diabetes: These products can mask signs of hypoglycemia (low blood sugar) and alter blood sugar levels. It may be necessary for your healthcare provider to alter your dose of diabetic medications while taking this medicine.

Spironolactone

(SPEER-oh-no-LAK-tone)

Alatone, Aldactone

A potassium-sparing diuretic or water pill. It is generally used to treat fluid accumulation and swelling, high blood pressure and to prevent or treat low potassium levels.

Precautions

DO NOT USE if you are allergic to this medicine or its relatives, or are breastfeeding.

BEFORE USING THIS MEDICINE, tell your healthcare provider if you are pregnant; or if you are taking, will be taking or stop taking any prescription or nonprescription medicine; or if you have any other medical conditions.

Side Effects

Every medicine can cause side effects, but many people have no, or minor, side effects. Tell your healthcare provider if any of the following occurs: stomach or intestinal pain; nausea; vomiting; diarrhea; constipation; gas; heartburn; loss of appetite; weakness, fatigue; drowsiness; confusion; tingling or numbness of hands or feet; depression; headache; dizziness or lightheadedness when arising from a seated or lying position; sleeplessness; nervousness; irregular pulse; chest pain; shortness of breath; cough; nasal congestion; rash; itching; yellowing of the skin or eyes; hair loss; muscle weakness or cramping; ringing in the ears; visual disturbances; changes in sex drive; dry mouth; deepening of the voice; breast enlargement in males; menstrual abnormalities.

Guidelines for Use

USE EXACTLY AS PRESCRIBED.

If a single dose is prescribed, generally take it in the morning.

May cause stomach upset. Take with food.

Use caution while driving or performing other tasks requiring alertness.

Avoid large quantities of potassium-rich food or salt substitutes.

Patients being treated for high blood pressure often feel tired for a few weeks. It takes time for the body to adjust to lowered blood pressure. Continue taking your medication and check with your healthcare provider regarding any new symptoms to assure that they are a normal consequence of changes in blood pressure.

Stavudine

(STAY-vyu-dine)

Zerit

This medicine is used for the treatment of advanced HIV/AIDS infection in adults.

Precautions

DO NOT USE if you are allergic to this medicine.

BEFORE USING THIS MEDICINE, tell your healthcare provider if you are pregnant or breastfeeding; if you are taking, will be taking or stop taking any prescription or nonprescription medicine; or if you have any other medical conditions.

Side Effects

Every medicine can cause side effects, but many people have no, or minor, side effects. Tell your healthcare provider if any of the following occurs: numbness; tingling or pain in feet and hands; headache; fever; chills; weakness; abdominal pain; general body discomfort; allergic reaction; flu; pelvic pain; chest pain; fainting; diarrhea; nausea; vomiting; loss of appetite; indigestion; constipation; sores in the mouth; weight loss; muscle/joint pain; sleeplessness; depression; nervousness; dizziness; confusion; migraine; drowsiness; tremor; nerve pain; memory impairment; difficulty breathing; pneumonia; asthma; rash; sweating; itching; scaling; hives; eye redness; abnormal vision; frequent, painful or difficult urination; genital pain; painful menstruation; vaginal infection/irritation; impotence; blood in urine.

Guidelines for Use

USE EXACTLY AS PRESCRIBED.

May be taken with or without food.

If a dose is missed, take it as soon as possible. If several hours have passed or if it is nearing time for the next dose, do not double the dose to "catch up," unless advised by your healthcare provider. If more than one dose is missed, contact your healthcare provider.

This medicine does not reduce the risk of transmitting HIV to others through sexual contact or blood contamination.

This medicine is NOT a cure and you may continue to acquire illnesses related to AIDS or ARC (AIDS-related complex). Tell your healthcare provider if any significant changes in your health occur.

Keep all appointments with your healthcare provider. Laboratory tests will be necessary.

Streptozocin

(STREP-toe-ZOE-sin)

Zanosar

Used to treat cancer of the pancreas.

Side Effects

Every medicine can cause side effects, but many people have no, or minor, side effects. Tell your healthcare provider if any of the following occurs: nausea; vomiting; confusion; drowsiness; depression; diarrhea; pain at the injection site.

Patient Information

Lab tests will be required to monitor therapy. Be sure to keep appointments.

Sucralfate

(sue-KRAL-fate)

Carafate Suspension, Carafate Tablets

An anti-ulcer medicine. It may occasionally be prescribed for other reasons.

Precautions

DO NOT USE if you are allergic to this medicine.

BEFORE USING THIS MEDICINE, tell your healthcare provider if you are pregnant or breastfeeding; if you are taking, will be taking or stop taking any prescription or nonprescription medicine; or if you have any other medical conditions.

Side Effects

Every medicine can cause side effects, but many people have no, or minor, side effects. Tell your healthcare provider if any of the following occurs: constipation; upset stomach; dry mouth; rash; dizziness; sleeplessness; hives; facial swelling; difficulty breathing.

Guidelines for Use

USE EXACTLY AS PRESCRIBED.

Take on an empty stomach at least 1 hour before meals and at bedtime.

Do not take antacids 30 minutes before or after taking sucralfate. If a dose is missed, take it as soon as possible.

If several hours have passed or if it is nearing time for the next dose, do not double the dose to "catch up," unless advised by your healthcare provider. If more than one dose is missed, contact your healthcare provider.

If you have red or black stools, or cough up or vomit bright red blood or coffee ground-like material, contact your doctor healthcare provider.

Ulcers are a chronic, recurrent disease. While a single course of therapy of 4 to 8 weeks may completely heal the ulcer, ulcers may occur again and may be more severe.

Suspension--Shake well before using.

Sulfasalazine

(SULL-fuh-SAL-uh-zeen)

Azulfidine EN-tabs, Azulfidine Suspension, Azulfidine Tablets

A medicine used to treat ulcerative colitis. It may occasionally be prescribed for rheumatoid arthritis, collagenous colitis and Crohn's disease.

Precautions

DO NOT USE if you are allergic to this medicine or its relatives (oral antidiabetic medicines or thiazide diuretics), salicylates or aspirin; if you are breastfeeding; during pregnancy at term; or if you have intestinal or urinary obstruction.

BEFORE USING THIS MEDICINE, tell your healthcare provider if you are pregnant; or if you are taking, will be taking or stop taking any prescription or nonprescription medicine; or if you have any other medical conditions.

Side Effects

Every medicine can cause side effects, but many people have no, or minor, side effects. Tell your healthcare provider if any of the following occurs: nausea; vomiting; diarrhea; appetite loss; stomach ache; headache; dizziness; depression; seizures; sleeplessness; drowsiness; rash; itching; hives; chills; unusual bleeding or bruising; yellowing of skin or eyes; numbness or tingling in hands or feet; ringing in ears; sensitivity to light; fever; joint pain; difficulty breathing; blue discoloration of skin; sore throat.

Guidelines for Use

USE EXACTLY AS PRESCRIBED.

Take this medicine at evenly spaced intervals, after meals.

Do not stop taking this medicine without talking to your healthcare provider.

If a dose is missed, take as soon as possible. If several hours have passed or if it is nearing time for the next dose, do not double the dose to "catch up," unless advised by your healthcare provider. If more than one dose is missed, contact your healthcare provider.

Avoid prolonged exposure to the sun. Use sunscreens and wear protective clothing until tolerance is determined.

This medicine may cause an orange-yellow discoloration of the urine or skin.

Notify your healthcare provider immediately if any of the following occurs: blood in urine; yellowing of skin or eyes; easy bruising; rash; ringing in ears; difficulty breathing; fever; sore throat or chills.

Sulfinpyrazone

(sul-fin-PEER-uh-zone)

Anturane, Novo-Pyrazone

Used for the prevention of gout attacks. It may occasionally be prescribed for other reasons.

Precautions

DO NOT USE aspirin or other salicylates, because these could make your condition worse. Do not use if you have an active peptic ulcer or are allergic to this medicine.

BEFORE USING THIS MEDICINE, tell your healthcare provider if you are pregnant or breastfeeding; or if you are taking, will be taking or stop taking any prescription or nonprescription medicine; or if you have any other medical conditions.

Side Effects

Every medicine can cause side effects, but many people have no, or minor, side effects. Tell your healthcare provider if any of the following occurs: stomach pain; nausea; vomiting; rash; trouble breathing; loss of appetite; diarrhea.

Guidelines for Use

USE EXACTLY AS PRESCRIBED.

The initial dose, for gout, is given twice daily and may be decreased or increased by your healthcare provider over time.

May cause stomach upset. Take with food, milk or antacids.

Drink plenty of water, at least 10 to 12 full glasses daily, to prevent kidney stones.

If a dose is missed, take it as soon as possible. If several hours have passed or if it is nearing time for the next dose, do not double the dose to catch up, unless advised by your healthcare provider. If more than one dose is missed, contact your healthcare provider.

Store at room temperature (below 89 degrees F). Protect from moisture.

Sulfisoxazole

(sull-fih-SOX-uh-zole)

Used to treat infections caused by various bacteria.

Precautions

DO NOT USE if you are allergic to this medicine or its relatives.

BEFORE USING THIS MEDICINE, tell your healthcare provider if you are pregnant or breastfeeding; or if you are taking, will be taking or stop taking any prescription or nonprescription medicine; or if you have any other medical conditions.

Side Effects

Every medicine can cause side effects, but many people have no, or minor, side effects. Tell your healthcare provider if any of the following occurs: vomiting; diarrhea; appetite loss; headache; feeling of a whirling motion (vertigo); depression; seizures; sleeplessness; drowsiness; rash; itching; hives; chills; unusual bleeding or bruising; yellowing of skin or eyes; numbness or tingling in hands or feet; ringing in the ears; sensitivity to light; fever; joint pain; difficult breathing.

Guidelines for Use

USE EXACTLY AS PRESCRIBED.

Oral — Complete full course of therapy for full benefit. Take on an empty stomach. Take with a full glass of water.

Oral Suspension — Shake well before using.

Tell your healthcare provider if any of the following occurs: blood in urine; yellowing of skin or eyes; easy bruising; rash; ringing in the ears; difficulty in breathing; fever; sore throat; chills.

Sulindac

(sull-IN-dak)

Clinoril, Apo-Sulin, Novo-Sundac

A nonsteroidal anti-inflammatory medicine (NSAID) used to relieve mild to moderate pain and inflammation of rheumatoid arthritis, osteoarthritis (degenerative joint disease) and acute gout. It may occasionally be prescribed for other reasons.

Precautions

DO NOT USE if you are allergic to this medicine or its relatives, aspirin or iodides.

BEFORE USING THIS MEDICINE, tell your healthcare provider if you are pregnant or breastfeeding; use alcohol chronically; are prone to fluid retention; or if you are taking, will be taking or stop taking any prescription or nonprescription medicines; or have any other medical conditions.

Side Effects

Every medicine can cause side effects, but many people have no, or minor, side effects. Tell your healthcare provider if any of the following occurs: allergic reaction (eg, rash, itching, fever); changes in vision; weight gain; fluid retention; stomach problems (eg, nausea, vomiting, diarrhea, pain); black stools; constipation; persistent headache; dizziness; nervousness; weakness; ringing in the ears; taste changes; unusual bruising or bleeding.

Guidelines for Use

USE EXACTLY AS PRESCRIBED.

Avoid aspirin and alcoholic beverages.

If stomach upset occurs, take with food, milk or antacids. If stomach pain continues, tell your healthcare provider.

If a dose is missed, take it as soon as possible. If several hours have passed or if it is nearing time for the next dose, do not double the dose to catch up, unless advised by your healthcare provider. If more than one dose is missed, contact your healthcare provider.

May cause drowsiness or dizziness. Observe caution while driving or performing other tasks requiring mental alertness, coordination and dexterity.

May cause sensitivity to sunlight. Avoid prolonged exposure to the sun. Use sunscreens and wear protective clothing until tolerance is determined.

Sumatriptan Succinate

(SUE-muh-TRIP-tan SOOS-in-ate)

Imitrex

A medicine used for the treatment of migraine headaches with or without aura.

Precautions

DO NOT USE if you are allergic to this medicine or with an ergotamine-containing preparation. This medication is not for intravenous administration.

BEFORE USING THIS MEDICINE, tell your healthcare provider if you are pregnant; or if you are taking, will be taking or stop taking any prescription or nonprescription medicines; or have any other medical conditions.

Side Effects

Every medicine can cause side effects, but many people have no, or minor, side effects. Tell your healthcare provider if any of the following occurs: difficulty swallowing; weakness; dizziness; drowsiness; fatigue; tightness or pressure in chest; flushing; sweating; throat discomfort; pain/redness at injection site; jaw discomfort; mouth/tongue discomfort; neck pain/stiffness; muscle pain/cramps; general body discomfort; atypical sensations (eg, tingling, burning, pressure, hot/cold, tightness).

Guidelines for Use

USE EXACTLY AS PRESCRIBED.

Patient information is available with product.

Usual dose is a single injection given just below the skin. It should be given as soon as the symptoms of your migraine appear, but it may be given at any time during an attack.

A second injection may be given if symptoms come back. Do not give more than two injections in any 24 hour period. Allow at least one hour between each dose.

If you experience pain or tightness in chest or throat, contact your healthcare provider before using again. If chest pain is severe or does not go away, contact your healthcare provider immediately.

Pain or redness at injection site usually lasts less than one hour.

Some people may experience atypical sensations, drowsiness, dizziness, tiredness or sickness. Discuss these symptoms with your healthcare provider.

If you have taken more than the prescribed dose of medicine, contact either your healthcare provider, hospital emergency department or your nearest poison control center immediately.

Store medicine away from heat and light.

Discard any unused portion.

Tacrine

(TAK-reen)

Cognex

A medicine used to treat mildly to moderately progressive mental deterioration of the Alzheimer's type. This medicine is not a cure, but it may slow the progressive memory loss associated with Alzheimer's disease.

Precautions

DO NOT USE if you are allergic to this medicine or any of its relatives, or if you have evidence of or a history of abnormal liver function.

BEFORE USING THIS MEDICINE, tell your healthcare provider if you are pregnant or breastfeeding; or if you are taking, will be taking or stop taking any prescription or nonprescription medicine; or if you have any other medical conditions.

Side Effects

Every medicine can cause side effects, but many people have no, or minor, side effects. Tell your healthcare provider if any of the following occurs: headache; fatigue; chest pain; weight loss; back pain; muscle stiffness; nausea; vomiting; loss of appetite; diarrhea; indigestion; abdominal pain; gas; constipation; chills; fever; general body discomfort; fluid retention; significant change in blood pressure; fracture; muscle and joint pain; arthritis; tight muscles; convulsions; dizziness; fainting; confusion; incoordination; sleeplessness; sleepiness; tremors; abnormal skin sensations; nervousness; sinus, lung or throat infections; difficulty breathing; coughing; increased sweating; eye infections; bleeding; agitation; depression; anxiety; hallucinations; feelings of hostility; rash; yellowing of the skin or eyes; color change in stool (very dark or very light); flushing; frequent urination; urinary tract infection; incontinence.

Guidelines for Use

USE EXACTLY AS PRESCRIBED.

This medicine should be taken between meals whenever possible; however, if stomach upset occurs, it may be taken with meals.

Do not stop taking this medicine or change the dose unless directed to do so by your healthcare provider. Discontinuing this medication abruptly or largely reducing the daily dose may cause serious side effects. Adjustments in the dose will be required during the course of therapy.

Lab testing to monitor serum levels will be required while taking this medicine. Be sure to keep appointments.

Tacrolimus (FK506)

(tack-CROW-lih-muss)

Prograf

An immunosuppressant used to prevent organ (liver) transplant rejection. It may be prescribed with adrenal corticosteroids.

Precautions

DO NOT USE if you are allergic to this medicine or if you are using cyclosporine, potassium-sparing diuretics or other immunosuppressives (except adrenal corticosteroids).

BEFORE USING THIS MEDICINE, tell your healthcare provider if you are pregnant, intend to become pregnant or if you are breastfeeding; if you are taking, will be taking or stop taking any prescription or nonprescription medicine (including vaccinations); or if you have any other medical conditions.

Side Effects

Every medicine can cause side effects, but many people have no, or minor, side effects. Tell your healthcare provider if any of the following occurs: diarrhea; nausea; constipation; appetite changes; vomiting; stomach pain; bloating; indigestion; gas; mood swings; stiffness; tremors; headache; sleep disorders; anxiety; confusion; depression; dizziness; hallucinations; abnormal dreams; incoordination; drowsiness; seizures; racing heartbeat; chest pain; difficulty breathing; cough; sore throat; voice alteration; sinus infection; bronchitis; itching; hives; rash; bruising; abnormal hair growth or loss; sweating; yellowing of the eyes or skin; weight loss; fever; weakness; swelling of the arms or legs; vision changes; ringing in the ears; speech impairment; infrequent urination; blood in the urine; chills; sensitivity to sunlight; general body pain; leg cramps; oral thrush; bleeding.

Guidelines for Use

USE EXACTLY AS PRESCRIBED.

The possibility of serious infection, nerve or kidney damage, diabetes and some cancers is increased with the use of this medicine.

Take in two divided doses every 12 hours on an empty stomach, or as directed by your healthcare provider.

If a dose is missed, take it as soon as possible. If several hours have passed or if it is nearing time for the next dose, do not double the dose to "catch up," unless advised by your healthcare provider. If more than one dose is missed, contact your healthcare provider.

Lab tests will be required to monitor therapy; keep appointments.

Notify your healthcare provider immediately if you experience any of the following: tremors, headache, dizziness, incoordination, abnormal sensations, suspected infections, changes in mental status or decreased urination.

May cause drowsiness, dizziness or visual problems. Use caution while driving or performing tasks requiring alertness or coordination.

Store at room temperature.

Tamoxifen Citrate

(ta-MOX-ih-fen SIH-trate)

Nolvadex

A chemotherapy agent used to treat certain cancers including breast, endometrial, prostate and kidney cancers. It may occasionally be prescribed for other reasons.

Precautions

DO NOT USE if you are allergic to this medicine; or if you are pregnant or breast-feeding.

BEFORE USING THIS MEDICINE, tell your healthcare provider if you are taking, will be taking or stop taking any prescription or nonprescription medicine; or if you have any other medical conditions.

Side Effects

Every medicine can cause side effects, but many people have no, or minor, side effects. Tell your healthcare provider if any of the following occurs: hot flashes, nausea; vomiting; fever, sore throat, rashes or chills; vision changes; marked weakness; sleepiness; mental confusion; pain/swelling of legs; shortness of breath; bone pain; weight gain; menstrual irregularities; dizziness; headache; appetite loss; stomach cramps; muscle pain; fluid retention; cough; skin changes; flushing; sexual function changes.

Guidelines for Use

USE EXACTLY AS PRESCRIBED.

Take twice daily (morning and evening) on an empty stomach (1 hour before or two hours after eating) with a full glass of water. However, if stomach upset occurs, take with food.

If a dose is missed, take as soon as possible. If several hours have passed or if it is nearing time for the next dose, do not double the dose to "catch up," unless advised by your healthcare provider. If more than one dose is missed, contact your healthcare provider.

Inform you healthcare provider if you are pregnant, become pregnant, are planning to become pregnant or if you are breastfeeding. Barrier or non-hormonal contraceptives are recommended during treatment to avoid birth defects.

Contact you healthcare provider if menstrual irregularities occur.

This medicine may lower your body's ability to fight infection. Notify your healthcare provider if any signs of infection occur, including fever, sore throat, rash or chills.

Gynecological exams and lab tests will be required to monitor treatment. Be sure to keep appointments.

Store at room temperture away from heat and light.

Temazepam

(tem-AZE-uh-pam)

Restoril

A benzodiazepine medicine that is a sleeping pill to treat insomnia for a short period of time (1 to 2 weeks). Long-term use generally is not recommended.

Precautions

DO NOT USE if you are allergic to this medicine or its relatives; or if you are pregnant.

BEFORE USING THIS MEDICINE, tell your healthcare provider if you are breastfeeding; or if you are taking, will be taking or stop taking any prescription or nonprescription medicine; or if you have any other medical conditions.

Side Effects

Every medicine can cause side effects, but many people have no, or minor, side effects. Tell your healthcare provider if any of the following occurs: vision changes; irregular heartbeat; headache; chest pain; yellowing of skin or eyes; rash; unusual bleeding or bruising; vomiting; heartburn; diarrhea; constipation; appetite loss; nervousness; irritability; memory loss; sleeplessness; ringing in the ears; sore throat; joint pain.

Guidelines for Use

USE EXACTLY AS PRESCRIBED.

Do not exceed prescribed dosage.

Take with a full glass of water.

Use caution while driving or performing other tasks requiring mental alertness, coordination and dexterity.

May cause morning drowsiness, unusual tiredness in the morning or daytime sleepiness after using these medications for sleep. The elderly are particularly sensitive to these effects.

Avoid alcohol and other medications that cause drowsiness (eg, pain relievers, sedatives, antihistamines).

Nighttime sleep may be disturbed for 1 or 2 nights following stopping of the medication.

May be habit-forming.

Do not discontinue medicine abruptly, especially if you have a history of seizures, regardless of other antiseizure medications you may be taking.

Long-term use may result in dependence.

Withdrawal symptoms may occur when the medication is stopped.

Teniposide

(TEN-ih-POE-side)

Vumon

Used in combination with other medicines to treat patients with refractory childhood acute lymphoblastic leukemia (ALL).

Precautions

DO NOT USE if you are allergic to this medicine.

BEFORE USING THIS MEDICINE, tell your healthcare provider if you are pregnant or breastfeeding; or if you are taking, will be taking or stop taking any prescription or nonprescription medicine; or if you have any other medical conditions.

Side Effects

Every medicine can cause side effects, but many people have no, or minor, side effects. Tell your healthcare provider if any of the following occurs: nausea; vomiting; diarrhea; stomach pain; inflammation of the mouth; loss of hair; weakness; unusual bleeding or bruising; chills; fever; flushing; difficulty breathing; dizziness; fainting; rash; pain at injection site.

Patient Information

Contraceptive (birth control) measures are recommended during treatment.

Tell your healthcare provider if any of the following occurs: fever, chills, rapid heartbeat, difficulty breathing.

Lab tests will be required to monitor therapy. Be sure to keep appointments.

Terazosin

(ter-AZE-oh-sin)

Hytrin

A medicine used to lower high blood pressure. It may occasionally be prescribed for other reasons.

Precautions

DO NOT USE if you are allergic to this medicine.

BEFORE USING THIS MEDICINE, tell your healthcare provider if you are pregnant or breastfeeding; or if you are taking, will be taking or stop taking any prescription or nonprescription medicine or if you have any other medical conditions.

Side Effects

Every medicine can cause side effects, but many people have no, or minor, side effects. Tell your healthcare provider if any of the following occurs: dizziness (especially when arising from a seated or lying position); lightheadedness; pounding in the chest; increased pulse; nausea; shortness of breath; nasal congestion; sinus inflammation; muscle pain; blurred vision; nervousness; numbness of fingers/toes; impotence; headache; swelling.

Guidelines for Use

USE EXACTLY AS PRESCRIBED.

Take the first dose at bedtime to reduce the risk of dizziness that may occur early in therapy.

If a dose is missed, take it as soon as possible. If several hours have passed or if it is nearing time for the next dose, do not double the dose to "catch up," unless advised by your healthcare provider. If more than one dose is missed, contact your healthcare provider.

Patients being treated for high blood pressure often feel tired and run down for a few weeks after beginning therapy. It takes time for the body to adjust.

Continue taking your medication even though you may not feel quite normal. Check with your healthcare provider if any new symptoms cause concern.

Use caution when driving or performing other tasks requiring mental alertness.

Avoid engaging in any hazardous tasks for at least 24 hours after taking the first dose of these medications, missing several doses, increasing the dose or taking other high blood pressure medications with these products.

Do not take nonprescription decongestants, weight loss products, cold or allergy medications without first consulting your healthcare provider.

Periodically see your healthcare provider to make certain that the medicine is working properly and to have routine laboratory tests.

Terbutaline Sulfate

(ter-BYOO-tuh-leen SULL-fate)

Brethaire, Brethine, Bricanyl

A medicine that makes breathing easier by widening breathing passages of the lung and by removing (expectorating) mucus and other debris causing congestion in the lungs.

Precautions

DO NOT USE if you have an allergy to this medicine or have heart rhythm disturbances associated with a rapid heart rate.

BEFORE USING THIS MEDICINE, tell your healthcare provider if you are pregnant or breastfeeding; or if you are taking, will be taking or stop taking any prescription or nonprescription medicine; or if you have any other medical conditions.

Side Effects

Every medicine can cause side effects, but many people have no, or minor, side effects. Tell your healthcare provider if any of the following occurs: nausea; vomiting; loss of appetite; heartburn; nervousness; restlessness; dizziness; lightheadedness; headache; anxiety; tension; tremor; drowsiness; weakness; sleeplessness; chest pain; pounding in chest; breathing problems; coughing; flushing; sweating; hives; muscle cramps; unusual or bad taste in mouth; drying or irritation of mouth.

Guidelines for Use

USE EXACTLY AS PRESCRIBED.

Tell your healthcare provider if pounding in the chest, chest pain, muscle tremors, dizziness, headache, flushing or difficult urination occurs, or if breathing difficulty or nervousness persists.

Do not exceed recommended dosage.

Excessive use may lead to side effects or loss of effectiveness.

Do not stop or adjust the dose except on the recommendation of your healthcare provider. If you do not get the usual relief from your normal dose, do not increase your dose, but call your healthcare provider immediately.

Oral: If stomach upset occurs, take with food.

Terconazole

(ter-CONE-uh-zole)

Terazol 3, Terazol 7

A medicine used to treat vaginal candida (yeast) infections.

Precautions

DO NOT USE if you have an allergy to this medicine.

BEFORE USING THIS MEDICINE, tell your healthcare provider if you are pregnant or breastfeeding; or if you are taking, will be taking or stop taking any prescription or nonprescription medicine; or if you have any other medical conditions.

Side Effects

Every medicine can cause side effects, but many people have no, or minor, side effects. Tell your healthcare provider if any of the following occurs: headache; body aches; local irritation; burning; rash; itching; sensitivity to light; vaginal discharge; vaginal swelling; soreness.

Guidelines for Use

USE EXACTLY AS PRESCRIBED.

Patient instructions for proper use are enclosed in each package. Insert high into the vagina, except during pregnancy.

Complete a full course of therapy.

Keep using, even during the menstrual period.

If the medicine causes burning or irritation, or if symptoms worsen, contact your healthcare provider.

Refrain from sexual intercourse during treatment or the male sexual partner should use a condom to avoid the risk of reinfection.

A sanitary napkin or mini-pad may be used to prevent staining of clothing due to seepage or leakage. Tampons should not be used.

If infection recurs, other factors may be involved. Factors that increase the risk of infection include AIDS, diabetes, chronic antibiotic therapy, pregnancy, chronic steroid use and oral contraceptive use.

Terfenadine

(ter-FEN-uh-deen)

Seldane

A medicine used for relief of allergy symptoms and symptoms associated with hives (mild and uncomplicated), some insect bites and stings and skin rash with mild to moderate itching.

Precautions

DO NOT USE if you are allergic to this medicine or its relatives; are breastfeeding; or are taking erythromycin or monoamine oxidase inhibitors (MAOIs) (eg, *Nardil*, *Parnate*).

BEFORE USING THIS MEDICINE, tell your healthcare provider if you are pregnant, or if you are taking, will be taking or stop taking any prescription or nonprescription medicine; or if you have any other medical conditions.

Side Effects

Every medicine can cause side effects, but many people have no, or minor, side effects. Tell your healthcare provider if any of the following occurs: drowsiness; dizziness; dry mouth; stomach upset; constipation; blurred vision; difficult urination; confusion; fainting; irregular heart beats.

Guidelines for Use

USE EXACTLY AS PRESCRIBED.

Take with food.

Avoid alcohol and drowsiness-causing medicines.

Use caution while driving or performing tasks requiring mental alertness.

Use alone when sneezing and runny nose exist, but nasal congestion is slight. When nasal congestion occurs with sneezing and runny nose, an oral or topical decongestant also may be used.

Do not take for several days before allergy skin testing.

Testolactone

(TESS-toe-lak-TONE)

Teslac

An anticancer drug used to treat breast cancer in postmenopausal women and women whose ovarian function has been terminated.

Precautions

DO NOT USE if you are allergic to this medicine; males should NOT take this medicine.

BEFORE USING THIS MEDICINE, tell your healthcare provider if you are pregnant or breastfeeding; or if you are taking, will be taking or stop taking any prescription or nonprescription medicine; or if you have any other medical conditions.

Side Effects

Every medicine can cause side effects, but many people have no, or minor, side effects. Tell your healthcare provider if any of the following occurs: nausea; vomiting; loss of appetite; numbness or tingling of fingers, toes or face; inflammation of the tongue; diarrhea; pain or swelling of the hands or lower legs; itching; rash; hair loss.

Guidelines for Use

USE EXACTLY AS PRESCRIBED.

Take on an empty somach (1 hour before or 2 hours after eating) with a full glass of water. However, if stomach upset occurs, take with food.

This medicine is usually taken 4 times daily. If a dose is missed, contact your healthcare provider.

Contraceptive measures (birth control) are recommended during treatment.

Notify your healthcare provider if numbness of fingers, toes or face occurs.

May cause diarrhea, loss of appetite, nausea, vomiting, loss of hair, swelling or redness of tongue; notify your healthcare provider if these problems become pronounced.

Lab test will be required during treatment. Be sure to keep appointments.

Store at room temperature. Avoid excessive heat.

Testosterone

(teh-STAHS-tuh-RONE)

Andro L.A. 200, Andropository-200, Delatestryl, depAndro 100 Injection, depAndro 200, Depotest 100, Depotest 200, Depo-Testosterone, Duratest-100, Duratest-200, Duratest-200 Injection, Durathate-200, Everone 200, Histerone 100, Tesamone, Testandro, Testoderm

A hormone used to treat testosterone deficiency. Prolonged treatment is required to maintain male sex characteristics. It is used for testes that fail to develop, to treat delayed male puberty (brief treatment with low doses), to treat male impotence caused by androgen deficiency, as secondary therapy for advanced, inoperable breast cancer that has spread to other areas, including bones, in women who are 1 to 5 years postmenopausal and as secondary therapy for breast pain and swelling immediately after childbirth.

Precautions

DO NOT USE if you are allergic to this medicine or its relatives.

BEFORE USING THIS MEDICINE, tell your healthcare provider if you are pregnant or breastfeeding; or if you are taking, will be taking or stop taking any prescription or nonprescription medicine; or if you have any other medical conditions. Use with caution in the elderly. Testosterone may increase risk of prostate enlargement or prostate cancer.

Side Effects

Every medicine can cause side effects, but many people have no, or minor, side effects. Tell your healthcare provider if any of the following occurs: headache; anxiety; depression; excessive growth of body hair; loss of scalp hair; acne; excessively oily skin, yellowing of skin; rash; edema; fluid retention; nausea; pain at injection site; increased cholesterol test; abnormal thyroid tests; liver problems; change in sex drive. Female: deepening of the voice, hair growth, acne, increased size of clitoris, menstrual irregularities. These symptoms usually follow high doses of androgens and should be tolerated during treatment for breast cancer. Male: Breast tenderness or swelling; decreased sperm count; erection problems (pain, frequency, increased duration).

Guidelines for Use

USE EXACTLY AS PRESCRIBED.

Injections provide therapeutic effects for about 4 weeks.

Tetracycline Hydrochloride

(teh-truh-SIGH-kleen HIGH-droe-KLOR-ide)

Achromycin V, Ala-Tet, Nor-Tet Capsules, Panmycin Capsules, Robitet Capsules, Sumycin Capsules, Sumycin 250, Sumycin 500, Teline, Teline-500 Capsules, Tetracap Capsules, Tetracyn 500 Capsules, Tetralan 250 Capsules, Tetralan-500 Capsules, Tetram Capsules

An anti-infection medicine used to treat a wide variety of infections caused by certain bacteria.

Precautions

DO NOT USE if you are allergic to this medicine or its relatives; if you are pregnant; or in children under 8 years of age; or if it is out of date.

BEFORE USING THIS MEDICINE, tell your healthcare provider if you are breastfeeding; or if you are taking, will be taking or stop taking any prescription or nonprescription medicine; or if you have any other medical conditions.

Side Effects

Every medicine can cause side effects, but many people have no, or minor, side effects. Tell your healthcare provider if any of the following occurs: headache; vomiting; nausea; diarrhea; vaginal infection; visual disturbances.

Guidelines for Use

USE EXACTLY AS PRESCRIBED.

Take on an empty stomach with a full glass of water or other fluid at least 1 hour before or 2 hours after a meal.

Avoid use with antacids, laxatives, dairy products or iron-containing products. If an antacid must be taken, take 2 to 3 hours before or after this medicine.

If a dose is missed, take it as soon as possible. If several hours have passed or if it is nearing time for the next dose, do not double the dose to "catch up," unless advised by your healthcare provider. If more than one dose is missed, contact your healthcare provider.

Continue to take until all the prescribed medicine is gone. Failure to take all of the medicine may prevent complete elimination of bacteria, causing the infection to return.

May cause sensitivity to sunlight. Avoid prolonged exposure to the sun and other ultraviolet light. Use sunscreens and wear protective clothing until tolerance is determined.

Do not use outdated medicine since it may be highly toxic.

Suspension: Shake well before using.

Theophylline

(thee-AHF-ih-lin)

Accurbron, Aerolate, Aquaphyllin, Asmalix, Bronkodyl, Constant-T, Elixomin, Elixophyllin, Elixophyllin SR, Lanophyllin, Quibron-T Dividose, Quibron-T/SR Dividose, Respbid, Slo-bid Gyrocaps, Slo-Phyllin, Slo-Phyllin Gyrocaps, Sustaire, Theo-24, Theobid Duracaps, Theobid Jr. Duracaps, Theochron, Theoclear L.A., Theoclear-80 Syrup, Theo-Dur, Theo-Dur Sprinkle, Theolair, Theolair-SR, Theo-Sav, Theospan-SR, Theostat 80, Theovent, T-Phyl, Uniphyl

A medicine that makes breathing easier. Used to prevent and relieve symptoms of bronchial asthma, and to treat chronic bronchitis and emphysema. It may occasionally be prescribed for other reasons.

Precautions

DO NOT USE if you have an allergy to this medicine or any xanthine (eg, caffeine, chocolate); or if you are breastfeeding.

BEFORE USING THIS MEDICINE, tell your healthcare provider if you are pregnant; or if you are taking, will be taking or stop taking any prescription or nonprescription medicine; or if you have any other medical conditions.

Side Effects

Every medicine can cause side effects, but many people have no, or minor, side effects. Tell your healthcare provider if any of the following occurs: nausea; vomiting; severe stomach pain; loss of appetite; sleeplessness; jitteriness; headache; rash; restlessness; convulsions; irregular heartbeat.

Guidelines for Use

USE EXACTLY AS PRESCRIBED.

If stomach upset occurs, take with food.

Take at regular intervals around the clock.

Avoid large amounts of caffeine-containing food or beverages, such as tea, coffee, cocoa and cola drinks or large amounts of chocolate. These products may increase side effects.

Do not change the dose of your medication without consulting your healthcare provider.

Do not use this medicine for an acute asthma attack.

Timed release: Swallow whole; do not crush or chew.

Solution: Shake well before using.

Thiabendazole

(THIGH-uh-BEND-uh-zole)

Mintezol

A medicine used to treat worm infections.

Precautions

DO NOT USE if you are allergic to this medicine.

BEFORE USING THIS MEDICINE, tell your healthcare provider if you are pregnant or breastfeeding; or if you are taking, will be taking or stop taking any prescription or nonprescription medicine; or if you have any other medical conditions.

Side Effects

Every medicine can cause side effects, but many people have no, or minor, side effects. Tell your healthcare provider if any of the following occurs: headache; dizziness; nausea; vomiting; fever; rash; seizures; yellowing of skin or eyes; loss of appetite; diarrhea; stomach pain; flushing; chills; trouble breathing; ringing in the ears; vision changes; fainting; blood in urine.

Guidelines for Use

USE EXACTLY AS PRESCRIBED.

This medicine is usually taken 2 times a day after meals. If a dose is missed, take it as soon as possible. If several hours have passed or if it is nearing time for the next dose, do not double the dose to "catch up," unless advised by your healthcare provider. If more than one dose is missed, contact your healthcare provider.

Continue use until all the prescribed medicine has been taken. Failure to take all of the medicine may prevent complete elimination of the worms, causing the infection to return.

May cause drowsiness or dizziness. Use caution while driving or performing other tasks requiring mental alertness, coordination and dexterity.

Strict hygiene is essential to prevent reinfection. Disinfect toilet facilities daily. Change and launder undergarments, bed linens, towels and nightclothes daily.

Store at room temperature.

Chewable tablets--Chew thoroughly before swallowing. Suspension--Shake well before using.

Thiamine (Vitamin B_1)

(THIGH-uh-min)

Biamine, Thiamilate

Used to treat or prevent thiamine deficiency (a severe form is called beriberi). It may occasionally be prescribed for other reasons.

Precautions

DO NOT USE if you are allergic to this medicine.

BEFORE USING THIS MEDICINE, tell your healthcare provider if you are pregnant or breastfeeding; or if you are taking, will be taking or stop taking any prescription or nonprescription medicine; or if you have any other medical conditions.

Side Effects

Every medicine can cause side effects, but many people have no, or minor, side effects. Tell your healthcare provider if any of the following occurs: weakness; restlessness; tightness of throat; shortness of breath; itching; hives; sweating; feeling of warmth; nausea; irritation at the injection site.

Guidelines for Use

USE EXACTLY AS PRESCRIBED.

Most people on a balanced diet do not need vitamin supplements. Recommended Dietary Allowance (RDA)—Adult males: 1.5 mg; Adult females: 1.1 mg; Pregnancy and lactation: 1.5 mg to 1.6 mg.

Common sources of thiamine—Pork, organ meats (liver, heart, kidney), whole-wheat flour, brewer's yeast, enriched and fortified grains and cereals, cooked dry beans and seeds/nuts.

Thioguanine

(THIGH-oh-GWAHN-een)

Thioguanine Tablets

An anticancer medicine used to treat chronic myelogenous leukemia and acute nonlymphocytic leukemias.

Precautions

DO NOT USE if you are pregnant or breastfeeding; or have shown prior resistance to this medicine or mercaptopurine.

BEFORE USING THIS MEDICINE, tell your healthcare provider if you are taking, will be taking or stop taking any prescription or nonprescription medicine; or if you have any other medical conditions.

Side Effects

Every medicine can cause side effects, but many people have no, or minor, side effects. Tell your healthcare provider if any of the following occurs: stomach discomfort; appetite loss; dizziness; headache; excessive uric acid in blood; yellowing of skin or eyes; unusual bleeding or bruising; chills; fever; sore throat; flu-like symptoms; joint pain; diarrhea; swelling of feet and legs; black tarry stools; dark or bloody urine.

Guidelines for Use

USE EXACTLY AS PRESCRIBED.

Drink plenty of liquids.

Practice effective birth control measures during therapy.

If a dose is missed, take it as soon as possible. If several hours have passed or if it is nearing time for the next dose, do not double the dose to "catch up," unless advised by your healthcare provider. If more than one dose is missed, contact your healthcare provider.

Thioridazine Hydrochloride

(THIGH-oh-RID-uh-zeen HIGH-droe-KLOR-ide)

Mellaril, Mellaril-S

A neuroleptic or major tranquilizer generally used to improve concentration and self-control in patients with psychotic behavior.

Precautions

DO NOT USE if you are allergic to this medicine or its relatives. Laboratory tests may be needed including eye exams, blood counts and kidney and liver tests.

BEFORE USING THIS MEDICINE, tell your healthcare provider if you are pregnant or breastfeeding; or if you are taking, will be taking or stop taking any prescription or nonprescription medicine; if you have any other medical conditions; or if you are allergic to tartrazine.

Side Effects

Every medicine can cause side effects, but many people have no, or minor, side effects. Tell your healthcare provider if any of the following occurs: tremors; drooling; shuffling gait; restlessness; muscle spasms; aching or numbness; sore throat; fever; unusual bleeding or bruising; skin rash; weakness; impaired vision; dark-colored urine; pale stools; yellowing of skin or eyes.

Guidelines for Use

USE EXACTLY AS PRESCRIBED.

Take routinely as directed; it controls illness symptoms and is not habit-forming.

Improvement may not be seen for several weeks.

May cause drowsiness. Use caution while driving or performing other tasks requiring mental alertness.

Avoid alcohol and medicines that cause drowsiness (eg, sleeping pills, antihistamines).

May cause sunlight sensitivity. Avoid long exposure to the sun. Use sunscreens and protective clothing until tolerance is known.

May discolor the urine pink or reddish brown. This is not harmful.

If dizziness or fainting occurs, avoid sudden changes in posture and use caution when climbing stairs, etc (more common during first week of therapy).

Caution in hot weather: May increase risk of heatstroke.

Suspension: Shake well before using.

Lab tests will be required to monitor therapy. Be sure to keep appointments.

Thiotepa

(thigh-oh-TEP-uh)

Thioplex

Used to treat cancer of the breast, ovary or bladder. It may occasionally be prescribed for other reasons.

Precautions

DO NOT USE if you are allergic to this medicine or if you have liver, kidney or bone marrow problems.

BEFORE USING THIS MEDICINE, tell your healthcare provider if you are pregnant or breastfeeding; or if you are taking, will be taking or stop taking any prescription or nonprescription medicine; or if you have any other medical conditions.

Side Effects

Every medicine can cause side effects, but many people have no, or minor, side effects. Tell your healthcare provider if any of the following occurs: pain at the injection site; loss of hair; skin discoloration; nausea; vomiting; stomach pain; loss of appetite; painful/ difficult urination; urinary retention; dizziness; headache; blurred vision; fatigue; weakness; eye irritation; painful periods; rash; difficulty breathing; wheezing.

Patient Information

Contraceptive (birth control) measures are recommended during treatment.

Lab tests will be required to monitor therapy. Be sure to keep appointments.

Thiothixene

(THIGH-oh-THIX-een)

Navane, Navane Concentrate

A medicine used in the treatment of mental disorders. It may occasionally be prescribed for other reasons.

Precautions

DO NOT USE if you are allergic to this medicine.

BEFORE USING THIS MEDICINE, tell your healthcare provider if you are pregnant or breastfeeding; or if you are taking, will be taking or stop taking any prescription or nonprescription medicine; or if you have any other medical conditions.

Side Effects

Every medicine can cause side effects, but many people have no, or minor, side effects. Tell your healthcare provider if any of the following occurs: lightheadedness; fainting; drowsiness; seizures; involuntary movements of the tongue, face, mouth or jaw; rash; trouble breathing; vision changes; nausea; vomiting; diarrhea; weight gain; swelling of the lower legs; dry mouth.

Guidelines for Use

USE EXACTLY AS PRESCRIBED.

May cause drowsiness, dizziness or blurred vision. Use caution when driving or performing other tasks requiring mental alertness.

Avoid alcohol and medicines (eg, tranquilizers, antihistamines, some pain medicines) that can cause drowsiness.

May cause sensitivity to sunlight. Avoid prolonged exposure to the sun. Use sunscreens and wear protective clothing until tolerance is determined.

Do not suddenly stop taking this medicine as this may cause serious health problems. Your doctor will instruct you on how to reduce the dosage safely over time.

Sucking on hard candy, drinking fluids or maintaining good dental hygiene can relieve dry mouth.

If constipation occurs, use stool softeners if necessary.

This medicine can reduce the ability to sweat, an important function by which overheating is prevented. Avoid excess sun or exercise, which may cause excessive heat buildup.

Concentrate and capsules: May be taken without regard to food.

Solution: May be diluted in fruit juice.

Thyroid Desiccated

(THIGH-royd, DESS-ih-KATE-uhd)

Armour Thyroid, S-P-T, Thyrar, Thyroid Strong

A thyroid hormone substitute used primarily for low thyroid hormone secretion and some other thyroid problems.

Precautions

DO NOT USE if you are allergic to thyroid hormones or as a treatment for obesity.

BEFORE USING THIS MEDICINE, tell your healthcare provider if you are pregnant or breastfeeding; or if you are taking, will be taking or stop taking any prescription or nonprescription medicine; if you have any other medical conditions; or if you are allergic to tartrazine.

Side Effects

Every medicine can cause side effects, but many people have no, or minor, side effects. Tell your healthcare provider if any of the following occurs: headache; nervousness; nausea; diarrhea; excessive sweating; heat intolerance; menstrual problems; chest pain; increased pulse rate; pounding in the chest; or any other unusual feeling or symptom. Partial loss of hair may be seen in children in the first few months of therapy, but this is usually temporary.

Guidelines for Use

USE EXACTLY AS PRESCRIBED.

Take as a single daily dose, usually before breakfast.

Do not stop medication except on advice of your healthcare provider. Dosage is intended to replace the low thyroid secretion.

Your response is evaluated by your healthcare provider with laboratory tests. It is important to keep regular appointments with your healthcare provider.

Replacement therapy is usually taken for life.

Ticarcillin

(TIE-car-sill-in)

Ticar

An antibiotic used to treat a variety of infections.

Precautions

DO NOT USE if you are allergic to this medicine.

BEFORE USING THIS MEDICINE, tell your healthcare provider if you are pregnant or breastfeeding; or if you are taking, will be taking or stop taking any prescription or nonprescription medicine; or if you have any other medical condition.

Side Effects

Every medicine can cause side effects, but many people have no, or minor, side effects. Tell your healthcare provider if any of the following occurs: rash; itching; convulsions; weakness; fever; nausea; vomiting; diarrhea; pain at the injection site; difficulty breathing.

Guidelines for Use

USE EXACTLY AS PRESCRIBED.

If symptoms of an allergic reaction develop (eg, difficulty breathing, facial swelling, rash, itching), stop the drug and contact your healthcare provider.

If a dose is missed, inject it as soon as possible. If several hours have passed or if it is nearing time for the next dose, do not double the dose to "catch up," unless advised by your healthcare provider. If more than one dose is missed, contact your healthcare provider.

Ticlopidine Hydrochloride

(tie-KLOE-pih-DEEN HIGH-droe-KLOR-ide)

Ticlid

An antiplatelet agent used to prevent blood clots by keeping platelets from clumping together. It also is used in prevention and treatment of stroke.

Precautions

DO NOT USE if you are allergic to this medicine; if you have severe liver disease; or if you have a blood clotting disorder or active bleeding.

BEFORE USING THIS MEDICINE, tell your healthcare provider if you are pregnant or breastfeeding; or if you are taking, will be taking or stop taking any prescription or nonprescription medicine; or if you have any other medical conditions.

Side Effects

Every medicine can cause side effects, but many people have no, or minor, side effects. Tell your healthcare provider if any of the following occurs: diarrhea; nausea; indigestion; stomach pain; vomiting; gas; appetite loss; rash; bruising; itching; dizziness.

Guidelines for Use

USE EXACTLY AS PRESCRIBED.

Take with food to minimize stomach discomfort.

Tell your healthcare provider immediately if you experience any signs of infection such as fever, chills or sore throat.

It may take longer than usual to stop bleeding when taking this medicine.

Report any unusual bleeding or dark colored stools to your healthcare provider.

Tell your dentist or healthcare provider that you are taking this medicine before any surgery is scheduled and before any new medicine is prescribed.

Tell your healthcare provider promptly if severe or persistent diarrhea, rashes or bleeding beneath the skin, or any signs of liver damage such as yellow skin or eyes, dark urine or light colored stools occurs.

Timolol Maleate Ophthalmic

(TI-moe-lahl MAL-ee-ate)

Timoptic, Timoptic Ocudose

An eye drop used to help lower the pressure inside of the eye in patients with chronic open-angle glaucoma and other conditions.

Precautions

DO NOT USE if you are allergic to this medicine or its relatives, are diabetic or are breastfeeding.

BEFORE USING THIS MEDICINE, tell your healthcare provider if you are pregnant; or if you are taking, will be taking or stop taking any prescription or nonprescription medicine; or if you have any other medical conditions.

Side Effects

Every medicine can cause side effects, but many people have no, or minor, side effects. Tell your healthcare provider if any of the following occurs: temporary stinging or pain when instilling drops; double vision; visual problems; irritation; inflammation; tearing, browache; light sensitivity; depression; confusion; hallucinations; dizziness; headache; pounding in the chest; stomach upset; nausea; breathing difficulty; rash.

Guidelines for Use

USE EXACTLY AS PRESCRIBED.

If a dose is missed, take it as soon as possible. If several hours have passed or if it is nearing time for the next dose, do not double the dose to "catch up," unless advised by your healthcare provider. If more than one dose is missed, contact your healthcare provider.

May cause stinging or pain when first put in the eye.

Eye pressure will have to be monitored periodically by your healthcare provider.

Tell your healthcare provider if you are using these eye drops and plan to have surgery. You may have to temporarily stop using them.

Timolol Maleate Oral

(TI-moe-lahl MAL-ee-ate)

Blocadren

A beta blocker medicine used to lower high blood pressure and to treat angina and heart attack.

Precautions

DO NOT USE if you are allergic to this medicine or its relatives, or if you are breastfeeding.

BEFORE USING THIS MEDICINE, tell your healthcare provider if you are pregnant; or if you are taking, will be taking or stop taking any prescription or nonprescription medicine; or if you have any other medical conditions.

Side Effects

Every medicine can cause side effects, but many people have no, or minor, side effects. Tell your healthcare provider if any of the following occurs: nausea; vomiting; stomach ache; diarrhea; constipation; appetite changes; indigestion; depression; anxiety; hallucinations; short-term memory loss; behavior changes; disorientation; fainting; dizziness; lightheadedness; tiredness; sleep disturbances; decreased concentration; headache; nightmares; emotional instability; changes in heart rate; chest pain; chills; cold or numb extremities; pounding of the chest; difficulty breathing; cough; nasal congestion; rash; hives; fluid retention; flushing or paleness; increased pigmentation; itching; hair loss; sweating; dry skin; psoriasis; painful and aching joints and muscles; painful, frequent or difficult urination; blurred vision; dry, burning or irritated eyes; ringing in the ears; taste changes; sore throat; dry mouth; slurred speech; fever; weight gain; changes in blood sugar levels.

Guidelines for Use

USE EXACTLY AS PRESCRIBED.

Ask your healthcare provider before using other medicines including nasal decongestants, diet aids or nonprescription cold preparations.

Do not stop this medicine suddenly, it could cause a worsening of disease including worse angina (chest pain), irregular heartbeats and increase risk of heart attack and death.

Withdraw these medications slowly over one to two weeks by gradually decreasing the dose.

Diabetes — These products can mask signs of low blood sugar and change blood sugar levels. It may be necessary for your healthcare provider to change your dose of diabetic medications.

Use caution while driving or performing other tasks requiring mental alertness, coordination and dexterity.

Tobramycin

(TOE-bruh-MY-sin)

AKTob, Tobrex

A medicine used to treat eye infections.

Precautions

DO NOT USE if you are allergic to this medicine.

BEFORE USING THIS MEDICINE, tell your healthcare provider if you are pregnant or breastfeeding; or if you are taking, will be taking or stop taking any prescription or nonprescription medicine; if you have any other medical conditions; or if you are allergic to sulfites.

Side Effects

Every medicine can cause side effects, but many people have no, or minor, side effects. Tell your healthcare provider if any of the following occurs: irritation; burning; stinging; itching; lid swelling; redness.

Guidelines for Use

USE EXACTLY AS PRESCRIBED.

Tilt head back and place medication in corner of the eye. Close eyes and apply light finger pressure for 1 minute following instillation.

May cause temporary blurring of vision or stinging following administration.

Contact your healthcare provider if stinging, burning or itching, redness, irritation, swelling, decreasing vision or pain persists or worsens.

Avoid contact between the dispensing container and the eye.

Tocainide Hydrochloride

(TOE-cane-ide HIGH-droe-KLOR-ide)

Tonocard

A heart medicine (antiarrhythmic) that reduces irregular heart beats to correct or prevent various types of heart rhythm disturbances.

Precautions

DO NOT USE if you are allergic to this medicine or amide-type local anesthetics.

BEFORE USING THIS MEDICINE, tell your healthcare provider if you are pregnant or breastfeeding; or if you are taking, will be taking or stop taking any prescription or nonprescription medicine; or if you have any other medical conditions.

Side Effects

Every medicine can cause side effects, but many people have no, or minor, side effects. Tell your healthcare provider if any of the following occurs: appetite loss; nausea; vomiting; diarrhea; numbness or tingling; dizziness; lightheadedness; tremor; slurred speech; confusion; change in mood or awareness; restlessness; anxiety; headache; sleepiness; irregular heartbeats or pounding in the chest; decreased blood pressure; chest pain; increased shortness of breath with physical activity; painful breathing; cough or wheezing; unusual bruising or bleeding; signs of infection such as fever, sore throat, chills; visual disturbances; ringing in the ears; hearing loss; sweating, clamminess; hot/cold feelings; rash; joint pain.

Guidelines for Use

USE EXACTLY AS PRESCRIBED.

Do not discontinue therapy unless instructed by your healthcare provider.

Take this medication at evenly spaced intervals around the clock.

May cause drowsiness or dizziness. Observe caution while driving or performing other tasks requiring mental alertness or physical dexterity.

May cause nausea, vomiting or diarrhea. Notify your healthcare provider if these persist or become severe.

Tolazamide

(tole-AZE-uh-mid)

Tolinase

An oral antidiabetic medicine that lowers blood sugar. It is used only in patients with non-insulin-dependent diabetes mellitus (Type II) who cannot manage blood sugar levels by diet and exercise alone.

Precautions

DO NOT USE if you have an allergy to this medicine or sulfa drugs.

BEFORE USING THIS MEDICINE, tell your healthcare provider if you are pregnant or breastfeeding; or if you are taking, will be taking or stop taking any prescription or nonprescription medicine; or if you have any other medical conditions.

Side Effects

Every medicine can cause side effects, but many people have no, or minor, side effects. Tell your healthcare provider if any of the following occurs: nausea; vomiting; heartburn; diarrhea; fever; sore throat; rash; itching; weakness; unusual bruising or bleeding.

Guidelines for Use

USE EXACTLY AS PRESCRIBED.

Take 30 minutes before a meal.

Take with food if nausea or stomach upset occurs.

Avoid alcohol, which can cause flushing, weakness, dizziness, a tingling sensation and headache.

Monitor blood sugar levels daily. Notify your healthcare provider if low blood sugar develops (eg, fatigue, nausea, confusion, agitation, excessive hunger, profuse sweating, numbness or tingling of lips, tongue or extremities) or if excessive thirst or urination, or other symptoms of high blood sugar levels occur (glucose or ketones in the urine or blood).

Proper diet and exercise are important.

To prevent low blood sugar:

1. Know the symptoms of low blood sugar.
2. Keep track of your blood sugar levels.
3. Keep a source of quick-acting sugar with you at all times.
4. Maintain an adequate diet.
5. Know how diet and exercise affect your blood sugar level.

Acute illness (eg, physical trauma, infection, fever, surgery) may require the temporary administration of insulin.

Tolbutamide

(tole-BYOO-tuh-mide)

Orinase

An oral antidiabetic medicine that lowers blood sugar. It is used only in patients with non-insulin-dependent diabetes mellitus (Type II) who cannot manage blood sugar levels by diet and exercise alone.

Precautions

DO NOT USE if you have an allergy to this medicine or sulfa drugs.

BEFORE USING THIS MEDICINE, tell your healthcare provider if you are pregnant or breastfeeding; or if you are taking, will be taking or stop taking any prescription or nonprescription medicine; or if you have any other medical conditions.

Side Effects

Every medicine can cause side effects, but many people have no, or minor, side effects. Tell your healthcare provider if any of the following occurs: nausea; vomiting; heartburn; diarrhea; fever; sore throat; rash; itching; weakness; unusual bruising or bleeding.

Guidelines for Use

USE EXACTLY AS PRESCRIBED.

Take 30 minutes before a meal.

Take with food if nausea or stomach upset occurs.

Avoid alcohol, which can cause flushing, weakness, dizziness, a tingling sensation and headache.

Monitor blood sugar levels daily. Notify your healthcare provider if low blood sugar develops (eg, fatigue, nausea, confusion, agitation, excessive hunger, profuse sweating, numbness or tingling of lips, tongue or extremities) or if excessive thirst or urination, or other symptoms of high blood sugar levels occur (glucose or ketones in the urine or blood).

Proper diet and exercise are important.

To prevent low blood sugar:

1. Know the symptoms of low blood sugar.
2. Keep track of your blood sugar levels.
3. Keep a source of quick-acting sugar with you at all times.
4. Maintain an adequate diet.
5. Know how diet and exercise affect your blood sugar level.

Acute illness (eg, physical trauma, infection, fever, surgery) may require the temporary administration of insulin.

Tolmetin Sodium

(TOLE-mee-tin SO-dee-uhm)

Tolectin 200 Tablets, Tolectin 600 Tablets, Tolectin DS Capsules

A nonsteroidal anti-inflammatory medicine (NSAID) generally used to treat osteoarthritis (degenerative joint disease), rheumatoid arthritis and juvenile rheumatoid arthritis. It may occasionally be prescribed for other reasons.

Precautions

DO NOT USE if you are allergic to this medicine or its relatives, aspirin or iodides.

BEFORE USING THIS MEDICINE, tell your healthcare provider if you are pregnant or breastfeeding; use alcohol; are prone to fluid retention; or if you are taking, will be taking or stop taking any prescription or nonprescription medicines; or have any other medical conditions.

Side Effects

Every medicine can cause side effects, but many people have no, or minor, side effects. Tell your healthcare provider if any of the following occurs: allergic reaction (eg, rash, itching, fever); changes in vision; weight gain; fluid retention; stomach problems (eg, nausea, vomiting, diarrhea, pain); black stools; constipation; persistent headache; dizziness; nervousness; weakness; ringing in the ears; taste changes; unusual bruising or bleeding.

Guidelines for Use

USE EXACTLY AS PRESCRIBED.

Avoid aspirin and alcoholic beverages.

If stomach upset occurs, take with food, milk or antacids. If stomach pain continues, tell your healthcare provider.

If a dose is missed, take it as soon as possible. If several hours have passed or if it is nearing time for the next dose, do not double the dose to "catch up," unless advised by your healthcare provider. If more than one dose is missed, contact your healthcare provider.

May cause drowsiness or dizziness.

Observe caution while driving or performing other tasks requiring mental alertness.

May cause sensitivity to sunlight. Avoid prolonged exposure to the sun. Use sunscreens and wear protective clothing until tolerance is determined.

Tolnaftate

(tahl-NAFF-tate)

Absorbine Antifungal, Absorbine Jr. Antifungal, Aftate for Athlete's Foot, Aftate for Jock Itch, Desenex, Genaspor, NP-27, Quinsana Plus, Tinactin, Tinactin for Jock Itch, Ting, Zeasorb-AF

A topical medicine used to treat fungal infections such as athlete's foot, jock itch, ringworm and tinea versicolor.

Precautions

DO NOT USE if you are allergic to this medicine.

BEFORE USING THIS MEDICINE, tell your healthcare provider if you are pregnant or breastfeeding; or if you are taking, will be taking or stop taking any prescription or nonprescription medicine; or if you have any other medical conditions.

Side Effects

Every medicine can cause side effects, but many people have no, or minor, side effects. Tell your healthcare provider if any of the following occurs: burning; hives; blistering; peeling; itching; stinging; redness; swelling; dryness.

Guidelines for Use

USE EXACTLY AS PRESCRIBED.

For external use only. Avoid contact with the eyes, nose, mouth or other mucous membranes.

Cleanse and dry the area to be treated before application.

Avoid inhalation.

Apply with caution to blistered or raw skin, oozing skin or skin over a deep puncture wound.

Avoid the use of tight dressings unless directed by your healthcare provider. Allergic reactions may occur.

If the condition being treated worsens or irritation, burning, redness, swelling or stinging persists, discontinue use.

Frequency of application and duration of therapy is dependent on the condition being treated, its location, the medicine, the strength of the medicine and the dosage guidelines; consult your healthcare provider.

For athlete's foot, wear well-fitting and ventilated shoes and change socks at least once a day.

Use these medications for the full treatment time, even if the symptoms improve. Tell your healthcare provider if there is no improvement after 4 weeks.

Torsemide

(TORE-suh-MIDE)

Demadex

A diuretic (water pill) that decreases excess water in the body and increases urine flow. This medicine is used to treat high blood pressure and edema (excess fluid) due to a variety of causes.

Precautions

DO NOT USE if you are allergic to this medicine or its relatives; oral diabetic medicines; sulfa antibiotics; or if you have severe kidney disease or loss of kidney function.

BEFORE USING THIS MEDICINE, tell your healthcare provider if you are pregnant or breastfeeding; or if you are taking, will be taking or stop taking any prescription or nonprescription medicine; or if you have any other medical conditions.

Side Effects

Every medicine can cause side effects, but many people have no, or minor, side effects. Tell your healthcare provider if any of the following occurs: excessive urination; sinus inflammation; weakness; diarrhea; cough; constipation; nausea; muscle and joint pain; indigestion; sore throat; chest pain; nervousness; rash.

Guidelines for Use

USE EXACTLY AS PRESCRIBED.

May be taken without regard to meals.

Increases urination; to avoid disruption of sleep at night, take early in the day, usually as a single dose.

Dizziness or lightheadedness may occur if you stand up too fast from a lying or sitting position. If this occurs, get up slowly and avoid sudden changes in posture.

Sensitivity to sunlight may occur. Use sunscreen and wear protective clothing until tolerance is determined.

Diabetes — May increase blood sugar levels.

May cause loss of potassium. If signs of potassium loss occur (weakness, cramps, nausea, dizziness, etc), contact your healthcare provider. Periodic monitoring of serum potassium and other electrolytes may be needed.

Tramadol Hydrochloride

(TRAM-uh-dole HIGH-droe-KLOR-ide)

Ultram

This medicine is used to relieve moderate to moderately severe pain in patients over 16 years of age.

Precautions

DO NOT USE if you are allergic to this medicine; if you have a drug or alcohol dependency; or have recently used depressants such as alcohol or narcotics.

BEFORE USING THIS MEDICINE, tell your healthcare provider if you are pregnant or breastfeeding; if you are taking, will be taking or stop taking any prescription or nonprescription medicine (eg, MAOIs); or if you have any other medical conditions.

Side Effects

Every medicine can cause side effects, but many people have no, or minor, side effects. Tell your healthcare provider if any of the following occurs: dizziness; feeling of whirling motion; nausea; constipation; headache; drowsiness; vomiting; rash; itching; nervousness; weakness; sweating; indigestion; dry mouth; diarrhea; general body discomfort; flushing; confusion; incoordination; sleep disorders; unstable emotions; appetite changes; gas; visual problems; urinary problems; menopausal symptoms; muscle stiffness.

Guidelines for Use

USE EXACTLY AS PRESCRIBED.

This medicine may be taken every 4-6 hours for pain relief as needed, not exceeding 400 mg per day.

Patients over 75 years of age may experience more side effects and require lower doses.

This medicine may be taken without regard to food.

Do not take this medicine more often than prescribed. This drug may be addicting and can cause breathing problems if taken in large doses.

This medicine may cause drowsiness, dizziness or confusion. Avoid driving or performing other tasks requiring alertness or coordination until effects are known, then use caution.

Do not use alcohol or other depressants (eg, tranquilizers) as they may cause increased drowsiness, dizziness, confusion or breathing problems.

Store at room temperature in a tight container.

Tranylcypromine Sulfate

(tran-il-SIP-row-meen SULL-fate)

Parnate

A monoamine oxidase inhibitor (MAOI) that generally is used to treat mental depression.

Precautions

DO NOT USE if you are allergic to this medicine. BEFORE USING THIS MEDICINE, tell your healthcare provider if you are pregnant or breastfeeding; or if you are taking, will be taking or stop taking any prescription or nonprescription medicines; or if you have any other medical conditions.

Tyramine-containing foods should be avoided including: any high protein food that is aged or undergoes breakdown by putrefaction process to improve flavor: many dairy products, some fish, alcohol products (especially beers, ales and red wines), some fruits/vegetables (eg, avocado, yeast extracts, bananas, figs, fava beans) and any caffeine-containing products or tyramine. Do not drink alcoholic beverages or self-medicate with cold, hay fever or weight-reducing preparations while undergoing therapy. Report promptly the occurrence of headache or other unusual symptoms.

Side Effects

Every medicine can cause side effects, but many people have no, or minor, side effects. Tell your healthcare provider if any of the following occurs: severe headache; skin rash; darkening of the urine; pale stools; yellowing of skin or eyes; dizziness; constipation; diarrhea; nausea; weight gain.

Guidelines for Use

USE EXACTLY AS PRESCRIBED.

May take a few weeks to work.

Do not discontinue this medication or take any other medication, except on the advice of your healthcare provider.

If a dose is missed, take it as soon as possible. If several hours have passed or if it is nearing time for the next dose, do not double the dose to "catch up," unless advised to do so by your healthcare provider. If more than one dose is missed, contact your healthcare provider.

May cause drowsiness or blurred vision. Use caution while driving or performing other tasks requiring mental alertness.

Initially, dizziness, weakness or fainting may occur when arising from a horizontal or sitting position. If this occurs, get up slowly.

Wear or carry identification saying that you take an MAOI.

Trazodone

(TRAY-zoe-dohn)

Desyrel, Desyrel Dividose

A mood elevating medicine used to relieve mental depression.

Precautions

DO NOT USE if you are allergic to this medicine.

BEFORE USING THIS MEDICINE, tell your healthcare provider if you are pregnant or breastfeeding; or if you are taking, will be taking or stop taking any prescription or nonprescription medicine; or if you have any other medical conditions.

Side Effects

Every medicine can cause side effects, but many people have no, or minor, side effects. Tell your healthcare provider if any of the following occurs: nausea; vomiting; diarrhea; constipation; dry mouth; drowsiness; anger; hostility; sleeplessness; nightmares/vivid dreams; confusion; decreased concentration; dizziness; fatigue; headache; tremors; impaired memory; nervousness; incoordination; blood pressure changes; irregular heart rhythm; pounding in the chest; chest pain; ringing in the ears; blurred vision; nasal congestion; rash; clamminess; sweating; blood in urine; incontinence of urine; prolonged painful erection; premature ejaculation; changes in sex drive; impotence; missed menstrual periods; breast enlargement; breathing difficulty; weight changes; swelling; aches and pains; fainting.

Guidelines for Use

USE EXACTLY AS PRESCRIBED.

Take with food.

If a dose is missed, take it as soon as possible. If several hours have passed or if it is nearing time for the next dose, do not double the dose to "catch up," unless advised by your healthcare provider. If more than one dose is missed, contact your healthcare provider.

May cause drowsiness or dizziness. Use caution while driving or performing other tasks requiring alertness and coordination.

Avoid alcohol or drowsiness-causing medications (eg, tranquilizers, pain medicine, antihistamines) while taking this medicine.

Male patients with prolonged and painful erections should immediately discontinue the medication and consult a healthcare provider.

May cause dry mouth, irregular heartbeat, shortness of breath, nausea and vomiting. Notify your healthcare provider if these become pronounced.

Tretinoin

(TREH-tih-NO-in)

Retin-A

A medicine used to treat acne. It may occasionally be prescribed for other reasons.

Precautions

DO NOT USE if you are allergic to this medicine.

BEFORE USING THIS MEDICINE, tell your healthcare provider if you are pregnant or breastfeeding; or if you are taking, will be taking or stop taking any prescription or nonprescription medicine or if you have any other medical conditions.

Side Effects

Every medicine can cause side effects, but many people have no, or minor, side effects. Tell your healthcare provider if any of the following occurs: red, irritated skin; blistered or crusted skin; increased or decreased skin pigmentation (color); increased sensitivity to sunlight and UV tanning lamps.

Guidelines for Use

USE EXACTLY AS PRESCRIBED.

For external use only.

Lightly apply to affected area at bedtime.

Wash hands immediately after use.

Application may cause a feeling of warmth and slight stinging.

Keep away from the eyes, mouth and nose.

Minimize exposure to sunlight and sunlamps. Use sunscreen products and wear protective clothing over treated areas.

May cause an unusual sensitivity to wind and cold. Avoid when possible.

Use of other acne agents is not recommended. Rest the skin for a few days before beginning therapy.

Use with caution on eczema (dry scaly skin).

If excessive medication is applied, redness, peeling and pain may occur. If these symptoms persist, use the medication less frequently or stop temporarily.

Thoroughly remove cosmetics before applying this medicine. Early in treatment, acne may appear worse due to the action of the medicine. Do not stop therapy.

Positive effects should be seen in 2 to 3 weeks, but may not be optimal for 6 weeks or more.

Triamcinolone Inhalation

(TRY-am-SIN-oh-lone)

Azmacort Aerosol

An anti-inflammatory medicine used to prevent or reduce the frequency and severity of bronchial asthma attacks. It is not used to treat an acute asthma attack.

Precautions

DO NOT USE if you are allergic to this medicine or are breastfeeding.

BEFORE USING THIS MEDICINE, tell your healthcare provider if you are pregnant; or if you are taking, will be taking or stop taking any prescription or nonprescription medicine; or if you have any other medical conditions.

Side Effects

Every medicine can cause side effects, but many people have no, or minor, side effects. Tell your healthcare provider if any of the following occurs: sore throat or mouth; hoarseness; cough; dry mouth; rash; facial swelling; difficult breathing.

Guidelines for Use

USE EXACTLY AS PRESCRIBED.

Read patient package insert carefully.

For preventive therapy only. Do NOT use for an acute asthma attack requiring rapid relief.

Use at regularly scheduled intervals as prescribed.

Do not exceed recommended dose.

Supplementary oral steroids may be necessary during periods of high stress or an asthma attack. Carry identification indicating this potential need.

If symptoms of steroid withdrawal occur when changing from oral to inhalant therapy (eg, joint or muscle pain, lack of energy, depression), contact your healthcare provider immediately for instructions.

Triamcinolone Injectable

(TRY-am-SIN-oh-lone)

Cenocort A-40, Kenaject-40, Kenalog 10, Kenalog-40, Tac-3, Tac-40, Triam-A, Triamonide 40, Tri-Kort, Trilog

A corticosteroid used to treat a variety of conditions.

Precautions

DO NOT USE if you are allergic this medicine.

BEFORE USING THIS MEDICINE, tell your healthcare provider if you are pregnant or breastfeeding; or if you are taking, will be taking or stop taking any prescription or nonprescription medicine; or if you have any other medical conditions.

Side Effects

Every medicine can cause side effects, but many people have no, or minor, side effects. Tell your healthcare provider if any of the following occurs: muscle weakness; stomach distention; nausea; vomiting; increased appetite and weight gain; thin fragile skin; loss of menstrual period; postmenopausal bleeding and other menstrual irregularities; headache; feeling of whirling motion; fatigue; sleeplessness; overall body aches.

Patient Information

Patients on chronic steroid therapy should wear or carry identification.

Tell your healthcare provider if unusual weight gain, swelling of the lower extermitites, muscle weakness, black tarry stools, vomiting of blood, puffing of the face, menstrual irregularities, prolonged sore throat, fever, cold or infection occurs.

Signs of adrenal insufficiency include fatigue, loss of appetite, nausea, vomiting, diarrhea, weight loss, weakness, dizziness and low blood sugar. Tell your healthcare provider immediately if these symptoms occur.

High-dose or long-term therapy: Avoid abrupt withdrawal of therapy.

Triamcinolone Nasal

(TRY-am-SIN-oh-lone)

Nasacort

Used for the treatment of seasonal and year-round allergic rhinitis symptoms.

Precautions

DO NOT USE if you are allergic to this medicine.

BEFORE USING THIS MEDICINE, tell your healthcare provider if you are pregnant or breastfeeding; or if you are taking, will be taking or stop taking any prescription or nonprescription medicine; or if you have any other medical conditions.

Side Effects

Every medicine can cause side effects, but many people have no, or minor, side effects. Tell your healthcare provider if any of the following occurs: burning; stinging; dryness; headache; lightheadedness.

Guidelines for Use

USE EXACTLY AS PRESCRIBED.

Patient instructions provided with the product.

Do not exceed recommended dosage.

May cause irritation and drying of nasal mucosa.

Tell your healthcare provider if symptoms do not improve, if the condition worsens or if sneezing or nasal irritation occurs.

Clear nasal passages of secretions prior to use. If nasal passages are blocked, use a decongestant just before administration to ensure adequate penetration of the spray. Effects are not immediate. Benefit requires regular use and usually occurs within a few days.

Triamcinolone Topical

(TRY-am-SIN-oh-lone)

Aristocort, Aristocort A, Delta-Tritex, Flutex, Kenalog, Kenalog-H, Kenonel, Triacet, Triderm

A topical anti-inflammatory agent used to treat rash or skin irritation.

Precautions

DO NOT USE near eyes or eyelids or if you have an allergy to this medicine.

BEFORE USING THIS MEDICINE, tell your healthcare provider if you are pregnant or breastfeeding; or if you are taking, will be taking or stop taking any prescription or nonprescription medicine; or if you have any other medical conditions.

Side Effects

Every medicine can cause side effects, but many people have no, or minor, side effects. Tell your healthcare provider if any of the following occurs: burning; itching; irritation; redness; dryness; acne; streaks in skin; stinging and cracking; elevated blood sugar; cataracts and glaucoma (prolonged use near eyes); numbness of fingers.

Guidelines for Use

USE EXACTLY AS PRESCRIBED.

Apply sparingly as a thin film. Rub in lightly.

Wash or soak the affected area before application as this may increase drug penetration.

Avoid contact with the eyes.

Avoid prolonged use, especially near the eyes, on the face, on genital and rectal areas, and in skin folds.

Do not use tight-fitting diapers or plastic pants on children being treated in the diaper area.

Do not wrap the treated area with bandages or tight-fitting clothing unless specifically directed by your physician. Skin infections may worsen.

It may be necessary to stop the corticosteroid and treat the infection.

Skin wasting may occur in 3 to 4 weeks.

Do not mix these products with other products. Allergic reactions may occur.

If the condition being treated gets worse or irritation, burning, redness, swelling or stinging persists, do not reapply the medicine. Contact your healthcare provider.

Alcohol-containing preparations may cause drying, burning or irritation of open lesions.

Triamterene

(try-AM-tur-een)

Dyrenium

A potassium-sparing diuretic or water pill. It is generally used to treat fluid accumulation and swelling, high blood pressure and to prevent or treat low potassium levels.

Precautions

DO NOT USE if you are allergic to this medicine or its relatives, or are breastfeeding.

BEFORE USING THIS DRUG, tell your healthcare provider if you are pregnant; or if you are taking, will be taking or stop taking any prescription or nonprescription medicine; or if you have any other medical conditions.

Side Effects

Every medicine can cause side effects, but many people have no, or minor, side effects. Tell your healthcare provider if any of the following occurs: stomach or intestinal pain; nausea; vomiting; diarrhea; constipation; gas; heartburn; loss of appetite; weakness, fatigue; drowsiness; confusion; tingling or numbness of hands or feet; depression; headache; dizziness or lightheadedness when arising from a seated or lying position; sleeplessness; nervousness; irregular pulse; chest pain; shortness of breath; cough; nasal congestion; rash; itching; yellowing of the skin or eyes; hair loss; muscle weakness or cramping; ringing in the ears; visual disturbances; changes in sex drive; dry mouth; sensitivity to sunlight; unusual bruising or bleeding.

Guidelines for Use

USE EXACTLY AS PRESCRIBED.

If a single dose is prescribed, generally take it in the morning.

May cause stomach upset. Take with food.

Use caution while driving or performing other tasks requiring mental alertness.

Avoid large quantities of potassium-rich food or salt substitutes.

Patients being treated for high blood pressure often feel tired for a few weeks. It takes time for the body to adjust to lowered blood pressure. Continue taking your medication and check with your healthcare provider regarding any new symptoms to assure that they are a normal consequence of changes in blood pressure.

Triazolam

(try-AZE-oh-lam)

Halcion

A benzodiazepine medicine that is a sleeping pill to treat insomnia for a short period of time (1 to 2 weeks). Long-term use generally is not recommended.

Precautions

DO NOT USE if you are allergic to this medicine or its relatives; or if you are pregnant.

BEFORE USING THIS MEDICINE, tell your healthcare provider if you are breastfeeding; or if you are taking, will be taking or stop taking any prescription or nonprescription medicine; or if you have any other medical conditions.

Side Effects

Every medicine can cause side effects, but many people have no, or minor, side effects. Tell your healthcare provider if any of the following occurs: vision changes; irregular heartbeat; headache; chest pain; yellowing of skin or eyes; rash; unusual bleeding or bruising; vomiting; heartburn; diarrhea; constipation; appetite loss; nervousness; irritability; memory loss; sleeplessness; ringing in the ears; sore throat; joint pain.

Short-term memory loss may occur.

Guidelines for Use

USE EXACTLY AS PRESCRIBED.

Do not exceed prescribed dosage. Take with a full glass of water.

Use caution while driving or performing other tasks requiring mental alertness, coordination and dexterity.

May cause morning drowsiness, unusual tiredness in the morning or daytime sleepiness after using these medications for sleep. The elderly are particularly sensitive to these effects.

Avoid alcohol and medications that cause drowsiness (eg, pain relievers, sedatives, antihistamines).

Nighttime sleep may be disturbed for 1 or 2 nights following stopping of the medication.

May be habit-forming.

Do not discontinue medication abruptly, especially if you have a history of seizures, regardless of other antiseizure medications you may be taking.

Long-term use may result in dependence.

Withdrawal symptoms may occur when the medication is stopped.

Trifluoperazine Hydrochloride

(try-flew-oh-PURR-uh-zeen HIGH-droe-KLOR-ide)

Stelazine, Stelazine Concentrate

A neuroleptic or major tranquilizer generally used to improve concentration and self-control in patients with psychotic behavior.

Precautions

DO NOT USE if you are allergic to this medicine or its relatives. Laboratory tests may be needed including eye exams, blood counts and kidney and liver tests.

BEFORE USING THIS MEDICINE, tell your healthcare provider if you are pregnant or breastfeeding; or if you are taking, will be taking or stop taking any prescription or nonprescription medicine; if you have any other medical conditions; or if you are allergic to tartrazine.

Side Effects

Every medicine can cause side effects, but many people have no, or minor, side effects. Tell your healthcare provider if any of the following occurs: tremors; drooling; shuffling gait; restlessness; muscle spasms; aching or numbness; sore throat; fever; unusual bleeding or bruising; skin rash; weakness; impaired vision; dark-colored urine; pale stools; yellowed skin or eyes.

Guidelines for Use

USE EXACTLY AS PRESCRIBED.

Take routinely as directed; it controls illness symptoms and is not habit-forming. Improvement may not be seen for several weeks.

May be diluted in distilled or acidified tap water or suitable juices.

If a dose is missed, take it as soon as possible. If several hours have passed or if it is nearing time for the next dose, do not double the dose to "catch up," unless advised by your healthcare provider. If more than one dose is missed, contact your healthcare provider.

May cause drowsiness. Use caution while driving or performing other tasks requiring mental alertness.

Avoid alcohol and medicines that cause drowsiness (eg, sleeping pills, antihistamines).

May cause sunlight sensitivity. Avoid long exposure to the sun. Use sunscreens and protective clothing until tolerance is known.

May discolor the urine pink or reddish brown. This is not harmful.

If dizziness or fainting occurs, avoid sudden changes in posture and use caution when climbing stairs.

Trihexyphenidyl Hydrochloride

(try-hex-ee-FEN-in-dill HIGH-droe-KLOR-ide)

Artane, Artane Sequels, Trihexy-2, Trihexy-5

A medicine used to reduce the symptoms of parkinsonism and to control medicine-induced parkinsonism-like disorders. This medicine does not cure the cause of these symptoms.

Precautions

DO NOT USE if you are breastfeeding or are allergic to this medicine or its relatives. Use caution in elderly patients.

BEFORE USING THIS MEDICINE, tell your healthcare provider if you are pregnant; or if you are taking, will be taking or stop taking any prescription or nonprescription medicines; or have any other medical conditions.

Side Effects

Every medicine can cause side effects, but many people have no, or minor, side effects. Tell your healthcare provider if any of the following occurs: nausea; vomiting; stomach pain; constipation; disorientation; confusion; memory loss; hallucinations; dizziness; weakness; agitation; nervousness; paranoia; delusions; delirium; excessive elation; excitement; depression; rapid heart rate; pounding in the chest; lightheadedness and dizziness upon rising quickly from a lying or sitting position; rash; flushing; decreased sweating; hives; visual disturbances; glaucoma; difficult/painful urination; muscle weakness; cramping; dry mouth; fever; numbness of fingers; difficulty achieving or maintaining an erection; swollen glands.

Guidelines for Use

USE EXACTLY AS PRESCRIBED.

Stomach upset may occur. Take with food.

May cause drowsiness, dizziness, or blurred vision. Use caution when driving or performing other tasks requiring alertness.

Avoid alcohol and medicines that cause drowsiness (eg, antihistamines, tranquilizers).

If dry mouth occurs, try sucking on hard candy, drinking fluids, and maintaining good dental hygiene.

Difficult urination and constipation can occur. Use stool softeners if necessary. Notify your healthcare provider if either difficult urination or constipation persists.

This medicine can reduce the ability to sweat and increase the possibility of heatstroke. Avoid excess sun or exercise, which may cause excessive sweating and overheating.

Sustained Release: Do not crush or chew.

Trimethobenzamide Hydrochloride

(try-meth-oh-BEN-zuh-mide HIGH-droe-KLOR-ide)

Arrestin, T-Gen, Tebamide, Ticon, Tigan, Tiject-20, Trimazide

A medicine used to control nausea and vomiting.

Precautions

DO NOT USE if you are allergic to this medicine.

BEFORE USING THIS MEDICINE, tell your healthcare provider if you are pregnant or breastfeeding; or if you are taking, will be taking or stop taking any prescription or nonprescription medicine; or if you have any other medical conditions.

Use this medicine in children only with specific instruction from your healthcare provider.

Side Effects

Every medicine can cause side effects, but many people have no, or minor, side effects. Tell your healthcare provider if any of the following occurs: appetite loss; nausea; vomiting; diarrhea; constipation; stomach upset; drowsiness; restlessness; sleeplessness; excitation (especially in children); headache; confusion; pounding in the chest; difficult urination; rash; yellowing of skin and eyes; blurred or double vision; dry eyes (contact lens wearers); visual and hearing hallucinations; ringing in the ears; dry mouth, nose and throat; muscle cramps; convulsions; depression; dizziness; muscle spasms.

Guidelines for Use

USE EXACTLY AS PRESCRIBED.

May cause drowsiness or blurred vision. Use caution while driving or performing other tasks requiring alertness, coordination and dexterity.

Avoid alcohol and other depressants (eg, sleeping pills, tranquilizers, antianxiety agents, narcotic pain relievers).

Capsules may be ineffective if expelled after vomiting has begun. Consider asking your healthcare provider for suppositories under such circumstances.

If used for motion sickness, the first dose should be taken 30 minutes before exposure to motion.

May cause dry mouth.

Suppository: If you do not know the correct way to insert the suppository, ask your healthcare provider.

Trimethoprim/Sulfamethoxazole Injection

Bactrim IV, Septra IV

A combination sulfa antibiotic medicine used to treat certain infections.

Precautions

DO NOT USE if you are allergic to any sulfonamide-related medicines (oral antidiabetic medicine or thiazide diuretics), trimethoprim or sulfites; are breastfeeding; or are a pregnant woman at term.

BEFORE USING THIS MEDICINE, tell your healthcare provider if you are pregnant; or if you are taking, will be taking or stop taking any prescription or nonprescription medicine; or if you have any other medical conditions.

Side Effects

Every medicine can cause side effects, but many people have no, or minor, side effects. Tell your healthcare provider if any of the following occurs: nausea; vomiting; appetite loss; sore throat; fever; chills; pale skin; yellowing of skin or eyes; rash; hives; wheezing; shortness of breath; dizziness; unusual bleeding or bruising.

Patient Information

Drink plenty of fluids during use.

Avoid products that may acidify the urine in large doses (eg, vitamin C, ammonium chloride).

Trimethoprim/Sulfamethoxazole Oral

(try-METH-oh-prim/suhl-fuh-meth-OX-uh-zole)

Bactrim DS, Cotrim D.S., Septra DS, Sulfamethoxazole/Trimethoprim DS, Sulfaprim DS, Sulfoxaprim DS

A combination sulfa antibiotic medicine used to treat certain infections.

Precautions

DO NOT USE if you are allergic to any sulfonamide-related medicines (oral antidiabetic medicines or thiazide diuretics) or trimethoprim; are breastfeeding; or are a pregnant woman at term.

BEFORE USING THIS MEDICINE, tell your healthcare provider if you are pregnant; or if you are taking, will be taking or stop taking any prescription or nonprescription medicine; if you have any other medical conditions; or if you are allergic to sulfites.

Side Effects

Every medicine can cause side effects, but many people have no, or minor, side effects. Tell your healthcare provider if any of the following occurs: nausea; vomiting; appetite loss; sore throat; fever; chills; pale skin; yellowing of skin or eyes; rash; hives; wheezing; shortness of breath; dizziness; unusual bleeding or bruising; sensitivity to sunlight or UV light; cough; joint or muscle pain.

Guidelines for Use

USE EXACTLY AS PRESCRIBED.

Take on an empty stomach. If upset stomach occurs, take with food.

Take with a full glass of fluid. Drink plenty of fluids during use.

If a dose is missed, take as soon as possible. If several hours have passed or if it is nearing time for the next dose, do not double the dose to "catch up," unless advised by your healthcare provider. If more than one dose is missed, contact your healthcare provider.

Complete the full course of therapy for best results and to decrease the risk of the infection returning.

Avoid products that may acidify the urine in large doses (eg, vitamin C, ammonium chloride).

Notify your healthcare provider immediatly if rash, sore throat or shortness of breath occurs.

May cause sensitivity to sunlight. Avoid prolonged exposure to the sun. Use sunscreen and wear protective clothing until tolerance is determined.

Suspension: Shake well before using.

Store at room temperature in a tight, light-resistant container.

Trimetrexate Glucuronate

(TRY-meh-TREK-sate glue-CURE-uh-nate)

Neutrexin

Used in combination with leucovorin to treat moderate-to-severe *Pneumocystis carinii pneumonia* (PCP). It may occasionally be prescribed for other reasons.

Precautions

DO NOT USE if you are allergic to this medicine, leucovorin or methotrexate.

BEFORE USING THIS MEDICINE, tell your healthcare provider if you are pregnant or breastfeeding; or if you are taking, will be taking or stop taking any prescription or nonprescription medicine; or if you have any other medical conditions.

Side Effects

Every medicine can cause side effects, but many people have no, or minor, side effects. Tell your healthcare provider if any of the following occurs: fever; rash; itching; nausea; vomiting; confusion; fatigue; weakness; pain at the injection site.

Patient Information

These drugs may lower your body's ability to fight infection. Notify your healthcare provider of any signs of infection including fever, sore throat, rashes or chills.

Lab tests may be required to monitor therapy. Be sure to keep appointments.

Triprolidine Hydrochloride

(try-PRO-lih-deen HIGH-droe-KLOR-ide)

Actidil, Myidyl

A medicine used for relief of allergy symptoms and symptoms associated with hives (mild and uncomplicated), some insect bites and stings and skin rash with mild to moderate itching.

Precautions

DO NOT USE if you are allergic to this medicine or its relatives, are breastfeeding or are taking monoamine oxidase inhibitors (MAOIs) (eg, *Nardil, Parnate*).

BEFORE USING THIS MEDICINE, tell your healthcare provider if you are pregnant; or if you are taking, will be taking or stop taking any prescription or nonprescription medicine; or if you have any other medical conditions.

Side Effects

Every medicine can cause side effects, but many people have no, or minor, side effects. Tell your healthcare provider if any of the following occurs: drowsiness; dizziness; dry mouth; stomach upset; constipation; blurred vision; difficult urination; confusion; fainting; irregular heartbeat.

Guidelines for Use

USE EXACTLY AS PRESCRIBED.

Take with food.

Avoid alcohol and drowsiness-causing medicines.

Use caution while driving or performing tasks requiring mental alertness.

Use when sneezing and runny nose exist but nasal congestion is slight. When more severe nasal congestion occurs with sneezing and runny nose, an oral or topical decongestant also may be used.

Do not take for several days before allergy skin testing.

Uracil Mustard

(YOU-ruh-sill mustard)

This medicine is used to treat certain leukemias, early polycythemia vera and mycosis fungoides. It may occasionally be prescribed for other reasons.

Precautions

DO NOT USE if you are allergic to this medicine or its relatives.

BEFORE USING THIS MEDICINE, tell your healthcare provider if you are pregnant or breastfeeding; or if you are taking, will be taking or stop taking any prescription or nonprescription medicine; or if you have any other medical conditions.

Side Effects

Every medicine can cause side effects, but many people have no, or minor, side effects. Tell your healthcare provider if any of the following occurs: nausea; vomiting; diarrhea; loss of appetite; stomach pain; unusual tiredness; mouth sores; sore throat; rash; yellow skin or eyes; nervousness; chills; cough; fever; seizures; abnormal menstrual periods; hair loss.

Guidelines for Use

USE EXACTLY AS PRESCRIBED.

Contraceptive measures (birth control) are recommended during treatment for both males and females.

Blood and urine tests will be required. Be sure to keep appointments.

This medicine may lower your body's ability to fight infection. Notify your healthcare provider of any signs of infection including fever, sore throat, rashes or chills.

May cause sensitivity to sunlight. Avoid prolonged exposure to the sun. Use sunscreens and wear protective clothing until tolerance is determined.

Avoid use of razors. Use soft toothbrushes.

Notify your healthcare provider if you experience tiredness or unexplained loss of weight.

Do not crush, chew or open capsules.

Even though this medication might cause nausea and vomiting, it is important that you continue to take it.

May cause nausea, vomiting or diarrhea; notify your healthcare provider if these effects persist.

Store at room temperature (below 86 degrees F). Protect from moisture.

Valacyclovir Hydrochloride

(val-lay-SIGH-kloe-vihr HIGH-droe-KLOR-ide)

Valtrex

An antiviral medicine to treat herpes zoster (shingles) in adults with healthy immune systems.

Precautions

DO NOT USE if you are allergic to this medicine or to acyclovir (Zovirax).

BEFORE USING THIS MEDICINE, tell your healthcare provider if you are pregnant or breastfeeding; if you are taking, will be taking or stop taking any prescription or nonprescription medicine; or if you have any other medical conditions.

Side Effects

Every medicine can cause side effects, but many people have no, or minor, side effects. Tell your healthcare provider if any of the following occurs: nausea; headache; vomiting; diarrhea; constipation; weakness; dizziness; stomach pain; appetite loss.

Guidelines for Use

USE EXACTLY AS PRESCRIBED.

It is important to start treatment as soon as possible after the first sign of shingles. This medicine is most effective when started within 48 hours of the onset of the rash. It may not work after 72 hours of onset.

This medicine may be taken without regard to meals.

The usual dose of this medicine is 1 g (2 capsules) 3 times daily for 7 days. Elderly patients may take a smaller dose.

Continue taking until all of the prescribed medicine has been used, even if the rash or other symptoms have disappeared. Failure to take all of the medicine may prevent complete elimination of the virus.

If a dose is missed, take it as soon as possible. If several hours have passed or if it is nearing time for the next dose, do not double the dose to "catch up," unless advised by your healthcare provider. If more than one dose is missed, contact your healthcare provider.

This medicine is not recommended for use if you are infected by the HIV virus or have had a bone marrow transplant or kidney transplant.

Store at room temperature.

Valproic Acid

(VAL-pro-ik acid)

Depakene, Depakote

A medicine that is used to treat epilepsy and seizures.

Precautions

DO NOT USE if you are allergic to this medicine or have liver disease.

BEFORE USING THIS MEDICINE, tell your healthcare provider if you are pregnant or breastfeeding; or if you are taking, will be taking or stop taking any prescription or nonprescription medicine; or if you have any other medical conditions.

Side Effects

Every medicine can cause side effects, but many people have no, or minor, side effects. Tell your healthcare provider if any of the following occurs: changes in appetite; nausea; vomiting; stomach cramps; indigestion; diarrhea; constipation; weakness; tiredness; clumsiness; drowsiness; behavior changes; depression; headache; yellowing of skin or eyes; unusual bleeding or bruising; rash; swelling of the face, hands and feet; double vision; unusual eye movements; weight gain or loss; changes in menstrual periods; hair loss.

Mania: nausea; drowsiness; dizziness; vomiting; accidental injury; weakness; abdominal pain; indigestion; rash.

Guidelines for Use

USE EXACTLY AS PRESCRIBED.

May cause stomach upset.

Take with food. Swallow whole; do not chew or crush. Chewing or crushing may cause irritation in the mouth or throat.

Do not take any medicine, especially those containing aspirin, without asking your healthcare provider.

May cause drowsiness or sleepiness. Use caution when driving or performing other tasks requiring mental alertness. Taking medicine at bedtime may help decrease drowsiness.

Do not stop taking this medicine without checking with your healthcare provider. If you stop taking it suddenly, your seizures may suddenly begin again.

See your healthcare provider regularly. The healthcare provider may want to adjust the dose for best results and to minimize side effects.

Laboratory tests may be required during treatment.

Diabetes — This medicine may interfere with urine tests for ketones and may give inaccurate test results.

Using this medicine with alcohol or other central nervous system depressants (eg, pain relievers, sedatives) may increase drowsiness.

Carry Medic-Alert identification indicating you are taking this medicine.

Vancomycin Injectable

(van-koe-MY-sin)

Lyphocin, Vancocin, Vancoled

This medicine is used to treat serious or severe infections. It may occasionally be prescribed for other reasons.

Precautions

DO NOT USE if you are allergic to this medicine or to benzyl alcohol.

BEFORE USING THIS MEDICINE, tell your healthcare provider if you are pregnant or breastfeeding; or if you are taking, will be taking or stop taking any prescription or nonprescription medicine; or if you have any other medical conditions.

Side Effects

Every medicine can cause side effects, but many people have no, or minor, side effects. Tell your healthcare provider if any of the following occurs: wheezing; difficulty breathing; rash; hives; irritation at the injection site; dizziness; itching; flushing; change in hearing; fever; nausea; chills; difficulty urinating; diarrhea; feeling of a whirling motion.

Guidelines for Use

USE EXACTLY AS PRESCRIBED.

Follow the administration and monitoring procedures taught to you by your healthcare provider.

If a dose is missed, inject it as soon as possible. If several hours have passed or if it is nearing time for the next dose, do not double the dose to "catch up," unless advised by your healthcare provider. If more than one dose is missed, contact your healthcare provider.

Continue use until all of the prescribed medicine has been used. Failure to use all of the medicine may prevent complete elimination of bacteria, allowing the infection to return.

If hearing problems, urination problems or symptoms of an allergic reaction (eg, difficulty breathing, facial swelling, rash, hives, itching) develop, stop using the drug immediately and contact your healthcare provider immediately.

Lab tests will be required to monitor therapy. Be sure to keep appointments.

Store IV bags ("piggybacks") in the refrigerator according to package instructions.

Vancomycin Oral

(van-koe-MY-sin)

Vancocin

Used to treat staphylococcal enterocolitis and antibiotic-associated pseudomembranous colitis.

Precautions

DO NOT USE if you are allergic to this medicine or to benzyl alcohol.

BEFORE USING THIS MEDICINE, tell your healthcare provider if you are pregnant or breastfeeding; or if you are taking, will be taking or stop taking any prescription or nonprescription medicine; or if you have any other medical conditions.

Side Effects

Every medicine can cause side effects, but many people have no, or minor, side effects. Tell your healthcare provider if any of the following occurs: hearing loss; feeling of a whirling motion; dizziness; fever; nausea; chills; rash.

Guidelines for Use

USE EXACTLY AS PRESCRIBED.

Complete full course of therapy. Do not discontinue this medicine without talking to your healthcare provider.

Vasopressin (8–Arginine-Vasopressin)

(VAY-so-PRESS-in)

Pitressin Synthetic

This medicine is used for the treatment of neurogenic diabetes insipidus; for the prevention and treatment of postoperative abdominal distention and in abdominal roentgenography to dispel interfering gas shadows.

Side Effects

Every medicine can cause side effects, but many people have no, or minor, side effects. Tell your healthcare provider if any of the following occurs: tremor; sweating; feeling of a whirling motion; pounding in the head; abdominal cramps; gas; nausea; vomiting; hives.

Guidelines for Use

USE EXACTLY AS PRESCRIBED.

Side effects such as skin blanching, abdominal cramps and nausea may be reduced by taking 1 or 2 glasses of water with the dose. These side effects usually are not serious and will probably disappear within a few minutes.

Venlafaxine

(VEN-luh-fax-EEN)

Effexor

A medicine used for the treatment of mental depression.

Precautions

DO NOT USE if you are allergic to this medicine, or if you are taking a monoamine oxidase inhibitor (MAOIs, eg, *Parnate*).

BEFORE USING THIS MEDICINE, tell your healthcare provider if you are pregnant or breastfeeding; or if you are taking, will be taking or stop taking any prescription or nonprescription medicine; or if you have any other medical conditions.

Side Effects

Every medicine can cause side effects, but many people have no, or minor, side effects. Tell your healthcare provider if any of the following occurs: general body discomfort; accidental injury; neck pain; migraine; difficulty swallowing; belching; bruising; weight gain; tightness in the jaw and mouth; mood swings; bronchitis; difficulty breathing; abnormal vision; ear pain; sexual problems; painful or difficult urination; blood in the urine; abnormal uterine bleeding; vaginal inflammation; sleepiness; anxiety; nervousness; sleeplessness; weakness; nausea; constipation; sweating; dry mouth; tremor; dizziness.

Guidelines for Use

USE EXACTLY AS PRESCRIBED.

Take with food.

Do not stop taking abruptly.

Avoid alcohol while taking this medicine.

If a dose is missed, take it as soon as possible. If several hours have passed or if it is nearing time for the next dose, do not double the dose to "catch up," unless advised by your healthcare provider. If more than one dose is missed, contact your healthcare provider.

This medicine may impair judgment, thinking or motor skills. Use caution when driving or performing other tasks requiring mental alertness or coordination.

Notify your healthcare provider if you develop a rash or hives.

Regular blood pressure monitoring may be needed.

Verapamil Hydrochloride Injectable

(veh-RAP-uh-mill HIGH-droe-KLOR-ide)

Isoptin

A calcium channel blocker that is used to treat supraventricular tachyarrhythmias. It also is used for temporary control of rapid ventricular rate.

Precautions

DO NOT USE if you are allergic to this medicine.

BEFORE USING THIS MEDICINE, tell your healthcare provider if you are pregnant or breastfeeding; or if you are taking, will be taking or stop taking any prescription or nonprescription medicine; or if you have any other medical conditions.

Side Effects

Every medicine can cause side effects, but many people have no, or minor, side effects. Tell your healthcare provider if any of the following occurs: irregular heartbeat; increased frequency/severity of angina; shortness of breath; swelling of hands and feet; dizziness; constipation; nausea; low blood pressure; symptoms of medicine allergy (eg, itching, rash, hives, difficult breathing); unusual bleeding or bruising; gum enlargement; irritation at the injection site.

Guidelines for Use

USE EXACTLY AS PRESCRIBED.

Verapamil Hydrochloride Oral

(veh-RAP-uh-mill HIGH-droe-KLOR-ide)

Calan, Isoptin

A calcium channel blocker medicine that is used to treat various types of angina, certain arrhythmias (irregular heartbeats) and high blood pressure. It may occasionally be prescribed for other reasons.

Precautions

DO NOT USE if you are allergic to this medicine.

BEFORE USING THIS MEDICINE, tell your healthcare provider if you are pregnant or breastfeeding; or if you are taking, will be taking or stop taking any prescription or nonprescription medicines; or if you have any other medical conditions.

Side Effects

Every medicine can cause side effects, but many people have no, or minor, side effects. Tell your healthcare provider if any of the following occurs: irregular heartbeat; increased frequency/severity of angina; shortness of breath; swelling of hands and feet; dizziness; constipation; nausea; low blood pressure; symptoms of a medicine allergy (eg, itching, rash, hives, difficult breathing); unusual bleeding or bruising; gum enlargement.

Guidelines for Use

USE EXACTLY AS PRESCRIBED.

If a dose is missed, take it as soon as possible. If several hours have passed or if it is nearing time for the next dose, do not double the dose to "catch up," unless advised by your healthcare provider. If more than one dose is missed, contact your healthcare provider.

Do not suddenly stop taking this medicine as this may cause serious chest pains. This can be minimized if the medicine is tapered slowly by your healthcare provider.

It is important to brush and floss your teeth and see your dentist regularly.

Verapamil Hydrochloride Oral Sustained-Release

(veh-RAP-uh-mill HIGH-droe-KLOR-ide)

Calan SR, Isoptin SR, Verelan

A calcium channel blocker medicine that is used to treat high blood pressure. It may occasionally be prescribed for other reasons.

Precautions

DO NOT USE if you are allergic to this medicine.

BEFORE USING THIS MEDICINE, tell your healthcare provider if you are pregnant or breastfeeding; or if you are taking, will be taking or stop taking any prescription or nonprescription medicines; or if you have any other medical conditions.

Side Effects

Every medicine can cause side effects, but many people have no, or minor, side effects. Tell your healthcare provider if any of the following occurs: irregular heartbeat; increased frequency/severity of angina; shortness of breath; swelling of hands and feet; dizziness; constipation; nausea; low blood pressure; symptoms of a medicine allergy (eg, itching, rash, hives, difficulty breathing); unusual bleeding or bruising; gum enlargement.

Guidelines for Use

USE EXACTLY AS PRESCRIBED.

Do not crush or chew this medicine.

If a dose is missed, take it as soon as possible. If several hours have passed or if it is nearing time for the next dose, do not double the dose to "catch up," unless advised by your healthcare provider. If more than one dose is missed, contact your healthcare provider.

Do not suddenly stop taking this medicine as this may cause serious chest pains. This can be minimized if the medicine is tapered slowly by your healthcare provider.

It is important to brush and floss your teeth and see your dentist regularly.

Vinblastine Sulfate (VLB)

(vin-BLAST-een SULL-fate)

Velban, Velsar

This medicine is used to treat certain types of cancers.

Side Effects

Every medicine can cause side effects, but many people have no, or minor, side effects. Tell your healthcare provider if any of the following occurs: nausea; vomiting; diarrhea; constipation; loss of appetite; abdominal pain; rectal bleeding; numbness in hands and feet; abnormal skin sensations; mental depression; headache; convulsions; overall body discomfort; weakness; dizziness; pain in tumor site; bone and jaw pain.

Guidelines for Use

USE EXACTLY AS PRESCRIBED.

Immediately report sore throat, fever, chill or sore mouth to your healthcare provider.

The following may occur: hair loss; jaw pain; pain in the organs containing the tumor; nausea and vomiting.

Scalp hair will regrow to its pretreatment condition.

Avoid constipation. Talk with your healthcare provider if you have problems with constipation.

Vincristine Sulfate (VCR; LCR)

(vin-KRISS-teen SULL-fate)

Oncovin, Vincasar PFS

This medicine is used to treat acute leukemia and in combination with other therapies to treat Hodgkin's disease, non-Hodgkin's malignant lymphomas, rhabdomyosarcoma, neuroblastoma and Wilms' tumor. It may occasionally be prescribed for other reasons.

Side Effects

Every medicine can cause side effects, but many people have no, or minor, side effects. Tell your healthcare provider if any of the following occurs: vision problems; acute shortness of breath; weight loss; fever; hair loss; rash; headache; urinary problems.

Warfarin

(WORE-fuh-rin)

Coumadin, Panwarfin, Sofarin

A medicine used to prevent unwanted blood clots in veins. It may occasionally be prescribed for other reasons.

Precautions

DO NOT USE if you are allergic to this medicine, pregnant, breastfeeding or planning to undergo surgery (including dental).

BEFORE USING THIS MEDICINE, tell your healthcare provider if you are menstruating; if you have recently given birth or had surgery; or if you are taking, will be taking or stop taking any prescription or nonprescription medicine; or if you have any other medical conditions.

Side Effects

Every medicine can cause side effects, but many people have no, or minor, side effects. Tell your healthcare provider if any of the following occurs: stomach upset; red-orange discoloration of urine; red or tar-black stools or diarrhea; skin rash; yellowing of skin or eyes; unusual bleeding or bruising.

Guidelines for Use

USE EXACTLY AS PRESCRIBED.

It is important to follow the prescribed schedule.

Dosage is highly individual and may have to be adjusted several times based on lab test results.

DO NOT take or discontinue any other medicine, except on advice of your healthcare provider.

Avoid alcohol, aspirin and drastic changes in dietary habits.

Zalcitabine (Dideoxycytidine; ddC)

(zal-SITE-uh-BEAN)

Hivid

An antiviral medicine used to treat HIV infection.

Precautions

DO NOT USE if you are allergic to this medicine.

BEFORE USING THIS MEDICINE, tell your healthcare provider if you are pregnant or breastfeeding; if you are taking, will be taking or stop taking any prescription or nonprescription medicines; or have any other medical conditions.

Side Effects

Every medicine can cause side effects, but many people have no, or minor, side effects. Tell your healthcare provider if any of the following occurs: peripheral neuropathy (numbness and burning feeling of arms or legs), which can progress to be very painful; severe abdominal pain; mouth ulcers; loss of appetite; vomiting; diarrhea; constipation; rash; itching; headache; dizziness; confusion; muscle ache; fatigue; sore throat; weight loss; difficult breathing.

Guidelines for Use

USE EXACTLY AS PRESCRIBED.

If a dose is missed, take it as soon as possible. If several hours have passed or if it is nearing time for the next dose, do not double the dose to "catch up," unless advised by your healthcare provider. If more than one dose is missed, contact your healthcare provider.

Peripheral neuropathy (numbness and burning feeling of the arms and legs) is the major toxicity of this medicine. If these symptoms develop, report them immediately to your healthcare provider.

Women of childbearing age should use effective birth control methods.

It is very important to keep regular appointments with your healthcare provider to watch your therapy and to do necessary laboratory tests.

Zidovudine

(zid-OH-vue-deen)

Retrovir

This medicine is used by HIV-positive persons to possibly delay the onset of AIDS and ARC (AIDS Related Complex). It may help prevent transmission of the HIV virus from pregnant mother to fetus.

Precautions

DO NOT USE if you are allergic to this medicine. HIV-infected women should not breastfeed. This medicine may cause liver damage, severe anemia, metabolic or muscular problems, especially in patients with advanced HIV disease. Prolonged use of this medicine may prompt symptoms similar to those produced by HIV.

BEFORE USING THIS MEDICINE, tell your healthcare provider if you are pregnant or breastfeeding; or if you are taking, will be taking or stop taking any prescription or nonprescription medicine; or if you have any other medical conditions.

Side Effects

Every medicine can cause side effects, but many people have no, or minor, side effects. Tell your healthcare provider if any of the following occurs: appetite loss; nausea; vomiting; diarrhea; indigestion; stomach pain; constipation; weakness; abnormal skin sensations; headache; confusion; mood swings; sleeplessness; dizziness; drowsiness; nervousness; anemia and other blood disorders; fever; sore throat; muscle, back or chest pain; sweating; feeling of numbness or tingling; difficulty breathing; rash; taste changes; general body discomfort; painful urination; blood in urine; slow reflexes; yellowing of skin or eyes; body odor; chills; lip swelling.

Guidelines for Use

USE EXACTLY AS PRESCRIBED.

Follow preparation and administration instructions exactly.

If a dose is missed, take it as soon as possible. If several hours have passed or if it is nearing time for the next dose, do not double the dose to "catch up," unless advised by your healthcare provider. If more than one dose is missed, contact your healthcare provider.

This medicine is not a cure for HIV infections and patients may continue to acquire illnesses associated with AIDS or ARC.

Tell your healthcare provider if changes in your health occur, especially infections. Symptoms such as fever, sore throat, shortness of breath, unusual weakness and dizziness should be reported to your healthcare provider immediately.

Contact your healthcare provider if you notice a rash, yellowing of the skin, abnormally dark urine or abdominal pain/swelling. Do not share this medicine with anyone else.

This medicine has NOT been shown to reduce the risk of transmitting HIV to others through sexual contact or blood contamination.

Lab tests will be necessary; be sure to keep appointments.

Zinc Sulfate Injection

(zink SULL-fate)

Zinca-Pak

A medicine used to treat zinc deficiency.

Precautions

DO NOT USE if you are allergic to this medicine.

BEFORE USING THIS MEDICINE, tell your healthcare provider if you are taking, will be taking or stop taking any prescription or nonprescription medicine; or if you have any other medical conditions.

Every medicine can cause side effects, but many people have no, or minor, side effects. Tell your healthcare provider if irritation at the injection site occurs.

Zinc Sulfate Ophthalmic Solution

(zink SULL-fate)

Eye-Sed

A medicine used for temporary relief of minor eye irritation.

Guidelines for Use

USE EXACTLY AS PRESCRIBED.

For use in eyes only.

Instill 1 to 2 drops into eye(s) up to 4 times daily.

Do not use if solution discolors or becomes cloudy.

If irritation persists or increases, or if eye pain or a change in vision occurs, discontinue use and consult your healthcare provider.

Zinc Sulfate Oral

(zink SULL-fate)

Orazinc, Verazinc

A medicine used to treat or prevent zinc deficiency. It may occasionally be prescribed for other reasons.

Precautions

DO NOT USE if you are pregnant or breastfeeding. Consult your healthcare provider before taking.

BEFORE USING THIS MEDICINE, tell your healthcare provider if you are taking, will be taking or stop taking any prescription or nonprescription medicine; or if you have any other medical conditions.

Side Effects

Every medicine can cause side effects, but many people have no, or minor, side effects. Tell your healthcare provider if any of the following occurs: nausea; vomiting; diarrhea; stomach pain; rash; restlessness.

Guidelines for Use

USE EXACTLY AS PRESCRIBED.

If stomach upset or nausea occurs, take with food.

Avoid foods high in calcium, phosphorus or phytate because they decrease absorption of zinc. Talk with your healthcare provider about which foods to avoid.

Do not exceed prescribed dose. Vomiting is likely to occur with doses over 2 g.

Recommended Dietary Allowances (RDA)—Males 15 mg, Females 12 mg.

Common sources of zinc—cooked dry beans, meat, eggs, liver, seafoods, whole grain products.

Use of Aerosol Metered Sprays

Precautions

BEFORE USING THIS MEDICINE, tell your healthcare provider if you are pregnant or breastfeeding; if you are taking, will be taking or stop taking any prescription or nonprescription medicine; or if you have any other medical conditions.

Side Effects

Every medicine can cause side effects, but many people have no, or minor, side effects. Tell your healthcare provider if any of the following occurs: mouth sores; sore throat; anxiety; cough; rash; dizziness; chest pain.

Guidelines for Use

USE EXACTLY AS PRESCRIBED.

Read all the patient information that comes with this medicine.

Not all inhalers can be used for asthma attacks. Be sure you know which one to use for an asthma attack.

Do not use more frequently than prescribed.

Store at room temperature (below 86° F). Protect from heat and cold. Avoid carrying your inhaler in a pocket close to your body.

Recommended Procedures for Administration:

Shake the inhaler before each use.

Take a drink of water to moisten your throat.

Place the inhaler mouthpiece two finger-widths away from your mouth.

Tilt head back slightly.

Breathe out as much air as possible.

While activating the inhaler, take a slow, deep breath for 3 to 5 seconds, hold your breath for about 10 seconds and breathe out slowly.

Allow at least 1 minute between puffs.

Rinse (do not swallow) your mouth with water or mouthwash after each use to help reduce dry mouth and hoarseness.

Clean the mouth piece as often as possible.

Use of Ophthalmic Products

Precautions

BEFORE USING THIS MEDICINE, tell your healthcare provider if you are pregnant or breastfeeding; if you are taking, will be taking or stop taking any prescription or nonprescription medicine; or if you have any other medical conditions.

Side Effects

Every medicine can cause side effects, but many people have no, or minor, side effects. Tell your healthcare provider if any of the following occurs: vision changes; burning, itching or other irritation not present before.

Guidelines for Use

USE EXACTLY AS PRESCRIBED.

For suspensions, shake well before each use.

For ointments, holding the tube in the hand for a few minutes will warm the ointment and make the flow easier. Also, temporary blurring of vision may occur. Avoid activities requiring clear vision until blurring clears.

Do not touch the dropper tip to any surface, including your eye, since this may contaminate the contents or damage/infect the eye.

Do not rub the eye. Minimize blinking.

Do not rinse the dropper.

Do not use eye drops that have changed color.

Recommended Procedures for Administration:

Wash hands thoroughly before use.

Tilt head backward or lie down and gaze upward. Gently grasp lower eyelid below eyelashes and pull the eyelid away from the eye to form a pouch. Place dropper directly over eye. Look upward just before applying a drop.

After instilling (releasing) the drop, look downward for several seconds. Release the lid slowly.

Close eyes gently for 1 to 2 minutes. For ointments, rotate the eye in all directions. Closing the eyes tightly after instillation may cause the drug to spill out of the eye.

Apply gentle pressure with fingers to the bridge of the nose (inside corner of eye). This prevents drainage of solution from the intended area.

Use of Oral Contraceptives

Quite often an unwanted pregnancy happens even when a woman is on the "pill." The main point of this is to help you take the medication properly, therefore preventing an unwanted pregnancy. It also has other valuable information about your medication.

Key Points:

- Take one tablet at the exact same time every day.
- If any tablets are missed take the tablet, and DO NOT forget to use additional birth control until you finish the pack.
- Tell your healthcare provider when certain side effects occur.

Pack Sizes:

The packs come with either 21 or 28 tablets. With the 21 tablets you will take 1 tablet at the same time each day for 21 days then not take any for 7 days. Quite often women will forget to start taking the medication again after the 7 "off" days. With the 28 tablets you take 1 tablet at the same time each day for 28 days then start a new pack, without skipping any days between. By missing the first tablet of the new pack, it is recommended you use additional birth control for the whole month. Because of this, the 28 tablet packs are prescribed. Ask your healthcare provider, about the 28 tablet packs, if you have problems remembering to start the new pack after the 7 off days.

Before Starting Your Birth Control:

Tell your healthcare provider if you have a family history of heart disease or cancer or high blood pressure; are over 35 years of age; have more than 10 years oral contraceptive use; if you smoke; if you are taking, will be taking or stop taking any prescription or nonprescription medicine; if you have any other medical conditions.

Starting Your Birth Control:

The most common way to start is to take the first tablet on the first Sunday after the menstrual period begins. If your menstrual period begins on Sunday, take the first tablet on that day. You can start taking the tablets on another day besides Sunday if it is more convenient. Talk to your healthcare provider if you prefer another day.

After starting the first pack, use additional birth control for at least the first week, but it is recommended that you use additional birth control for the whole first month. By doing this it decreases the chances of an unwanted pregnancy.

How to Take:

Take once a day at the same time each day. It is important that the tablet is taken at the same time each day, because any deviation can lead to spotting or an unwanted pregnancy. A good way to remember to take it would be to take a tablet before doing an activity that you do at the same time each day (eg, eating, bedtime, brushing teeth).

Missed Tablets:

Pregnancy or spotting is not likely to occur if one tablet is missed, but it can happen. The more tablets you miss in one month, the more likely you are to become pregnant.

Any time a tablet is missed, additional birth control should be used for at least 7 to 14 days, but it is recommended until you finish the pack, because pregnancy is still possible 14 days after 1 missed tablet.

If 1 tablet is missed, take it as soon as remembered or take 2 tablets the next day. If 2 tablets are missed, take 2 tablets as soon as remembered, with the next tablet at the usual time or take 2 tablets daily for the next 2 days, then resume regular schedule. DO NOT forget to use additional birth control until you finish the pack.

(cont.)▶

Side Effects:

Every medicine can cause side effects, but many people have no, or minor, side effects. Tell your healthcare provider if any of the following occurs: nausea; vomiting; headaches; breast tenderness; swelling in the lower legs; spotting; heavy or painful periods; vision changes; rash.

Caution:

Birth control can increase the risk of breast cancer. However, it can provide some protection against ovarian and endometrial cancer.

Use of Otic Products

Precautions

DO NOT USE if you have a perforated ear drum.

BEFORE USING THIS MEDICINE, tell your healthcare provider if you are pregnant or breastfeeding; if you are taking, will be taking or stop taking any prescription or nonprescription medicine; or if you have any other medical conditions.

Side Effects

Every medicine can cause side effects, but many people have no, or minor, side effects. Tell your healthcare provider if any of the following occurs: hearing changes; dizziness; burning, itching or other irritation not present before.

Guidelines for Use

USE EXACTLY AS PRESCRIBED.

For suspensions, shake well before each use.

Avoid touching the dropper to the ear.

If symptoms do not improve, contact your healthcare provider.

Hold the container in your hand for a few minutes to warm the container if it has been refrigerated.

Have another person instill the ear drops when possible.

Recommended Procedures for Administration:

Wash hands thoroughly before use.

Lie on your side or tilt the affected ear up prior to administering the drug. Administer the prescribed number of drops.

Keep the ear tilted for about 2 minutes. May insert a soft cotton plug, unless directed otherwise.

To assist the drops reaching the external ear canal, gently pull the earlobe up and back in adults and down and back in children.

Use of Rectal Products

Precautions

BEFORE USING THIS MEDICINE, tell your healthcare provider if you are pregnant or breastfeeding; if you are taking, will be taking or stop taking any prescription or nonprescription medicine; or if you have any other medical conditions.

Side Effects

Every medicine can cause side effects, but many people have no, or minor, side effects. Tell your healthcare provider if any of the following occurs: burning, itching or other irritation not present before.

Guidelines for Use

USE EXACTLY AS PRESCRIBED.

Read all the patient information that comes with this medicine.

Some products will need to be shaken well before each use.

Maintain normal bowel movements by proper diet, adequate fluid intake and regular exercise.

Washing or soaking the affected area before application is encouraged, as this may increase drug absorption.

Avoid excessive laxative use.

Notify your healthcare provider if symptoms do not improve in 7 days, or if bleeding, protrusion or seepage occurs.

Use caution when using tight-fitting diapers or plastic pants on children.

Avoid contact with eyes.

Recommended Procedures for Administration:

Wash hands thoroughly before each use.

Apply a thin layer. Rub in lightly.

Wash hands thoroughly after use.

This information is advisory only; it does not contain all information about this medicine. If you have any questions about your medicine, ask your healthcare provider.

Use of Rectal Suppositories

Precautions

BEFORE USING THIS MEDICINE, tell your healthcare provider if you are pregnant or breastfeeding; if you are taking, will be taking or stop taking any prescription or nonprescription medicine; or if you have any other medical conditions.

Side Effects

Every medicine can cause side effects, but many people have no, or minor, side effects. Tell your healthcare provider if any of the following occurs: rectal bleeding or other irritation not present before.

Guidelines for Use

USE EXACTLY AS PRESCRIBED.

Do not use adult size suppositories for children; be sure to use the correct dosage.

Do not use any gels or ointments for lubrication.

Store in refrigerator if directed.

Recommended Procedures for Administration:

Wash hands thoroughly before use.

Unwrap the suppository. If the suppository has been in the refrigerator you may let the suppository come to room temperature before inserting.

Lay on your side. Using your middle finger push the suppository into the rectum.

Wash hands thoroughly after use.

This information is advisory only; it does not contain all information about this medicine. If you have any questions about your medicine, ask your healthcare provider.

Use of Respiratory Nebulizers

Precautions

BEFORE USING THIS MEDICINE, tell your healthcare provider if you are pregnant or breastfeeding; if you are taking, will be taking or stop taking any prescription or nonprescription medicine; or if you have any other medical conditions.

Side Effects

Every medicine can cause side effects, but many people have no, or minor, side effects. Tell your healthcare provider if any of the following occurs: nervousness; headache; dizziness; weakness; nausea; vomiting; pounding heartbeat; flushing; tremors; increase in sweating; difficulty breathing; coughing; nasal congestion; sneezing; wheezing; drowsiness; nasal itching or burning; nose bleeds; stomach pain; chest pain; voice changes; rash; eye congestion.

Guidelines for Use

USE EXACTLY AS PRESCRIBED.

Read all the patient information that is provided with this product.

If the unit is stored in a cool area, let it warm to room temperature before using it.

Keep in mind the tubing, nebulizer and mouthpiece/mask are disposable, and need to be replaced often. They are sold separately from the compressor.

Recommended Procedures for Administration:

Wash hands thoroughly before use.

Place the unit on a table where it will not fall off, but where it can be reached during use.

Remove the mouthpiece/mask, nebulizer and tubing from the storage compartment.

Attach the tubing.

Add the prescribed amount of medication to the nebulizer.

Attach the mouthpiece/mask to the nebulizer.

Plug the compressor into a wall socket that has high enough voltage for this unit.

Turn the compressor on with the on/off switch.

To use the mouthpiece, keep your mouth closed, and hold the mouthpiece with your teeth. If using a mask, place it over the mouth and nose, but, if possible, breathe through your mouth.

Inhale slowly through your mouth, hold your breath for at least 10 seconds. Exhale completely through your mouth. Continue to breathe for the prescribed amount of time.

When finished, turn the compressor off and unplug it. Remove the tubing, mouthpiece/mask and nebulizer.

After each use, wash the mouthpiece/mask and nebulizer. The tubing does not need to be washed.

Wash in dishwashing detergent and warm water. Rinse well with warm water. Soak in 1 part vinegar and 3 parts warm water for 30 minutes.

Wash hands thoroughly before removing unit.

Rinse unit well with warm water.

Let air dry. Be sure the pieces are completely dry before placing back into the storage compartment of the unit.

Store the unit in a dry area.

This information is advisory only; it does not contain all information about this medicine. If you have any questions about your medicine, ask your healthcare provider.

Use of Topical Products

Precautions

BEFORE USING THIS MEDICINE, tell your healthcare provider if you are pregnant or breastfeeding; if you are taking, will be taking or stop taking any prescription or nonprescription medicine; or if you have any other medical conditions.

Side Effects

Every medicine can cause side effects, but many people have no, or minor, side effects. Tell your healthcare provider if any of the following occurs: burning, itching or other irritation not present before.

Guidelines for Use

USE EXACTLY AS PRESCRIBED.

For external use only.

Avoid contact with eyes.

Do not bandage, unless directed otherwise.

If irritation develops, discontinue use and notify healthcare provider.

Recommended Procedures for Administration:

Wash hands thoroughly before use.

Clean and dry the area to be treated thoroughly before use.

Apply a thin layer of the medicine.

Wash hands thoroughly after use.

This information is advisory only; it does not contain all information about this medicine. If you have any questions about your medicine, ask your healthcare provider.

Use of Transdermal Patches

Precautions

BEFORE USING THIS MEDICINE, tell your healthcare provider if you are pregnant, become pregnant, are planning to become pregnant or breastfeeding; if you are taking, will be taking or stop taking any prescription or nonprescription medicine; or if you have any other medical conditions.

Side Effects

Every medicine can cause side effects, but many people have no, or minor, side effects. Tell your healthcare provider if any of the following occurs: burning, itching, rash or other irritation not present before.

Guidelines for Use

USE EXACTLY AS PRESCRIBED.

If a patch falls off, you may reapply the same patch or use a new one.

Rotate application sites on the body with at least 1 week between applications to one site.

Recommended Procedures for Administration:

Wash hands thoroughly before use.

Remove the patch from its protective pouch. Use only if pouch is intact.

Place adhesive side of the system on non-hairy, clean, dry skin.

Press firmly in place with the palm of the hand for about 10 seconds.

Make sure there is good contact, especially around the edges.

Wash hands thoroughly after application.

Leave on the prescribed amount of time.

Remove patch.

Wash hands thoroughly after removal.

Use of Vaginal Creams

Precautions

BEFORE USING THIS MEDICINE, tell your healthcare provider if you are pregnant, become pregnant, are planning to become pregnant, or breastfeeding; if you are taking, will be taking or stop taking any prescription or nonprescription medicine; or if you have any other medical conditions.

Side Effects

Every medicine can cause side effects, but many people have no, or minor, side effects. Tell your healthcare provider if any of the following occurs: stomach pain; fever; vaginal discharge that smells bad; burning, itching or other irritation not present before.

Guidelines for Use

USE EXACTLY AS PRESCRIBED.

Read all the patient information that comes with this medicine.

If symptoms do not improve in 3 days, contact your healthcare provider.

Continue use until all the prescribed medicine has been used.

Failure to use all of the medicine may prevent complete elimination of the yeast, allowing the infection to return.

This medicine is best used at bedtime.

You may wear a mini pad, but do not use a tampon.

Recommended Procedures for Administration:

Wash hands thoroughly before use.

Break the seal on the tube by removing the lid and turning it upside down and pressing.

Screw the applicator onto the tube.

Squeeze the tube until the applicator is full.

Lay down, on your back, and bend your knees.

Insert the applicator into the vagina as far as it can comfortably go.

Push the inside piece of the applicator, slowly, until the applicator is empty.

Remove the applicator.

If the applicator is disposable, throw it away.

If the applicator is not disposable, clean it after each use.

Pull the applicator apart.

Wash in lukewarm water and soap.

Dry thoroughly before putting the applicator back together.

Wash hands thoroughly after use.

This information is advisory only; it does not contain all information about this medicine. If you have any questions about your medicine, ask your healthcare provider.

Use of Vaginal Suppositories

Precautions

BEFORE USING THIS MEDICINE, tell your healthcare provider if you are pregnant, become pregnant, are planning to become pregnant or breastfeeding; if you are taking, will be taking or stop taking any prescription or nonprescription medicine; or if you have any other medical conditions.

Side Effects

Every medicine can cause side effects, but many people have no, or minor, side effects. Tell your healthcare provider if any of the following occurs: stomach pain; fever; vaginal discharge that smells bad; burning; itching or other irritation not present before.

Guidelines for Use

USE EXACTLY AS PRESCRIBED.

Read all the information provided with this product.

If symptoms do not improve in 3 days, contact your healthcare provider.

Continue use until all the prescribed medicine has been used.

Failure to use all of the medicine may prevent complete elimination of the yeast, allowing the infection to return.

This medicine is best used at bedtime.

You may wear a mini pad, but do not use a tampon.

Recommended Procedures for Administration:

Wash hands thoroughly before use.

Unwrap one suppository.

Place the suppository in the applicator.

Lay down, on your back, and bend your knees.

Insert the applicator into the vagina as far as it can comfortably go.

Push the inside piece of the applicator, slowly, until the applicator is empty.

Remove the applicator.

Clean the applicator after each use.

Pull the applicator apart.

Wash applicator in lukewarm water and soap.

Dry thoroughly before putting the applicator back together.

Wash hands thoroughly after use.

INDEX

A

Abitrexate, 397
Absorbine Antifungal Foot Powder, 441
Absorbine Antifungal, 608
Absorbine Jr. Antifungal, 608
Acarbose, 1
Accupril, 578
Accurbron, 591
Accutane, 332
Acebutolol HCl, 2
Acel-Imune, 213
Acephen, 3
Aceta w/Codeine, 4
Acetaminophen, 3
Acetaminophen/Butalbital/Caffeine, 72
Acetaminophen/Butalbital/Caffeine/Codeine, 73
Acetaminophen/Codeine, 4
Acetaminophen/Hydrocodone, 322
Acetaminophen/Isometheptene Mucate/Dichloral phenazone, 356
Acetaminophen/Propoxyphene Napsylate, 567
Acetaminophen/Oxycodone, 467
Acetazolamide, 5
Acetohexamide, 6
Acetylcysteine, 7
Aches-N-Pain, 302
Achromycin V, 590
ACTH, 155
ACTH-40, 155
ACTH-80, 155
Acthar, 155
Actidil, 626
Actidose-Aqua, 115
Actidose with Sorbitol, 115
Actimmune, 319
Actinex, 377
Acular, 344
Acutrim, 530
Acyclovir, 8
Adalat, 440
Adalat CC, 441
Adapin, 208
Adrenalin Chloride, 218
Adriamycin, 209
Adriamycin PFS, 209
Adrucil, 256
Adsorbocarpine, 535
Advil, 302
AeroBid, 255
AeroBid-M, 255
Aerolate, 590
Aeroseb-Dex, 179
Aerosol Metered Sprays, Use of, 645
Afrin, 533
Aftate, 608
Aftate for Jock Itch, 608
AH-chew D, 529
A-hydrocort, 296
Akarpine, 535
AK-Dex, 178
AK-Dilate, 493
Akineton, 60
AK-Chlor, 120
AK-Mycin, 243
AKne-mycin, 223
AK-Nefrin, 512
AK-Pred, 550
AK-Tab, 603
AK-Zol, 5
Alatone, 520
Ala-Tet, 590
Albumin, Normal Serum, 9
Albuterol, 9
Alconefrin, 494
Aldactone, 570
Aldomet, 398
Alendronate, 10
Aleve, 430
Alferon LDO, 317
Alferon N, 317
Alka-Mints, 81
Alkeran, 384
Aller-Chlor, 127
Allermax, 198
Allermed, 572
Allopurinol, 11
Alophen, 491
AlphaNine, 260
AlphaNine SD, 260
Alprazolam, 12
Alprostadil, 13
Altace, 583
Alterna-Gel, 15
Altretamine, 14
Alu-Cap, 15
Aluminum Salts, 15
Alupent, 389
Alu-Tab, 15
Amacodone, 294
Amantadine, 16
Amaphen, 72
Amaryl, 272
Amen, 381
A-Methapred, 431
Amicar, 19
Amifostine, 17
Amiloride, 18
Aminocaproic Acid, 19
Aminophylline, 20
Aminosalicylate Sodium, 21
Amio-Aqueous, 25
Amiodarone, 22
Ami-Tex LA, 531
Amitone, 81
Amitriptyline, 23
Amitriptyline/Chlordiazepoxide, 129
Amitriptyline/Perphenazine, 521
Amlodipine, 24
Amobarbital, 25
Amobarbital/Secobarbital, 26
Amodopa, 398
Amonidrin, 284
Amoxapine, 27
Amoxicillin, 28
Amoxicillin/Potassium Clavula nate, 29
Amoxil, 28
Amoxil Pediatric, 28
Amphetamine, 30
Amphojel, 15
Amphotericin B Injection, 31
Amphotericin B Topical, 32
Ampicillin, 33
Ampicillin/Sulbactam, 34
Amyl Nitrite, 35
Amyl Nitrite Aspirols, 35
Amyl Nitrite Vaporole, 35
Amytal Sodium, 25
Anafranil, 144
Analpram-HC, 295
Anaprox, 430
Anastrozole, 36
Ancef, 95
Ancobon, 253
Andro L.A. 200, 589
Andropository-200, 589
Ane-mycin, 222
Anergan, 525
Anestacon, 359
Anexsia, 294
Anodynos DHC, 294
Anoquan, 72
Ansaid, 261
Ansamycin, 544
Antabuse, 203
Antispas, 188
Anti-Tuss, 284
Antivert/25 Chewable Tablets, 379
Antivert/25 Tablets, 379
Antivert/50 Tablets, 379
Antivert, 379
Antrizine, 379

Trade names appear in italics.

Anturane, 575
Anucort, 295
Anucort-HC, 295
Anumed HC, 295
Anuprep HC, 295
Anusol-HC, 295
Anxanil, 301
Apacet, 3
APAP *w/Codeine*, 4
Apo-Sulin, 577
Apresoline, 291
Aquachloral Supprettes, 116
AquaMEPHYTON, 498
Aquaphyllin, 591
Aralen, 125
Arcet, 72
Aredia, 470
Arimidex, 36
Aristocort, 659
Aristocort A, 659
Arm-a-Med Isoetharine HCl, 325
Arm-a-Med Metaproterenol Sul fate, 389
Armour Thyroid, 641
Arrestin, 664
Artane, 663
Arthritis Pain Formula Aspirin Free, 3
Articulose, 551
Asacol Delayed-Release Tablets, 388
Ascorbic Acid (Vitamin C), 37
Ascorbicap, 37
Ascriptin A/D, 38
Asendin, 27
Aspergum, 38
Asmalix, 591
Aspirin, 38
Aspirin/Butalbital/Caffeine, 74
Aspirin/Butalbital/Caffeine/ Codeine, 75
Astemizole, 39
Asthma-Nefrin, 218
Astromorph, 421
Atabrine HCl, 577
Atarax, 301
Atarax 100, 301
Atenolol, 40
Atenolol/Chlorthalidone, 41
A/T/S, 223
Ativan Tablets, 368
Atovaquone, 42
Atretol, 85
Atromid-S, 142
Atropine Care, 48
Atropine/Diphenoxylate, 212
Atropine-1, 43
Atropine Care, 43
Atropine Ophthalmic, 43
Atropine Oral, 44
Atropine/Scopolamine/ Hyoscyamine/ Phenobarbital, 45
Atropine Sulfate S.O.P., 43
Atropisol, 43
Atrovent, 324
Augmentin, 29
Auranofin, 46
Aventyl, 448
Aurolate, 281
Axid, 446
Azathioprine, 47
Azithromycin, 48
Azmacort Aerosol, 614
Azo-Standard, 488
Azulfidine, 574

B

B-A-C, 74
Baclofen, 49
Bactocill, 462
Bactrim DS, 624
Bactrim IV, 623
Bactroban, 422
Bancap HC, 294
Banesin, 3
Banflex, 461
Banophen, 198
Barbidonna, 50
Baridium, 488
Basaljel, 15
Bayer, 38
Bayer Childrens, 38
Beclomethasone Dipropionate Aerosol, 50
Beclomethasone Dipropionate Nasal Spray, 51
Beclovent, 50
Beconase, 51
Beconase AQ, 51
Beepen-VK, 478
Beesix, 535
Belix, 198
Belladonna Alkaloids w/Pheno barbital, 50
Bell/ans, 564
Bemote, 188
Benadryl, 198
Benahist,, 198
Ben-Allergin-50, 198
Benazepril HCl, 52
Benemid, 577
Benoject, 198
Bentyl, 188
Benylin Cough, 198
Benzphetamine, 53
Benztropine Mesylate, 54
Beta-2, 355
Betachron E-R, 568
Betagan Liquifilm, 353
Betamethasone, 55
Betamethasone/Clotrimazole, 56
Betapace Tablets, 404
Betapen-VK, 478
Betaseron, 318
Betaxolol Ophthalmic, 57
Betaxolol Oral, 58
Bethanechol Chloride, 59
Betoptic, 57
Betoptic S, 57
Biaxin, 137
Bicillin L-A, 477
BiCNU, 88
Biltricide, 510
Biomox, 28
Biotropin, 608
Biperiden, 60
Bisacodyl, 61
Biscolax, 61
Bismatrol, 62
Bismatrol Extra-Strength, 62
Bismuth Subsalicylate, 62
Bisoprolol, 63
Bitolterol Mesylate, 64
Black-Draught, 560
Blocadren, 602
Bonine Chewable Tablets, 379
Breezee Mist Antifungal, 652
Breonesin, 284
Brethaire, 585
Brethine, 585
Brevicon 21-day, 28-day, 459
Bricanyl, 585
Bromocriptine, 65
Bromphen, 66
Brompheniramine, 66
Bronitin, 218
Bronkaid Mist, 218
Bronkodyl, 591
Bronkosol, 325
Bucet, 72
Budesonide, 67
Bufferin, 38
Bumetanide, 68
Bumex, 68
Bupropion Hydrochloride, 69
BuSpar, 70
Buspirone, 70
Busulfan, 71
Butace, 72
Butalbital/Acetaminophen/ Caffeine, 72
Butalbital/Acetaminophen/ Caffeine/Codeine, 73
Butalbital/Aspirin/Caffeine, 74
Butalbital/Aspirin/Caffeine/ Codeine, 75
Butalbital Compound, 82
Butoconazole, 76
Butorphanol, 77
Byclomine, 188
Bydramine Cough, 198

C

Caffeine/Butalbital/Aceta- minophen, 72
Caffeine/Butalbital/Aceta- minophen/Codeine, 73
Caffeine/Butalbital/Aspirin, 74
Caffeine/Butalbital/Aspirin/ Codeine, 75

Calan, 679
Calan SR, 680
Cal Carb-HD, 81
Calci-Chew, 81
Calciday-667, 81
Calcimar, 79
Calci-Mix, 81
Calcitonin-Human, 78
Calcitonin-Salmon, 79
Calcium 600, 81
Calcium Injectable, 80
Calcium Oral, 81
CaldeCort, 297
Calphosan, 88
Caltrate 600, 81
Caltrate Jr., 81
Cama Arthritis Pain Reliever, 38
Capital w/codeine, 4
Capoten, 83
Cal Plus, 81
Capsaicin, 82
Captopril, 83
Carafate, 573
Carbachol, 500
Carbamazepine Suspension, 84
Carbamazepine Tablets, 85
Carbenicillin, 86
Carbidopa/Levodopa, 384
Cardene, 437
Cardene I.V., 436
Cardioquin, 579
Cardizem, 196
Cardura, 207
Carisoprodol, 87
Carmustine, 88
Carteolol Ophthalmic, 89
Carteolol Oral, 90
Cartrol, 190
Castor Oil, 91
Castor Oil, 91
Cataflam, 186
Catapres, 146
Caverject, 13
Cebid, 41
Cebid Timecelles, 37
Ceclor, 92
Cecon, 37
Cee Nu, 365
Cedax, 106
Cefaclor, 92
Cefadroxil, 93
Cefadyl, 113
Cefamandole, 94
Cefazolin, 95
Cefixime, 96
Cefizox, 107
Cefmetazole, 97
Cefobid, 99
Cefonicid, 98
Cefoperazone, 99
Cefotan, 101
Cefotaxime, 100
Cefotetan, 101
Cefoxitin, 102
Cefpodoxime, 103
Cefprozil, 104
Ceftazidime, 105
Ceftibuten, 106
Ceftin, 110
Ceftizoxime, 107
Ceftriaxone, 108
Cefuroxime Oral, 110
Cefuroxime Injectable, 109
Cefzil, 104
Celestone, 55
Cell Cept, 424
Cenafed, 572
Cena-K, 546
Cenocort, 615
Cephalexin, 111
Cephalothin, 112
Cephapirin, 113
Cephradine, 114
Cephulac, 347
Ceptaz, 105
Cerespan, 472
Cerezyme, 693
Cerozyme, 306
Cetane, 37
Cevalin, 37
Cevi-Bid, 37
Ce-Vi-Sol, 37
Charcoaid, 115
Charcoal, Activated, 115
Chibroxin, 447
Children's Congestion Relief, 572
Children's Feverall, 3
Children's Hold, 181
Children's Nostril, 529
Chlo-Amine, 134
Chloral Hydrate, 116
Chlorambucil, 117
Chloramphenicol Ophthalmic, 120
Chloramphenicol Oral, 118
Chloramphenicol Otic, 119
Chloramphenicol Topical, 121
Chlorate, 127
Chlordiazepoxide, 122
Chlordiazepoxide/Amitriptyline, 123
Chlorhexidine Gluconate, 124
Chloromycetin Oral, 118
Chloromycetin Otic, 119
Chloroptic, 120
Chloroptic SOP, 120
Chloroquine, 125
Chlorotrianisene, 126
Chlorpheniramine Oral, 127
Chlorpromazine, 128
Chlorpropamide, 129
Chlorspan-12, 127
Chlorthalidone, 130
Chlorthalidone/Atenolol, 46
Chlor-Trimeton, 127
Chlortab-4, 127
Chlortab-8, 127
Chlor-Tripolon, 127
Chlor-Tripolon Repetabs, 127
Chlorzoxazone, 131
Cholac, 347
Cholestyramine, 132
Choline Magnesium Trisalicylate, 593
Chooz, 81
Chronulac, 347
Cibacalcin, 78
Cibalith-S Syrup, 363
Cilastatin/Imipenem IM, 334
Cilastatin/Imipenem IV, 335
Ciloxan, 134
Cimetidine, 133
Cipro, 135
Cipro IV, 135
Ciprofloxacin Ophthalmic, 134
Ciprofloxacin Systemic, 135
Cisapride, 136
Citracal, 81
Citrate of Magnesia, 372
Citro Carbonate, 564
Citro-Nesia, 372
Claforan, 100
Clarithromycin, 137
Claritin, 367
Clavulanate Potassium/Ticarcillin, 643
Clemastine, 138
Cleocin, 139, 141
Cleocin Pediatric, 139
Cleocin T, 140
Clindamycin Oral, 139
Clindamycin Topical, 140
Clindamycin Vaginal, 141
Clinoril, 577
Clo-Amine, 127
Clofibrate, 142
Clomid, 143
Clomiphene Citrate, 143
Clomipramine, 144
Clonazepam, 145
Clonidine, 146
Clorazepate Dipotassium, 147
Clotrimazole Oral, 148
Clotrimazole Topical, 149
Clotrimazole Vaginal, 150
Clotrimazole/Betamethasone, 63
Clozapine, 151
Clozaril, 151
Codaphen, 4
Codeine, 152
Codeine/Acetaminophen, 4
Codeine/Butalbital/Acetaminophen/Caffeine, 73
Codeine/Butalbital/Aspirin/Caffeine, 75
Codimal-A, 66
Cogentin, 54
Co-Gesic, 294
Cognex, 579
Colace, 204
Colchicine, 153

Trade names appear in italics.

Colestid, 154
Colestipol Hydrochloride, 154
Colovage, 507
CoLyte, 507
Compazine, 521
Compoz Nighttime Sleep Aid, 198
Congestion Relief, 532
Constilac, 347
Constulose, 347
Constant-T, 591
Control, 530
Cophene-B, 66
Cordarone, 22
Corgard, 426
Cortaid with Aloe, 297
Cort-Dome High Potency, 295
Corticaine, 297
Cortef, 296
Corticotropin, 155
Cortisone Oral, 156
Cortone Acetate, 156
Cortrosyn, 157
Cosyntropin, 157
Cotazym, 471
Cotazym-S, 471
Cotrim D.S., 624
Coumadin, 684
Cozaar, 369
Creon, 471
Crixivan, 33
Crolom, 160
Cromolyn Sodium Inhalation, 158
Cromolyn Sodium Nasal, 159
Cromolyn Sodium Ophthalmic, 160
Cromolyn Sodium Oral, 161
Crystamine, 162
Crysticillin, 477
Crystodigin, 193
Curretab, 381
Cyanocobalamin Injectable, 162
Cyanocobalamin, 163
Cyanoject, 162
Cylert, 475
Cyclobenzaprine, 164
Cyclophosphamide, 165
Cycloserine, 166
Cyclosporine, 167
Cycrin, 381
Cyomin, 162
Cyproheptadine, 168
Cystagon, 169
Cysteamine Bitartrate, 169
Cytomel, 361
Cytotec, 415
Cytovene, 269
Cytoxan, 165

D

Dacarbazine, 170
Dalmane, 259
Dalteparin Sodium, 171
D-Amp, 33
Danazol, 172
Danocrine, 172
Dantrium, 174
Dantrium Intravenous, 173
Dantrolene Injectable, 173
Dantrolene Oral, 174
Darvocet-N, 528
Dapa, 3
Darvon, 527
Darvon-N, 527
Datril Extra Strength, 3
Daypro, 463
Dazamide, 5
DC Softgels, 204
DDAVP, 176
Decadron, 179
Decadron Phosphate, 178
Decofed, 572
Decaspray, 179
DeFed-60, 572
Dehist, 66
Delatestryl, 589
Del-mycin, 222
Delsym, 181
Delta-Cortef, 513
Deltasone, 514
Delaxin, 396
Delta-Tritex, 617
Demadex, 609
Demerol HCl Syrup, 385
Demerol HCl Tablets, 385
Depakene, 672
Depakote, 672
depAndro, 589
Depitol, 85
depMedalone, 431
Depoject, 431
Depo-Medrol, 431
Deponit, 445
Depopred, 431
Depo-Provera, 411
Depotest, 629
Depo-Testosterone, 629
DES, 191
Desenex, 608
Desipramine, 175
Desmopressin, 177
Desmopressin Acetate, 176
Desogen, 459
Desoxyn, 392
Desoxyn Gradumets, 392
Desyrel, 612
Dexameth, 189
Dexamethasone Ophthalmic, 178
Dexamethasone, 179
Dexatrim, 530
Dexedrine, 180
Dexone, 179
Dextroamphetamine, 180
Dextromethorphan, 181
D.H.E. 45, 195
DiaBeta, 276
Diabetic Tussin EX, 284
Diabinese, 129
Dialose, 204
Dialume, 15
Diamine T.D., 66
Diamox, 5
Diamox Sequels, 5
Diastat, 192
Diazepam, 182
Diazoxide Oral, 183
Dibent, 188
Dibenzyline, 492
Dicarbosil, 81
Dichloralphenazone/Isometheptene Mucate/Acetaminophen, 356
Diclofenac Ophthalmic, 184
Diclofenac Oral, 185
Diclofenac Potassium, 186
Dicloxacillin, 187
Dicyclomine, 188
Didanosine (ddI; dideoxyinosine), 189
Didrex, 53
Didronel, 235
Diethylpropion Hydrochloride, 190
Diethylstilbestrol (DES), 191
Diflucan, 252
Diflunisal, 192
Digitoxin, 193
Digoxin, 194
Dihydroergotamine, 195
Dilacor XR, 196
Dilantin, 497
Dilatrate-SR, 329
Dilaudid, 298
Dilaudid HP, 298
Diltiazem, 196
Dimenhydrinate, 197
Dimetabs, 197
Dimetane, 66
Dimetane Extentabs, 66
Diocto, 204
Diocto-K, 204
Dioeze, 204
Dipentum, 456
Diphen Cough, 198
Diphenacen-50, 198
Diphenatol Hydrochloride, 199
Diphenhydramine, 198
Diphenoxylate/Atropine, 199
Diphenylan, 497
Diprolene, 55
Diprosone, 55
Dipyridamole, 200
Dirithromycin, 201
Disonate, 204
Disopyramide, 202
Dispos-a-Med Isoproterenol HCl, 328
Disulfiram, 203
Ditropan, 465
Dizymes, 471

Trade names appear in italics.

D-Med, 431
Docusate, 204
DOK, 204
Dolacet, 294
Dolanex, 3
Dolene, 527
Dolobid, 192
Dolophine HCl Tablets, 391
Dommanate, 197
Donnapine, 50
Donnatal, 45
Donnazyme, 471
Dopar Capsules, 354
Doral, 576
Dorcol Children's Decongestant, 572
Doriden, 275
Dornase Alfa, 205
Doryx, 210
Dorzolamide, 206
DOS Softgel, 204
Doxazosin, 207
Doxepin, 208
Doxinate, 204
Doxorubicin Hydrochloride (ADR), 209
Doxy 100, 210
Doxy 200, 210
Doxy Caps, 210
Doxychel Hyclate, 210
Doxycycline, 210
Dr. Caldwell Senna Laxative, 560
Dramamine, 197
Dramamine II, 409
Dramanate, 197
Dramoject, 197
Drixoral Non-Drowsy, 533
Dronabinol, 211
DSS, 204
DTIC-Dome, 170
DTwP, 214
Dulcagen, 61
Dulcolax, 61
Dull-C, 37
Duocet, 294
Duphalac, 347
Duradyne DHC, 284
Duragesic-100, 245
Duragesic-25, 245
Duragesic-50, 245
Duragesic-76, 245
Dura-Gest, 496
Duralone, 431
Duramorph, 421
Duratest, 589
Durathate-200, 589
Dura-Vent, 531
Duricef, 93
Duvoid, 59
Dyazide, 293
Dycill, 187
Dymelor, 6
Dymenate, 197
Dynabac, 201
Dynacin, 412
DynaCirc, 334
Dyna-Hex, 124
Dynapen, 187
Dyrenium, 618

E

Easprin, 38
E-Base, 222
EC-Naprosyn, 430
Econazole, 212
Econopred, 512
Econopred Plus, 512
Ecotrin, 38
Edecrin, 232
Edecrin Sodium, 254
E.E.S., 244
Effer-K, 508
Effexor, 677
Efudex, 256
Elavil, 23
Eldepryl, 559
Elixomin, 591
Elixophyllin, 591
Elocon Cream, 420
Elocon Lotion, 420
Elocon Ointment, 420
Eltroxin, 387
Emcyt, 228
Empirin, 38
Emulsoil, 91
E-Mycin, 222
Enalapril, 213
Enalapril/Hydrochlorothiazide, 214
Endep, 23
Endolor, 72
Ener-B, 163
Enomine, 496
Enovil, 23
Enoxacin, 215
Enoxaparin Sodium Injection, 216
Entex LA, 496
Entozyme, 471
Enulose, 347
En-Vert, 379
En-Vert Tablets, 379
Ephedrine, 217
Epifrin, 218
Epinal, 218
Epinephrine Pediatric, 218
Epitol, 85
Epivir, 348
Epoetin Alfa, 219
Epogen, 219
Eppy/N, 218
Epsom Salt, 375
Equilet, 81
Equanil, 386
Eramycin, 222
Ergamisol, 352
Ergoloid Mesylates, 220
Eridium, 488
Eryc, 222
Erygel, 222
EryPed, 222
Ery-Tab, 222
Erythrityl Tetranitrate (Discontinued), 242
*Erythrocin Stearate*222
Erythromycin Ophthalmic, 221
Erythromycin Systemic, 222
Erythromycin/Sulfisoxazole, 224
Erythromycin Topical, 223
Eryzole Granules, 224
Esgic, 72
Esidrix, 292
Eskalith Capsules, 363
Eskalith CR Timed Release Tablets, 363
Eskalith Tablets, 363
Espotabs, 491
Estrace, 225
Estrace Vaginal Cream, 227
Estraderm Transdermal, 226
Estradiol Oral, 225
Estradiol Transdermal, 226
Estradiol Vaginal, 227
Estramustine, 228
Estrogen, Conjugated, 229
Estropipate Oral, 230
Estropipate Vaginal, 231
Ethacrynate and Ethacrynic Acid, 232
Ethclorvynol, 233
Ethinyl Estradiol/Norethindrone, 459
Ethosuximide, 234
Ethyol, 17
Etidronate, 235
Etodolac, 236
Etoposide, 237
Etrafon, 487
Ethyol, 17
Eulexin, 262
Evac-U-Gen, 491
Evac-U-Lax, 491
Evalose, 347
Everone 200, 589
Excedrin IB, 302
Exgest, 531
Exidine, 124
Ex-Lax, 491
Eye-Sed, 688
Ezide, 292

F

5-FC, 253
5-Fluorocytosine, 253
Famciclovir, 238
Famotidine, 239
Famvir, 238
FDUR, 251
Feen-a-mint, 491
Felbamate, 240
Felbatol, 240

Feldene, 505
Felodipine, 241
Femcare, 150
Femcet, 72
Femiron, 246
Femstat, 76
Fenesin, 284
Fenfluramine, 242
Fenoprofen, 243
Fentanyl, 244
Fentanyl Citrate Oral, 244
Fentanyl Oralet, 244
Fentanyl Transdermal System, 245
Feosol, 246
Feostat, 268
Feratab, 246
Fergon, 246
Fer-In-Sol, 246
Fer-Iron, 246
Ferndex, 180
Fero-Gradumet Filmtab, 246
Ferospace, 246
Ferralet, 246
Ferralet S.R., 246
Ferralyn Lancaps, 246
Ferra-TD, 246
Ferrous Salts, 246
Ferrous Sulfate, 246
Filgrastim, 247
Finasteride, 248
Fiorgen PF, 74
Fioricet, 72
Fioricet w/Codeine, 75
Fiorinal, 74
Fiorinal w/Codeine, 75
Flagyl, 406
Flatulex, 562
Flavorcee, 37
Flavoxate, 249
Flecainide, 250
Fleet, 61
Fleet Babylax, 278
Fleet Flavored Castor Oil, 91
Fleet Laxative, 68
Fleet Phospho-soda, 565
Fletcher's Castoria, 560
Flexeril, 164
Flexoject, 461
Flexon, 461
Florical, 81
Florinef Acetate, 254
Floxin, 455
Floxuridine, 251
Fluconazole, 252
Flucytosine, 253
Fludrocortisone, 254
Flu-Immune, 313
Flumadine, 590
Flunisolide, 255
Fluogen, 313
Fluoroplex, 256
Fluorouracil, 256
Fluoxetine, 257
Fluphenazine, 258
Flurazepam, 259
Flurbiprofen Ophthalmic, 260
Flurbiprofen Oral, 261
Flu-Shield, 313
Flutamide, 262
Flutex, 617
Fluvastatin, 263
Fluvoxamine Maleate, 264
Fluzone, 313
Folex PFS, 428
Formula Q Capsules, 540
Fortaz, 105
Fosamax, 10
Foscarnet, 265
Foscavir, 265
Fosinopril, 266
Fragmin, 171
FUDR, 273
Fulvicin P/G, 283
Fulvicin U/F, 283
Fumasorb, 246
Fumerin, 246
Fungizone, 32
Fungizone Intravenous, 31
Fungoid, 441
Furadantin, 443
Furosemide, 267
Furalan, 443
Furanite,443

G

Gabapentin, 268
Ganciclovir, 269
Gantrisin, 617
Garamycin, 271
Gas Relief, 562
Gastrocrom, 161
Gas-X, 602
Gee-Gee, 284
Gemfibrozil, 270
Genabid, 507
Genahist, 198
Genapap Extra Strength, 3
Genaphed, 572
Genaspor, 608
Genatuss, 284
Gencalc 600, 81
Gen-D-Phen, 198
Genebs, 3
Gen-K, 546
Genoptic, 271
Genoptic S.O.P., 271
Genora, 459
Genpril, 302
Gentacidin, 271
Gentak, 271
Gentamicin, 271
Gentlax, 580
Genprin, 38
Genuine Bayer, 38
Gen-Xene, 147
Geocillin, 86
Gerimal, 220
Geridium, 488
Gesterol, 523
GG-Cen, 284
Glaucon, 218
Glimepiride, 272
Glipizide, 273
Glucagon, 274
Glucophage, 390
Glucotrol, 273
Glutethimide, 275
Glyate, 284
Glyburide, 276
Glycerin Oral, 277
Glycerin RectaL, 278
Glycopyrrolate Injectable, 279
Glycopyrrolate Oral, 280
Glycotuss, 284
Glynase PresTab, 276
Glytuss, 306
G-myticin, 271
Gold Sodium Thiomalate, 281
GoLYTELY, 507
Goserelin, 282
Grifulvin, 283
Grisactin Ultra, 283
Griseofulvin, 283
Gris-PEG, 283
Guaifenesin, 284
Guaifenesin/Phenyl propanolamine, 531
Guaipax, 531
Guanabenz, 285
Guanadrel, 286
Guanethidine, 287
Guanfacine, 288
GuiaCough CF, 284
GuiaCough PF, 284
Guiatuss, 284
Gynecort 10 (Extra Strength), 297
Gynecort-5, 297
Gyne-Lotrimin, 150
Gyne-Lotrimin Combination Pack, 150

H

Habitrol, 439
Haemophilus B Vaccine, 311
Halazepam (Discontinued), 312
Halcion, 619
Haldol, 289
Halfprin, 38
Halofed, 532
Halenol, 3
Haloperidol, 289
Halotussin, 284
Haltran, 302
HCTZ/Triamterene, 293
Hemocyte, 246
Hemorrhoidal HC, 295
Heparin, 290
Heparin Sodium, 290
Heparin Sodium Lock Flush, 290

Hep-Lock, 290
Hep-Lock U/P, 290
Heptalac, 347
Herplex, 304
Hexadrol, 179
Hexalen, 14
Hibiclens, 124
Hibistat, 124
HibTITER, 311
Hiprex, 393
Hismanal, 39
Histaject, 66
Histerone 100, 629
Hi-Vegi-Lip, 471
Hivid, 685
Hold, Children's, 191
Hold DM, 181
Humatin, 473
Humatrope, 568
Humibid L.A., 284
Humibid Sprinkle, 284
Humulin 70/30, 314
Humulin L, 314
Humulin N, 314
Humulin R, 314
Humulin U, 314
Hydeltrasol, 513
Hydeltra-T.B.A., 513
Hydergine, 220
Hydergine LC, 220
Hydralazine, 291
Hydramine, 198
Hydramyn, 198
Hydrate, 197
Hydrea, 300
Hydrocet, 294
Hydrochlorothiazide, 292
Hydrochlorothiazide/Enalapril, 214
Hydrochlorothiazide/Triamterene, 293
Hydrocodone/Acetaminophen, 294
Hydrocortisone Anorectal, 295
Hydrocortisone Systemic, 296
Hydrocortisone Topical, 297
Hydrocortone, 296
HydroDIURIL, 292
Hydrogesic, 294
Hydromorphone, 298
Hydro-Par, 292
Hydroxacen, 301
Hydroxychloroquine, 299
Hydroxyurea, 300
Hydroxyzine, 301
Hygroton, 130
Hylorel, 286
Hyoscyamine/Atropine/Scopolamine/Phenobarbital, 50
Hyosophen, 50
HY-PHEN, 294
Hyrexin-50, 198
Hytrin, 584
Hytuss, 284
Hyzine-50, 301

I

Ibuprin, 302
Ibuprofen, 302
Ibu-Tab, 302
Idamycin, 303
Idarubicin, 303
Idoxuridine, 304
Ifex, 305
Ifosfamide, 305
Iletin Lente, 314
Iletin I NPH, 314
Iletin I Regular, 314
Iletin II Lente (Pork), 314
Iletin II NPH, 314
Iletin II Regular, 314
Iletin II Regular Concentrate, 314
Ilosone, 244
Ilotycin Ophthalmic, 221
Ilotycin Gluceptate, 244
Ilozyme, 471
ImDur, 331
Imiglucerase, 306
Imipenem/Cilastatin IM, 307
Imipenem/Cilastatin IV, 308
Imipramine, 309
Imipramine Pamoate, 309
Imitrex, 578
Imodium A-D Caplets, 366
Imodium A-D Liquid, 366
Imodium Capsules, 366
Imuran, 47
Indapamide, 310
Inderal, 529
Inderal LA, 529
Indinavir Sulfate, 311
Indochron E-R, 312
Indocin, 312
Indocin IV, SR Suppositories, 312
Indocin IV, 312
Indocin SR, 312
Indocin Suppositories, 312
Indocin Suspension, 312
Indomethacin Capsules, 312
Indomethacin Sustained Release Capsules, 312
Inflamase Forte, 512
Inflamase Mild, 512
Infumorph, 454
Insulin, 314
Insultard NPH, 314
Intal, 158
Intensol, 514
Interferon alfa-2a, 315
Interferon alfa-2b, 316
Interferon alfa-n3, 317
Interferon beta-1b, 318
Interferon gamma-1B, 319
Intron A, 316
Intropin, 220
Invirase, 553
Iodine Antiseptic, 320
Iodine Expectorant, 321
Iodine (Lugol's Solution), 320, 322
Iodine Thyroid, 322
Iodine Tincture, 320
Ipecac Syrup, 323
Ipratropium Bromide, 324
Ircon, 246
Ismelin, 287
ISMO *Tablets*, 331
Isocom, 326
Isoetharine Hydrochloride, 325
Isollyl Improved, 74
Isometheptene/Dichloralphenazone/Acetaminophen, 326
Isoniazid, 327
Isopan, 371
Isopap, 326
Isoproterenol, 328
Isoptin (Injection), 634
Isoptin (Oral), 635
Isoptin SR (Oral), 636
Isopto Atropine, 43
Isopto Carpine, 535
Isopto Frin, 493
Isopto Hyoscine, 555, 556, 557
Isordil, 330
Isordil Tembids, 329
Isordil Titradose, 329
Isosorbide Dinitrate Sublingual, 330
Isosorbide Dinitrate Oral, 329
Isosorbide Mononitrate, 331
Isotretinoin, 332
Isoxsuprine, 333
Isradipine, 334
Isuprel Glossets, 328
Isuprel Mistometer, 328
Itraconazole, 293

J

Janimine, 309
Jenamicin, 293
Jenest, 459

K

Kanamycin Injectable, 336
Kanamycin Oral, 337
Kantrex (Injectable), 336
Kantrex (Oral), 337
Kaochlor, 546
Kaolin with Pectin, 338
Kaon-Cl, 508
Kaopectate II, 396
Kao-Spen, 368
Kapectolin, 338
Kasof, 204
Kay Ciel, 546
Kayexalate, 566
K + Care, 546
K-Dur, 508

Keflet, 111
Keflex, 111
Keflin, 112
Keftab, 111
Kefurox, 110
Kefzol, 95
Kemadrin, 522
Kenaject-40, 615
Kenalog, 615, 617
Kenalog-H, 617
Kenonel, 617
Kerlone, 58
Ketalar, 369
Ketoconazole Cream, 339
Ketoconazole Oral, 340
Ketoconazole Shampoo, 341
Ketoprofen Capsules, 342
Ketoprofen Sustained Release, 343
Ketorolac Ophthalmic, 344
Ketorolac Systemic, 345
Key-Pred, 513
Kinesed, 50
K-Lease, 508
Klonopin, 145
K-Lor, 546
Klor-Con, 508
Klor-Con/EF, 508
Klotrix, 508
KLyte/Cl, 508
K-Norm, 508
Konakion, 498
Kondon's, 217
K-Phen-50, 525
K-Tab, 508
K + 10, 508
Ku-Zyme HP, 471

L

Labetalol, 346
Lactulose, 347
Lanacourt 5, 297
Lanacourt 10, 297
Legetrin Tablets, 540
Lamivudine, 348
Laniazid, 327
Lannett, 30
Lanophyllin, 591
Lanorinal, 74
Lanoxicaps, 194
Lanoxin, 194
Lansoprazole, 349
Larodopa Tablets, 354
Lasix, 267
Lax Pills, 491
Laxative Pills, 491
Ledercillin VK, 478
Lente Ilentin, 314
Lente L, 314
Lescol, 263
Leucovorin Calcium, 350
Leukeran, 117
Leukine, 554
Leuprolide, 351
Levamisole, 352
Levatol, 476
Levlen, 459
Levobunolol, 353
Levodopa, 354
Levodopa/Carbidopa, 355
Levomethadyl, 356
Levonorgestrel Implants, 357
Levora, 493
Levothroid, 358
Levothyroxine, 358
Levoxine, 358
Levoxyl, 387
Libritabs, 122
Librium, 122
Lidocaine Mucosal, 359
Lidocaine Topical, 360
Limbitrol DS 10-25, 123
Lioresal, 49
Liothyronine Sodium, 361
Liquaemin Sodium, 290
Liqui-Char, 115
Liquiprin, 3
Liquid Pred, 514
Lisinopril, 362
Lithane Tablets, 363
Lithium, 363
Lithobid Timed Release Tablets, 363
Lithonate Capsules, 363
Lithotabs Tablets, 363
Lodine, 236
Loestrin, 459
Logen, 212
Lomanate, 199
Lomefloxacin, 364
Lomotil, 199
Lomustine, 365
Loniten, 414
Lonox, 199
Lo/Ovral, 459
Loperamide, 366
Lopid, 270
Lopressor Tablets, 404
Lopurin, 11
Lorabid Capsules, 120
Loratadine, 378
Lorazepam, 368
Lorazepam Intensol Liquid, 368
Lorazepam Tablets, 368
Lorcet-HD, 294
Lorcet Plus, 322
Lorelco, 518
Lortab, 294
Losartan Potassium, 369
Lotensin, 52
Lotrimin, 149
Lotrimin AF Cream, 149
Lotrimin AF Lotion, 149
Lotrimin AF Solution, 149
Lotrimin AF Spray Liquid, 441
Lotrimin AF Spray Powder, 441
Lotrisone, 56
Lo-Trol, 199
Lovastatin, 370
Lovenox, 216
Lozol, 310
Ludiomil, 376
Lugol's Solution, 320, 322
Luminal, 490
Lupron, 351
Lupron Depot, 351
Lupron Depot-Ped, 351
Luvox, 263
Lyphocin, 673
Lysodren, 417

M

Maalox Anti-Diarrheal, 396
Magaldrate, 371
Magnaprin, 38
Magnesium Citrate, 372
Magnesium Oxide, 373
Magnesium Sulfate, 374
Magnesium Sulfate Injectable, 374
Magnesium Sulfate Oral, 375
Mag-Ox 400, 373
Major-Con, 602
Malatal, 45
Mallamint, 81
Malotuss, 284
Mandelamine, 424
Mandol, 94
Maox, 373, 420
Maprotiline, 376
Marezine Tablets, 379
Margesic, 80
Margesic H, 294
Marnal, 74
Marinol, 211
Masoprocol, 377
Matulane, 520
Maxair, 504
Maxaquin, 364
Maxolon, 402
Maxidex Ointment, 178
Maxzide, 293
Maxzide-25 MG, 293
Mebendazole, 378
Meclizine, 379
Meclofenamate, 380
Meclomen, 380
Meda Cap, 3
Medigesic, 72
Medihaler ISO, 328
Medilax, 491
Medipren, 302
Medralone, 400
Medrol, 400
Medroxyprogesterone, 381
Mefenamic Acid, 382
Mefoxin, 102
Megace, 383
Megestrol, 383
Mellaril, 638
Melphalan, 384
Meni-D, 379

Trade names appear in italics.

Meperidine, 385
Mephyton, 499
Meprobamate, 386
Mepron, 42
Meprospan, 386
Mercaptopurine, 387
Mesalamine, 388
Metaprel, 389
Metaproterenol, 389
Metformin, 390
Methadone, 391
Methamphetamine, 392
Methenamine, 393
Methicillin, 394
Methimazole, 395
Methocarbamol, 396
Methotrexate, 397
Methyldopa, 398
Methylphenidate, 399
Methylprednisolone, 400
Methysergide, 401
Meticorten, 514
Metoclopramide, 402
Metolazone, 403
Metoprolol, 404
MetroGel, 405
MetroGel-Vaginal, 407
Metro I.V., 406
Metronidazole Gel, 405
Metronidazole Systemic, 406
Metronidazole Vaginal, 407
Mevacor, 370
Mevinolin, 370
Mexiletine, 408
Mexitil, 408
Mezlin, 409
Mezlocillin, 408
Miacalcin, 79
Micatin, 410
Miconazole, 410
Micro-K, 508
Micronase, 276
MicroNefrin, 218
Micronor, 460
Midamor, 18
Midchlor, 326
Midol IB, 302
Midrin, 326
Migratine, 326
Milk of Magnesia, 411
Milophene, 143
Miltown, 386
Minipress, 511
Minitran, 445
Minocin, 412
Minocycline, 412
Minoxidil Oral, 413
Minoxidil Topical, 414
Mintezol, 592
Miochol, 500
Miostat, 500
Misoprostol, 415
Mithracin, 541
Mitomycin, 416
Mitotane, 417
Mitoxantrone, 418
Mitran, 122
M-KYA 580
Modane, 491
Modane Soft, 204
Modicon, 459
Moexipril Hydrochloride, 419
Mol-Iron, 246
Mometasone, 420
Monistat, 441
Monocid, 98
Monodox, 210
Monoket, 361
Mononine, 260
Monopril, 266
Morphine, 421
Motrin, 302
Motrin IB, 302
M-Prednisol, 431
MS Contin, 454
MSIR, 454
Mucomyst, 7
Mucosil-10, 7
Mucosil-20, 7
Mupirocin, 422
Muromonab-CD3, 423
Mutamycin, 448
Myapap, 3
Mycelex, 149
Mycelex-7, 159
Mycelex-G, 159
Mycelex OTC, 149
Mycelex Troches, 148
Mycobutin, 588
Mycophenolate Mofetil, 424
Mycostatin, 449, 450, 451, 452
Mydfrin, 493
Myidyl, 626
Mykrox, 403
Mylanta Gas, 562
Myleran, 71
Mylicon, 562
Myochrysine, 281
Myolin, 461
Myotonachol, 59
Mysoline, 516
Mytussin, 284

N

Nabumetone, 425
Nadolol, 426
Nafarelin Acetate, 427
Nalbuphine, 428
Naldecon Senior EX, 284
Nalfon, 243
Nalidixic Acid, 429
Naprosyn, 430
Naproxen, 430
Nardil, 489
Nasacort, 616
Nasahist B, 66
Nasalcrom, 159
Nasalide, 255
Natacyn, 431
Natamycin, 431
Navane, 597
Nebcin, 647
NebuPent, 480
Nedocromil Sodium, 432
N.E.E., 493
Nefazodone Hydrochloride, 433
NegGram, 429
Nelova, 459
Nelulen, 459
Nembutal, 482
Neo-Calglucon, 81
Neoral, 167
Neoquess, 188
Neosar, 165
Neostigmine, 434
Neo-Synephrine, 493
Nephro-Calci, 81
Nephro-Fer, 246
Nephron, 218
Nestrex, 535
Neupogen, 247
Neuralgon, 55
Neurontin, 268
Neut, 564
Neutrexin, 625
Nia-Bid, 466
Niac, 466
Niacels, 466
Niacin (Vitamin B3), 435
Niacor, 466
Nicardipine Injectable, 436
Nicardipine Oral, 437
N'ice Vitamin C Drops, 37
Nico-400, 466
Nicobid, 466
Nicoderm, 439
Nicolar, 466
Nicorette, 438
Nicotine Gum, 438
Nicotine Transdermal, 439
Nicotinex, 466
Nicotinic Acid, 466
Nicotrol, 439
Nico-Vert, 197
Nidryl, 198
Nifedipine (GITS), 441
Nifedipine Capsules, 440
Nifedipine Sustained Release, 441
Niloric, 220
Nilstat, 449, 450, 451
Nimodipine, 442
Nimotop, 442
Nipent, 483
Nitro-Bid, 445
Nitro-Bid Plateau Caps, 476
Nitro-Bid SR, 444
Nitrocine, 444
Nitrodisc, 445
Nitro-Dur, 445
Nitrofan, 443
Nitrofurantion, 443

Nitrogard, 444
Nitroglycerin Oral, 444
Nitroglycerin Topical, 445
Nitroglyn, 444
Nitrol, 445
Nitrolingual, 444
Nitrong, 444
Nitrostat, 444
Nizatidine, 446
Nizoral, 370, 371, 372
Nolvadex, 581
Norcept, 459
Norcet, 294
Nordette, 459
Norditropin, 608
Norethin, 459
Norethindrone (mini-pill), 460
Norflex, 461
Norfloxacin, 447
Norgestimate Ethinyl Estradiol, 459
Norgestrel, 460
Norinyl, 459
Norlestrin, 459
Normodyne, 346
Noroxin, 447
Norpace, 202
Norpace CR, 202
Norplant, 357
Norpramin, 175
Nor-Q.D., 460
Nor-Tet, 590
Nortriptyline, 448
Norvasc, 24
Novafed, 532
Novo-Pyrazone, 575
Novo-Sundac, 577
Novolin 70/30, 314
Novolin 70/30 Penfill, 314
Novolin L, 314
Novolin N, 314
Novolin N Penfill, 314
Novolin R, 314
Novolin R Penfill, 314
Novantrone, 418
NPH Iletin I, 314
NPH-N, 314
NP 27, 608
Nubain, 428
Nuprin, 302
Nutropin, 568
Nydrazid, 327
Nystat, 449
Nystatin Mouth and Throat, 449
Nystatin Oral, 450
Nystatin Topical, 451
Nystatin Vaginal, 452
Nystex, 451
Nytol, 198

O

OCL, 507
Octamide PFS, 402
Octreotide Acetate, 453
Ocufen, 260
Ocuflox Ophthalmic, 454
Ocupress, 89
Ocusert Pilo, 535
Ofloxacin Ophthalmic, 454
Ofloxacin Oral, 455
Ogen (Oral), 230
Ogen (Vaginal), 231
Olsalazine, 456
Omeprazole, 457
OmniHIB, 311
Omnipen, 33
Omnipen-N, 33
Oncovin, 683
Ondansetron HCl, 458
Ophthalmic Products, Use of, 647
Oral Contraceptives, Combination Products, 459
Oral Contraceptives, Progestin-Only, 460
Oral Contraceptives, Use of, 646
Oramorp SR, 421
Oraphen-PD, 3
Orasone, 514
Orazinc, 689
Oretic, 292
Orinase, 606
ORLAAM, 356
Ormazine, 128
Orphenadrine Citrate, 461
Ortho-Cept, 459
Orthoclone OKT3, 423
Ortho-Cyclen, 459
Ortho-Est, 230
Ortho-Novum, 459
Ortho Tri-Cyclen, 459
Orudis, 373
Oruvail, 374
Os-Cal 500, 81
Osmoglyn, 277
Osteocalcin, 79
Otic Products, Use of, 648
Ovcon, 459
Ovral, 459
Ovrette, 460
Oxacillin, 462
Oxaprozin463
Oxazepam, 464
Oxybutynin Chloride, 465
Oxycodone HCl, 466
Oxycodone/Acetaminophen, 467
OxydessII, 180
Oxytocin Nasal Spray, 468
Oysco 500, 81
Oystercal 500, 81

P

Paclitaxel Injection, 469
Pamelor, 448
Pamidronate, 470
Panadol, 3
Panasol-S, 514
Pancrease, 471
Pancreatin, 471
Pancrelipase, 471
Panex, 3
Panmycin, 590
Papaverine, 472
Paraflex, 131
Parafon Forte DSC, 131
Parlodel, 65
Parnate, 611
Paromomycin, 473
Paroxetine, 474
Partuss LA, 531
Pathocil, 187
Pavabid, 472
Pavased, 472
Pavasule, 472
Pavatine, 472
Pavatym, 472
Paverolan, 472
Paxil, 474
PCE Dispertab, 222
Pectin/Kaolin, 368
PediaCare Decongestant, 532
Pediapred, 513
Pedia-Profen, 302
Pediazole, 224
PEG, 507
Pemoline, 475
Penetrex, 215
Penicillin G, 477
Penicillin V, 478
Penicillin VK, 511
Pentacarinat, 479, 480
Pentam 300, 479
Pentamidine Injectable, 479
Pentamidine Inhalation, 480
Pentasa Delayed-Release, 388
Pentazine, 525
Pentazocine Oral, 481
Pentids, 477
Pentobarbital, 482
Pentostatin, 483
Pentoxifylline, 484
Pen-VK, 478
Pen-Vee K, 478
Pepcid, 239
Pepcid AC, 239
Pepto-Bismol,
Pepto-Bismol Maximum Stregnth, 62
Pepto Diarrhea Control, 366
Percocet, 467
Perestan, 204
Pergolide Mesylate, 485
Periactin, 168
Peridex, 124
Permapen, 477
Permax, 485
Permitil, 258
Perphenazine, 486

Perphenazine/Amitriptyline, 487
Persantine, 200
Persanting IV, 200
Pertofrane, 175
Pertussin CS, 181
Pfeiffer's Allergy, 127
Pfizerpen, 477
Pfizerpen-AS, 477
Phazyme, 562
Phenameth, 525
Phenphen, 3
Phenaphen w/Codeine No. 2, 4
Phenaphen w/Codeine No. 3, 4
Phenaphen w/Codeine No. 4, 4
Phenaphen-650 w/Codeine, 4
Phenaphen w/Codeine, 3
Phenazine, 563
Phenazodine, 488
Phenazopyridine, 488
Phencen-50, 525
Phendry, 198
Phenelzine, 489
Phenergan, 525
Phenetron, 127
Phenobarbital, 490
Phenobarbital/Atropine/Scopolamine/Hyoscyamine, 50
Phenoject-50, 525
Phenolax, 491
Phenolphthalein, 491
Phenoptic, 493
Phenoxybenzamine, 492
Phenyldrine, 530
Phenylephrine Ophthalmic, 493
Phenylephrine Systemic, 494
Phenylfenesin L.A., 531
Phenylpropanolamine, 495
Phenylpropanolamine/Guaifenesin, 496
Phenytoin, 497
Phillips Milk of Magnesia, 411
Phyllocontin, 20
Phytonadione (Vitamin K1) Injection, 498
Phytonadione (Vitamin K1) Oral, 499
Pilagan, 535
Pilocar, 535
Pilocarpine Ophthalmic, 500
Pilocarpine Systemic, 501
Pilopine HS, 500
Piloptic, 500
Pilopto-Carpine, 535
Pilostat, 500
Pima, 321
Pindolol, 502
Pink Bismuth, 62
Piperacillin, 503
Pipracil, 503
Pirbuterol, 504
Piroxicam, 505
Pitressin Synthetic, 675
Placidyl, 233
Plaquenil Sulfate, 327
Plendil, 241
Plicamycin, 506
Pneumomist, 284
Pneumopent, 513
Polycillin, 33
Polycillin-N, 33
Polycillin Pediatric, 33
Polycillin PRB (with probenecid), 33
Polyethylene Glycol Solution, 507
Polymox, 28
Pondimin, 242
Ponstel, 382
Potasalan, 546
Potassium Chloride, 508
Potassium Iodide, 349
Pramoxine HC, 295
Pravachol, 509
Pravastatin, 509
Praziquantel, 510
Prazosin, 511
Precose, 1
Pred Forte, 512
Pred Mild, 512
Predaject, 551
Predalone, 551
Predcor,, 513
Predicort, 513
Predlone T.B.A., 513
Prednicen-M, 514
Prednisol TBA, 551
Prednisolone Ophthalmic, 512
Prednisolone Systemic, 513
Prednisone, 514
Prefrin Liquifilm, 493
Prelone, 513
Premarin, 229
Premarin IV, 229
Prevacid, 349
Pretz-D, 217
Prilosec, 457
Primaquine, 515
Primatene Mist, 218
Primaxin IM, 307
Primaxin IV, 308
Primidone, 516
Principen, 33
Prinivil, 362
Pro-50, 525
Probalan, 517
Probampacin (with probenecid), 33
Pro-Banthine, 526
Probenecid, 517
Probucol, 518
Procainamide, 519
Pro-Cal-Sof, 204
Procan, SR, 519
Procarbazine, 520
Procardia, 440
Procardia XL, 441
Prochlorperazine, 521
Procrit, 219
Proctocort, 323
ProctoFoam-HC, 295
Procyclidine, 522
Progestaject, 523
Progestasert, 524
Progesterone Intrauterine System, 524
Progesterone Injectable, 523
Proglycem, 183
Prograf, 580
ProHIBiT, 311
Prolixin, 258
Prolixin Decanoate, 258
Prolixin Enanthate, 258
Prometa, 389
Prometh 50, 525
Promethazine, 525
Pronestyl, 519
Propacet, 528
Propagest, 495
Propantheline Bromide, 526
Propoxyphene, 527
Propoxyphene/Acetaminophen, 528
Propoxyphene Napsylate, 566
Propoxyphene Napsylate/Acetaminophen, 528
Propranolol, 529
Propulsid, 136
Propylthiouracil, 530
Propyl-Thyracil, 530
Prorex, 525
Proscar, 248
Pro-Sof, 204
Prostaphlin, 462
ProStep, 439
Prostigmin, 434
Prothazine, 525
Protilase, 471
Protostat, 406
Protriptyline, 531
Protropin, 567
Protropin II, 608
Proventil, 9
Proventil Repetabs, 9
Provera, 381
Prozac, 257
Prulet, 491
Pseudo, 572
Pseudoephedrine HCl, 532
Pseudoephedrine Sulfate, 533
Pseudo-Gest, 532
Pulmozyme, 205
Purge, 91
Purinethol, 387
Pyrazinamide, 534
Pyridiate, 488
Pyridium, 488
Pyridoxine, 575
Pyridoxine (Vitamin B6), 535

Trade names appear in italics.

Q

Quazepam, 536
Questran, 132
Questran Light, 132
Quibron-T, 591
Quiess, 301
Quinacrine, 537
Quinaglute, 579
Quinalan, 579
Quinamm, 580
Quinapril, 538
Quinidex, 579
Quinidine, 539
Quinine Sulfate, 540
Quinora, 579
Quinsana Plus, 608
Quiphile, 580
Q-vel, 580

R

Racepinephrine, 218
Ramipril, 541
Ranitidine, 542
RDF, 209
Rectacort, 295
Rectal Products, Use of, 649
Rectal Suppositories, Use of, 650
Reglan, 402
Regular Ilentin I, 314
Regular Insulin, 314
Regulax SS, 204
Regutol, 204
Rela, 87
Relafen, 425
Relaxadon, 50
Relief, 493
Remular-S, 131
Repan, 72
Reposans-10, 122
Respid, 591
Respiratory Nebulizers, Use of, 651
Restoril, 582
Retin-A, 613
Retrovir, 686
Rheumatrex Dose Pack, 397
Rhinall, 494
Rhinocort, 67
RhoD Immune Globulin, 585
RhoGAM, 585
Ribavirin, 586
Riboflavin, 543
Ridaura, 46
Rifabutin, 544
Rifadin, 589
Rifampin, 545
Riluzole, 546
Rimactane, 589
Rimantadine, 547
Riopan, 371
Risperdal, 591
Risperidone, 548
Ritalin, 399
Ritalin-SR, 399
Ritodrine, 549
Ritonavir, 550
RMS, 421
Robaxin, 396
Robicillin VK, 478
Robimycin, 222
Robinul (Injection), 279
Robinul (Tablets), 280
Robinul Forte, 280
Robitet, 590
Robitussin, 284
Robitussin Cough Calmers, 191
Robitussin Pediatric, 181
Rocephin, 108
Roferon-A, 315
Rogaine, 414
Rolaids, 15
Rolaids Calcium Rich, 81
Rowasa Rectal Suspension, 388
Roxanol, 421
Roxanol SR Timed Released Tablets, 421
Roxanol UD Solution, 421
Roxanol 100, 421
Roxicet, 467
Roxicodone, 466
Roxilox, 467
Rubesol-1000, 162
Rubex, 209
Rubramin PC, 162
Rufen, 302
Rum-K, 546
Ru-Vert-M, 379
Rymed-TR, 531

S

S-2, 218
Saizen, 608
Salagen, 501
Saleto-200, 302
Salicylate Combination, 551
Salmonine, 79
Salmeterol Xinafoate, 552
Sal-Tropine, 44
Saquinavir Mesylate, 553
Sandimmune, 167
Sandostatin, 453
Sani-Supp, 278
Sansert, 401
Saquinavir Mesylate, 553
Sargramostim, 554
Scopolamine Injectable, 555
Scopolamine Ophthalmic, 556
Scopolamine Transdermal, 557
Scopolamine/Atropine/Hyoscyamine/Phenobarbital, 50
Scot-Tussin DM Cough Chasers, 181
Scot-tussin Expectorant, 284
Secobarbital, 558
Secobarbital/Amobarbital, 29
Seconal, 558
Sectral, 2
Seldane, 587
Selegiline, 559
Senexon, 560
Senna, 560
Senna-Gen, 560
Senokot, 560
Senokotxtra, 560
Senolax, 560
Septra DS, 624
Septra IV, 623
Serax, 464
Serevent, 552
Seromycin, 166
Serophene, 143
Sertraline, 561
Serzone, 433
Seudotabs, 572
Silace, 219
Simethicone, 562
Simron, 246
Simvastatin, 563
Sinemet, 355
Sinequan, 208
Sinequan Concentrate, 208
Sinex, 529
Sinustop Pro, 572
SINUvent, 531
Sleep-eze 3, 198
Sleepinal (Maximum Strength), 198
Sleepwell 2-nite, 198
Slo-bid, 591
Slo-Niacin, 466
Slo-Phyllin, 633
Slow FE 246
Snaplets-FR, 3
Sodium Bicarbonate, 564
Sodium P.A.S., 21
Sodium Polystyrene Sulfonate, 566
Sodium Phosphates, 565
Sodium Phosphate/Sodium Biphosphate, 565
Solarcaine, 360
Soldol, 87
Solfoton, 490
Solu-Cortef, 296
Solu-Medrol, 431
Soma, 87
Somatrem, 567
Somatropin, 568
Sominex, 198
Somaphyllin-DF, 20
Soprodol, 87
Sorbitrate, 329, 330
Sotalol, 569
Sotalol Tablets (Metoprolol), 404
Spancap No. 1, 180
Span-FF, 246
Spasmoject, 188
Spasmolin, 45
Spasmophen, 50

Trade names appear in italics.

Spectazole, 212
Spironolactone, 570
Sporanox, 335
SPS, 566
S-P-T, 598
SSKI, 321
Stadol, 77
Stadol NS, 77
Stagesic, 294
Staphcillin, 394
Stavudine, 571
Stelazine, 620
Sterapred, 514
Sterapred DS, 514
Stimate, 292
Storzolamide, 5
St. Joseph Cough Suppressant, 181
Streptozocin, 572
Sublimaze, 266
Sucralfate, 573
Sucrets Cough Control, 181
Sudafed, 532
Sudafed 12-Hour, 532
Sulbactam/Ampicillin, 37
Sulfalax Calcium, 204
Sulfamethoxazole/Trimethoprim Injection, 623
Sulfamethoxazole/Trimethoprim Oral, 624
Sulfaprim DS, 624
Sulfasalazine, 574
Sulfinpyrazone, 575
Sulfisoxazole, 576
Sulfisoxazole/Erythromycin, 245
Sulfoxaprim DS, 625
Sulindac, 577
Sumatriptan, 578
Sumycin, 590
Super Char, 115
Suppress, 191
Suprax, 96
Surfak Liquigels, 204
SusPhrine, 218
Susano, 50
Sustaire, 591
Symadine, 16
Symmetrel, 16
Synarel, 427
Synthroid, 358
Syntocinon, 468
Syroxine, 358

T

Tac-3, 615
Tac-40, 615
Tace, 126
Tacrine, 579
Tacrolimus (FK506), 580
Tagamet HB, 133
Tagamet, 133
Talwin NX, 481
Tambocor, 250
Tamoxifen Citrate, 581
Tapanol Extra Strength, 3
Tapazole, 395
Tavist, 138
Tavist-1, 138
Taxol, 469
Tazicef, 105
Tazidime, 105
Tebamide, 622
Tebrazid, 534
Tegretol, 85
Tegretol Chewable, 85
Tegretol (Suspension), 84
Telachlor, 127
Teldrin, 127
Teline, 590
Temazepam, 582
Tempra, 3
Tencet, 72
Tenex, 288
Teniposide, 583
Ten-K, 508
Tenoretic, 41
Tenormin, 40
Tenuate, 190
Tenuate Dospan, 190
Tepanil, 190
Tepanil Ten-Tab, 190
Terazol 3, 586
Terazol 7, 586
Terazosin, 584
Terbutaline Sulfate, 585
Terconazole, 586
Terfenadine, 587
Tesamone, 589
Teslac, 588
Testandro, 589
Testoderm, 589
Testolactone, 588
Testosterone, 589
Tetracap, 590
Tetracyn, 590
Tetracycline, 590
Tetralan, 590
Tetram, 590
T-Gen, 622
T-Gesic, 294
Thalitone, 130
Theobid, 591
Theochron, 591
Theoclear, 591
Theo-Dur, 591
Theolair, 591
Theophylline, 591
Theoplex, 596
Theo-Sav, 591
Theospan SR, 591
Theostat, 591
Theo-24, 591
Theovent, 591
Thiabendazole, 592
Thiamilate, 593
Thiamine (Vitamin B1), 593
Thioguanine, 594
Thioridazine, 595
Thiotepa, 596
Thiothixene, 597
Thorazine, 128
Thyrar, 641
Thyro-Block, 322
Thyroid, Desiccated, 598
Thyroid Strong, 598
Ticar, 599
Ticarcillin, 599
Ticlid, 600
Ticlopidine, 600
Ticon, 622
Tigan, 622
Tiject-20, 622
Tilade, 432
Timolol Ophthalmic, 601
Timolol Oral, 602
Timoptic, 601
Tinactin, 608
Ting, 608
Tipramine, 309
Tobramycin, 603
Tobrex, 603
Tocainide Hydrochloride, 604
Tofranil, 309
Tofranil-P.M., 309
Tolazamide, 605
Tolbutamide, 606
Tolectin, 607
Tolinase, 605
Tolmetin, 607
Tolnaftate, 608
Tonocard, 604
Topical Products, Use of, 651
Toprol XL Tablets, 404
Toradol, 376
Tornalate, 64
Torsemide, 609
Totacillin, 33
Totacillin-N, 33
T-Phyl, 591
Tramadol Hydrochloride, 610
Trandate, 346
Transdermal Patches, Use of, 652
Transderm-Nitro, 445
Transderm-Scop, 557
Tranxene, 147
Tranxene-SD, 147
Tranxene-SD Half Strength, 147
Tranylcypromine Sulfate, 611
Trazodone, 612
Trendar, 302
Trental, 484
Tretinoin, 613
Triacet, 617
Triad, 72
Triam-A, 615
Triamcinolone Inhalation, 614
Triamcinolone Injection, 615
Triamcinolone Nasal, 616
Triamcinolone Topical, 617
Triamonide 40, 615
Triamterene, 618

Trade names appear in italics.

Triamterene/Hydrochlorothiazide, 321
Triavil, 487
Triazolam, 619
Triderm, 617
Trifluoperazine, 620
Trihexy-2, 621
Trihexy-5, 621
Trihexyphenidyl, 621
Tri-Immunol, 214
Tri-Kort, 657
Trilafon, 486
Tri-Levlen, 459
Trilisate, 593
Trilog, 615
Trimazide, 622
Trimethobenzamide, 622
Trimethoprim/Sulfamethoxazole Injection, 623
Trimethoprim/Sulfamethoxazole Oral, 624
Trimetrexate, 625
Trimox, 31
Tri-Norinyl, 459
Triostat, 361
Tripedia, 213
Triphasil, 459
Triprolidine, 626
Triptone, 197
Trisilate, 551
Trocal, 181
Truphylline, 20
Trusopt, 206
Tuinal, 29
Tuinal Pulvules, 26
Tums, 81
Tums EX Extra Strength, 81
Tusstat, 198
Twilite, 198
Two-Dyne, 72
Tylenol, 3
Tylenol w/codeine, 4
Tylenol w/codeine #2, 4
Tylenol w/codeine #3, 4
Tylenol w/codeine #4, 4
Tylox, 467
Ty Tab #3, 4

U

U-Cort, 297
ULR-LA, 531
Ultracef, 103
Ultram, 610
Ultrase, 471
Unasyn, 34
Uni-Bent Cough, 198
Uniphyl, 591
Unisome SleepGels, 198
Unitrol, 530
Uni-tussin, 284
Univasc, 419
Urabeth, 59
Uracil Mustard, 627
Urecholine, 66
Urex, 393
Urispas, 249
Urodine, 488
Urogesic, 488
Uro-Mag, 373
Uticort, 55

V

V-Cillin K, 478
Vaginal Creams, Use of, 653
Vaginal Suppositories, Use of, 654
Valacyclovir Hydrochloride, 628
Valium, 182
Valproic Acid and Derivatives, 629
Valrelease, 182
Vancenase, 51
Vancenase AQ, 51
Vanceril, 50
Vancocin, 673, 674
Vancoled, 673
Vancomycin Injectable, 630
Vancomycin Oral, 631
Vanex LA, 496
Vantin Suspension, 103
Vaponefrin, 218
Vaseretic 10-25 Tablets, 214
Vasodilan, 333
Vasopressin, 632
Vasotec, 213
Veetids, 478
Velban, 682
Velosef, 114
Velosulin Human Insulin, 314
Venlafaxine, 633
Ventolin, 9
Ventolin Rotacaps, 9
VePesid, 237
Verapamil Injectable, 634
Verapamil Oral, 635
Verapamil Oral Sustained Release, 636
Verazinc, 689
Verelan, 680
Vergon, 409
Vermox, 378
Vertab, 197
V-Gan, 525
Vibramycin, 210
Vibramycin IV, 210
Vibra-Tabs, 210
Vicks Vatronol, 217
Vicodin, 294
Vicodin ES, 294
Videx, 189
Vinblastine Sulfate (VLB), 637
Vincasar PFS, 683
Vincristine, 638
Viokase, 471
Visken, 502
Vistacon, 301
Vistaject, 301
Vistaject-25, 301
Vistaject-50, 301
Vistaquel, 301
Vistaril, 301
Vistazine 50, 301
Vistaril, 329
Vita-C, 37
Vitamin B12, 163
Vitamin B6, 575
Vitamin C, 37
Vivactil, 531
Volteran (Ophthalmic), 184
Volteran (Oral), 185
Voxsuprine, 333
Vumon, 583

W

Warfarin, 639
Wehamine, 197
Wehdryl, 198
Wellbutrin, 69
Wellcovorin, 350
Westcort, 297
Wycillin, 477
Wymox, 28
Wytensin, 285

X

Xanax, 12
X-prep, 560
Xylocaine, 359, 360

Y

Yutopar, 592

Z

Zalcitabine, 640
Zanosar, 572
Zantac, 584
Zarontin, 234
Zaroxolyn, 403
Zeasorb-AF, 608
Zebeta, 63
Zefazone, 97
Zerit, 571
Zestril, 362
Zetran, 182
Ziac, 70
Zidovudine, 641
Zinacef Injection, 109
Zinacef Oral, 110
Zinc Sulfate Injectable, 642
Zinc Sulfate Ophthalmic, 643
Zinc Sulfate Oral, 644
Zinca-Pak, 687
Zincate, 689
Zithromax, 48
Zocor, 563
Zofran, 458
Zoladex, 282
Zolicef, 95
Zoloft, 561

Trade names appear in italics.

Zonalon, 208
ZORprin, 38
Zostrix, 82
Zostrix-HP, 82
Zovirax, 8
Zydone, 294
Zyloprim, 11
Zymase, 471